Antiviral Chemotherapy

Antiviral Chemotherapy

Edited by

D. J. JEFFRIES
St Bartholomew's Hospital, London, UK

E. DE CLERCQ
Katholieke Universiteit Leuven, Belgium

JOHN WILEY & SONS
Chichester · New York · Brisbane · Toronto · Singapore

Telephone: National (01243) 779777
International +44 1243 779777

Other Wiley Editorial Offices

John Wiley & Sons, Inc., 605 Third Avenue,
New York, NY 10158-0012, USA

Jacaranda Wiley Ltd, 33 Park Road, Milton,
Queensland, 4064, Australia

John Wiley & Sons (Canada) Ltd, 22 Worcester Road,
Rexdale, Ontario M9W 1L1, Canada

John Wiley & Sons (SEA) Pte Ltd, 37 Jalan Pemimpin #05-04,
Block B, Union Industrial Building, Singapore 2057

Library of Congress Cataloging-in-Publication Data

Antiviral chemotherapy/edited by D. J. Jeffries and E. De Clercq.
p. cm.
Includes bibliographical references and index.
ISBN 0-471-93040-7
1. Antiviral agents. I. Jeffries, D. J. II. De Clercq, Erik.
[DNLM: 1. Virus Diseases-drug therapy. 2. Antiviral Agents-therapeutic use. WC 500 A6334 1994]
RM411.A568 1994
616.9'25061-dc20
DNLM/DLC
for Library of Congress 94-30007
CIP

British Library Cataloguing in Publication Data

A catalogue record for this book is available from the British Library

ISBN 0 471 93040 7

Typeset in 10/12 pt Palatino by Photo·graphics, Honiton, Devon
Printed and bound in Great Britain by Biddles Ltd, Guildford

Contents

Contributors

Dr Koen Andries
Jamsen Research Foundation, Turnhoutseweg 30, B-2340 Beerse, Belgium.

Dr Eurico Arruda
Department of Internal Medicine, University of Virginia Health Sciences Center, Charlottesville, VA 22908, USA.

Dr M. Atkins
Department of Thoracic Medicine, Royal Free Hospital, Pond Street, London, NW3 2QG, UK.

Dr Jan Balzarini
Rega Institute for Medical Research, Katholieke Universiteit Leuven, Minderbroederstraat 10, B-3000 Leuven, Belgium.

Dr E. F. Bowen
Department of Thoracic Medicine, Royal Free Hospital, Pond Street, London, NW3 2QG, UK.

Dr Peter Brocklehurst
Academic Department of Genitourinary Medicine, The Middlesex Hospital, Mortimer Street, London W1N 8AA, UK. Present address: NPEU, Radcliffe Infirmary, Oxford OX2 6HE, UK.

Dr Mary Ann Carmack
Department of Pediatrics, Division of Infectious Diseases, Stanford University School of Medicine, Stanford, CA 94305, USA.

Professor Anthony L. Cunningham
Head, Virology Department, Westmead Hospital, Institute of Clinical Pathology and Medical Research, Westmead, NSW 2145, Australia.

Dr Erik De Clercq
Rega Institute for Medical Research, Katholieke Universiteit Leuven, Minderbroederstraat 10, B-3000 Leuven, Belgium.

Dr V. C. Emery
Department of Virology, The Royal Free Hospital Medical School, Rowland Hill Street, London NW3 2QG, UK.

Dr A. Kirk Field
Hybridon Inc., 1 Innovation Drive, Worcester, MA 017605, USA.

Dr Hugh J. Field
Department of Clinical Veterinary Medicine, University of Cambridge, Madingley Road, Cambridge CB3 0ES, UK.

Dr Susan Fisher-Hoch
Department of Health and Human Services, Centers for Disease Control, Atlanta, GA 30333, USA. Present address: Department of Pathology, Aga Khan University, Karachi 74 800, Pakistan.

Dr Siân E. Goldthorpe
Department of Clinical Veterinary Medicine, University of Cambridge, Madingley Road, Cambridge CB3 0ES, UK.

Professor P. D. Griffiths
Department of Virology, The Royal Free Hospital Medical School, Rowland Hill Street, London NW3 2QG, UK.

Dr Mary L. Haffey
Bristol-Myers Squibb Pharmaceutical Group, PO Box 4000, Princeton, NJ 08543-4000, USA.

Dr Tim J. Harrison
University Department of Medicine, The Royal Free Hospital School of Medicine, Rowland Hill Street, London NW3 2PF, UK.

Professor Frederick G. Hayden
Department of Internal Medicine, University of Virginia Health Sciences Center, Charlottesville, VA 22908, USA.

Professor Donald J. Jeffries
Department of Virology, The Medical College of St Bartholomew's Hospital, 51–53 Bartholomew Close, London EC1A 7BE, UK.

Dr M. A. Johnson
Department of Thoracic Medicine, Royal Free Hospital, Pond Street, London, NW3 2QG, UK.

Dr Hillar O. Kangro
Department of Virology, The Medical College of St Bartholomew's Hospital, 51–53 Bartholomew Close, London EC1A 7BE, UK. Present address: Statens Seruminstitut, 5, Artilleriveg, DK-2300 Copenhagen, Denmark.

Dr Derek Kinchington
Department of Virology, The Medical College of St Bartholomew's Hospital, 51–53 Bartholomew Close, London EC1A 7BE, UK.

Dr Mikaël A. Le Moal

Unité des Virus Oncogènes, Département de Biotechnologies, Institut Pasteur, F-75724 Paris, France.

Professor Stephen A. Locarnini
Director, Virology Department, Fairfield Hospital, Fairfield, Victoria 3078, Australia.

Dr Adrian Mindel
Academic Department of Genitourinary Medicine, The Middlesex Hospital, Mortimer Street, London W1N 8AA, UK. Present address: Academic Unit of Sexual Health Medicine, Nightingale Wing, Sydney Hospital, Sydney NSW 2001, Australia.

Dr Joseph S. Pagano
Director, UNC Lineberger Comprehensive Cancer Center, University of North Carolina, Chapel Hill, NC 27514, USA.

Dr D. Pillay
Department of Virology, The Royal Free Hospital Medical School, Rowland Hill Street, London NW3 2QG, UK. Present address: Regional Virus Laboratory, PHLS, Birmingham Heartlands Hospital, Bordsley Green East, Birmingham B9 5FT, UK.

Dr Charles G. Prober
Department of Pediatrics, Division of Infectious Diseases, Stanford University School of Medicine, Stanford, CA 94305, USA.

Dr Sally Redshaw
Roche Products Ltd, Broadwater Road, Welwyn Garden City, Herts AL7 5AY, UK.

Dr Françoise Thierry
Unité des Virus Oncogènes, Département de Biotechnologies, Institut Pasteur, F-75724 Paris, France.

Professor Ian Weller
Academic Department of Genitourinary Medicine, University College London Medical School, The Mortimer Market Centre, Mortimer Market, London WC1E 6AU and *Camden and Islington Community Health Services NHS Trust, 112 Hampstead Road, London NW1 2LT, UK.*

Professor Arie J. Zuckerman
Department of Medical Microbiology, The Royal Free Hospital School of Medicine, Rowland Hill Street, London NW3 2PF, UK.

Introduction

DONALD J. JEFFRIES
The Medical College of St. Bartholomew's Hospital, London, UK

ERIK DE CLERCQ
Rega Institute for Medical Research, Katholieke Universiteit Leuven, Belgium

In recent years, much attention has been focused on the development of specific antiviral drugs. The fortuitous discovery of the anti-herpes drug, acyclovir, provided an important precedent in demonstrating the possibility of inhibiting a virus-specific target with the achievement of a high chemotherapeutic index. The need for further knowledge of virus replication, identification of potential chemotherapeutic targets and development of drugs has been accelerated by the increase in viral diseases, accompanying the increasing incidence of immunocompromise generated by organ transplantation and the AIDS pandemic. Demonstration of the emergence of resistant viruses to most currently available antiviral drugs highlights the need for alternative strategies which may allow the possibility of combination therapy.

In this book, we present information on the current status of specific antiviral treatment for most of the important human pathogenic viruses. The chapters are arranged to provide information on basic research alongside details of clinical trials and licensed use of drugs. Although some information is of necessity included in passing, we have not attempted to cover the important aspects of general management and support, immunotherapy or, in the case of HIV infection, the treatment of opportunistic infection. We realize that some important topics have not been covered, including basic research on a number of compounds active against retroviruses, influenza and arboviruses. Rather than prolong the book's gestation period by seeking further authors, in an attempt to produce an all-inclusive volume, we considered it more important to proceed to publication while the information is still valid and topical.

In Chapter 1 D. Kinchington and S. Redshaw focus on a very specific protein, the HIV proteinase, as a target enzyme for anti-HIV agents. The HIV proteinase functions as a homodimer, with each monomer containing the Asp-Thr-Gly triad that is typical of aspartic proteinases. The HIV proteinase is responsible for the proteolytic cleavage of the *gag* precursor protein Pr 55 and *gag-pol* precursor protein Pr 160 to the capsid proteins p17,

Antiviral Chemotherapy. Edited by D.J. Jeffries and E. De Clercq

p24, p7, p6, as well as the proteinase itself (p11), the reverse transcriptase (p51), ribonuclease H (p15) and integrase (p34). The design of HIV protease inhibitors has been based on the 'transition state mimetics', the rationale being that the transition state binds more tightly to the enzyme than either the substrate or the products. Thus were created HIV-1 proteinase inhibitors based on phosphinate dipeptide mimetics, reduced amide dipeptide mimetics, statine-type dipeptide mimetics, hydroxyethylene dipeptide mimetics, dihydroxyethylene dipeptide mimetics, difluoromethyl ketone dipeptide mimetics, hydroxyethylamine dipeptide mimetics and hydroxymethylcarbonyl dipeptide mimetics. Symmetrical inhibitors of HIV proteinase, exploiting the two-fold rotational symmetry of the native enzyme, have also been synthesized. Among the most potent inhibitors were the hydroxyethylene dipeptide mimetic L-687,908, the hydroxymethylcarbonyl dipeptide mimetic Ro 31-8959 and the symmetrical inhibitor L-700,417, which all inhibited the HIV-1 proteinase at a concentration below 1 nM and blocked the spread of HIV-1 infection (or expression of viral proteins) at nanomolar concentrations. While a range of highly potent and selective inhibitors of HIV-1 proteinase is now available, problems of poor oral absorption and short half-life still had to be overcome before these compounds could be turned into clinically useful drugs. However, recent work with renin inhibitors has indicated that with adequate chemical modifications oral bioavailability of these transition state peptidomimetics can be significantly increased (H. D. Kleinert, S. H. Rosenberg, W. R. Baker, H. H. Stein, V. Klinghofer, J. Barlow, K. Spina, J. Polakowski, P. Kovar, J. Cohen and J. Denissen: Discovery of a peptide-based renin inhibitor with oral bioavailability and efficacy, *Science* **257**: 1940–1943 (1992)).

At present, the only compounds that have been formally licensed for the treatment of HIV infections are the dideoxynucleosides AZT, ddI and ddC. In addition, various other 2′,3′-dideoxynucleoside analogues, e.g. 2′,3′-didehydro-2′,3′-dideoxythymidine (D4T), 3′-fluoro-2′,3′-dideoxythymidine (FLT), 5-chloro-3′-fluoro-2′,3′-dideoxyuridine (FddClUrd), 3′-thia-2′,3′-dideoxycytidine (3TC) and its 5-fluoro derivative (FTC) have been found to achieve selective inhibition of HIV replication. These compounds are now in a more or less advanced stage of development, and their anti-HIV properties have been the subject of recent review articles (E. De Clercq: HIV inhibitors targeted at the reverse transcriptase, *Aids Res. Human Retrovir.* **8**: 119–134 (1992); M. J. M. Hitchcock: 2′,3′-Didehydro-2′,3′-dideoxythymidine (D4T), an anti-HIV agent, *Antiviral Chem. Chemother.* **2**: 125–132 (1991); K. J. Connolly and S. M. Hammer: Antiretroviral therapy: reverse transcriptase inhibition, *Antimicrob. Agents Chemother.* **36**: 245–254 (1992)). These different dideoxynucleoside analogues are assumed to interact in a similar fashion to AZT, that is as chain terminators of the HIV-associated reverse transcriptase (RT) reaction following their intracellular phosphorylation to the 5′-triphosphate form. This means that they are targeted at the substrate binding site of RT. In this respect they differ fundamentally from the so-called HIV-1-specific RT inhibitors which are targeted at a non-substrate binding site (E. De Clercq: HIV-1-specific RT inhibitors: highly selective inhibitors of human immunodeficiency virus type 1 that are specifically targeted at the viral reverse transcriptase, *Med. Res. Rev.* **13**: 229–258 (1993)) and can be considered as allosteric inhibitors of HIV-1 RT (Z. Debyser, R. Pauwels, K. Andries, J. Desmyter, Y. Engelborghs, P. A. J. Janssen and E. De Clercq: Allosteric inhibition of human immunodeficiency virus type 1 reverse transcriptase by tetrahydroimidazo[4,5,1-*jk*][1,4]benzodiazepin-2(1*H*)-one and -thione compounds, *Mol. Pharmacol.* **41**: 203–208 (1992)). Various other approaches towards the chemotherapy of HIV infections have been the subject of multi-authored treatises (see *Design of Anti-AIDS Drugs* (ed. E. De Clercq), Elsevier Science Publishers, Amsterdam, The Netherlands, 371 pp. (1990); and *Anti-AIDS Drug Development: Challenge, Strategies and Prospects* (eds P. Mohan and M. Baba), Harwood Academic Publishers, Chur, Switzerland, in press (1994)).

Chapter 2 by J. Balzarini and E. De Clercq highlights the potential of acyclic nucleoside phosphonates as retrovirus inhibitors. Foremost among this class of acyclic nucleotide analogues are PMEA, PMEDAP, FPMPA, PMPA and PMPDAP. Following their intracellular phosphorylation to the diphosphoryl derivatives these compounds act, akin to the 2′,3′-dideoxynucleoside 5′-triphosphates, as chain terminators of the RT reaction. PMEA and its congeners have demonstrated a remarkable efficacy in several animal models for HIV infection, for example in murine AIDS, feline AIDS and simian AIDS models. Of particular importance is that these compounds provide a prolonged antiviral response, lasting for up to one week or even longer after a single-dose administration. This long-lasting antiviral action would allow these compounds to be administered as single doses in the prophylaxis and/or infrequent doses in the therapy of retrovirus infections.

In Chapter 3, E. F. Bowen, M. Atkins, I. A. V. Weller and M. A. Johnson provide a brief introductory summary of the main targets for HIV chemotherapy and then summarize the results of the major clinical trials of drugs active against HIV. With the relentless expansion of the AIDS pandemic the urgency of the need for developments in HIV therapy cannot be overemphasized. Although encouragement may be derived from the short-term delays in disease progression achieved by nucleoside analogues, the rapid emergence of resistance to drugs used in monotherapy has led to a series of trials of combination regimens. This chapter is likely to be the first to become outdated but the editors and the authors considered it important to record the state of play at the time of publication.

In Chapter 4 M. L. Haffey and A. K. Field discuss the possible targets for chemotherapeutic intervention within the replicative cycle of human cytomegalovirus (HCMV) as well as the currently available armamentarium of anti-HCMV therapeutics in clinical use and in development. A number of specific viral proteins and/or processors could be considered as possible targets for chemotherapeutic intervention; e.g. the attachment/penetration of the HCMV virions, which appears to be a multi-faceted process in which participate the interaction of the viral glycoprotein gB with the 30 kDa cell membrane glycoprotein, the interaction of the viral glycoprotein gH with the 92 kDa cell membrane glycoprotein, and the interaction of the viral UL18 gene product with the cellular β_2-microglobulin. The initial interaction of the HCMV virions with the cell receptor(s) would be based on recognition by heparan sulphate at the outer cell membrane—a target that is approachable by sulphated polysaccharides such as dextran sulphate (J. Neyts, R. Snoeck, D. Schols, J. Balzarini, J. D. Esko, A. Van Schepdael and E. De Clercq: Sulfated polymers inhibit the interaction of human cytomegalovirus with cell surface heparan sulfate, *Virology* **189**: 48–58 (1992)). Various other events in the HCMV replicative cycle could be considered as targets for intervention, e.g. the IE ('immediate–early') gene expression machinery, the various proteins (DNA polymerase, DNA binding protein, origin-of-replication binding protein, helicase, primase) involved in viral DNA synthesis and the proteins (e.g. the proteinase assemblin and the putative protein kinases) involved in the assembly process. The fact that the permissiveness of the cells for HCMV can be substantially enhanced following differentiation (or, in the case of T cells, activation) points to the interplay of cellular factors, which may, in turn, also serve as targets for chemotherapeutic intervention. Also, HCMV is by itself immunosuppressive and enhances HIV replication, and this adds another dimension to the design of antiviral strategies in the treatment of HCMV infections in immunosuppressed (e.g. AIDS) patients. At present, only ganciclovir and foscarnet have been approved for limited use, e.g. intravenous treatment of HCMV retinitis in AIDS patients. Both compounds are targeted at the viral DNA polymerase. To interact with the viral DNA polymerase, ganciclovir needs to be phosphorylated (e.g. by a protein kinase encoded by HCMV) (E. Littler, A. S. Stuart and M. S. Chee: Human cytomegalovirus UL97 open reading frame encodes a protein that phosphorylates the antiviral nucleoside analogue ganciclovir, *Nature* **358**: 160–162 (1992); V. Sullivan, C. L. Talarico, S. C. Stanat, M. Davis, D. M. Coen and K. K. Biron: A protein kinase homologue controls phosphorylation of ganciclovir in human cytomegalovirus-infected cells, *Nature* **358**: 162–164 (1992)). HCMV mutants that have developed resistance to ganciclovir because of a deficient phosphorylation may still be sensitive to compounds (e.g. foscarnet) that are not dependent on this phosphorylation. In addition to ganciclovir and foscarnet, several other compounds have been identified as potential anti-HCMV drugs, e.g. DHPC, 2′-nor-cGMP, FIAC and HPMC. All these compounds can be considered as phosphorylation-dependent DNA polymerase inhibitors, the most potent of the series being HPMPC ((*S*)-1-(3-hydroxy-2-phosphonylmethoxypropyl)cytosine). An attractive feature of HPMPC is its prolonged antiviral action, which permits infrequent dosing. HPMPC has proved highly efficacious in a variety of animal models for HCMV infection (E. De Clercq: Therapeutic potential of HPMPC as an antiviral drug, *Rev. Med. Virol.* **3**: 85–96 (1993)), including murine cytomegalovirus infection in the severely immunosuppressed SCID mouse (J. Neyts, J. Balzarini, L. Naesens and E. De Clercq: Efficacy of (*S*)-1-(3-hydroxy-2-phosphonylmethoxypropyl)cytosine and 9-(1,3-dihydroxy-2-propoxymethyl) guanine for the treatment of murine cytomegalovirus infection in severe combined immunodeficiency mice, *J. Med. Virol.* **37**: 67–71 (1992)). HPMPC is now in phase I/II clinical trials in AIDS patients with HCMV infection.

As discussed in Chapter 5 by H. J. Field and S. E. Goldthorpe, of all virus diseases those caused by herpes simplex virus (HSV) have proved most amenable to chemotherapy, one of the reasons being the induction within the infected cells of virus-specific enzymes (i.e. thymidine kinase and DNA polymerase) which then serve as suitable targets for chemotherapeutic intervention. In fact, the 'second-generation' nucleoside analogues (such as acyclovir, penciclovir and bromovinyldeoxyuridine), which, in contrast to the 'first-generation' nucleoside analogues (such as idoxuridine and trifluorothymidine) are highly selective inhibitors of HSV replication, take advantage of these virus-induced enzymes: they are specifically phosphorylated by the viral thymidine kinase and in their active (triphosphorylated) form they show greater affinity for the viral DNA polymerase than for the cellular DNA polymerase. This means that their anti-HSV selectivity is accomplished at two levels: thymidine kinase and DNA polymerase (E. De Clercq: Biochemical aspects of the selective antiherpes activity of nucleoside analogues, *Biochem. Pharmacol.* **33**: 2159–2169 (1984)). In addition to the compounds discussed here, some other compounds have been found specifically to inhibit either the HSV thymidine kinase (e.g. (±)-9-[[(*Z*)-2-(hydroxymethyl)cyclohexyl]methyl]guanine) or HSV DNA polymerase (e.g. acyclic nucleoside phosphonates such as HPMPC) (for review see E. De Clercq: Therapy for herpesvirus infections, *Curr. Opin. Infect. Dis.* **4**: 795–803 (1991); J. Neyts, R. Snoeck and E. De Clercq: Therapy for herpesvirus infections, *Curr. Opin. Infect. Dis.* **5**: 816–826 (1992)). The major problems associated with HSV chemotherapy are resistance development and latency. Quite predictably, development of virus resistance to the drugs is based on mutations in the viral thymidine kinase gene or viral DNA polymerase gene. Virus–drug resistance has not emerged as a major problem in man, except in immunocompromised (i.e. AIDS) patients, the likely explanation being that most resistant mutants show reduced pathogenicity. Latency is a problem inherent to HSV infections. As there are no virus-induced enzymes, with which the known antiviral agents could interact, expressed in the latently infected cells (i.e. neurones), latent HSV is 'immune' from elimination by these antiviral agents.

In Chapter 6 J. S. Pagano reviews critical events in the replication of

Epstein–Barr virus (EBV), diseases associated with EBV infection, antiviral compounds that interfere with EBV replication, and possible approaches to treat EBV-associated diseases. EBV infection shows a characteristic duality: (1) latent infection, whereby the EBV DNA occurs as episomes and replicates through the normal cellular DNA polymerase machinery; and (2) productive infection, whereby the EBV DNA occurs as linear DNA and replicates via the viral DNA polymerase. The outcome of EBV infection is either (1) cell proliferation, usually in B lymphocytes that harbour the latent infection or (2) cytolysis, usually in epithelial cells, the seat of productive infection. Episomal DNA replication starts at *ori*-P as a point of origin following binding of the *trans*-acting viral latency protein EBNA-1 (Epstein–Barr nuclear antigen 1), which is essential for the initiation and maintenance of replication of the EBV episomes and thus an ideal target for chemotherapeutic intervention. Linear DNA replication starts at *ori*-Lyt as point of origin following binding of BZLF-1, a *trans*-acting immediate-early viral protein, which triggers reactivation of EBV in latently infected cells and, again, would occur as a suitable target for chemotherapy. All the compounds that have so far been found to inhibit EBV replication are targeted at the viral DNA polymerase and thus interfere with the productive infection. These compounds include acyclovir, ganciclovir, BVDU, BVaraU, FIAC, FIAU, HPMPA, PMEA, PMEDAP and HPMPC. These compounds do not affect the replication of EBV episomes yet they are able to inhibit a productive EBV infection at a concentration as low as 0.005 μM (FIAC), with a selectivity index as high as 5000 (HPMPC) or 6500 (BVDU). To shut off EBV episomal replication, an antisense oligonucleotide directed to EBNA-1 mRNA could be envisaged. Other chemotherapeutic target proteins that could be considered are the (virus-encoded) ribonucleotide reductase and the viral envelope glycoprotein gp340. Depending on the nature of the EBV-associated disease, different strategies may be considered: for the treatment of hairy leukoplakia, a viral DNA polymerase (pol) inhibitor; for the treatment of infectious mononucleosis, a viral DNA pol inhibitor in combination with an immunomodulator; for the treatment of nasopharyngeal carcinoma, a viral DNA pol inhibitor (during the phase of active viral replication) together with cytokines and/or differentiation promoters; for the treatment of polyclonal B cell lymphomas, any means that lead to episomal disruption, in combination with cytokines; and for the treatment of Burkitt's lymphoma, primarily inhibitors of *c-myc* gene product expression.

In Chapter 7 A. Mindel and P. Brocklehurst present a detailed and critical analysis of all published clinical trials of herpes simplex virus infection. The fortuitous discovery of acyclovir was a major milestone in antiviral drug research. From the clinical viewpoint, its remarkably low toxicity renders it sufficiently safe to consider for long-term prophylaxis in any patient group. In severe or potentially life-threatening manifestations of herpes simplex such as encephalitis its low toxicity profile leads most practitioners to initiate treatment on suspicion of infection and often without laboratory confirmation, which may be difficult to achieve. The success of acyclovir therapy has other significance which acts as a major stimulus for continuing research; it provides a clear demonstration that inhibition of a virus-encoded enzyme will lead to the very high order of chemotherapeutic index that might be anticipated on theoretical grounds. It is hardly surprising that the vast majority of the clinical trials reviewed by Mindel and Brocklehurst have related to acyclovir and it is opportune that the drug became available during the 1980s when the numbers of individuals, vulnerable through immunocompromise, increased as a result of the HIV epidemic and the increase in organ transplantation. They also document the current status of other therapies, including the toxic nucleoside analogues (idoxuridine, trifluorothymidine and vidarabine) which predated acyclovir and the alternatives (specifically foscarnet) that can be used in patients with resistant virus. The summary to this chapter should be welcomed as it provides detailed recommendations for treatment of each of the recognized manifestations of herpes simplex infection. Some of the minor details may be contested but the experience of these authors, coupled with their careful analysis of data from controlled trials, renders this unlikely.

In Chapter 8 H. O. Kangro and D. J. Jeffries present a brief review of the clinical features, complications and pathogenesis of varicella zoster virus infection together with details of possible targets for therapy. They also review the current status of therapy in various clinical situations with indications of the appropriate use of specific antiviral drugs. It is important to consider all aspects of management of patients with viral diseases and, therefore, a short section on specific immunoglobulin use is included. Varicella and herpes zoster (shingles) are important causes of morbidity, mortality and, in a minority, chronic problems such as eye disease and persistent neuralgia. It is not surprising therefore that clinical trials, informed discussion and basic research are leading to consensus views on treatment and the introduction of potentially useful new drugs. One new drug for shingles treatment, famciclovir, has recently been licensed in the UK and there is the promise of others to come. The likely introduction of valaciclovir, a prodrug of acyclovir, will allow increased oral bioavailability of acyclovir and, hopefully, increased efficacy in herpesvirus infections in general and varicella zoster in particular. Initial fears that the widespread use of acyclovir might lead to the emergence of viral resistance have not been realized in the immunocompetent although this is of some concern in those with severe immunocompromise. Firm data on the burden of eye disease generated by ophthalmic zoster and the debility of zoster-associated pain highlight the need to consider prompt treatment with a specific antiviral drug at the earliest opportunity after diagnosis of the acute attack. Concern over the costs of acute-phase treatment should be viewed initially in the context of an overall cost–benefit analysis which includes the cost of hospitalization, follow-up visits and long-term pain control.

In Chapter 9 D. Pillay, V. C. Emery and P. D. Griffiths present the current status of cytomegalovirus (CMV) therapy, which is almost totally focused on the two licensed drugs, ganciclovir and foscarnet. Both have significant toxicities and leave much to be desired, particularly if therapy is to be considered for neonates and in combination with other potentially toxic drugs. Although, understandably and correctly, the authors of this chapter stress the need for new, less toxic drugs and the importance of placebo-controlled trials, the ethical dilemmas posed by attempting to include a placebo in the treatment of sight- and/or life-threatening infections should not be underestimated. The evidence for different pathogenic mechanisms in CMV infection complicating immunosuppressive conditions is reasonably convincing and this has been presented in previous publications from this group. Some may be slightly nervous to accept that their compelling arguments apply to every case and particularly in the management of AIDS patients. There is no doubt that CMV pneumonia is much less common in AIDS than in other immunocompromised patients and this may be explained by the hypothesis that it is normally generated by the patient's immune response. This discounts the possibility, however, that CMV is able to produce sufficient lung destruction by itself to produce a clinically apparent pneumonia. It is conceivable that certain strains of CMV may be more virulent in the lung than others. CMV pneumonitis is recognized as a rare, but definite, disease entity in AIDS patients with low CD4 cell counts, and with increased longevity the condition may become more common. Thus the advice given in the text of this chapter and in Table 9.4, indicating no treatment for lung infection in AIDS patients, may be disputed by some clinicians. Other topics discussed by Pillay, Emery and Griffiths are also controversial. The SOCA group's findings on mortality in patients with AIDS treated with ganciclovir or foscarnet showed a survival benefit in the foscarnet group. Despite reservations expressed about the nature of this study, the authors have used it as a basis for recommending foscarnet for first-line therapy of CMV retinitis in AIDS patients. On the evidence presented in this study population this advice may be appropriate but other factors involved in treatment, particularly the preference of ganciclovir for maintenance therapy, mean that many still regard ganciclovir as the first-line treatment.

In Chapter 10 K. Andries reviews the various compounds that are active against picornaviruses, particularly rhinoviruses. Most of these compounds bind to the viral capsid and are therefore referred to as capsid-binding compounds. They probably bind into the same hydrophobic pocket beneath the floor of the canyon formed by the viral protein VP1, as originally shown for disoxaril (WIN 51711) (T. J. Smith, M. J. Kremer, M. Lou, G. Vriend, E. Arnold, G. Kamer, M. G. Rossmann, M. A. McKinlay, G. D. Diana and M. J.

Otto: The site of attachment in human rhinovirus 14 for antiviral agents that inhibit uncoating, *Science* **233**: 1286–1293 (1986)). The evaluation of a panel of structurally different capsid-binding compounds against all 100 different rhinovirus serotypes has enabled the identification of two groups of rhinoviruses, designated group A (33 serotypes) and group B (67 serotypes) (K. Andries, B. Dewindt, J. Snoecks, L. Wouters, H. Moereels, P. J. Lewi and P. A. J. Janssen: Two groups of rhinoviruses revealed by a panel of antiviral compounds present sequence divergence and differential pathogenicity, *J. Virol.* **64**: 1117–1123 (1990)). Most of the capsid-binding compounds are mainly active against group B rhinoviruses: i.e. 4′,6-dichloroflavan (BW 683C), 4′-ethoxy-2′-hydroxy-4,6′-dimethoxychalcone (Ro 09-410), 5-[5-[2,6-dichloro-4-(4,5-dihydro-2-oxazolyl)phenoxy]pentyl]-3-methylisoxazole (WIN 54954), and 3-methoxy-6-[4-(3-methylphenyl)-1-piperazinyl] pyridazine (R 61837). In contrast, the predecessor of WIN 54954, namely WIN 51711 (disoxaril), is mainly active against group A rhinoviruses. However, the broadest spectrum is demonstrated by the phenoxypyridazinamine Pirodavir (R77975), which is highly active against both group A and group B rhinoviruses (K. Andries, B. Dewindt, J. Snoecks, R. Willebrords, K. Van Eemeren, R. Stokbroekx and P. A. J. Janssen: In vitro activity of pirodavir (R77975), a substituted phenoxypyridazinamine with broad-spectrum antipicornaviral activity, *Antimicrob. Agents Chemother.* **36**: 100–107 (1992)). Pirodavir, because of its broad-spectrum anti-rhinovirus activity, may seem a promising candidate drug for treatment of rhinovirus infections. Capsid-binding compounds have generally been assumed to act as uncoating inhibitors. However, depending on both the viral serotype and the nature of the compound, capsid-binding compounds may affect viral adsorption and/or penetration as well as uncoating. Not all picornavirus inhibitors can be considered as capsid-binding agents. Some of these compounds (e.g. guanidine) seem to act primarily at the RNA synthesis step, whereas for others which are not actively pursued (such as enviroxime) the precise mechanism of action has remained unclear.

The adverse effects of virus infections are not confined to individuals and their immediate contacts. In the introduction to Chapter 11 on picornaviruses, E. Arruda and F. G. Hayden highlight the scale of the impact of rhinovirus infection on absenteeism, general practitioner attendances and antibiotic usage. To the individual, the unpleasant effects and inconvenience of a head cold would induce the majority to seek specific therapy if one could be found. Thus the humanitarian and financial rewards to be gained from the discovery of an anti-picornaviral or anti-rhinoviral agent have long been realized. Some of the viruses grouped in this family present much greater threats than minor respiratory tract disease. The obvious example is poliomyelitis but other enteroviruses may, on occasion, induce severe, potentially fatal, central nervous system, cardiac or neonatal disease. With more than 170 different serotypes of picornaviruses the prospects of specific vaccines remain bleak, although this approach has proved to be successful with the polioviruses and recently with hepatitis A virus. Apart from the strain variability of picornaviruses an obstacle to acute-phase chemotherapy may be the nature of the diseases themselves. As Arruda and Hayden indicate, the main symptoms of rhinovirus infection may result from the inflammatory response to the infection rather than direct mucosal damage. Attempts at specific chemotherapy may thus be ineffective unless applied at the prodromal phase, or even earlier. In this comprehensive, fully referenced review chapter Arruda and Hayden describe the different strategies identified for targeting of antiviral drugs. They provide a detailed account of each of the candidate compounds considered for further development, most of which have been abandoned for either lack of efficacy or unacceptable toxicity. Although some are still undergoing assessment nothing, as yet, has achieved a product licence.

In Chapter 12 M. A. Carmack and C. G. Prober provide a comprehensive review of the history, epidemiology, clinical spectrum and pathogenesis of respiratory syncytial virus (RSV) infection. They then assess, critically, the clinical efficacy and toxicity profile of ribavirin. This is a very controversial area and this carefully prepared account should be of great assistance to paediatricians who are undecided about the merit of ribavirin either in general or in specific cases. In 1986, the Food and Drug Administration (FDA) in the USA approved the licensing of ribavirin for the treatment of RSV infection in spontaneously breathing infants on the basis of three small controlled trials. These trials and a further five trials involving collectively over 170 ribavirin-treated patients have been criticized by the authors in terms of subjective endpoints and small numbers. Although all the studies showed modest benefit from the drug the real issue is whether the benefits demonstrated are meaningful in patient care. One suspects that some paediatricians may tend to over-prescribe ribavirin with an eye to the medico-legal implications of a fatality in an untreated baby. Details of the current costs of therapy render this an expensive exercise. There are some clear conclusions to be drawn from this review which will be of value to the reader. Most now agree that severely ill children and those with underlying cardiac or pulmonary disease should be treated with ribavirin. The FDA approval of ribavirin did not include patients undergoing mechanical ventilation due to the risk of precipitation in the equipment although there is some evidence that the severely ill, intubated patients may be the most likely to benefit from treatment. A detailed assessment of the possible implications of inhalation, by staff, of a compound with teratogenic, carcinogenic and mutagenic potential is presented particularly in the context of health care workers of reproductive age. One is left with the impression, however, that although the risk should be recognized and countered as far as possible, the current lack of evidence of long-term effects and the limited evidence for pulmonary uptake by staff attendants renders the problem theoretical rather than real. What is not defined is the possible effect of ribavirin on future pulmonary disease in infants treated for RSV. The answer to this question, together with information on any delayed toxicity and details of any benefits of treatment of infants who are less than critically ill, will need to come from larger, well-controlled studies.

The term 'exotic viruses' is unsatisfactory but useful to describe the diverse, usually dangerous, pathogens which are usually zoonotic and mainly prevalent in tropical areas. The word 'exotic' is defined as 'unusual' or 'from abroad' and its use in the present context reveals a North American/Western European perspective of diseases which may be very common and far from exotic in some other regions. The choice of title for Chapter 13 was the editors', not that of S. Fisher-Hoch, who has produced a valuable account of the current approaches to therapy. Is it by chance that all the potentially dangerous exotic virus infections are caused by RNA viruses? Probably not, and although the DNA viruses of smallpox and monkey pox have been regarded as exotic in the past, in general DNA viruses behave in a more species-specific manner than RNA. As most strategies (and successes) with antiviral chemotherapy in general have been directed at DNA viruses or, in the case of HIV, DNA provirus formation, few candidate drugs have been available for clinical trials in exotic virus infections. The excellent results from the trials and subsequent use of ribavirin in lassa fever demonstrate the feasibility of a chemotherapeutic approach in this type of acute and potentially fatal infection and, as indicated by the laboratory data, other infections may be amenable to treatment. As stressed by Dr Fisher-Hoch, pharmaceutical companies are most unlikely at present to invest major resources into attempts to develop antiviral drugs for diseases which are mainly confined to areas of extreme poverty. There may be cause for optimism as a result of intense interest in the newly characterized virus of hepatitis C. This virus is clearly recognized as an important target for antiviral chemotherapy and, as it is classified as a flavivirus, it will be important to screen all novel candidate antiviral drugs for activity against yellow fever and other members of the family. Rabies remains stunning and terrifying in its total lethality. The benefits of post-exposure prophylaxis have been demonstrated throughout the world. Recent trials of dissemination of baits seeded with recombinant vaccinia-based rabies vaccines are highly promising and, particularly if there is a predominant carnivore vector such as the fox, may offer the best hope for control of the virus.

In Chapter 14 T. J. Harrison and A. J. Zuckerman describe the causative agents of hepatitis A, B, C, D and E, being HAV, HBV, HCV, HDV and HEV, respectively. From the functional organization of the viral genomes, it appears that several proteins could serve as adequate targets for possible chemotherapeutic attack. The enterovirus 72, HAV, encodes at least two proteinases (within the 2A and C3 domain, respectively), which are responsible for the processing of the HAV polyprotein; the 3C domain encodes the viral replicase which contains the Gly-Asp-Asp motif common to viral RNA-dependent RNA polymerases. The calicivirus HEV also encodes an RNA-dependent RNA polymerase in addition to some other functional viral proteins that remain to be characterized. Whereas both HAV and HEV are (+)RNA viruses, the hepadnavirus HBV genome is composed of two linear DNA strands held together in a circular configuration by base-pairing at the 5′- ends. A motif of 12 base pairs is directly repeated near to the 5′-ends of the two strands, and these sequences may play an important role in the replication of the genome. The most obvious target protein encoded by the HBV genome is the viral (RNA- and DNA-dependent) DNA polymerase, which can act with either RNA or DNA as template. Also encoded by the HBV genome is the x protein, which may well act as a transcriptional transactivator. So-called precore HBV mutants (with a point mutation in the penultimate codon of the precore region) may be associated with increased pathogenicity (i.e. fulminant hepatitis B). HBV is notorious for its propensity to lead, via the chronic carrier state, to hepatocellular carcinoma (HCC). However, the mechanism of HBV oncogenesis has remained obscure. Like many other cancers, development of HCC is likely to be a multi-step process involving a number of factors (possibly including the aforementioned x protein). HDV is known to require the help of HBV (more specifically, HBsAg) for its transmission. The HDV genome is composed of closed circular RNA, resembling that of the satellite viroids of plants, and encodes at least one protein that seems to be required for replication of the genome. HCV is regarded as a flavivirus. Its (+)RNA genome encodes several functional proteins, including a proteinase (involved in the cleavage of the non-structural portion of the polyprotein), a helicase (presumably involved in RNA replication) and a replicase (containing the Gly-Asp-Asp motif common to viral RNA-dependent RNA polymerases). At least 50% of HCV infections progress to chronicity, and HCV infection also is associated with progression to HCC.

On a global basis, the hepatitis viruses collectively contribute significantly to morbidity and mortality. In the comprehensive chapter by S. A. Locarnini and A. L. Cunningham (Chapter 15), all aspects of the clinical features and general and specific management of infections are presented. The editors were aware of overlap of information with Chapter 14 on basic research by T. J. Harrison and A. J. Zuckerman but decided to present the information from both groups in full. Knowledge about hepatitis viruses is still incomplete and there is clearly a need for new therapies which are more effective, cheaper and less cumbersome to administer than interferons. This type of therapy may be of value in selected patients in developed countries but, even then, not all authorities agree about the use of interferons in certain groups. There is still much to learn about the pathogenesis and true clinical importance of hepatitis C virus infection in different regions. The facts that the virus frequently establishes a persistent infectious carrier state and can cause fulminant hepatitis and chronic liver disease are indisputable. The long-term implications of localized liver damage, with or without demonstration of persistent viraemia, are not clearly defined and prolonged studies are necessary to answer this question and to assess the benefits of therapy in different patient groups. Early work on the development of molecular genetic techniques to identify strain differences in hepatitis C isolates (Simmonds *et al.*: *J. Gen. Virol.* **74**: 661–668 (1993)) may prove to be a useful basis for characterizing different biological effects of the viruses and particularly the demonstration of types most likely to produce severe liver disease and those most amenable to treatment.

In Chapter 16 M. A. Le Moal and F. Thierry provide a detailed account on the organization and functioning of the human papillomavirus (HPV) genome. Papillomaviruses demonstrate a marked epitheliotropism: they infect undifferentiated cells of the basal layer of the squamous epidermis, but their eventual (vegetative) replication and maturation only occur within the upper cornified layers. With standard culture methods it is impossible to reproduce the various stages of epithelial differentiation *in vitro*, and this explains why it has proved so difficult to establish cellular models for the propagation of HPVs. Yet, several viral proteins could be considered as putative targets for anti-HPV chemotherapy: e.g. E1, which binds to the viral origin-of-replication (ORI) DNA site and thus regulates the initiation of viral DNA replication; E2, which is also involved in replication initiation, and, in addition, acts as a transcriptional transactivator through binding to a specific DNA sequence; and E5, E6 and E7, which are endowed with oncogenic function as they are apparently involved in cell transformation. Proteins E6 and E7 can also act as transcriptional activators; they contain zinc-finger motifs and are found in the nucleus of cervical carcinoma cells originating from infection with HPV16 or HPV18. Integration of the viral DNA in the host genome is required for malignancy, but the role of E6 and E7 in the oncogenic potential of HPVs remains to be further assessed. Integration of the viral DNA thus also seems to be an adequate target for therapeutic intervention. Considering the fact that the final (vegetative) replication of papillomaviruses occurs only following terminal differentiation of the keratinocytes, and thus depends on cellular factors generated during this terminal differentiation, any drugs that interfere with the terminal differentiation of the epithelial cells may be expected to suppress viral proliferation as well.

Part A

RETROVIRUSES

1 Inhibitors of HIV Proteinase

DEREK KINCHINGTON
The Medical College of St Bartholomew's Hospital, London, UK

SALLY REDSHAW
Roche Products Ltd, Welwyn Garden City, UK

INTRODUCTION

The acquired immune deficiency syndrome (AIDS) was first described in two reports from the Centers for Disease Control in 1981 (1,2), and since then an unprecedented scientific and clinical effort has been made to overcome this devastating disease. By 1984, the causative agent was recognized to be a lentivirus (3–7), and by analogy with other viruses of this group was called the human immunodeficiency virus (HIV). Two genetically distinct viruses (8–10), termed HIV-1 and HIV-2, which occur in different geographical regions have since been identified. Early work showed that HIV infected the CD4 lymphocytes (5,11), which declined in number as the infection progressed. However, it is now clear that HIV can infect a large number of other cell types: these include macrophages and monocytes (12), cells of the brain (13–16), gastrointestinal tract (17), kidney (18), liver (19), lung (20) and skin (21). This complex pattern of infection by HIV may lead to opportunistic infections, neurological disorders, neoplasia and, ultimately, death. The rapid progress made in elucidating the replication cycle of HIV (Figure 1.1) has allowed identification of several molecular targets for chemotherapeutic intervention, amongst them a virally encoded proteinase.

IDENTIFICATION OF HIV PROTEINASE

In the mid-1980s, molecular cloning and sequence determination of the HIV genome revealed putative *gag* and *pol* open reading frames. Previous work with other retroviruses had shown that these open reading frames were first translated into *gag* and *gag-pol* fusion proteins which were further processed to the mature forms. This process was known to be mediated, at least in part, by a virally encoded proteinase. It was suggested (22), on the basis of the nucleotide sequence of HIV, that the *pol* open reading frame might encode a proteinase similar to those of other retroviruses.

Antiviral Chemotherapy. Edited by D.J. Jeffries and E. De Clercq

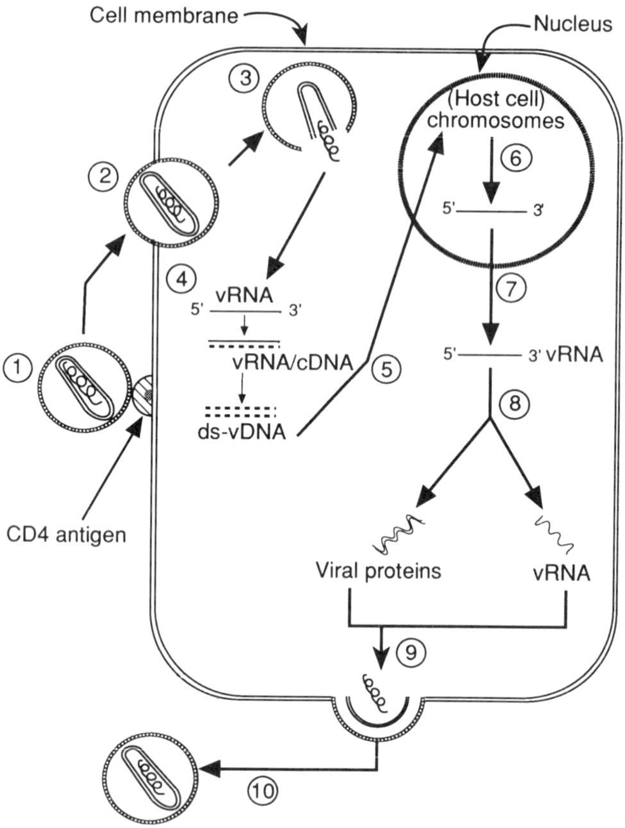

Figure 1.1. Schematic diagram of the replication cycle of HIV. (1) gp120-mediated binding of virion to $CD4^+$ receptor on cell surface. (2) Fusion of membrane portion of viral envelope with cell membrane. (3) Uncoating of virion and release of HIV RNA–nucleocapsid complex and viral enzymes into cytoplasm. (4) Transcription of viral RNA into DNA by reverse transcriptase. (5) Viral DNA incorporated into host cell genome by the viral enzyme integrase. (6) Transcription of viral DNA. (7) Primary RNA transcript of provirus made by host cell RNA polymerase II. (8) Translation of proviral mRNA into viral polyproteins. (9) Post-translational modification and assembly. (10) Processing and maturation

The proteinase in HIV *pol* was first shown to be essential for the processing of the *gag* polyprotein by a frameshift mutation in the proteinase region of *pol* (23). Recombinant HIV *gag-pol* was expressed in yeast cells and processing of the *gag* polyprotein was observed. However, when the frameshift mutation was made, *gag* processing was lost, indicating that at least in yeast, cellular enzymes could not take over the function of the viral proteinase.

It was further recognized (24) that the highly conserved Asp-Thr-Gly triad in the putative retroviral proteinase was reminiscent of the catalytic centre of aspartic proteinases, and it was suggested that the HIV enzyme might belong to this family. Despite this sequence homology, there seemed to be significant differences between the classical aspartic proteinases and the viral enzyme. The former all comprise more than 200 amino acids and consist of two homologous domains (25). The Asp-Thr-Gly motif occurs in each domain, and the two aspartic acids must come together to form the catalytic centre. The viral enzyme, in contrast, has only 99 amino acids and a single Asp-Thr-Gly triad.

These observations led to the suggestion (26) that the retroviral proteinase must function as a homodimer, with each monomer contributing one conserved aspartate to the active site. Site-directed mutagenesis of the putative active site aspartate, which completely abolished catalytic activity (27–29), confirmed the mechanistic class of the enzyme. Further biological and crystallographic studies subsequently established that HIV proteinase does indeed function as a homodimer of 198 amino acids.

ROLE OF THE PROTEINASE

Host cell ribosomes translate the proviral messenger RNA into viral polyproteins. The *gag* open reading frame is translated as a 55 kDa precursor protein, $Pr55^{gag}$, which includes the nucleocapsid and core proteins of the virion (30). The *pol* open reading frame is translated only as a *gag-pol* fusion protein, $Pr160^{gag\text{-}pol}$. This latter protein, which arises as the result of a ribosomal frameshift (31), encompasses the viral enzymes reverse transcriptase, integrase and proteinase (32), as well as the *gag* proteins. Cellular enzymes carry out post-translational modifications of the viral polyproteins including myristoylation (33–35) and glycosylation. The proteins then aggregate at the cell membrane where they are specifically further processed by the virally encoded proteinase. Newly budded virions appear to lack assembled nucleocapsid cores, suggesting that *gag* and *gag-pol* processing occurs during or after virion formation (3,5,7,36,37).

The proteinase was shown to be essential for viral replication by site-directed mutagenesis of the active site aspartate. Such mutagenesis does not prevent viral assembly and budding, but the resulting mutants retain their immature morphology and are non-infectious (27,28,35,38).

HIV proteinase, then, acts primarily at a late stage in the viral replication cycle and inhibition of this enzyme was seen to offer a novel point of intervention to limit virus growth.

CHARACTERIZATION OF HIV PROTEINASE

PURIFICATION OF THE PROTEINASE

Although Lillehoj *et al.* (39) managed to purify minute amounts of the proteinase directly from HIV, sufficient quantities for further biochemical analysis have been prepared either by total synthesis or using recombinant DNA technology. Several syntheses of both HIV-1 (40–42) and HIV-2 (42,43) proteinases have been reported. Constructs expressing only the HIV-1 (44–46) or HIV-2 (47) proteinase sequence have been cloned and expressed in yeast. Expression of constructs of the *gag-pol* fusion products (45,48–55) resulted in autoprocessing of these proteins to give the mature 11 kDa form of HIV proteinase. Several protocols for the purification of the enzyme have been reported, including ligand-affinity chromatography (47,56), high-performance liquid chromatography (HPLC)–size exclusion chromatography (57) and reversed-phase (RP)-HPLC (58).

ASSAY SYSTEMS

Assays developed for HIV proteinase activity can be divided into two categories depending upon whether they are continuous or discontinuous. Continuous assays based on spectrophotometric (59,60) or fluorimetric (61,62) determination have been developed. Discontinuous assays are, in general, more sensitive since the conditions for detection can be optimized independently from the conditions needed for enzyme activity.

Samples taken during the course of the reaction may be analysed colorimetrically (63), by thin-layer chromatography (TLC) or HPLC (64–68) (for peptide substrates) or by gel electrophoresis (69) or immunoblot assay (29,40,45,50,51,70) (for protein substrates). Many of the substrates used for these assays take advantage of the unusual ability of HIV proteinase to cleave between an aromatic amino acid and proline, the observed cleavage frequently being between Tyrosine and Proline.

Direct comparisons of IC_{50} values determined by different laboratories should be made with caution since these values can be affected by substrate concentration and also by effects such as mutual depletion.

SUBSTRATE SPECIFICITY

Aspartic proteinases, including HIV-1 proteinase, bind substrates in an extended conformation forming multiple hydrogen bonds with the backbone amide groups. HIV-1 proteinase has been shown to be responsible for specific cleavage at eight distinct sites in the viral *gag* and *pol* polyproteins (Figure 1.2). The scissile bond at three of these cleavage sites (sites 1, 5 and 6) is between an aromatic amino acid and proline: P_1 and P_1' residues at

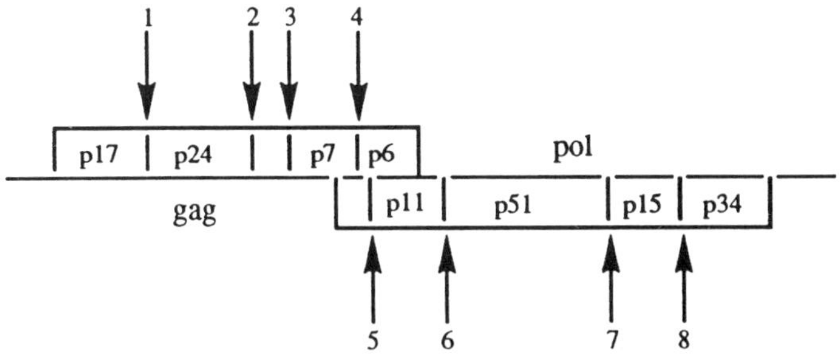

1:	Gln .Asn.Tyr	Pro .Ile.Val
2:	Arg .Val.Leu	Ala .Gln.Ala
3:	Thr .Ile.Met	Met .Gln.Arg
4:	Gly .Asn.Phe	Leu .Gln.Ser
5:	Phe.Asn.Phe	Pro .Gln.Ile
6:	Leu.Asn.Phe	Pro .Ile.Ser
7:	Glu .Thr.Phe	Tyr .Val.Asp
8:	Lys .Ile.Leu	Phe.Leu.Asp

Figure 1.2. Figure 1.2. Schematic representation of sites cleaved by HIV-1 proteinase within the *gag* and *gag-pol* polyprotein

the remaining cleavage sites are more heterogeneous, but are generally lipophilic in character. How the enzyme is able to effect these highly specific cleavages in such disparate amino acid sequences remains an enigma, although it is likely that conformational factors as well as sequence are important (43,52).

In general, if a particular amide bond is cleaved by HIV-1 proteinase in a protein substrate, it will also be cleaved in a synthetic peptide of sufficient length based on the same sequence. Using both synthetic and recombinant HIV-1 proteinase, Darke *et al.* (71) have demonstrated the specific cleavage of oligopeptides corresponding to all the proposed processing sites in the *gag* and *pol* gene products. The minimum size for efficient and specific cleavage was found to be a heptapeptide spanning P_4 to P'_3.

STRUCTURE OF HIV PROTEINASE

The structure of HIV-1 proteinase, both as the native enzyme and in complexes with inhibitors, has been extensively studied. The X-ray crystallographic structure of the apoenzyme was solved almost simultaneously by a number of groups (72–74), confirming modelling studies (75) based on the crystal structure of respiratory syncytial virus (RSV) proteinase bound to an inhibitor of *Rhizopus* pepsin. The native enzyme has been shown to

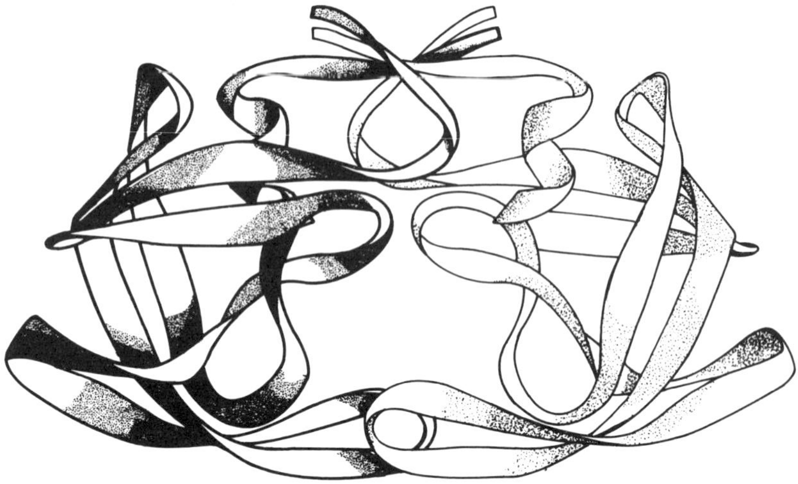

Figure 1.3. Ribbon diagram of native HIV-1 proteinase showing two-fold rotational (C_2) symmetry

exist as a homodimer (Figure 1.3) whose structure and properties are similar to the two-domain mammalian and fungal aspartic proteinases.

The protein comprises four interdigitated strands of β-sheet, a projecting loop from each monomer enclosing the catalytic cleft. The active site triad Asp^{25}-Thr^{26}-Gly^{27} is located within a loop whose structure is stabilized by a network of hydrogen bonds. The loops of each monomer are then interlinked by four hydrogen bonds forming the 'fireman's grip' arrangement (76) which is characteristic of aspartic proteinases.

X-ray crystallographic structures of several enzyme–inhibitor complexes have now been reported and doubtless many more have been determined but not yet published. The published structures include complexes with acetyl pepstatin (77), and with inhibitors incorporating the reduced amide (65), hydroxyethylamine (78) and hydroxyethylene (79) transition state mimetics, as well as with C_2 symmetric inhibitors (80,81). In each case, the structure of the enzyme is similar to that of the uncomplexed dimer, the main difference being in the 'flap' region. The native dimer symmetry is disturbed as the tips of the flaps close over the inhibitor. The flaps thus form the top half of a pocketed hydrophobic tunnel where the pockets serve as subsites (80). The main chain torsion angles of all bound inhibitors correspond to an extended conformation except around the P_1 and P_1' residues. Hydrogen bonds are formed between the inhibitor and the 'floor' of the catalytic cleft in the other direction. The S_2 and S_2' pockets comprise mainly hydrophobic residues and make extensive van der Waals' contacts with the side-chains of inhibitors. When the inhibitor contains a hydroxyl group,

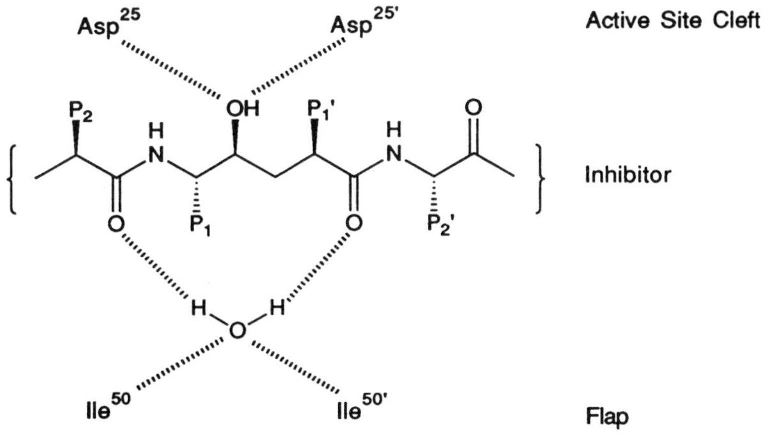

Figure 1.4. Partial schematic representation of the hydrogen bonding interactions between a hydroxyethylene inhibitor and HIV-1 proteinase, showing the position of the water molecule

this is positioned between the side-chain carboxyl groups of the two active site aspartates and is within hydrogen bonding distance.

A major difference between the structures of complexes of HIV-1 proteinase with inhibitors and those of the archetypal aspartic proteinases lies in the role of a tightly bound water molecule which mediates hydrogen bonds between the Ile^{50} and $Ile^{50'}$ amide hydrogens of the flaps and the P_2 and P_1' carbonyl oxygens of the inhibitor (Figure 1.4).

If this water molecule is also present in the enzyme–substrate complex, it would establish hydrogen bonds between the enzyme flaps and the substrate. These hydrogen bonds would exert strain on the scissile amide bond, thereby substantially increasing its vulnerability to hydrolysis (78).

DESIGN OF INHIBITORS

Catalysis by aspartic proteinases is generally considered not to involve an acyl enzyme intermediate, but to proceed via a high-energy tetrahedral transition state formed by addition of water to the scissile amide bond of the substrate (79,82–85) (Figure 1.5).

Since the (unstable) transition state binds to the enzyme more tightly than either the substrate or the products, a successful strategem for the inhibition of aspartic proteinases, notably renin, has been to incorporate a stable transition state mimetic into a substrate analogue. Dreyer *et al.* (86) investigated the effectiveness against HIV-1 proteinase of a number of transition state mimetics of P_1–P_1' Phe-Gly (Figure 1.6) inserted into an analogue of a heptapeptide substrate with a sequence similar to that around the cleavage site between p17 and p24 in the natural substrate $Pr55^{gag}$ (Table 1.1).

The most potent inhibitors in this series incorporated the (*S*)-hydroxyethylene dipeptide isostere (II); inhibitors incorporating the (*R*)-hydroxyethylene dipeptide isostere (III) were much less effective (compound 2 versus compound 3). The statine analogue (I) afforded an inhibitor with moderate potency (compound 1), whilst the phosphinic acid transition state mimetics (IV and V) were less effective when incorporated into this particular heptapeptide analogue (compounds 4 and 5). The difluoromethylketone (VI) was also an effective transition state mimetic in this series (compound 6). Dreyer *et al.* (86) also explored replacement of scissile Phe-Pro by transition state mimetics (Figure 1.7).

The hydroxyethylene isostere again afforded the most potent inhibitor, compound 8 (Table 1.2), although this peptide mimetic was less potent than the unsubstituted analogue (compound 2). It is suggested that this is because the cyclopentane ring may not be an optimal mimetic for a prolyl residue undergoing pyramidalization at nitrogen during proteolysis. The reduced amide dipeptide isostere (VII) afforded a relatively weak inhibitor (compound 7) and the phosphinate transition state mimetic (IX) again gave only moderate potency (compound 9).

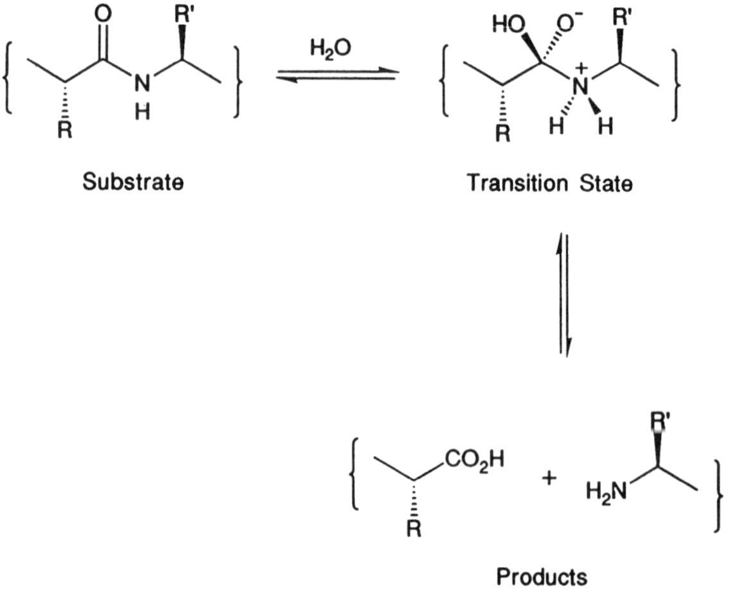

Figure 1.5. Hydrolysis of amide bond, showing tetrahedral transition state

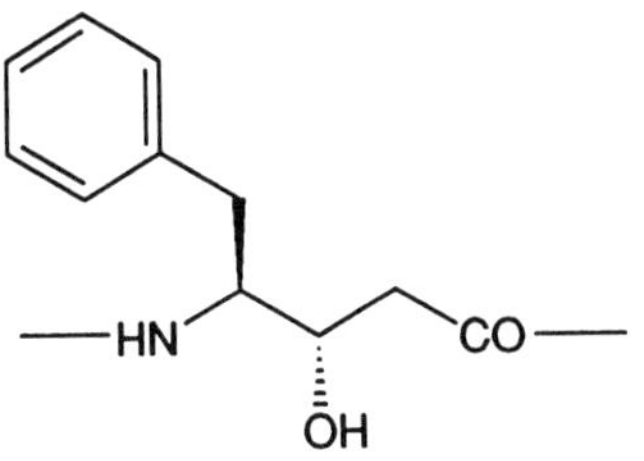

(I)

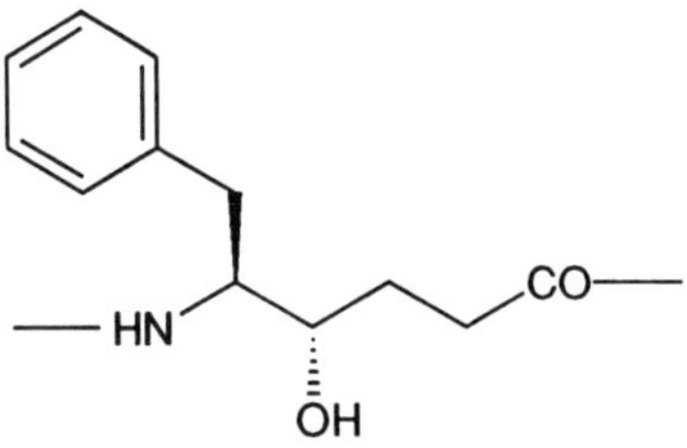

(II)

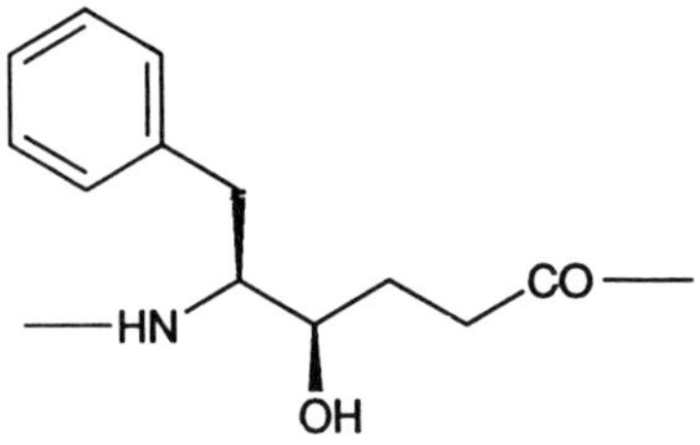

(III)

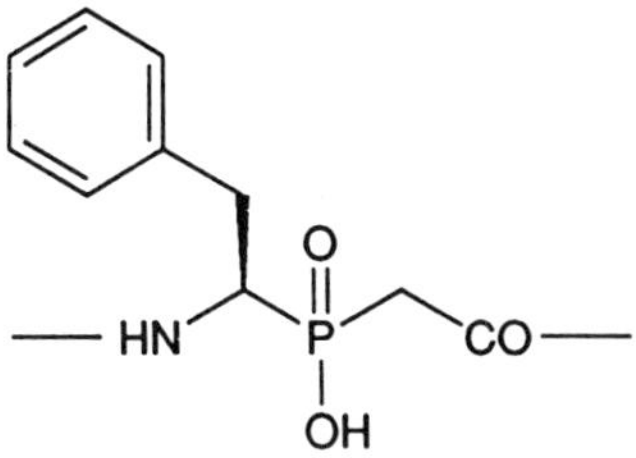

(IV)

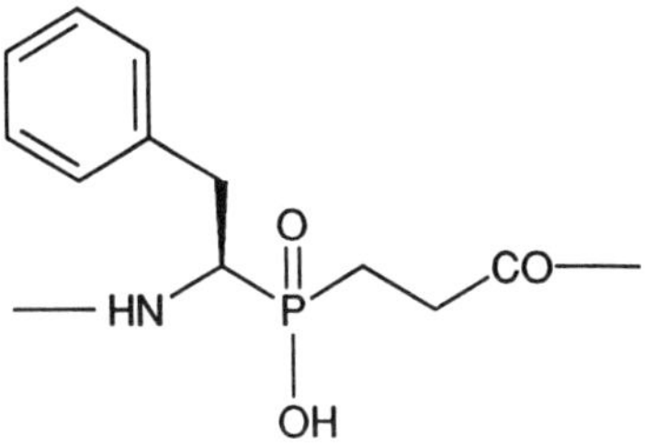

(V)

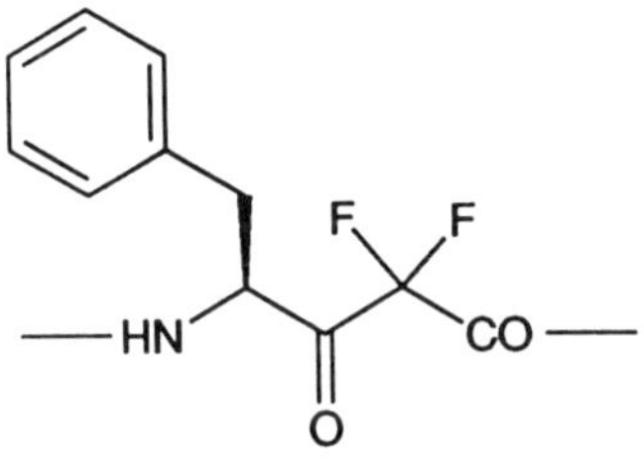

(VI)

Figure 1.6. Hydrolytically stable transition state mimetics of scissile Phe-Gly

It was later shown by Grobelny and co-workers (87) that the potency of inhibitors incorporating the phosphinic acid isostere is very sensitive to changes in the P_1 and P_1' positions (Table 1.3). In agreement with Dreyer *et al*. (86), Grobelny found that phosphinates based on scissile Phe-Pro had poor affinity for the viral enzyme (compound 10). Replacement of the Phe^P-^CPro isostere by a Phe^P-^CPhe isostere decreased the K_i by a factor of some 6000-fold at pH 6.5 (compound 11). Further extension of this inhibitor to include residues in the P_3-P_2 positions gave an extremely potent inhibitor

Table 1.1. Substrate analogue inhibitors of HIV-1 proteinase based on scissile Phe-Gly

no.	structure	K_i(nM)	Ref.
1	H.Ser.Ala.Ala --I-- Val.Val.OMe	810	86
2	H.Ser.Ala.Ala --II-- Val.Val.OMe	62	86
3	H.Ser.Ala.Ala --III-- Val.Val.OMe	4900	86
4	H.Ser.Ala.Ala --IV-- Val.Val.OMe	4500	86
5	H.Ser.Ala.Ala --V-- Val.Val.OMe	4400	86
6	Boc.Ser.Ala.Ala--VI-- Val.Val.OMe	160	86

Boc = ^{t}butyloxycarbonyl

(compound 12). The binding affinity of less potent inhibitors was found to be strongly pH dependent, the affinity increasing with lowered pH.

In general, compounds incorporating the reduced amide dipeptide isostere show only weak inhibitory potency (Table 1.4). Representative examples of inhibitors based on the natural cleavage sequences of the viral enzyme show inhibitory potencies in the micromolar range (compounds 13 (65), 14 (66,88) and 15 (89,90)). The weak activity of these inhibitors may be due to the fact that they are unable to form a direct interaction with the catalytic aspartates in the enzyme active site (92).

Recently Urban *et al.* (91) have described a series of reduced amide tight binding inhibitors of HIV-1 proteinase based on synthetic substrates which bind to the enzyme with much higher affinities than the natural substrates. In particular, incorporation of a glutamic acid residue at P_2' dramatically decreased the K_i value (compound 17 versus compound 16). The hydroxylamine derivative (compound 18) showed an improvement in potency similar to that achieved by incorporating a hydroxyethylene isostere, suggesting that the hydroxyl group of the hydroxylamine binds between the two catalytic aspartates and excludes the water molecule from the enzyme active site.

Iva.Val.Val.Sta.Ala.Sta.OH (compound 19)

The classic aspartic proteinase inhibitor, pepstatin A (compound 19), has a relatively poor affinity for HIV-1 proteinase. IC_{50} values between 0.4 and 1.4 μM have been reported (92–95).

Ac.Val.Val.Sta.Ala.Sta.OH (compound 20)

Acetyl pepstatin (compound 20) is a substantially more potent inhibitor (K_i = 20 nM) (96). Other potent inhibitors of HIV-1 proteinase incorporating the naturally occurring amino acid statine were identified by Hui *et al.* (97).

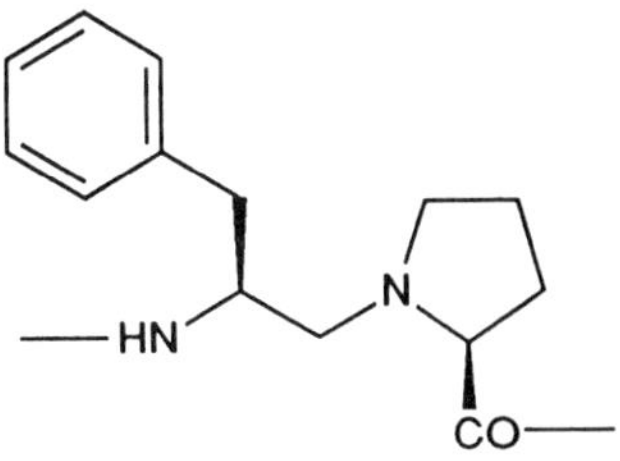

(VII)

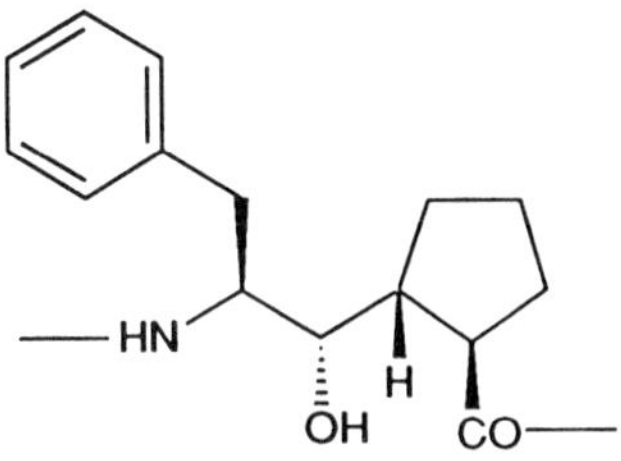

(VIII)

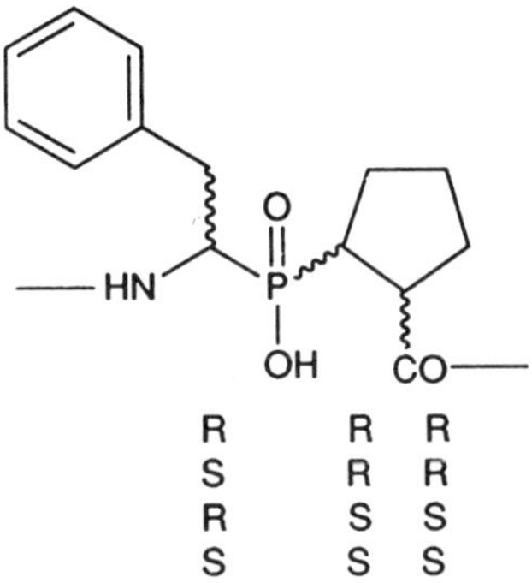

(IX)

Figure 1.7. Hydrolytically stable transition state mimetics of scissile Phe-Pro

Table 1.2. Substrate analogue inhibitors of HIV-1 proteinase based on scissile Phe-Pro

no.	structure	K_i(nM)	Ref.
7	H.Ser.Ala.Ala-VII-- Val.Val.OMe	19 000	86
8	H.Ser.Ala.Ala-VIII-- Val.Val.OMe	500	86
9	H.Ser.Ala.Ala--IX-- Val.Val.OMe	4 000	86

Compounds 21–24 (Table 1.5) which were originally described as dog renin inhibitors show encouraging activity against the viral enzyme.

Compound 24 is a potent inhibitor of HIV proteinase but does not show antiviral activity. The authors suggest (97) that this might be attributable to the presence of a free amino group which could hinder cell penetration

Table 1.3. Inhibitors of HIV-1 proteinase based on phosphinate dipeptide mimetics

no.	structure	K_i(nM) pH 6.5	pH 4.5	Ref.
10	Bz.Phe[P]--[C]Pro.Val.Val.NH_2	13 000	450	87
11	Bz.Phe[P]--[C]Phe.Val.Val.NH_2	2	0.6	87
12	Boc.Val.Val.Phe[P]--[C]Phe.Val.Val.NH_2	0.4	0.04	87

C atoms in P_1 and P_1' positions are racemic

Table 1.4. Inhibitors of HIV-1 proteinase based on reduced amide dipeptide mimetics

no.	structure	IC_{50}(nM)	Ref.
13	Ac.Ser.Gin.Asn.Phe.Ψ[CH_2N]Pro.Val.Val.NH_2	14 000	65
14	Val.Ser.Gin.Asn.Phe.Ψ[CH_2N]Pro.Ile.Val.OH	3 520	66,88
U-84645E			
15	Ac.Thr.Ile.Nle.Ψ[CH_2N]Nle.Gln.Arg.NH_2	789	89,90
MVT-101	Boc.Phe.Ψ[CH_2N]Phe.Ile.Phe.OMe		
16	Boc.Phe.Ψ[CH_2N]Phe.Glu.Phe.OMe	23	91
17	Boc.Phe.Ψ[CH_2N]Phe.Ile.Phe.OMe	0.2	91
18	|	0.5	91
	OH		

or facilitate metabolism of the compound. Compounds 21 and 22 both showed good antiviral efficacy, the activity of compound 21 being comparable to that of AZT or ddC in MT-2 cells infected with HIV.

Raju and Deshpande (98) have more recently described a series of phenylnorstatine derivatives based on the class C substrate type. Compound 25 is the most potent of this series of inhibitors, with an IC_{50} value of 63 nM. Kahn *et al.* (99) set out to explore the importance of secondary structure in proteolytic processing by HIV proteinase. Incorporation of their previously reported β-turn mimetics (A) and (B) into substrate analogues containing a statine-type dipeptide replacement afforded compounds with modest to good inhibitory potencies (Table 1.6).

Molecular dynamics analysis suggested that the *N*-benzyl substituent of β-turn mimetic (A) was outside the HIV proteinase binding pocket and, indeed, compound 28 which lacks this benzyl group was the most potent inhibitor of the series. Incorporation of the β-turn mimetic (B) at P_3-P_2 thus gives a potent inhibitor of HIV proteinase even with a non-optimal transition state mimetic.

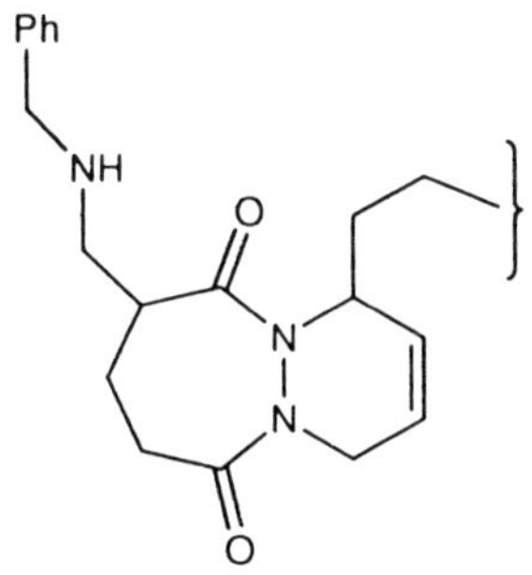

(A)

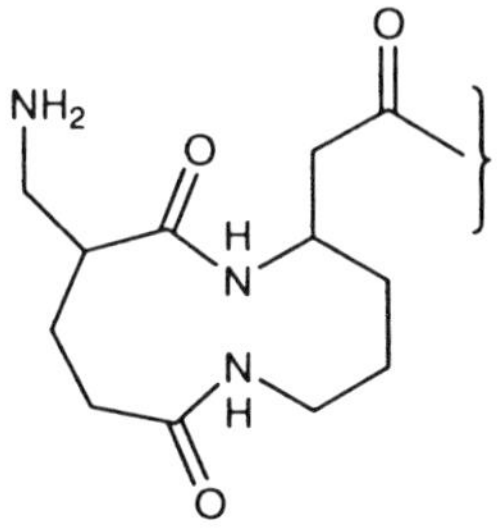

(B)

Of the transition state mimetics which have been used to generate inhibitors of HIV proteinase, the hydroxyethylene dipeptide mimetic has received most attention. The ready availability of renin inhibitors allowed many groups to consider screening these compounds, or close analogues, as inhibitors of HIV proteinase. Leads derived from these studies have been developed to afford very potent inhibitors. Some examples of hydroxyethylene-containing inhibitors which have arisen in this way and of those which have been designed specifically as inhibitors of HIV proteinase are shown in Table 1.7.

As well as high affinity for the viral enzyme, many of these compounds have been reported to show good antiviral activity in cell culture. At a concentration of 100 μM, the hexapeptide analogue 30 completely blocked $p55^{gag}$ and $p160^{gag\text{-}pol}$ processing in CEM_{IIIB} cells and also prevented infection in naive T lymphocytes (100).

The octapeptide analogue, U-85548E (compound 31) (101), did not inhibit HIV replication in cell culture (102), but U-81749 (compound 32) (101) was found to suppress replication of the virus in human peripheral blood lymphocytes with an IC_{50} of 0.1–1.0 μM (102).

Two reports from workers at Merck (103, 104) describe compounds derived from the renin inhibitor L-364,505 (compound 33). Vacca *et al.* (103) deleted two amino acid residues (Phe-Phe) from the N-terminus of this heptapeptide, thereby improving the affinity for HIV proteinase and also destroying renin inhibitory activity. Optimization of the P_1' and P_3' residues then gave the tripeptide derivatives 34 and 35 (L-687,908), which completely blocked the spread of HIV-1_{IIIB} infection in H9 human T lymphoid cells at concentrations of 200 nM and 12 nM, respectively. Using a slightly different strategy, Lyle *et al.* (104) modified the lead compound by incorpor-

Table 1.5. Inhibitors of HIV-1 proteinase based on statine-like dipeptide mimetics

no.	structure	IC_{50} (nM)	Ref.
21	Ac.NA.Pro.Phe.Val.NH 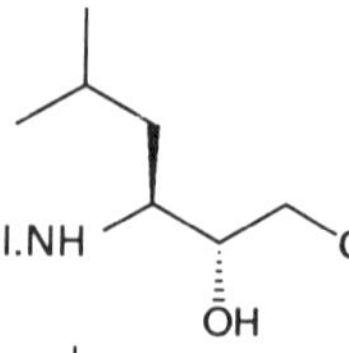 CO.Leu.Phe.NH_2	400	97
22	Ac.YOM.Pro.Phe.Val.NH 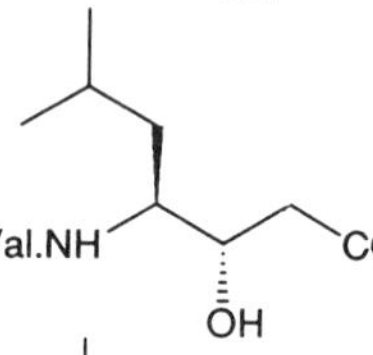 CO.Leu.Phe.NH_2	170	97
23	Ac.paF.Pro.paF.Val.NH 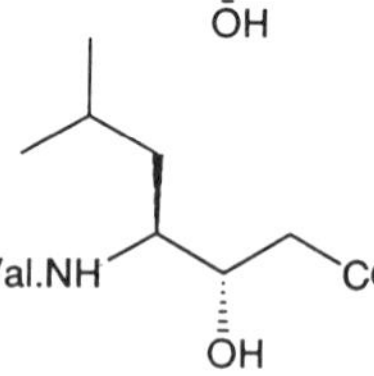 CO.Leu.Phe.paF.NH_2	80	97
24	Pro.paF.Pro.Phe.Val.NH 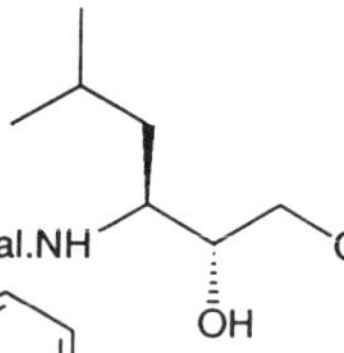 CO.Leu.Phe.paF.NH_2	50	97
25	Boc.NH 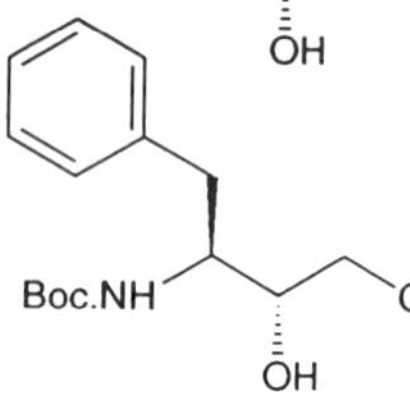 CO.Glu.Phe.OH	63	98

YOM = *O* - methyltyrosine; paF = *para* - aminophenylalanine;
NA = 3 - (1'- naphthyl)alanine.

ating conformationally restricted amines at the C-terminus. This approach also led to high-affinity inhibitors of the viral enzyme. Compounds 36 (L-685,434) and 37 completely inhibited the spread of HIV-1 in human T lymphoid cell culture at concentrations of 400 nM and 100 nM, respectively.

Attempts to improve the solubility and hence cell penetration and antiviral activity of L-685,434 have concentrated on modifications of the phenyl

Table 1.6. Inhibitors of HIV-1 proteinase based on statine-like dipeptide mimetics which incorporate a β-turn mimetic at the N-terminus

no.	structure	IC_{50}(nM)	Ref.
26	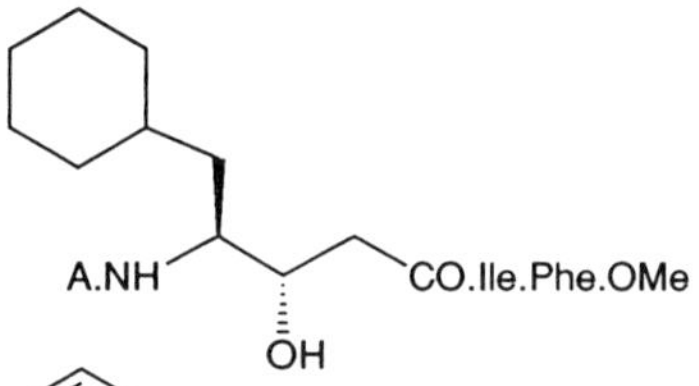	360 000	99
27	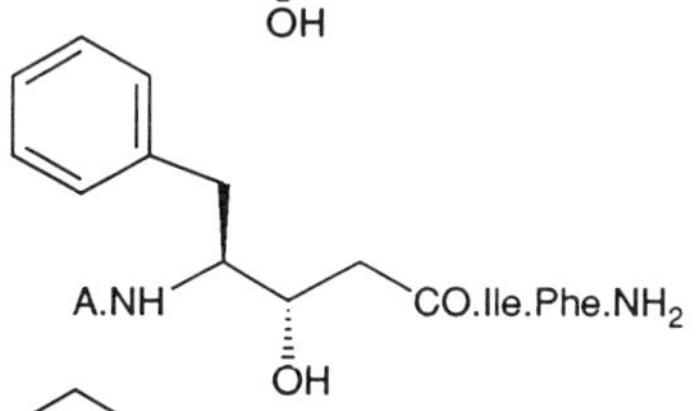	350 000	99
28	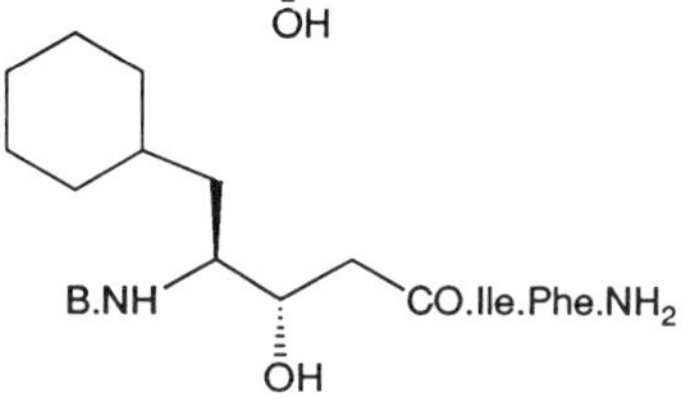	26	99

ring at P_1'. Substitution of the P_1' phenyl ring with a 3-hydroxypropyl led to L-693,549 (compound 38) (105), which is some 8–16-fold more potent as an antiviral agent than L-685,434. Incorporation of a morpholine moiety to give L-689,502 (compound 39) (106) also resulted in enhanced antiviral activity despite a slight decrease in its effect on enzyme inhibition. In general, for this series of compounds, the presence of a weakly basic group was found to increase antiviral activity and, by implication, cell penetration, whereas the presence of more strongly basic groups tended to decrease both enzyme inhibitory and antiviral activity.

Lingham *et al.* (107) investigated microbial biotransformation of the potent HIV-1 proteinase inhibitor L-689,502 (compound 39) as a way to generate novel but closely related compounds. Incubation with *Streptomyces lavendulae* resulted in oxidative cleavage of the morpholino group to give L-694,746 (compound 40), a potent and specific inhibitor of HIV proteinase. Other isolatable products of the microbial biotransformation of L-689,502 were a β-hydroxyindane derivative and a metabolite which had been hydroxylated on the *tert*-butyloxycarbonyl group.

Workers at Pfizer (108) have reported on the antiviral activity of the tetra-

Table 1.7. Inhibitors of HIV-1 proteinase based on hydroxyethylene dipeptide mimetics

no.	structure	K_i (nM)	Ref.
29	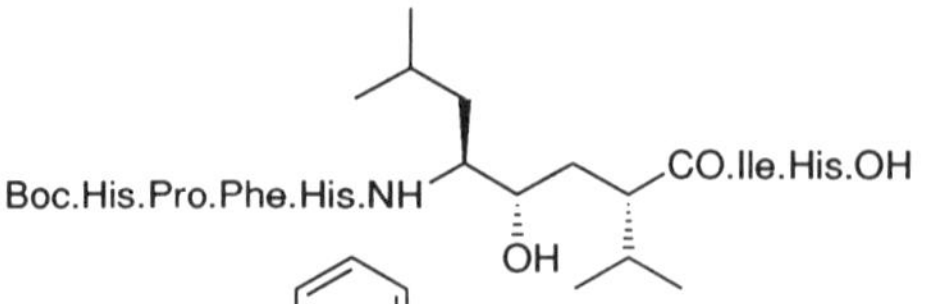	5	96
30	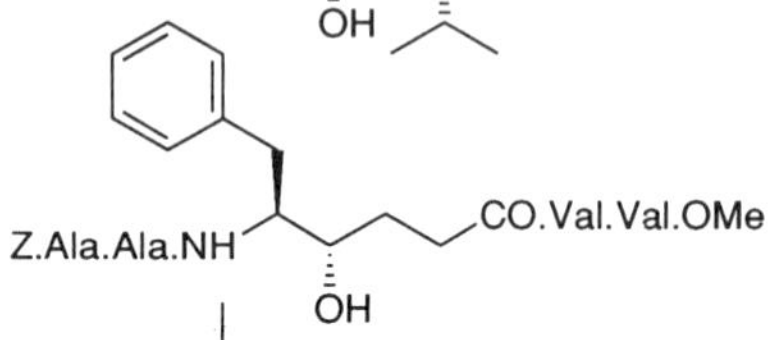	48	100
31 U 85548E	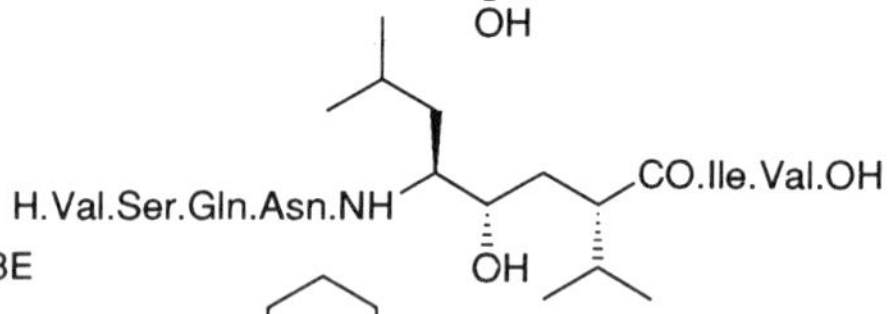	<1	101
32 U 81749	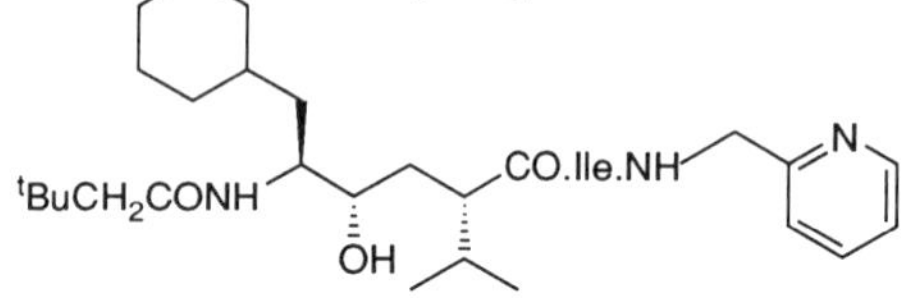	80	101
33 L-364,505	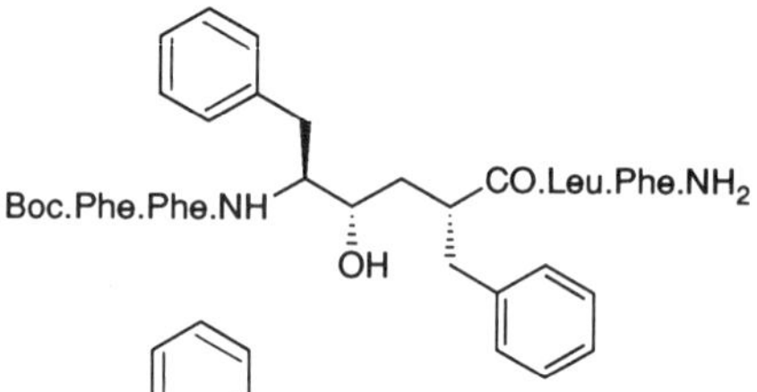	1	103
34	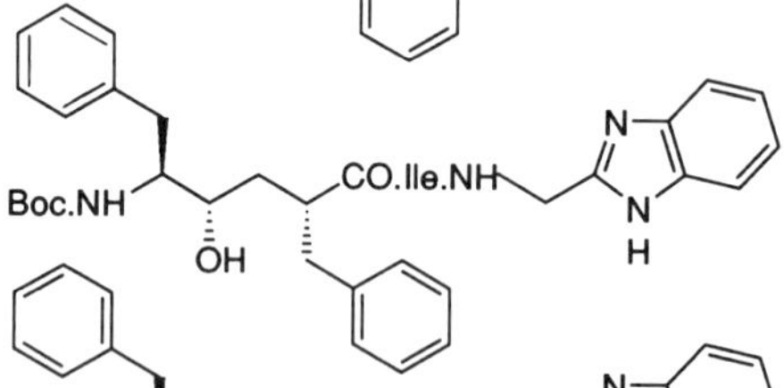	0.07 (IC_{50})	103
35 L-687,908	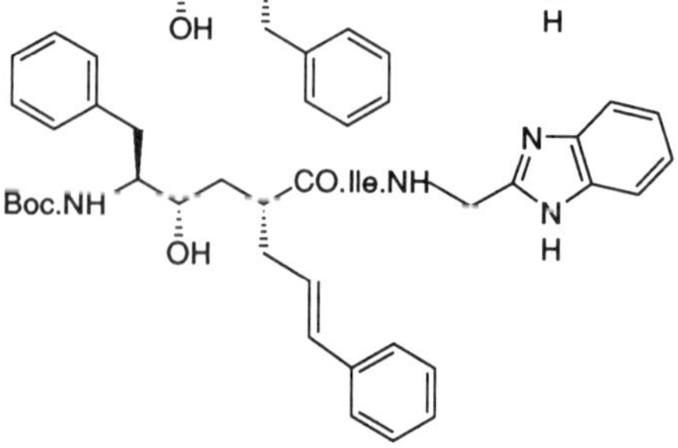	0.03 (IC_{50})	103

Table 1.7. Continued

36 L-685,434	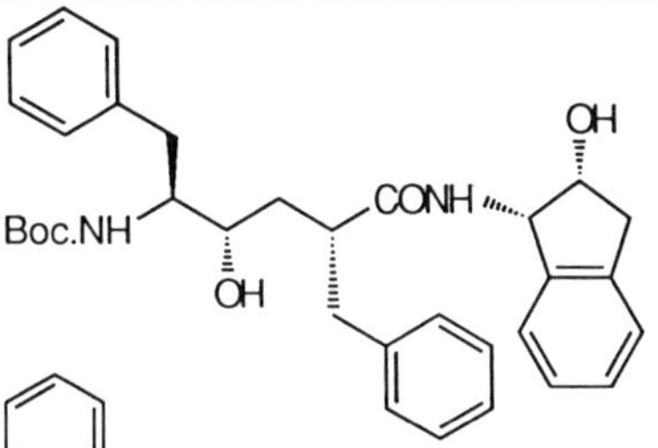	0.3 (IC_{50})	104
37	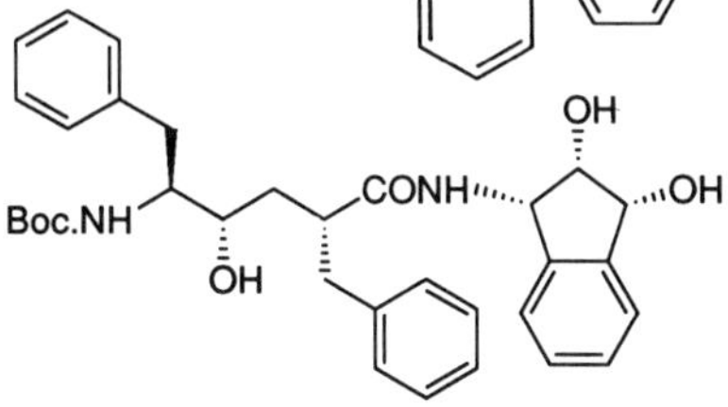	0.1 (IC_{50})	104
38 L-693,549	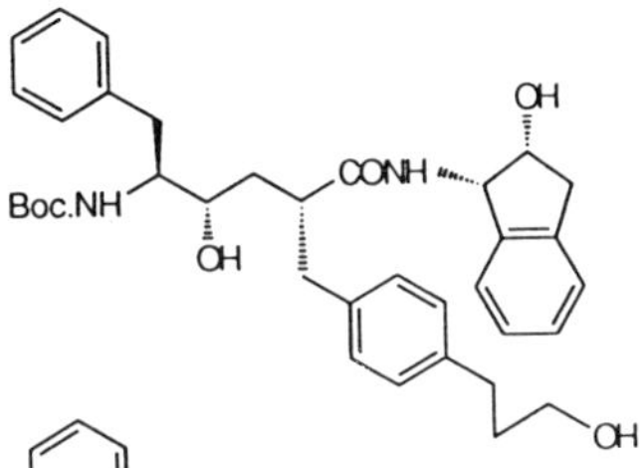	0.1 (IC_{50})	105
39 L-689,502	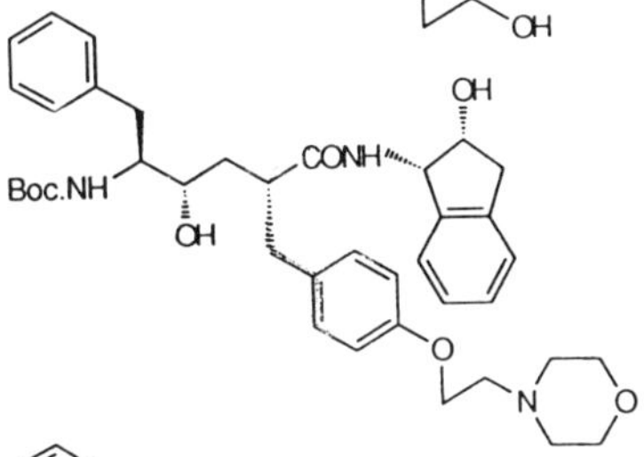	1 (IC_{50})	106
40 L-694,746	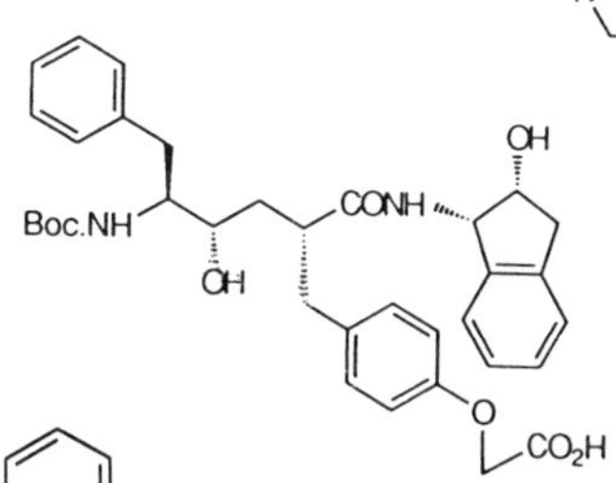	1 (IC_{50})	107
41 UK 88,947	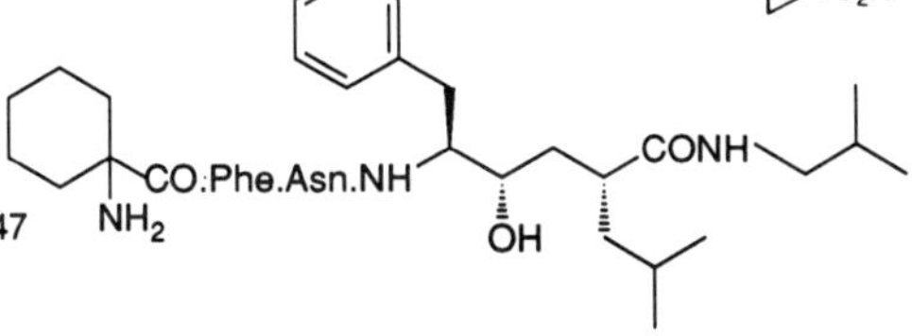	12 (IC_{50})	108

peptide analogue UK 88,947 (compound 41). At a concentration of 6 μM, UK 88,947 blocked the production of infectious virus in H9 cells infected with HIV-1_{IIIB}.

A series of hexapeptide analogues containing the dihydroxyethylene isostere has also been reported (109) to inhibit HIV-1 proteinase with high affinity (Table 1.8). The most potent of these inhibitors, U-75875 (compound 44), was examined in H9 cells chronically infected with HIV-1_{IIIB}. At a concentration of 1 μM, U-75875 completely blocked the processing of p55 to p24. Virus particles produced in the presence of the drug were morphologically immature and non-infectious. In cultures of peripheral blood mononuclear cells infected with HIV_{LAV}, 1 μM U-75875 completely blocked the spread of infection as measured by supernatant p24 and reverse transcriptase levels.

The difluoromethyl ketone transition state mimetic has been incorporated (110) into low-molecular-weight inhibitors which are relatively non-peptidic in nature (Table 1.9). The aqueous solubility of these compounds could be enhanced without loss of enzyme inhibitory activity by incorporation of a pyridyl moiety either in the P_1' position (compound 46) or at the N-terminus (compound 47). The parent compound of this series (45) did not

Table 1.8. Inhibitors of HIV-1 proteinase based on dihydroxyethylene dipeptide mimetics

no.	structure	K_i (nM)	Ref.
42	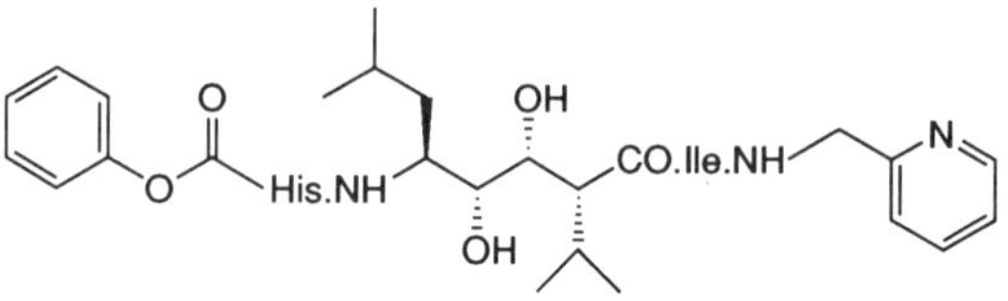	3	109
43	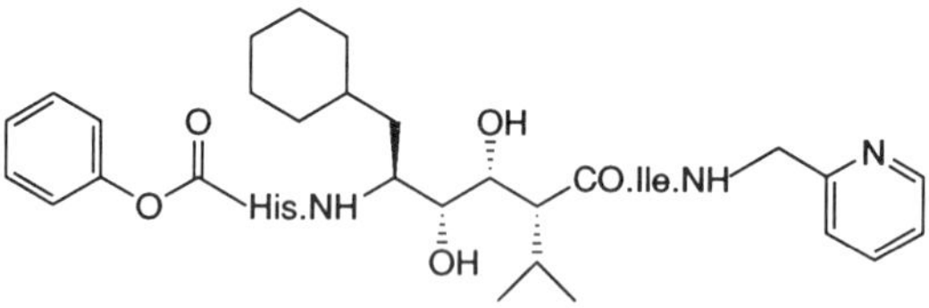	2	109
44 U75875	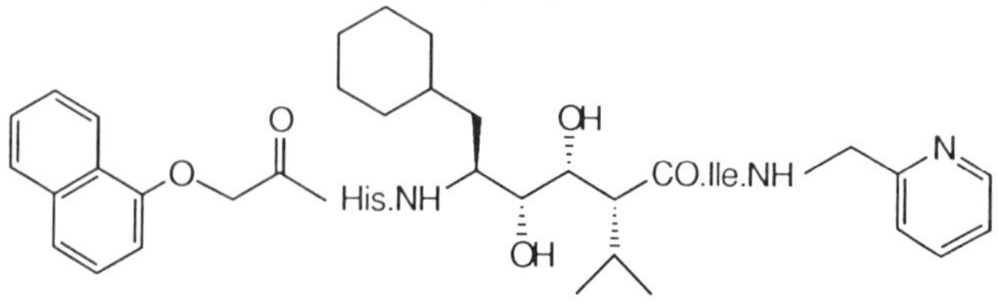		109

Table 1.9. Inhibitors of HIV-1 proteinase based on difluoromethyl ketone dipeptide mimetics

no.	structure	IC_{50} (nM)	Ref.
45	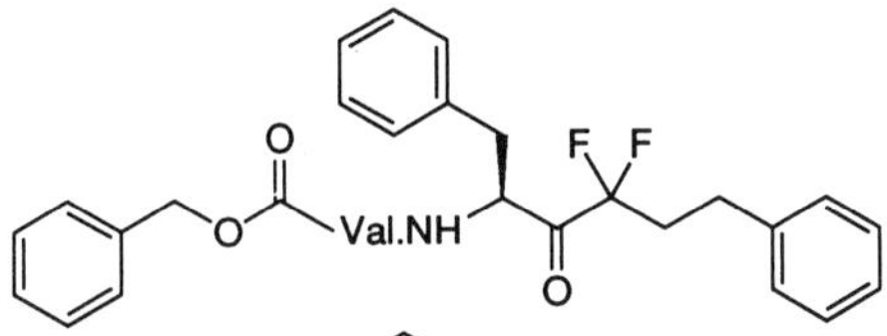	5.0	110
46	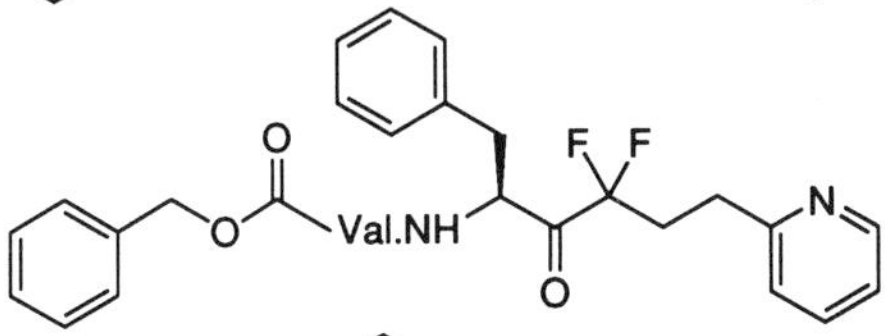	14.0	110
47	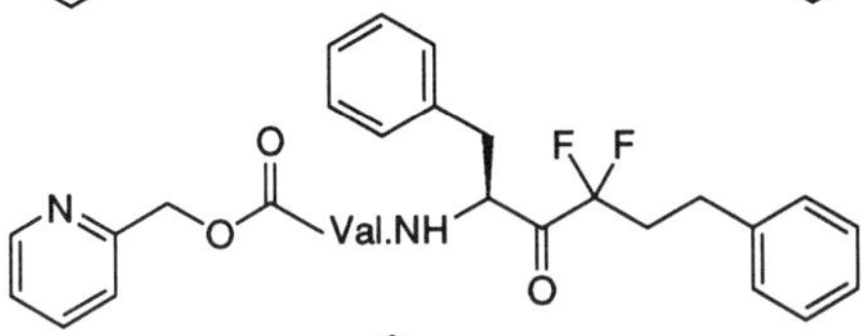	2.2	110
48	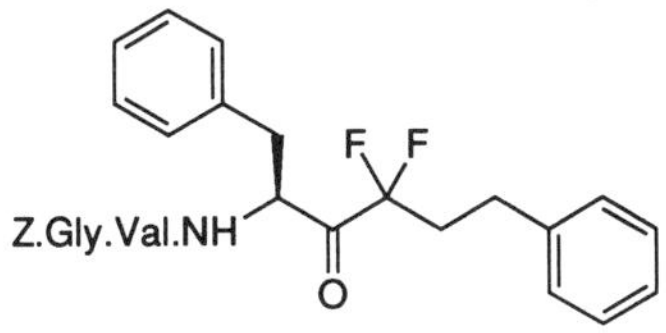	1.0	110

show any antiviral activity, possibly because of its very low solubility in the aqueous culture medium. Compounds 46, 47 and 48 all showed good antiviral efficacy, the most potent, compound 48, having an IC_{50} value of 1.9 μM when examined in MT-4 cells infected with $HIV\text{-}1_{IIIB}$.

Although incorporation of the hydroxyethylamine transition state mimetic into substrate analogues leads to compounds which contain an extra carbon atom compared with the corresponding substrates, this approach has nevertheless given very potent inhibitors of HIV proteinase (Table 1.10). In this type of inhibitor, the stereochemical requirement at the carbon centre bearing the hydroxyl group appears to depend critically both upon the length of the inhibitor and upon the nature of individual residues. This is in sharp contrast to inhibitors which use either the hydroxyethylene dipeptide isostere or a statine analogue as the transition state mimetic, since in these compounds the *S*- stereochemistry is clearly preferred.

In heptapeptide analogues spanning P_4 to P_3' and in pentapeptide

Table 1.10. Inhibitors of HIV-1 proteinase based on hydroxyethylamine dipeptide mimetics

no.	structure	IC_{50} (nM)	Ref.
49	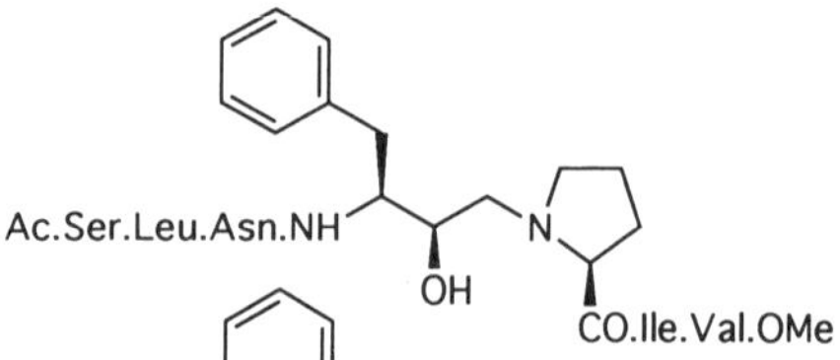	65	112
50	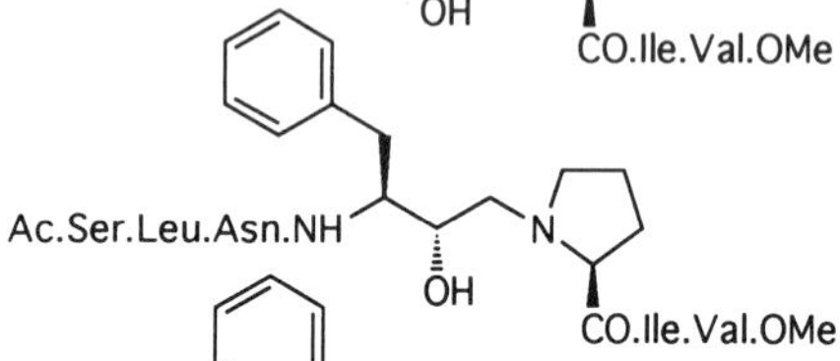	3.4 (K_i 0.24)	111, 112
51	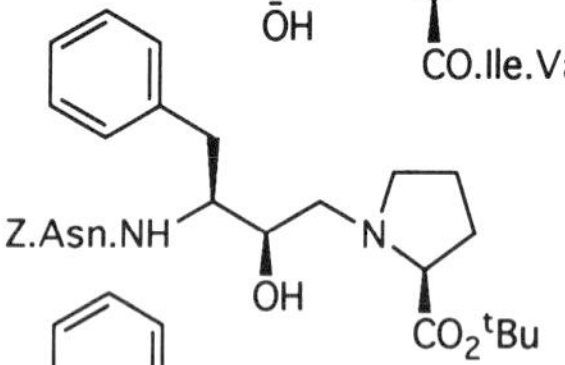	140 (51)	114 (112)
52	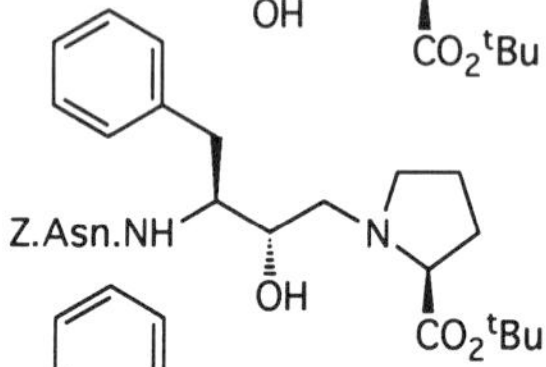	300 (450)	114 (112)
53	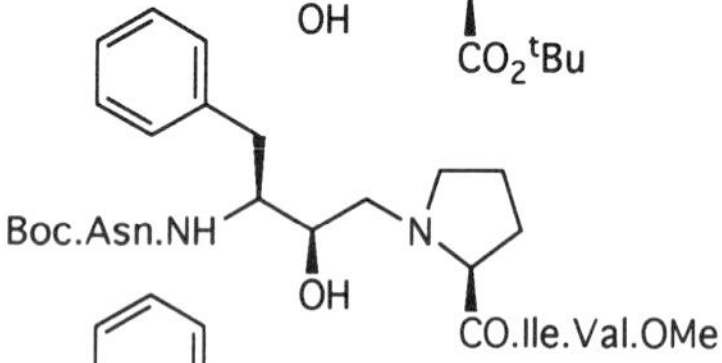	850	112
54	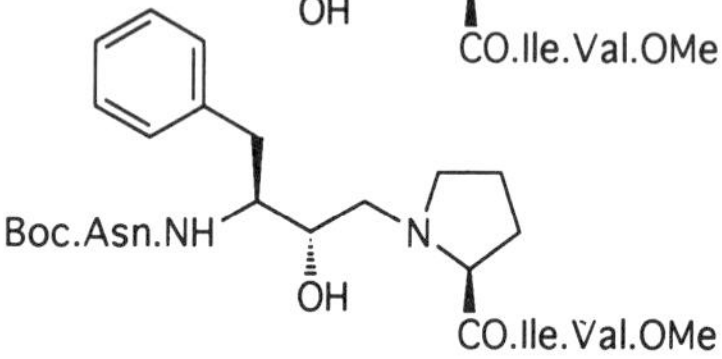	16	112
55	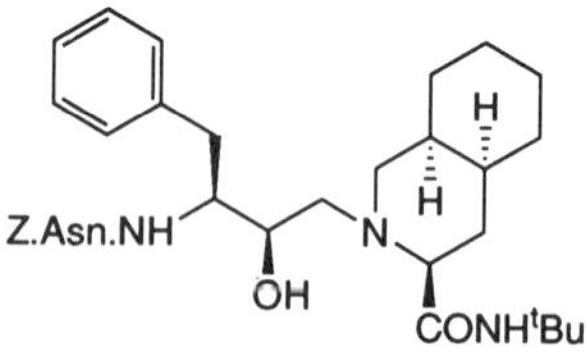	<2.7	114
56	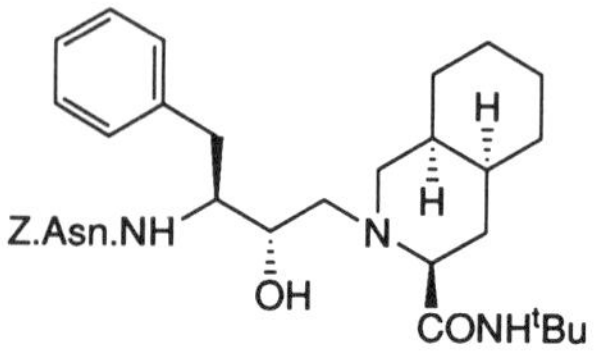	>100	114

Table 1.10. Continued

no.	structure	IC_{50} (nM)	Ref.
57 Ro 31-8959	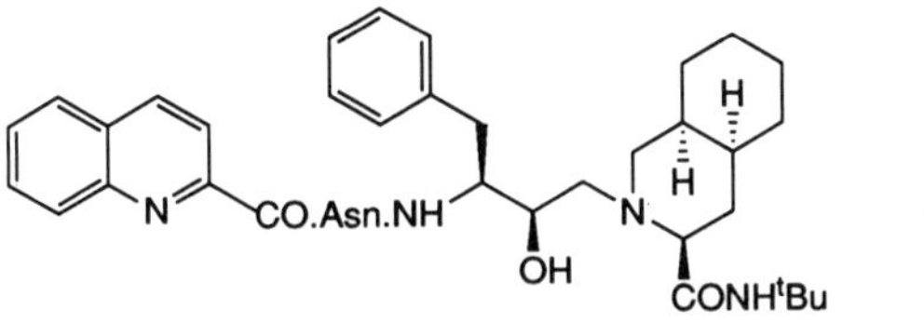	<0.4 (K_i 0.12)	113,114
58	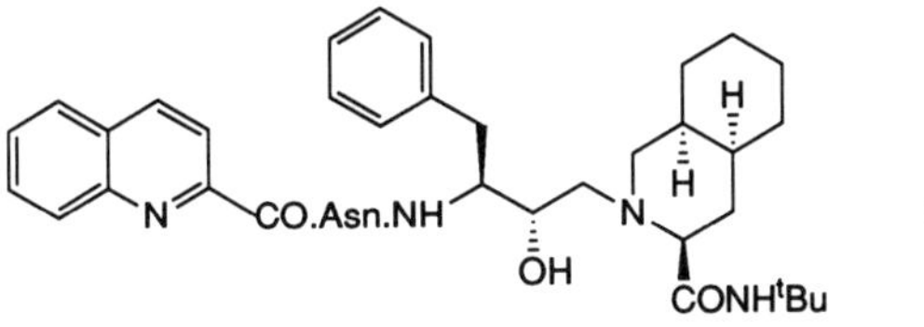	>100	114
59	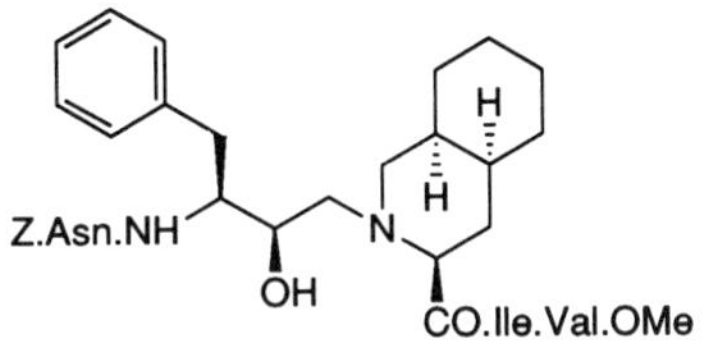	>>100	114
60	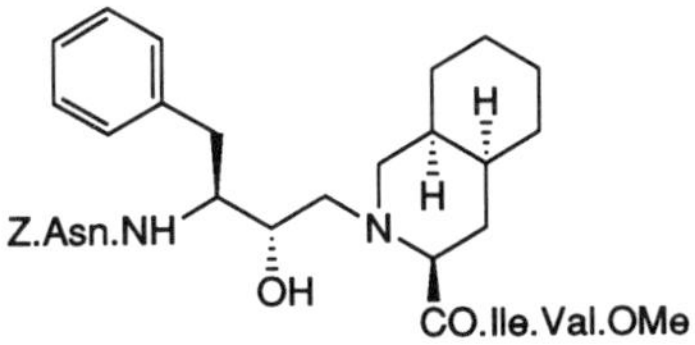	>>100	114
61	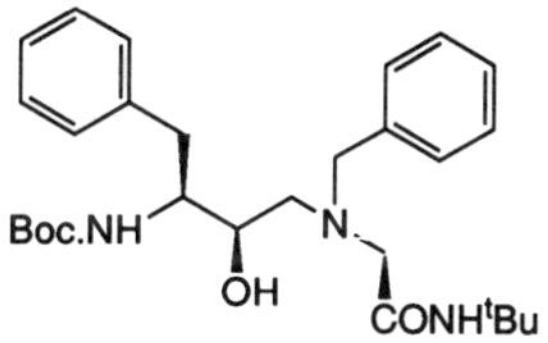	>100 000	115
62	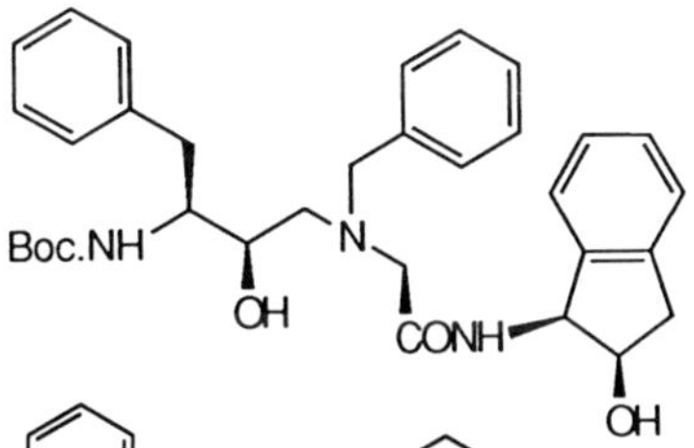	252	115
63	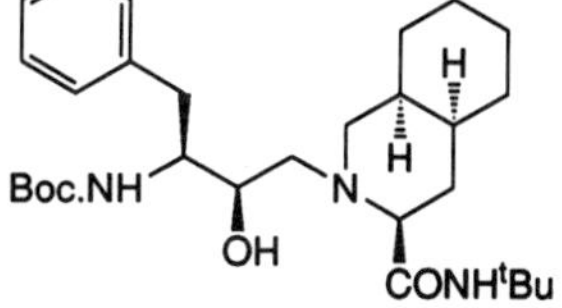	>3000	115

Table 1.10. Continued

no.	structure	IC_{50} (nM)	Ref.
64	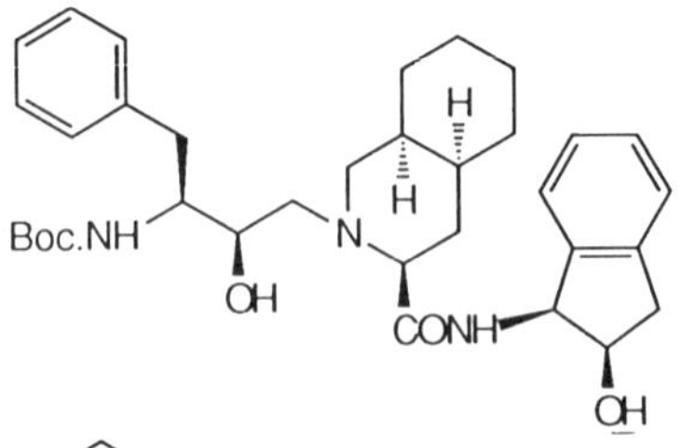		115
65 L-704,325	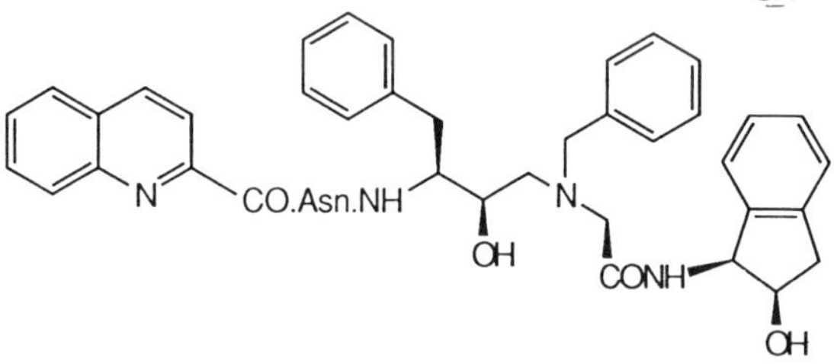	5.4	115

analogues spanning P_2 to P'_3 the *S*- diastereomer has higher affinity for the enzyme (compound 50 versus compound 49 and compound 54 versus compound 53) (112). Truncated inhibitors, spanning only P_2 to P'_1, show a weak preference for the *R*- stereochemistry at the hydroxyl group when the P'_1 residue is proline (compound 51 versus compound 52) (112–114). When the prolyl residue at P'_1 is replaced by the [(4a*S*,8a*S*)-decahydroisoquinoline-3(*S*)-yl]carbonyl (DIQ) group, there is a large increase in potency (compound 55 versus compound 51) (114) and a strong preference for the *R*- diastereomer emerges (compound 55 versus compound 56 and compound 57 versus compound 58). Inhibitors which incorporate a DIQ group at P'_1 become substantially less potent if extended towards the C-terminus to include P'_2 and P'_3 residues (compound 59 and compound 60) (114). It has been proposed (112,114) that, whilst binding at the S_3 to S_1 subsites is similar for the two classes of inhibitor, binding at the S'_1 and S' subsites is substantially different, with the *tert*-butyl group of compounds such as 55 and 57 occupying the S'_2 subsite rather than following the path of the substrate backbone.

The most potent compound of this series, Ro 31-8959 (compound 57) (113), shows excellent selectivity for the viral enzyme over a range of other human aspartic proteinases. Ro 31-8959 showed antiviral activity in C8166 cells infected with HIV_{RF} ($IC_{50} = 2$ nM determined by p24 antigen) and in

JM cells infected with HIV-1_{GB} ($IC_{50} = 2.5$ nM determined by syncytium counts).

Inhibitors incorporating the hydroxyethylamine transition state mimetic which use a non-cyclic secondary amine at P_1' have been reported by Tucker *et al.* (115). These compounds also demonstrate a clear preference for the *R*- configuration at the carbon atom bearing the transition state alcohol. Compound 62, which lacks the P_1 and P_2 residues, shows good enzyme inhibitory potency ($IC_{50} = 252$ nM) and is at least 13 times more potent than the inhibitors 63 and 64 which incorporate the decahydroisoquinoline moiety at P_1'. Interestingly, use of the 1(*S*)-amino-2-(*R*)-hydroxyindan group does not lead to significantly enhanced activity in these latter compounds (compare compounds 64 and 63 versus compounds 62 and 61), indicating distinct differences in the way the P_1-P_1' region of these compounds interact with the enzyme active site relative to inhibitors incorporating a non-cyclic secondary amine at P_1'.

N-terminal extension of compound 62 to include the P_2 and P_3 residues gave L-704,325 (compound 65) with an IC_{50} value of 5.4 nM. Somewhat surprisingly, this enhancement of potency is very much smaller than that achieved by corresponding N-terminal extension of compound 63 to give compound 57 (55-fold versus 8000-fold enhancement of potency) despite the fact that in their truncated form the non-cyclic inhibitors are more potent. It is suggested that these differences may arise because of the tighter binding of the secondary amine transition state isostere which reduces the freedom of movement of the P_2-P_3 region or induces changes in the overall conformation of the enzyme. Again, two closely related classes of inhibitor appear to bind to the enzyme in quite different ways. Compound 65 inhibited the spread of HIV-1 in MT-4 human T lymphoid cells at a concentration of 200 nM compared with 12.5 nM for compound 57 in the same assay.

Mimoto *et al.* (116,117) have recently described incorporation of the hydroxymethylcarbonyl transition state mimetic into HIV proteinase inhibitors (Table 1.11). In this series of compounds, the *S*-(*syn*) diastereomer appears to be preferred in inhibitors incorporating P_1' and P_2' residues (compound 66 versus compound 67).

The heptapeptide analogue KNI-93 (compound 67) is a very potent inhibitor of HIV proteinase. Deletion of the P_4 serine residue substantially reduces inhibitory potency (KNI-81, compound 68), although somewhat surprisingly, potency is restored in the tripeptide analogue KNI-102 (compound 69). Although the longer-chain peptide analogues have little antiviral activity, KNI-102 is reported to exhibit complete anti-HIV activity at 2 μM (117).

Modifications of the P_1' residue of KNI-102 produced interesting results (118). In this series, replacement of proline by pipecolinic acid (compound 70 versus compound 69) gave decreased enzyme inhibitory activity, in

Table 1.11. Inhibitors of HIV-1 proteinase based on hydroxymethylcarbonyl dipeptide mimetics

no.	structure	IC_{50} (nM)	Ref.
66 KNI-122	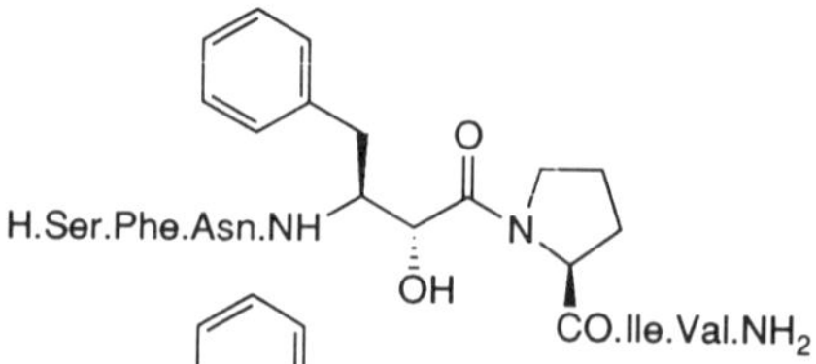	100	116
67 KNI-93	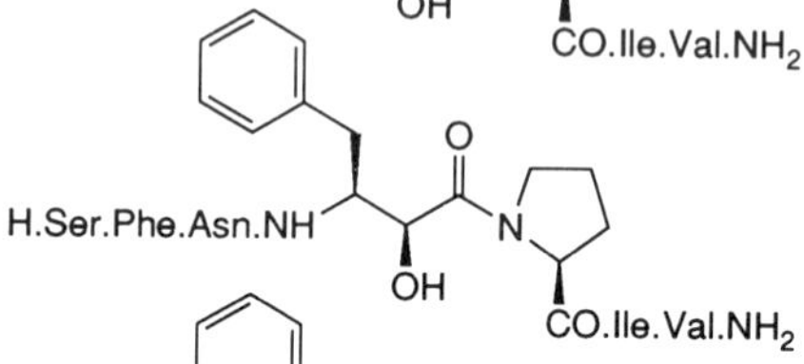	5	116
68 KNI-81	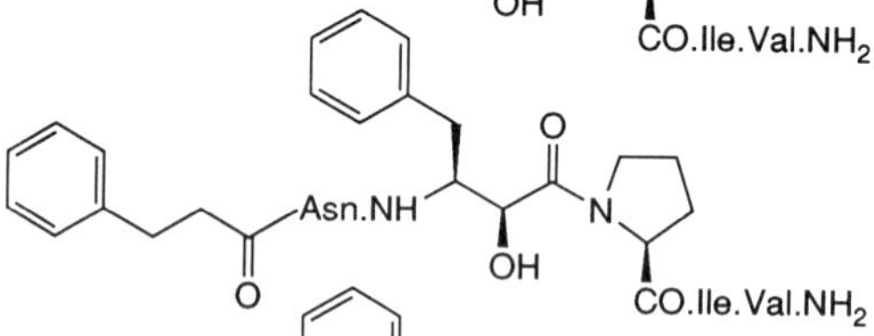	468	117
69 KNI-102	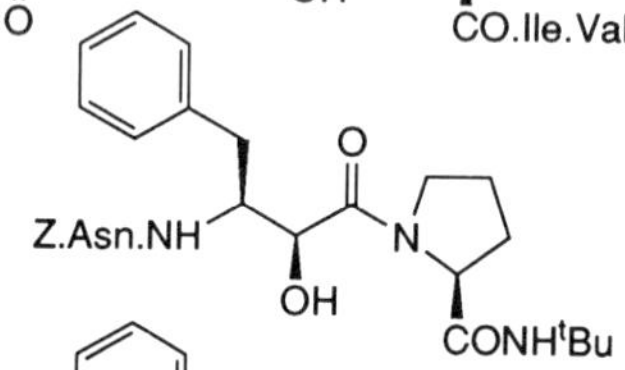	89 (7.4)	117 (120)
70	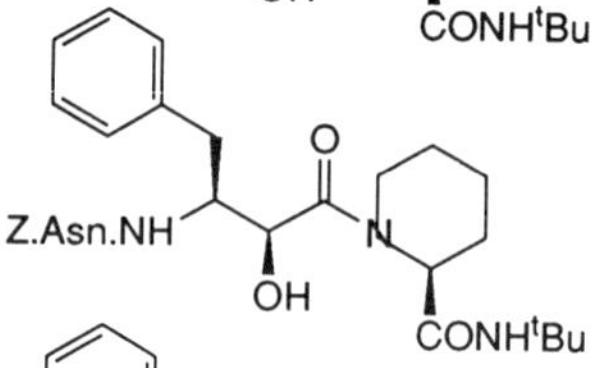	450 (26)	118 (120)
71 KNI - 272	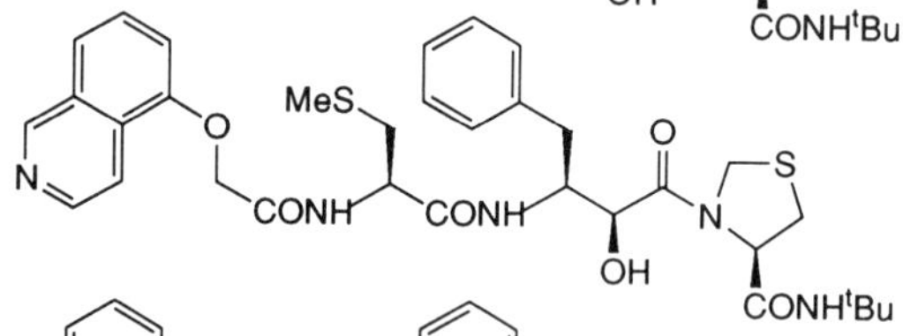	6.5	118
72 KNI - 272	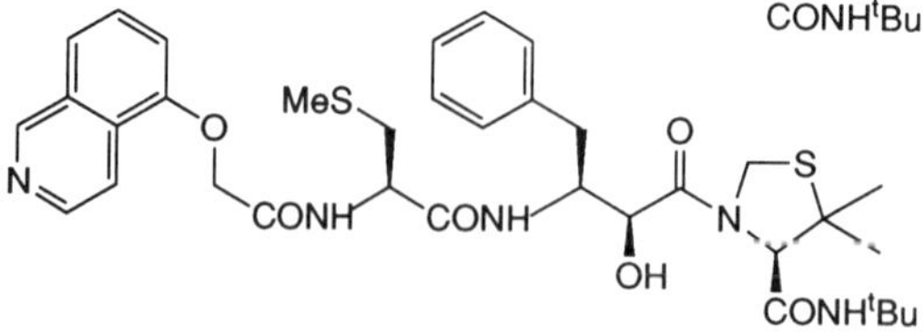	2.3	118
73	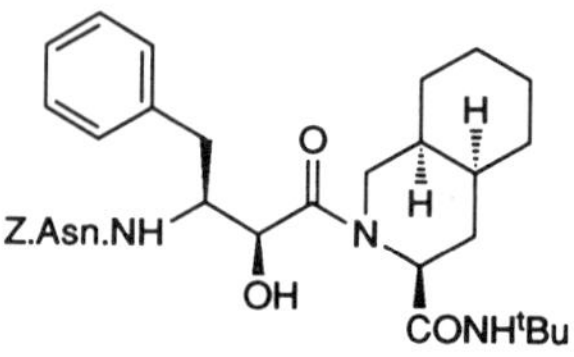	84	120

Table 1.11. Continued

no.	structure	IC_{50} (nM)	Ref.
74	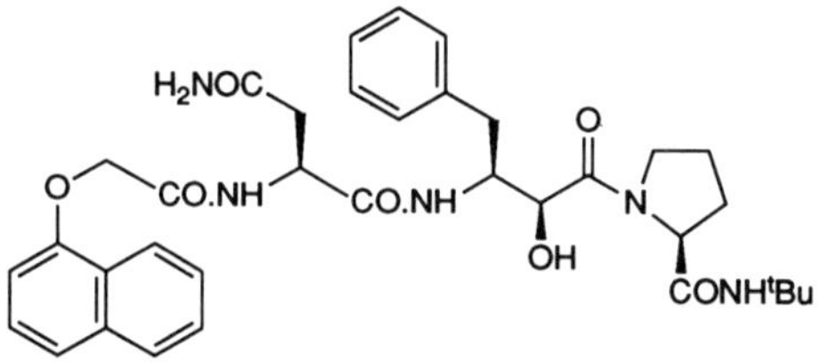	0.58 (K_i 0.4)	120

contrast to the case of the hydroxyethylamine-type inhibitors (114). Replacement of the pyrrolidine ring of proline by heterocyclic five-membered rings, especially thiazolidine or dimethyl thiazolidine, however, led to significantly improved activity. Further modifications of the P_2 and P_3 residues resulted in the potent and selective inhibitors, KNI-272 (compound 71) and KNI-227 (compound 72). Both compounds are active (IC_{50} = 20–100 nM) against a wide spectrum of HIV strains, including AZT-resistant clinical isolates. KNI-227 also shows moderate bioavailability (4%) in the rat (119).

A second series of hydroxymethylcarbonyl transition state mimetics has been described by Krantz *et al.* (120). They extended the observations of Mimoto and co-workers, reporting a decrease in activity for residues at P_1' in the order proline > pipecolinic acid > decahydroisoquinoline carboxylic acid (compounds 69, 70 and 73), which is opposite to that observed for inhibitors incorporating the hydroxyethylamine transition state mimetic. The effect of extension towards the C-terminus is also different in this series: activity is improved in the less active (*R*)- diastereomer but remains unchanged in the more active (*S*)- diastereomer. The need for specific interactions with the P_1 carbonyl or intrinsic conformational effects may explain the intriguing differences in structure–activity relationships between these inhibitors and the seemingly closely related hydroxyethylamine derivatives. The most potent inhibitor reported by Krantz *et al.* is compound 74, with a K_i of 0.4 nM.

An elegant approach to the design of HIV proteinase inhibitors which exploits the two-fold rotational (C_2) symmetry of the native enzyme was taken by Kempf *et al.* (80,121). A hypothetical axis of symmetry in the substrate was defined, based on the C_2 axis of the enzyme. The P′ portion of the substrate was deleted and a C_2 operation performed on the remaining P residues to generate a symmetrical inhibitor. This procedure gives rise to either a diamino alcohol (compounds 75 and 76) or a diaminodiol

Table 1.12. Symmetrical inhibitors of HIV-1 proteinase

no.	structure	IC_{50} (nM)	Ref.
75	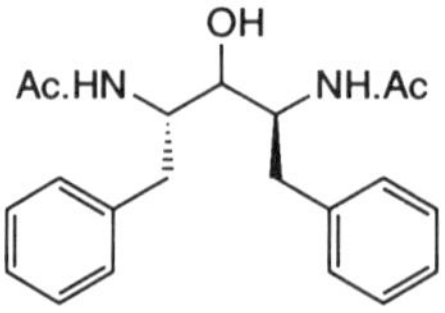	>10 000	121
76 A 74704	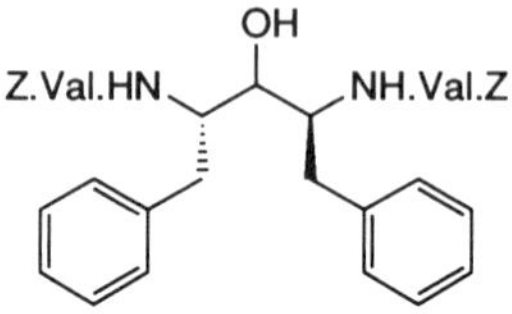	3	121
77 (3*R*,4*S*) 78 (3*R*,4*S*) 79 (3*R*,4*S*)	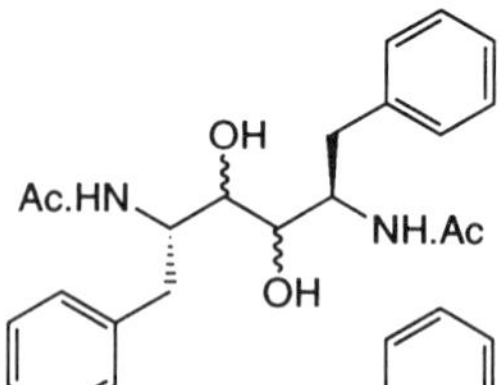	40 280 12	121
80 (3*R*,4*S*) 81 (3*R*,4*S*) 82 (3*R*,4*S*)	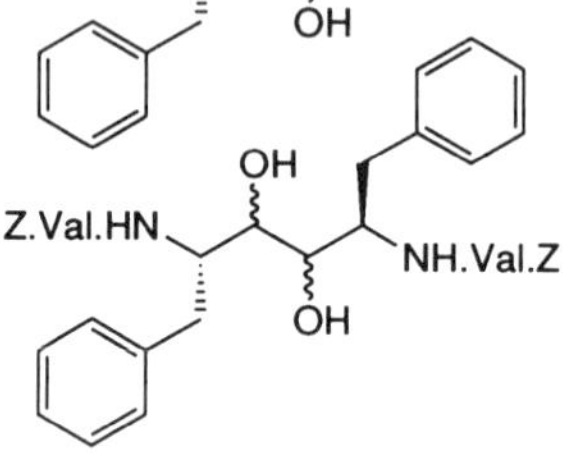	0.22 0.38 0.22	121
83 A-77003	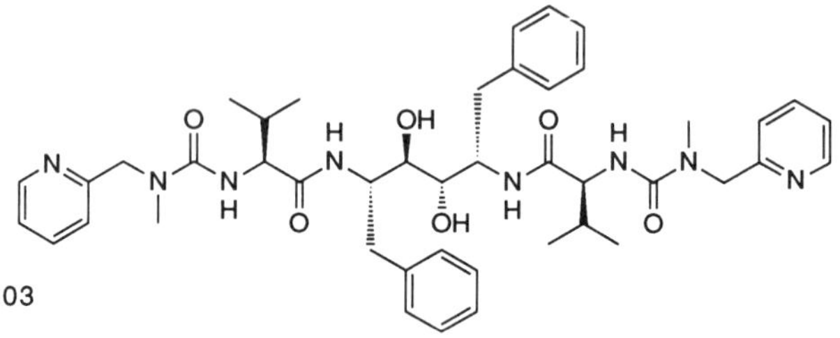	<1	122
84 A-80987	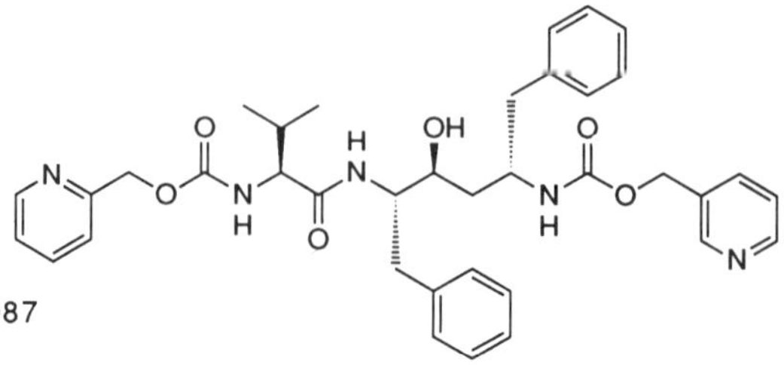	0.25 (K_i)	123

Table 1.12. Continued

no.	structure	IC_{50} (nM)	Ref.
85 L-700,417	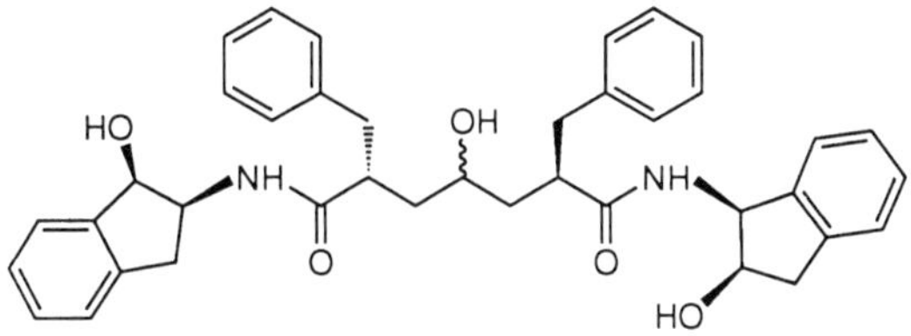	0.67	81

(compounds 77–82), depending on whether the C_2 axis is orientated through the carbonyl carbon atom or through the middle of the scissile bond (Table 1.12).

Compound 75, which can interact only with S_1 and S_1' subsites, shows only weak activity; incorporation of the P_2 and P_2' residues gives the nanomolar inhibitor, A74704 (compound 76). Inhibitors derived from the alternative C_2 axis intepretation were in general around 10-fold more potent and, surprisingly, showed little dependency on the stereochemistry of the two hydroxyl groups (compounds 77–79 and compounds 80–82). Compounds 80–82 blocked the spread of HIV-1_{IIIB} in both H9 cells and MT-4 cells (IC_{50} 20–150 nM) as measured by p24 antigen levels or cytopathic effects.

The poor aqueous solubility of such inhibitors posed difficulties for evaluation *in vivo* and more soluble compounds were obtained by modifying the terminal phenyl groups to pyridyl groups and by modifying the carbamate linkages to *N*-methyl ureas (122). This approach afforded, *inter alia*, A-77003 (compound 83) with an $IC_{50} < 1$ nM. A-77003 inhibited the formation of HIV p24 antigen production in H9 and CEM cells and also prevented the spread of HIV in MT-4 cells at submicromolar concentrations. The antiviral EC_{50} ranged from 30 to 300 nM depending on the cell line, virus strain, viral load and assay method. Despite reasonable aqueous solubility (~ 100 mg/ml), the bioavailability of A-77003 in rats, dogs and monkeys was disappointingly low at <3%.

Further studies identified A-80987 (compound 84) as a potent inhibitor of HIV proteinase (K_i 0.25 nM) which was active against laboratory strains of HIV as well as clinical isolates including AZT-resistant strains, with an ED_{50} of approximately 130 nM (123). Moreover, the oral bioavailability of A-80987 ranged from 13% to 26%, and with improved formulation has been increased to over 50% in the dog. In view of its good *in vitro* antiviral activity and favourable pharmacodynamic profile, A-80987 has been selected as a candidate for oral treatment of HIV-infected persons.

Using a similar strategy to that of Kempf, Bone *et al.* (81) have designed a series of pseudosymmetric inhibitors based on L-685,434 (compound 36). One of these, L-700,417 (compound 85) inhibited HIV proteinase with an IC_{50} of 0.67 nM and completely blocked the spread of HIV-1_{IIIB} infection in human T lymphoid cell culture at a concentration of 100 nM.

Recently, a number of non-peptidic inhibitors of HIV proteinase have been described (Table 1.13). A boronated porphyrin (compound 86) has been reported (124) with an IC_{50} of 185 nM against HIV-1 proteinase. Removal of all four carborane moieties significantly reduced activity. Compound 86 was also shown to prevent processing of HIV polyproteins in cell culture at micromolar concentrations.

A screening programme (125) identified the penicillin-derived C_2 symmetric dimers as potent inhibitors of HIV-1 proteinase. Although the diester (compound 87) failed to block the cytopathic effects of HIV-1 in MT-4 cells, the diamides (compounds 89 and 90) were both effective (ED_{50} values of 5.4 nM and 0.29 nM, respectively). The more hydrophilic diamide (compound 88) failed to show an antiviral effect, possibly because of poor cell penetration. Compounds 89 and 90 inhibited syncytia formation in HIV-1-infected C8166 cells (ED_{50} 1.11 μM and 0.06 μM) and also inhibited the expression of p24 antigen in H9 cells (ED_{50} 0.42 μM and 0.025 μM). Neither compound showed cytotoxicity in any of the cellular assays and neither showed any inhibition of other aspartic proteinases (renin, pepsin or cathepsin D) at concentrations up to 100 mg/ml. An X-ray structure of the diamide (compound 89) complexed to recombinant enzyme has shown that the interaction with the inhibitor is indeed symmetrical, as had been speculated. Studies are in progress to investigate the potential of this novel series of compounds as chemotherapeutic agents for the treatment of AIDS.

Another novel inhibitor of HIV proteinase was purified from *Hypoxylon fragiforme*, a fungus isolated from the bark of the American beech tree (126). L-696,474 (compound 91) (127), a novel cytochalasin, was found to be a competitive inhibitor of HIV-1 proteinase, with an IC_{50} of 3 μM (128). L-696,474 did not inhibit stromelysin, papain or human leucocyte elastase, although it did inhibit another aspartic proteinase, pepsin, with an IC_{50} of 52 μM.

The identification of novel non-peptidic natural product inhibitors may prove very useful in offering lead compounds which could be used to develop more efficacious treatments and managements for AIDS.

CONCLUSION

If present estimates of the spread of HIV are accurate, then the next decade will see a continued increase in the number of individuals infected by HIV

Table 1.13. Non-peptidic inhibitors of HIV proteinase

no.	structure	IC_{50} (nM)	Ref.
86	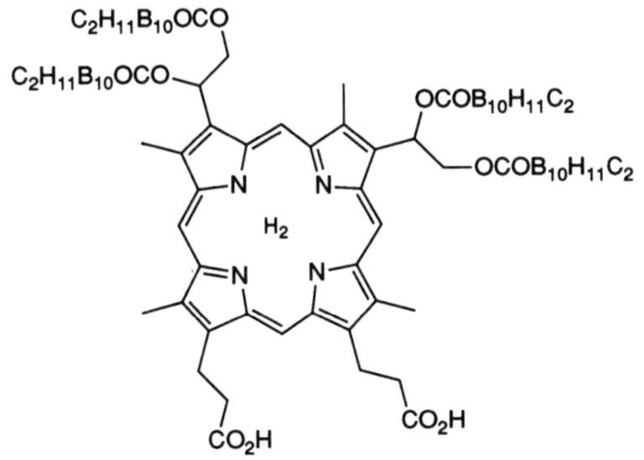	185	124
87 R = OCH_3	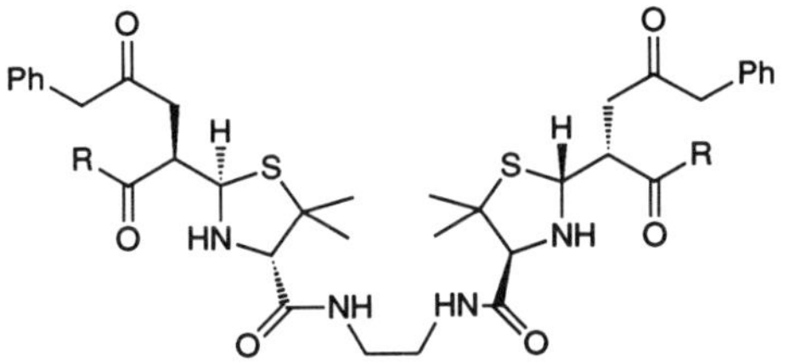	60	125
88 R = NH_2		3	125
89 R = NHEt		4.8	125
90 R = $NHCH_2Ph$		0.9	125
91 L-696,474	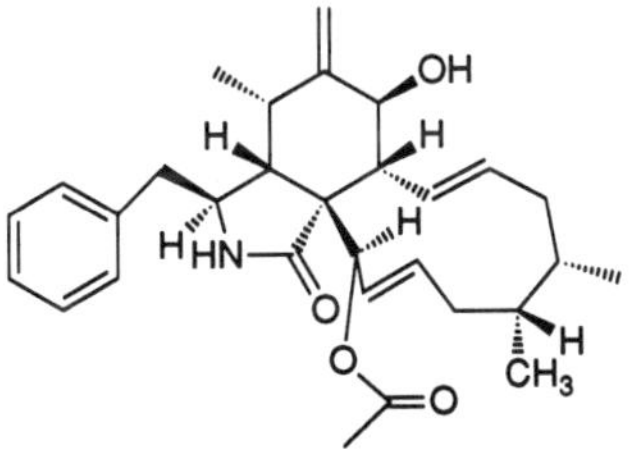	3000	128

and in the number of cases of AIDS. The urgency of finding treatments is self-evident, and unfortunately the currently available nucleoside-based inhibitors of reverse transcriptase can show significant toxicity. Perhaps more importantly, mutations in the genome of HIV can lead to drug resistance (129). Notable progress has been made towards the development of an inhibitor of the virally encoded proteinase as a viable alternative therapy. A range of highly potent and selective inhibitors, many of which strongly attenuate viral replication in cell culture, is now available.

Recent studies have also demonstrated favourable interactions (synergy or additive effects) between reverse transcriptase inhibitors and proteinase inhibitors. Synergy occurs when the combined effect of the compounds given simultaneously is greater than that predicted from the sum of the individual drug effects. SKF 108922 has been shown (130) to exhibit either additivity or potent synergy with AZT depending upon the assay conditions used. A-77003 (compound 83) and other C_2 symmetric inhibitors have been shown (131) to be synergistic with AZT, although the interactions with ddI were essentially additive.

Additive to synergistic effects have also been demonstrated (132) when Ro 31-8959 (compound 57) was combined with AZT, ddC or rIFN-aA in acutely infected peripheral blood mononuclear cells. In a second study (133), Ro 31-8959 was shown to interact synergistically with AZT, ddC and 2′-FddC. Compared with concentrations needed when inhibitors were used individually, reductions of between 2- and 30-fold were seen for the combinations, depending on the nucleoside analogue and the ratio of concentrations employed.

There are a number of theoretical advantages to treatment with both a reverse transcriptase and a proteinase inhibitor. Reverse transcriptase inhibitors act early in the viral replication cycle and can prevent the virus genome from becoming incorporated into newly infected cells. The effect of AZT is thus manifest in acute infections. Chronically infected cells, however, can continue to proliferate and shed virus even in the presence of a reverse transcriptase inhibitor. Proteinase inhibitors, on the other hand, act late in the replication cycle and are effective in both acute and chronic infections. Although proteinase inhibitors do not prevent the formation of virus antigen by cells already chronically infected with HIV-1, the virus produced is not infectious. It has been further speculated (133) that the antigen produced during such treatment might act as a potential stimulus to the immune system.

The range of potential benefits of treatment with a proteinase inhibitor together with a reverse transcriptase inhibitor justifies full examination of combination therapies. Whilst there are still problems to be overcome with the oral bioavailability of many of the proteinase inhibitors, there are encouraging indications both from work in this area (123) and from work on renin inhibitors (134) that appropriate structural modifications can lead to compounds with acceptable pharmacological properties.

REFERENCES

1. Centers for Disease Control (1981). Kaposi's sarcoma and *Pneumocystis* pneumonia among homosexual men: New York City and California. *MMWR*, **30**, 305–308.

2. Centres for Disease Control (1981). *Pneumocystis* pneumonia: Los Angeles. *MMWR*, **30**, 250–252.
3. Barre-Sinoussi, F., Chermann, J. C., Rey, F. *et al.* (1983). Isolation of a T-lymphotropic retrovirus from a patient at risk for acquired immune deficiency syndrome (AIDS). *Science*, **220**, 868–871.
4. Coffin, J., Haase, A., Levy, J. A. *et al.* (1986). Human immunodeficiency viruses (letter). *Science*, **232**, 697.
5. Gallo, R. C., Salahuddin, S. Z., Popovic, M. *et al.* (1984). Frequent detection and isolation of cytopathic retroviruses (HTLV-III) from patients with AIDS and at risk for AIDS. *Science*, **224**, 500–503.
6. Gallo, R. C. and Montagnier, L. (1988). AIDS in 1988. *Sci. Am.*, **259**, 25–32.
7. Popovic, M., Sarngadharan, M. G., Read, E. and Gallo, R. C. (1984). Detection and continuous production of cytopathic retroviruses (HTLV-III) from patients with AIDS and pre-AIDS. *Science*, **224**, 497–500.
8. Clavel, F., Guyader, M., Guetard, D. *et al.* (1986). Molecular cloning and polymorphism of the human immune deficiency virus type 2. *Nature*, **324**, 691–695.
9. Guyader, M., Emerman, M., Sonigo, P. *et al.* (1987). Genome organization and transactivation of the human immunodeficiency virus type 2. *Nature*, **326**, 662–669.
10. Levy, J. A. (1989). Human immunodeficiency viruses and the pathogenesis of AIDS. *JAMA*, **261**, 2997–3006.
11. Klatzmann, D., Barre-Sinoussi, F., Nugeyre, M. T. *et al.* (1984). Selective tropism of lymphadenopathy associated virus (LAV) for helper-inducer T lymphocytes. *Science*, **225**, 59–63.
12. Levy, J. A., Shimabukuro, J., McHugh, T. *et al.* (1985). AIDS-associated retroviruses (ARV) can productively infect other cells besides human T helper cells. *Virology*, **147**, 441–448.
13. Shaw, G. M., Harper, M. E. and Hahn, B. H. (1985). HTLV-III infection in brains of children and adults with AIDS encephalopathy. *Science*, **227**, 177–182.
14. Wiley, C. A., Schrier, R. D., Nelson, J. A. *et al.* (1986). Cellular localization of human immunodeficiency virus infection within the brains of acquired immune deficiency syndrome patients. *Proc. Natl Acad. Sci. USA*, **83**, 7089–7093.
15. Levy, J. A., Shimabukuro, J., Hollander, H. *et al.* (1985). Isolation of AIDS-associated retroviruses from cerebrospinal fluid and brain of patients with neurological symptoms. *Lancet*, **ii**, 586–588.
16. Harouse, J. M., Kunsch, C., Hartle, H. T. *et al.* (1989). CD4-independent infection of human neural cells by human immunodeficiency virus type 1. *J. Virol.*, **63**, 2527–2533.
17. Nelson, J. A., Wiley, C. A., Reynolds, K. C. *et al.* (1988). Human immunodeficiency virus detected in bowel epithelium from patients with gastrointestinal symptoms. *Lancet*, **i**, 259–262.
18. Cohen, A. H., Sun, N. C., Shapshak, P. and Imagawa, D. T. (1989). Demonstration of human immunodeficiency virus in renal epithelium in HIV-associated nephropathy. *Med. Pathol.* **2**, 125–128.
19. Cao, Y. Z., Friedman-Kien, A. E., Huang, Y. X. *et al.* (1990). CD4-independent, productive human immunodeficiency virus type 1 infection of hepatoma cell lines in vitro. *J. Virol.*, **64**, 2553–2559.
20. Plata, F., Garcia, P. F., Ryter, A. *et al.* (1990). HIV-1 infection of lung alveolar fibroblasts and macrophages in humans. *Aids. Res. Hum. Retroviruses*, **6**, 979–986.
21. Tateno, M., Gonzalez, S. F. and Levy, J. A. (1989). Human immunodeficiency virus can infect CD4-negative human fibroblastoid cells. *Proc. Natl Acad. Sci. USA*, **86**, 4287–4290.

22. Ratner, L., Haseltine, W., Patarca, R. *et al.* (1985). Complete nucleotide sequence of the AIDS virus, HTLV-III. *Nature*, **313**, 277–284.
23. Kramer, R. A., Schaber, M. D., Skalka, A. M. *et al.* (1986). HTLV-III gag protein is processed in yeast cells by the virus pol-protease. *Science*, **231**, 1580–1584.
24. Toh, H., Ono, M., Saigo, K. and Miyata, T. (1985). Retroviral protease-like sequence in the yeast transposon Ty *1*. *Nature*, **315**, 691–692.
25. Tang, J., James, M. N. G., Hsu, I. N. *et al.* (1977). Structural evidence for gene duplication in the evolution of the acid proteases. *Nature*, **271**, 618–621.
26. Pearl, L. H. and Taylor, W. R. (1987). A structural model for the retroviral proteases. *Nature*, **329**, 351–354.
27. Kohl, N. E., Emini, E. A., Schleif, W. A. *et al.* (1988). Active human immunodeficiency virus protease is required for viral infectivity. *Proc. Natl Acad. Sci. USA*, **85**, 4686–4690.
28. Le-Grice, S. F., Mills, J. and Mous, J. (1988). Active site mutagenesis of the AIDS virus protease and its alleviation by trans complementation. *EMBO J.*, **7**, 2547–2553.
29. Seelmeier, S., Schmidt, H., Turk, V. and von der Helm, K. (1988). Human immunodeficiency virus has an aspartic-type protease that can be inhibited by pepstatin A. *Proc. Natl Acad. Sci. USA*, **85**, 6612–6616.
30. Leis, J., Baltimore, D., Bishop, J. M. *et al.* (1988). Standardized and simplified nomenclature for proteins common to all retroviruses. *J. Virol.*, **62**, 1808–1809.
31. Jacks, T., Power, M. D., Masiarz, F. R. *et al.* (1988). Characterization of ribosomal frameshifting in HIV-1 *gag-pol* expression. *Nature*, **331**, 280–283.
32. Farmerie, W. G., Loeb, D. D., Casavant, N. C. *et al.* (1987). Expression and processing of the AIDS virus reverse transcriptase in *Escherichia coli*. *Science*, **236**, 305–308.
33. Veronese, F. D., Copeland, T. D., Oroszlan, S. *et al.* (1988). Biochemical and immunological analysis of human immunodeficiency virus *gag* gene products p17 and p24. *J. Virol.*, **62**, 795–801.
34. Bathurst, I. C., Chester, N., Gibson, H. L. *et al.* (1989). *N*-Myristoylation of the human immunodeficiency virus type 1 *gag* polyprotein precursor in *Saccharomyces cerevisiae*. *J. Virol.*, **63**, 3176–3179.
35. Gottlinger, H. G., Sodroski, J. G. and Haseltine, W. A. (1989). Role of capsid precursor processing and myristoylation in morphogenesis and infectivity of human immunodeficiency virus type 1. *Proc. Natl Acad. Sci. USA*, **86**, 5781–5795.
36. Witte, O. N. and Baltimore, D. (1978). Relationship of retrovirus polyprotein cleavages to virion maturation studied with temperature-sensitive murine leukemia virus mutants. *J. Virol.*, **26**, 750–761.
37. Katsumoto, T., Hattori, N., Yamada, O. and Kurimura, T. (1988). Intermediate virions in maturation of human immunodeficiency virus, strain LAV. *J. Electron. Microsc. Tokyo*, **37**, 205–207.
38. Peng, C., Ho, B. K., Chang, T. W. and Chang, N. T. (1989). Role of human immunodeficiency virus type 1-specific protease in core protein maturation and viral infectivity. *J. Virol.*, **63**, 2550–2556.
39. Lillehoj, E. P., Salazar, F. H., Mervis, R. J. *et al.* (1988). Purification and structural characterization of the putative gag-pol protease of human immunodeficiency virus. *J. Virol.*, **62**, 3053–3058.
40. Schneider, J. and Kent, S. B. (1988). Enzymatic activity of a synthetic 99 residue protein corresponding to the putative HIV-1 protease. *Cell*, **54**, 363–368.
41. Nutt, R. F., Brady, S. F., Darke, P. L. *et al.* (1988). Chemical synthesis and enzymatic activity of a 99-residue peptide with a sequence proposed for the human immunodeficiency virus protease. *Proc. Natl Acad. Sci. USA*, **85**, 7129–7133.

42. Copeland, T. D. and Oroszlan, S. (1988). Genetic locus, primary structure, and chemical synthesis of human immunodeficiency virus protease. *Gene Anal. Tech.*, **5**, 109–115.
43. Wu, J. C., Carr, S. F., Jarnagin, S. *et al.* (1990). Synthetic HIV-2 protease cleaves the GAG precursor of HIV-1 with the same specificity as HIV-1 protease. *Arch. Biochem. Biophys.*, **277**, 306–311.
44. Darke, P. L., Leu, C.-T., Davis, L. J. *et al.* (1989). Human immunodeficiency virus protease. *J. Biol. Chem.*, **264**, 2307–2312.
45. Graves, M. C., Lim, J. J., Heimer, E. P. and Kramer, R. A. (1988). An 11-kDa form of human immunodeficiency virus protease expressed in *Escherichia coli* is sufficient for enzymatic activity. *Proc. Natl Acad. Sci. USA*, **85**, 2449–2453.
46. Cheng, Y. S., McGowan, M. H., Kettner, C. A. *et al.* (1990). High-level synthesis of recombinant HIV-1 protease and the recovery of active enzyme from inclusion bodies. *Gene*, **87**, 243–248.
47. Rittenhouse, J., Turon, M. C., Helfrich, R. J. *et al.* (1990). Affinity purification of HIV-1 and HIV-2 proteases from recombinant *E. coli* strains using pepstatin-agarose. *Biochem. Biophys. Res. Commun.*, **171**, 60–66.
48. Lapatto, R., Blundell, T., Hemmings, A. *et al.* (1989). X-ray analysis of HIV-1 proteinase at 2.7 A resolution confirms structural homology among retroviral enzymes. *Nature*, **342**, 299–302.
49. Billich, S., Knoop, M. T., Hansen, J. *et al.* (1988). Synthetic peptides as substrates and inhibitors of human immune deficiency virus-1 protease. *J. Biol. Chem.*, **263**, 17905–17908.
50. Debouck, C., Gorniak, J. G., Strickle, J. E. *et al.* (1987). Human immunodeficiency virus protease expressed in *Escherichia coli* exhibits autoprocessing and specific maturation of the *gag* precursor. *Proc. Natl Acad. Sci. USA*, **84**, 8903–8906.
51. Hansen, J., Billich, S., Schulze, T. *et al.* (1988). Partial purification and substrate analysis of bacterially expressed HIV protease by means of monoclonal antibody. *EMBO J.*, **7**, 1785–1791.
52. Hostomsky, Z., Appelt, K. and Ogden, R. C. (1989). High-level expression of self-processed HIV-1 protease in *Escherichia coli* using a synthetic gene. *Biochem. Biophys. Res. Commun.*, **161**, 1056–1063.
53. Korant, B. D. and Rizzo, C. J. (1990). Expression in *Escherichia coli* of the AIDS virus aspartic protease through a protein fusion. *Biol. Chem. Hoppe Seyler*, **371**, 271–275.
54. Hirel, Ph-H., Parker, F., Boiziau, J. *et al.* (1990). HIV-1 aspartic proteinase: high-level production and automated fluorometric screening assay of inhibitors. *Antiviral Chem. Chemother.*, **1**, 9–15.
55. Danley, D. E., Geoghegan, K. F., Scheld, K. G. *et al.* (1989). Crystallizable HIV-1 protease derived from expression of the viral *pol* gene in *Escherichia coli. Biochem. Biophys. Res. Commun.*, **165**, 1043–1050.
56. Heimbach, J. C., Garsky, V. M., Michelson, S. R. *et al.* (1989). Affinity purification of the HIV-1 protease. *Biochem. Biophys. Res. Commun.*, **164**, 955–960.
57. Strickler, J. E., Gorniak, J., Dayton, B. *et al.* (1989). Characterization and autoprocessing of precursor and mature forms of human immunodeficiency virus type 1 (HIV-1) protease purified from *Escherichia coli. Proteins*, **6**, 139–154.
58. Tomasselli, A. G., Hui, J. O., Sawyer, T. K. *et al.* (1990). Interdomain hydrolysis of a truncated *Pseudomonas* exotoxin by the human immunodeficiency virus-1 protease. *J. Biol. Chem.*, **265**, 408–413.
59. Richards, A. D., Phylip, L. H., Farmerie, W. G. *et al.* (1990). Sensitive soluble chromogenic substrates for HIV-1 proteinase. *J. Biol. Chem.*, **265**, 7733–7736.
60. Nashed, N. T., Louis, J. M., Sayer, J. M. *et al.* (1989). Continuous spectrophoto-

metric assay for retroviral proteases of HIV-1 and AMV. *Biochem. Biophys. Res. Commun.*, **163**, 1079–1085.

61. Matayoshi, E. D., Wang, G. T., Krafft, G. A. and Erickson, J. (1990). Novel fluorogenic substrates for assaying retroviral proteases by resonance energy transfer. *Science*, **247**, 954–958.
62. Geohegan, K. F., Spencer, R. W., Danley, D. E. *et al.* (1990). Fluorescence-based continuous assay for the aspartyl protease of human immunodeficiency virus-1. *FEBS Lett.*, **262**, 119–122.
63. Broadhurst, A. V., Roberts, N. A., Ritchie, A. J. *et al.* (1991). Assay of HIV-1 proteinase: a colorimetric method using small peptide substrates. *Anal. Biochem.*, **193**, 280–286.
64. Darke, P. L., Nutt, R. F., Brady, S. F. *et al.* (1988). HIV-1 protease specificity of peptide cleavage is sufficient for processing of *gag* and *pol* polyproteins. *Biochem. Biophys. Res. Commun.*, **156**, 297–303.
65. Moore, M. L., Bryan, W. M., Fakhoury, S. A. *et al.* (1989). Peptide substrates and inhibitors of the HIV-1 protease. *Biochem. Biophys. Res. Commun.*, **159**, 420–425.
66. Tomasselli, A. G., Olsen, M. K., Hui, J. O. *et al.* (1990). Substrate analogue inhibition and active site titration of purified recombinant HIV-1 protease. *Biochemistry*, **29**, 264–269.
67. Krausslich, H. G., Ingraham, R. H., Skoog, M. T. *et al.* (1989). Activity of purified biosynthetic proteinase of human immunodeficiency virus on natural substrates and synthetic peptides. *Proc. Natl Acad. Sci. USA*, **86**, 807–811.
68. Meek, T. D., Dayton, B. D., Metcalf, B. W. *et al.* (1989). Human immunodeficiency virus 1 protease expressed in *Escherichia coli* behaves as a dimeric aspartic protease. *Proc. Natl Acad. Sci. USA*, **86**, 1841–1845.
69. Tomasselli, A. G., Hui, J. O., Sawyer, T. K. *et al.* (1990). Interdomain hydrolysis of a truncated *Pseudomonas* exotoxin by the human immunodeficiency virus-1 protease. *J. Biol. Chem.*, **265**, 408–413.
70. Giam, C. Z. and Boros, I. (1988). *In vivo* and *in vitro* autoprocessing of human immunodeficiency virus protease expressed in *Escherichia coli*. *J. Biol. Chem.*, **263**, 14617–14620.
71. Darke, P. L., Nutt, R. F., Brady, S. F. *et al.* (1988). HIV-1 protease specificity of peptide cleavage is sufficient for processing of gag and pol polyproteins. *Biochem. Biophys. Res. Commun.*, **156**, 297–303.
72. Navis, M. A., Fitzgerald, P. M. D., McKeever, B. M. *et al.* (1989). Three-dimensional structure of aspartyl protease from human immunodeficiency virus HIV-1. *Nature*, **337**, 615–620.
73. Wlodawer, A., Miller, M., Jaskolski, M. *et al.* (1989). Conserved folding in retroviral proteases: crystal structure of a synthetic HIV-1 protease. *Science*, **245**, 616–621.
74. Lapatto, R., Blundell, T., Hemmings, A. *et al.* (1989). X-ray analysis of HIV-1 proteinase at 2.7A resolution confirms structural homology among retroviral enzymes. *Nature*, **342**, 299–302.
75. Weber, I. T., Miller, M., Jaskolski, M. *et al.* (1989). Molecular modelling of the HIV-1 protease and its substrate binding site. *Science*, **243**, 928–931.
76. Pearl, L. and Blundell, T. L. (1984). The active site of aspartic proteinases. *FEBS Lett.*, **174**, 96–101.
77. Fitzgerald, P. M. D., McKeever, B. M., Van Middlesworth, J. F. *et al.* (1990). Crystallographic analysis of a complex between human immunodeficiency virus type 1 protease and acetyl-pepstatin at 2.0-A resolution. *J. Biol. Chem.*, **265**, 14209–14219.
78. Swain, A. L., Miller, M. M., Green, J. *et al.* (1990). X-ray crystallographic struc-

ture of a complex between a synthetic protease of human immunodeficiency virus 1 and a substrate-based hydroxyethylamine inhibitor. *Proc. Natl Acad. Sci. USA*, **87**, 8805–8809.

79. Jaskolski, M., Tomasselli, A. G., Sawyer, T. K. *et al.* (1991). Structure at 2.5-A resolution of chemically synthesised human immunodeficiency virus type 1 protease complexed with a hydroxyethylene-based inhibitor. *Biochemistry*, **30**, 1600–1609.
80. Erickson, J., Neidhart, D. J., Vandrie, J. *et al.* (1991). Design, activity, and 2.8 A crystal structure of a C_2 symmetric inhibitor complexed to HIV-1 protease. *Science*, **249**, 527–533.
81. Bone, R., Vacca, J. P., Anderson, P. S. and Holloway, M. K. (1991). X-ray crystal structure of the HIV protease complex with L-700,417, an inhibitor with pseudo C_2 symmetry. *J. Am. Chem. Soc.*, **113**, 9382–9384.
82. Suguna, K., Paldan, E. A., Smith, C. W. *et al.* (1987). Binding of a reduced peptide inhibitor to the aspartic proteinase from *Rhizopus chinesis*: implications for a mechanism of action. *Proc. Natl Acad. Sci. USA*, **84**, 7009–7013.
83. Pearl, L. H. (1987). The catalytic mechanism of aspartic proteinases. *FEBS Lett.*, **214**, 8–12.
84. Rich, D. H. (1985). Pepstatin-derived inhibitors of aspartic proteinases: a close look at an apparent transition-state analogue inhibitor. *J. Med. Chem.*, **28**, 263–273.
85. James, M. N. G. and Sielecki, A. R. (1985). Stereochemical analysis of peptide bond hydrolysis catalysed by the aspartic proteinase penicillopepsin. *Biochemistry*, **24**, 3701–3713.
86. Dreyer, G. B., Metcalf, B. W., Tomaszek, T. A., Jr *et al.* (1989). Inhibition of human immunodeficiency virus 1 protease *in vitro*: rational design of substrate analogue inhibitors. *Proc. Natl Acad. Sci. USA*, **86**, 9752–9756.
87. Grobelny, D., Wondrak, E. M., Garlady, R. E. and Oroszlan, S. (1990). Selective phosphinate transition-state analogue inhibitors of the protease of human immunodeficiency virus. *Biochem. Biophys. Res. Commun.*, **169**, 1111–1116.
88. Sawyer, T. K., Tomasselli, A. G., Poorman, R. A. *et al.* (1990). Design, structure–activity and specificity of highly potent P_1-P_1'-modified pseudopeptidyl inhibitors of HIV-1 aspartyl protease. In *Peptides: Chemistry, Structure and Biology. Proceedings of the Eleventh American Peptide Symposium*, J. E. Rivier and G. R. Marshall (eds), ESCOM, Leiden, pp. 855–857.
89. Miller, M., Schneider, J., Sathyanarayana, B. K. *et al.* (1989). Structure of complex of synthetic HIV-1 protease with a substrate-based inhibitor at 2.3A resolution. *Science*, **246**, 1149–1152.
90. Toth, M. V., Chiu, F., Glover, G. *et al.* (1990). Inhibitors of HIV protease based on modified peptide substrates. In *Peptides: Chemistry, Structure and Biology. Proceedings of the Eleventh American Peptide Symposium*, J. E. Rivier and G. R. Marshall (eds), ESCOM, Leiden, pp. 835–838.
91. Urban, J., Konvalinka, J., Stehlikova, J. *et al.* (1992). Reduced-bond tight-binding inhibitors of HIV-1 protease. *FEBS Lett.*, **298**, 9–13.
92. Darke, P. L., Leu, C.-T., Davis, L. J. *et al.* (1989). Human immunodeficiency virus protease. *J. Biol. Chem.*, **264**, 2307–2312.
93. Nutt, R. F., Brady, S. F., Darke, P. L. *et al.* (1988). Chemical synthesis and enzymatic activity of a 99-residue peptide with a sequence proposed for the human immunodeficiency virus protease. *Proc. Natl Acad. Sci. USA*, **85**, 7129–7133.
94. Krausslich, H.-G., Ingraham, R. H., Skoog, M. T. *et al.* (1989). Activity of purified biosynthetic proteinase of human immunodeficiency virus on natural substrates and synthetic peptides. *Proc. Natl Acad. Sci. USA*, **86**, 807–811.

95. Krausslich, H. G., Schneider, H., Zybarth, G. *et al.* (1988). Processing of in vitro-synthesised *gag* precursor proteins of human immunodeficiency virus (HIV) type 1 by HIV proteinase generated in *Escherichia coli. J. Virol.*, **62**, 4393–4397.
96. Richards, A. D., Roberts, R., Dunn, B. M. *et al.* (1989). Effective blocking of HIV-1 proteinase activity by characteristic inhibitors of aspartic proteinases. *FEBS Lett.*, **247**, 113–117.
97. Hui, K. Y., Manetta, J. V., Gygi, T. *et al.* (1991). A rational approach in the search for potent inhibitors against HIV proteinase. *FASEB J.*, **5**, 2606–2610.
98. Raju, B. and Deshpande, M. S. (1991). Investigating the stereochemistry of binding to HIV-1 protease with inhibitors containing isomers of 4-amino-3-hydroxy-5-phenylpentanoic acid. *Biochem. Biophys. Res. Commun.*, **180**, 187–190.
99. Kahn, M., Nakanishi, H., Chrusciel, R. A. *et al.* (1991). Examination of HIV-1 protease secondary structure specificity using conformationally constrained inhibitors. *J. Med. Chem.*, **34**, 3395–3399.
100. Meek, T. D., Lambert, D. M., Dreyer, G. B. *et al.* (1990). Inhibition of HIV-1 protease in infected T-lymphocytes by synthetic peptide analogues. *Nature*, **343**, 90–92.
101. Tomasselli, A. G., Hui, J. O., Sawyer, T. K. *et al.* (1990). Specificity and inhibition of proteases from human immunodeficiency viruses 1 and 2. *J. Biol. Chem.*, **265**, 14675–14683.
102. McQuade, T. J., Tomasselli, A. G., Liu, L. *et al.* (1990). A synthetic HIV-1 protease inhibitor with antiviral activity arrests HIV-like particle maturation. *Science*, **247**, 454–456.
103. Vacca, J. P., Guare, J. P., de Solms, S. J. *et al.* (1991). L-687,908, a potent hydroxyethylene-containing HIV protease inhibitor. *J. Med. Chem.*, **34**, 1225–1228.
104. Lyle, T. A., Wiscount, C. M., Guare, J. P. *et al.* (1991). Benzocycloalkyl amines as novel C-termini for HIV protease inhibitors. *J. Med. Chem.*, **34**, 1228–1230.
105. Young, S. D., Payne, L. S., Thompson, W. J. *et al.* (1992). HIV-1 protease inhibitors based on hydroxyethylene dipeptide isosteres: an investigation into the role of the P_1' side chain on structure–activity. *J. Med. Chem.*, **35**, 1702–1709.
106. Thompson, W. J., Fitzgerald, P. M. D., Holloway, M. K. *et al.* (1992). Synthesis and antiviral activity of a series of HIV-1 protease inhibitors with functionality tethered to the P_1 or P_1' phenyl substituents: X-ray crystal structure assisted design. *J. Med. Chem.*, **35**, 1685–1701.
107. Lingham, R. B., Arison, B. H., Colwell, L. F. *et al.* (1991). HIV-1 protease inhibitory activity of L-694,746, a novel metabolite of L-689,502. *Biochem. Biophys. Res. Commun.*, **181**, 1456–1461.
108. Baboonian, C., Dalgleish, A., Bountiff, L. *et al.* (1991). HIV-1 proteinase is required for synthesis of pro-viral DNA. *Biochem. Biophys. Res. Commun.*, **179**, 17–24.
109. Ashorn, P., McQuade, T. J., Thaisrivongs, S. *et al.* (1990). An inhibitor of the protease blocks maturation of human and simian immunodeficiency viruses and spread of infection. *Proc. Natl Acad. Sci. USA*, **87**, 7472–7476.
110. Sham, H. L., Betebenner, D. A., Wideburg, N. E. *et al.* (1991). Potent HIV-1 protease inhibitors with antiviral activities *in vitro. Biochem. Biophys. Res. Commun.*, **175**, 914–919.
111. Rich, D. H., Green, J., Toth, M. V. *et al.* (1990). Hydroxyethylamine analogues of the p17/p24 substrate cleavage sites are tight-binding inhibitors of HIV protease. *J. Med. Chem.*, **33**, 1285–1288.
112. Rich, D. H., Sun, Q.-C., Prasad, J.V. N. V. *et al.* (1991). Effect of hydroxyl group configuration in hydroxyethylamine dipeptide isosteres on HIV protease inhibition: evidence for multiple binding modes. *J. Med. Chem.*, **34**, 1222–1225.

113. Roberts, N. A., Martin, J. A., Kinchington, D. *et al.* (1990). Rational design of peptide-based HIV proteinase inhibitors. *Science*, **248**, 358–361.
114. Krohn, A., Redshaw, S., Ritchie, J. C. *et al.* (1991). Novel binding mode of highly potent HIV-proteinase inhibitors incorporating the (*R*)-hydroxyethylamine isostere. *J. Med. Chem.*, **34**, 3340–3342.
115. Tucker, T. J., Lumma, W. C. Jr, Payne, L. S. *et al.* (1992). A series of potent HIV-1 protease inhibitors containing a hydroxyethyl secondary amine transition state isostere: synthesis enzyme inhibition and antiviral activity. *J. Med. Chem.*, **35**, 2525–2533.
116. Mimoto, T., Imai, J., Tanaka, S. *et al.* (1991). Rational design and synthesis of a novel class of active-site targeted HIV protease inhibitors containing a hydroxymethylcarbonyl isostere: use of phenylnorstatine or allophenylnorstatine as a transition-state mimetic. *Chem. Pharm. Bull.*, **39**, 2465–2467.
117. Mimoto, T., Imai, J., Tanaka, S. *et al.* (1991). KNI-102, a novel tripeptide HIV protease inhibitor containing allophenylnorstatine as a transition-state mimetic. *Chem. Pharm. Bull.*, **39**, 3088–3090.
118. Mimoto, T., Imai, J., Kisanuki, S. *et al.* (1992). Kynostatin (KNI)-227 and -272, highly potent anti-HIV agents: conformationally constrained tripeptide inhibitors of HIV protease containing allophenylnorstatine. *Chem. Pharm. Bull.*, **40**, 2251–2253.
119. Kageyama, T., Mimoto, T., Murakawa, Y. *et al.* (1992). Activities of HIV protease inhibitors, KNI-227 and -272, against HIV *in vitro*. *Program Abstr. Intersci. Conf. Antimicrob. Agents Chemother.*, **32 (0)**, 163, Abstr. 318.
120. Tam, T. F., Carriere, J., MacDonald, D. *et al.* (1992). Intriguing structure–activity relations underlie the potent inhibition of HIV protease by norstatine-based peptides. *J. Med. Chem.*, **35**, 1318–1320.
121. Kempf, D. J., Norbeck, D. W., Codacovi, L. M. *et al.* (1990). Structure-based, C_2 symmetric inhibitors of HIV protease. *J. Med. Chem.*, **33**, 2687–2689.
122. Kempf, D. J., Marsh, K. C., Paul, D. A. *et al.* (1992). Antiviral and pharmacokinetic properties of C_2 symmetric inhibitors of the human immunodeficiency virus type 1 protease. *Antimicrob. Agents Chemother.*, **35**, 2209–2214.
123. Norbeck, D. W., Kempf, D. J., Marsh, K. C. *et al.* (1992). Orally bioavailable HIV proteinase inhibitors for experimental AIDS therapy. *Program Abstr. Intersci. Conf. Antimicrob. Agents Chemother.*, **32 (0)**, 410.
124. Decamp, D. L., Babe, L. M., Salto, R. *et al.* (1992). Specific inhibition of HIV-1 protease by boronated porphyrins. *J. Med. Chem.*, **35**, 3426–3428.
125. Humber, D. C., Cammack, N., Coates, J. A. V. *et al.* (1992). Penicillin derived C_2-symmetric dimers as novel inhibitors of HIV-1 proteinase. *J. Med. Chem.*, **35**, 3080–3081.
126. Dombrowski, A. W., Bills, G. F., Sabnis, G. *et al.* (1992). L-696,474, a novel cytochalasin as an inhibitor of HIV-1 protease. I. The producing organism and its fermentation. *J. Antibiotics*, **45**, 671–678.
127. Ondeyka, J., Hensens, O. D., Zink, D. *et al.* (1992). L-696,474, a novel cytochalasin as an inhibitor of HIV-1 proteinase. II. Isolation and structure. *J. Antibiotics*, **45**, 679–685.
128. Lingham, R. B., Hsu, A., Silverman, K. C. *et al.* (1992). L-696,474, a novel cytochalasin as an inhibitor of HIV-1 proteinase. III. Biological activity. *J. Antibiotics*, **45**, 686–691.
129. Boucher, C. A. B., Tersmette, M., Lange, J. M. A. *et al.* (1990). Zidovudine sensitivity of human immunodeficiency viruses from high-risk, symptom-free individuals during therapy. *Lancet*, **336**, 585–590.
130. Lambert, D. M., Bartus, H., Dreyer, G. B. *et al.* (1992). Cooperativity of an HIV-

1 protease inhibitor (SKF 108922) with AZT in acute and chronic HIV-1 infections *in vitro*. *Antiviral Res.*, **17** (Suppl. 1), 47.

131. Kageyama, S., Weinstein, J. N., Shirasaka, T. *et al.* (1992). In vitro inhibition of human immunodeficiency virus (HIV) type 1 replication by C_2 symmetry-based HIV proteinase inhibitors as single agents or in combinations. *Antimicrob. Agents Chemother.*, **36**, 926–933.
132. Johnson, V. A., Merrill, D. P., Chou, T.-C. and Hirsch, M. S. (1992). Human immunodeficiency virus type 1 (HIV-1) inhibitory interactions between protease inhibitor Ro 31-8959 and zidovudine, 2′,3′-dideoxycytidine, or recombinant interferon-aA against zidovudine-sensitive or -resistant HIV-1 in vitro. *J. Infect. Dis.*, **166**, 1143–1146.
133. Craig, J. C., Duncan, I. B., Whittaker, L. and Roberts, N. A. (1993). Antiviral synergy between inhibitors of HIV proteinase and reverse transcriptase. *Antiviral Chem. Chemother.*, **4**, 161–166.
134. Rosenberg, S. H., Kleinert, H. D., Stein, H. H. *et al.* (1991). Design of a well-absorbed renin inhibitor. *J. Med. Chem.*, **34**, 469–471.

2 Acyclic Purine Nucleoside Phosphonates as Retrovirus Inhibitors

JAN BALZARINI and ERIK DE CLERCQ
Rega Institute for Medical Research, Katholieke Universiteit Leuven, Belgium

ANTIVIRAL ACTIVITY OF ACYCLIC PURINE NUCLEOSIDE PHOSPHONATE DERIVATIVES

Acyclic nucleoside phosphonates represent a novel class of antiviral agents first described in 1986 by De Clercq, Holy and their co-workers (1). Members of this class contain a phosphonate group linked to the acyclic (alkyl) side-chain of purine or pyrimidine bases. Unlike the natural nucleotides, the acyclic nucleoside phosphonates are resistant to phosphorolytic cleavage by cellular esterases and are, as such, in an unaltered (intact) form, taken up by the cells. Among the cyclic nucleoside phosphonates several subclasses have been identified (Figure 2.1): HPMP derivatives (prototype: (*S*)-9-(3-hydroxy-2-phosphonylmethoxypropyl)adenine (HPMPA)), PME derivatives (prototype: 9-(2-phosphonylmethoxyethyl)adenine (PMEA)), FPMP derivatives (prototype: (*S*)-9-(3-fluoro-2-phosphonylmethoxy- propyl) adenine (FPMPA)) and PMP derivatives (prototype: (*R*)-9-(2-phosphonylmethoxypropyl)adenine (PMPA)), each subclass of compounds displaying a particular antiviral activity spectrum.

HPMP DERIVATIVES

The prototype compound HPMPA may be regarded as a hybrid molecule between (*S*)-9-(2,3-dihydroxypropyl)adenine (DHPA) and phosphonoacetic acid (PAA), which have been shown to exert inhibitory activity against RNA/DNA viruses and herpesviruses, respectively (2,3). HPMPA is active against a broad spectrum of DNA viruses, including the herpesviruses (herpes simplex virus type 1 (HSV-1) and type 2 (HSV-2)), thymidine kinase (TK)-deficient mutants thereof (TK^- HSV-1), cytomegalovirus (CMV), varicella zoster virus (VZV), Epstein–Barr virus (EBV), human herpes virus type 6 (HHV-6), adenoviruses, poxviruses and iridoviruses (1,4,5; and our unpublished observations). HPMPA is not effective against RNA viruses

Antiviral Chemotherapy. Edited by D.J. Jeffries and E. De Clercq

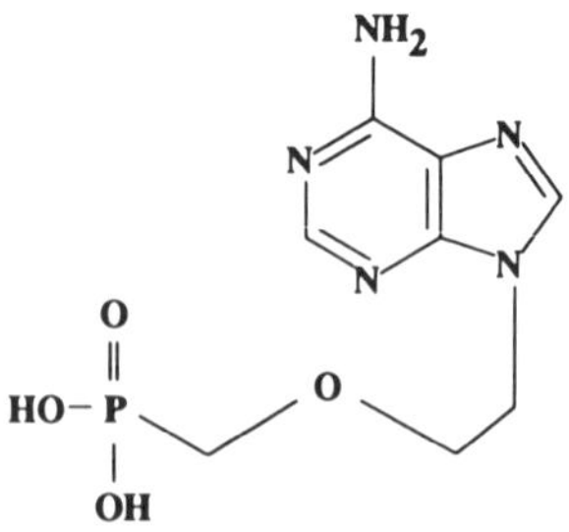

(PMEA)

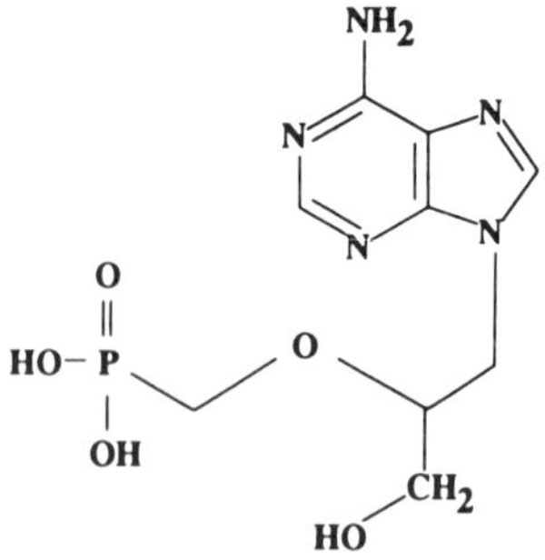

(HPMPA)

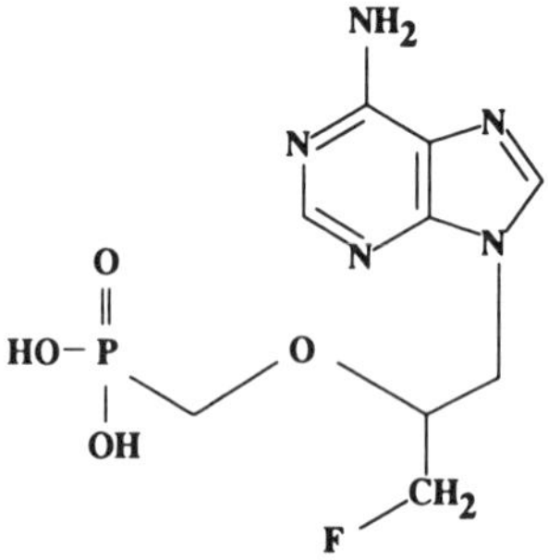

(FPMPA)

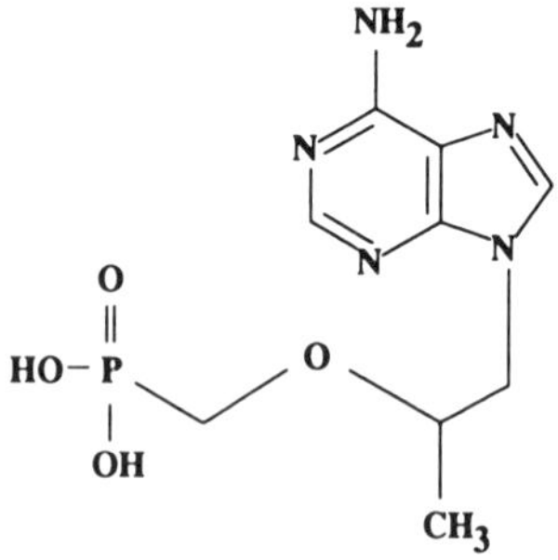

(PMPA)

Figure 2.1. Formulae of 9-(3-hydroxy-2-phosphonylmethoxypropyl)adenine (HPMPA), 9-(2-phosphonylmethoxyethyl)adenine (PMEA), 9-(3-fluoro-2-phosphonylmethoxypropyl) adenine (FPMPA) and 9-(2-phosphonylmethoxypropyl) adenine (PMPA)

(1,4,5) and little, if any, inhibitory activity has been noted with HPMPA against retroviruses, its 50% effective concentration (EC_{50}) for human immunodeficiency virus (HIV) being close to the toxicity threshold (4,5) (Table 2.1).

PME DERIVATIVES

In vitro antiviral activity

PME derivatives are endowed with activity against both DNA viruses (e.g. HSV) and retroviruses (4–7). Whereas the anti-herpes virus activity of the prototype compound PMEA is less pronounced than that of HPMPA (particularly against VZV and CMV), its anti-retrovirus activity is quite

Table 2.1. *In vitro* antiviral activity of HPMPA, PMEA, FPMPA and PMPA

Virus	Cell culture	EC_{50}[a,b] (μg/ml)			
		HPMPA	PMEA	FPMPA	PMPA
HSV-1	PRK	1–3	7	330	> 600
TK^- HSV-1	PRK, E_6SM	0.7–1	7	—	> 600
HSV-2	PRK	1–3	7	20	> 600
CMV	HEL	0.3	25	150	> 300
VZV	HEL	0.004	10	90	> 100
EBV	P3HR-1	0.08	1.1	—	—
Adenovirus	HeLa	0.6–2.5	> 125	—	—
Vaccinia virus	PRK	0.3	150	> 200	> 100
African swine fever virus	Vero	0.01	—	—	—
HIV-1 (III_B)	MT-4	> 20	5.9	23	5.9
(III_B)	PBL	> 20	3.7	3.9	—
(Ba-L)	M/M	3.2	0.022	0.95	—
HIV-2 (ROD)	MT-4	> 20	5.5	11	4.9
SIV (MAC_{251})	MT-4	> 20	9.2	13	—
SRV	Raji	> 100	0.7	2	—
MSV	C3H/3T3	12	1.2	5.9	3.4

[a] 50% effective concentration, or compound concentration required to inhibit virus-induced cytopathicity by 50%.
[b] Data taken from references 1, 4, 26 and 27.

prominent. In this sense, the antiviral activity spectrum of PMEA differs from that of HPMPA.

PMEA can be regarded as a broad-spectrum anti-retroviral agent. It has proved to be inhibitory to the replication of human immunodeficiency virus type 1 (HIV-1) and type 2 (HIV-2), simian immunodeficiency virus (SIV), simian AIDS-related virus (SRV), feline immunodeficiency virus (FIV), feline leukaemia virus (FeLV), Moloney murine sarcoma virus (MSV), Rauscher murine leukaemia virus (RLV), Friend murine leukaemia virus (FLV), murine LP-BM-5 retrovirus complex and Visna virus (8–17). Against all these viruses PMEA shows a similar potency irrespective of the nature of the cell line used for the determination of antiviral activity (i.e. human T lymphocyte cell lines (MT-4, CEM), or peripheral blood lymphocytes (PBL) for HIV and SIV, feline Crandell kidney cells and feline thymocytes for FIV, murine C3H/3T3 embryo fibroblasts for MSV, sheep choroid plexus cells for Visna virus)) or the parameter used to monitor the anti-retrovirus activity (i.e. HIV-induced cytopathicity in MT-4 cells, HIV-induced syncytium formation in CEM cells, HIV-specific antigen expression in MT-4 cells (Figure 2.2) or HIV-1-specified p24 release in the culture medium of PBL). These observations suggest that in all these cell lines PMEA is metabolized to a comparable extent and that its active metabolite

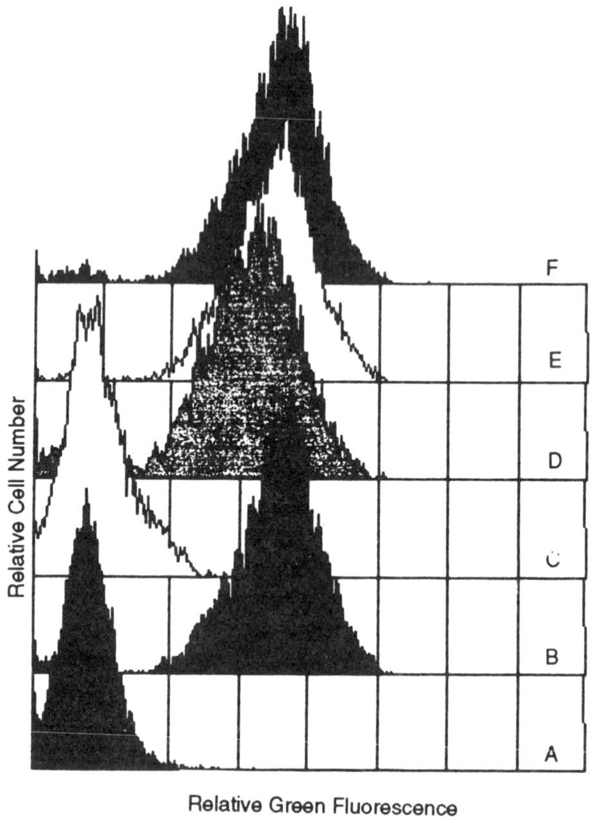

Figure 2.2. Fluorescence histogram of HIV-1(III_B)-infected MT-4 cells. Row A represents the non-specific fluorescence of uninfected cells. Row B represents the fluorescence of cells infected with 100 $CCID_{50}$ (50% cell culture infectious doses) of HIV-1(III_B). Rows C, D, E and F correspond to HIV-1(III_B)-infected MT-4 cells treated with PMEA at 20, 4, 0.8 and 0.16 μM, respectively. (Courtesy of Dr D. Schols, Rega Institute for Medical Research, Leuven, Belgium)

is an equipotent inhibitor of the different retrovirus-associated reverse transcriptases.

Within the PME series different congeners containing as purine base adenine (A), 2-monoaminopurine (MAP), 2,6-diaminopurine (DAP), hypoxanthine (Hx) or guanine (G) have been synthesized and evaluated for their anti-HIV and anti-MSV activity *in vitro* (6). As a rule, PMEDAP is more active than PMEA but also more toxic. Consequently, its selectivity index (ratio of cytotoxic concentration to antivirally effective concentration) is comparable to that of PMEA. PMEG is by far the most active PME derivative but also the most toxic, and its antiviral activity is achieved at concentrations that are close to its toxicity threshold. Thus, PMEG has a very small selectivity index. PMEMAP shows little anti-retroviral activity and PMEHx is devoid of anti-retroviral activity. In this respect, the structure–activity relationship of the PME purine derivatives differs from that of the purine 2′,3′-dideoxynucleoside derivatives (ddN). Indeed, the different purine ddN derivatives (i.e. ddA, ddDAP, ddI and ddG) show a similar activity to anti-retrovirus agents irrespective of the nature of the purine base. This difference in the structure–function relationship of the PME and ddN derivatives suggests that, while their active metabolites may interact in the same fashion with the target enzyme (reverse transcriptase), considerable differences must exist in the enzymatic processes that lead to the active forms of these compounds.

In vivo antiviral activity

PMEA and its closely related derivative PMEDAP have been extensively investigated for their anti-retroviral properties in several animal models. Marked efficacy has been demonstrated with both PMEA and PMEDAP in a variety of experimental retrovirus infections: SIV infection in rhesus monkeys (PMEA) (8), FIV infection in cats (11,12) and FeLV infection in cats (PMEA) (12,14), MSV infection in mice (PMEA, PMEDAP) (9,10,18–21), FLV infection in mice (PMEA, PMEDAP) (20,22), RLV infection in mice (22), LP-BM-5 retrovirus complex infection in mice (PMEA) (15). In all these animal models, PMEA and PMEDAP proved at least as effective as, if not more effective than, AZT. Further investigations with different treatment schedules in MSV-infected or FLV-infected NMRI mice revealed that PMEA, and also PMEDAP, were markedly more efficient in suppressing MSV-induced tumour formation or FLV-induced splenomegaly when administered as a single dose on the day of infection than when the total dose was spread over two, four or seven administrations within one week after virus infection (18,19). Moreover, while the infrequent dosing regimen increased the anti-retrovirus potency of PMEA, it did not increase its toxicity for the host. This unique behaviour to confer a long-lasting antiviral response apparently extends to other acyclic nucleoside phosphonates (e.g. the potent anti-herpesvirus agent HPMPC) (23–25), and makes these compounds attractive candidates for the long-term treatment of virus infections, including HIV infections.

Due to their high polar nature the oral bioavailability of the acyclic nucleoside phosphonates is very low. For PMEA, it has been estimated that less than 5% of the drug given orally may be absorbed. However, we recently demonstrated that PMEDAP is highly efficacious when given orally to mice infected with either MSV, FLV or even CMV (20). PMEDAP markedly delayed MSV-induced tumour initiation when administered orally at 50, 100 or 250 mg/kg per day during five subsequent days. At the highest dose tested (i.e. 250 mg/kg per day), PMEDAP completely prevented tumour formation in the MSV-infected animals and caused about 90% inhibition of FLV-induced splenomegaly in FLV-infected mice. It has not been revealed yet whether PMEDAP is better absorbed orally than PMEA, or whether the marked efficacy found for PMEDAP following oral administration is simply due to the fact that it is intrinsically more potent than PMEA as an anti-retroviral agent. Thus, with the doses of PMEDAP that were given orally, even if the compound were to be poorly absorbed, sufficient plasma drug levels may be attained to achieve a pronounced antiviral effect.

FPMP AND PMP DERIVATIVES

In vitro antiviral activity

Among the acyclic nucleoside phosphonates the FPMP and PMP derivatives differ from the aforementioned HPMP and PME derivatives in that they are virtually devoid of anti-herpetic activity, yet exhibit pronounced anti-retroviral activity. In this respect, the FPMP and PMP derivatives should be considered as the most selective anti-retroviral agents among the acyclic nucleoside phosphonates (26). It is also clear that the PMP derivatives may be substituted at the 3-methyl group of the propyl side-chain by an atom or group other than hydroxyl and keep an antiviral activity spectrum similar to that of the unsubstituted PMP derivatives. This is exemplified by the FPMP derivative FPMPA, where a hydrogen atom of the 3-methyl group was replaced by a fluorine (27). Thus, FPMPA and PMPA proved to be as potent inhibitors of HIV and MSV as PMEA; but, in contrast to PMEA, both FPMPA and PMPA proved much less toxic to T lymphocytes and human bone marrow cells (26,27). Thus, the selectivity index of FPMPA and PMPA was substantially higher than that of PMEA. The (*S*)-enantiomer of FPMPA and the (*R*)- enantiomer of PMPA were 30- to 100-fold more active against HIV and MSV than their enantiomeric counterparts (26). In this context it should be mentioned that, although the designation differs, the conformation of the (*S*)- enantiomer of FPMPA is identical to that of the (*R*)- enantiomer of PMPA. For PMPG, both (*S*)- and (*R*)- enantiomers were equally active against retrovirus replication. For PMPDAP, the (*R*)- enantiomer was at least 15- to 40-fold more active than the (*S*)- enantiomer. Reflections on the reason(s) for the differential anti-retroviral effects of the (*S*)- and (*R*)- enantiomers of the FPMP and PMP congeners will be provided below, under 'Mechanism of anti-retroviral action'.

Of all acyclic nucleoside phosphonates that have so far been evaluated PMPDAP emerged as the most potent and selective inhibitor of retrovirus replication (26) (Table 2.2). Its EC_{50} for HIV-1 and HIV-2 replication in MT-4 cells and MSV-induced transformation of murine C3H/3T3 cells ranged between 0.1 and 0.6 μM. Its selectivity index was 1500 in MT-4 and 1000

Table 2.2. Anti-HIV-1 activity of acyclic nucleoside phosphonates in MT-4 cells

Compound	EC_{50} (μM)[a]	CC_{50} (μM)[b]	SI[c]
HPMPA[d] ((*S*)- enantiomer)	> 13	26	< 2
HPMPDAP[d] ((*S*)- enantiomer)	⩾ 62	56	⩽ 0.9
PMEA[a]	5.6	67	12
PMEDAP[e]	1.4	18	13
FPMPA[d] ((*S*)- enantiomer)	8.9	> 300	> 34
FPMPDAP[d] ((*S*)- enantiomer)	15	> 300	20
PMPA[d] ((*R*)- enantiomer)	5.9	> 300	> 51
PMPDAP[d] ((*R*)- enantiomer)	0.17	> 300	> 1765

[a] 50% effective concentration, or compound concentration required to inhibit HIV-1-induced cytopathicity in MT-4 cells by 50%.
[b] 50% cytotoxic concentration, or compound concentration required to reduce MT-4 cell viability by 50%.
[c] Selectivity index, or ratio of CC_{50} to EC_{50}.
[d] Data taken from reference 26.
[e] Data taken from reference 27.

in C3H/3T3 cells (as compared to 33 and 200 for PMEA in MT-4 and C3H/3T3 cells, respectively) (6,26).

In vivo antiviral activity

When evaluated for its antiviral efficacy in MSV-infected newborn NMRI mice, PMPDAP efficiently decreased MSV-induced tumour formation and significantly increased the survival time of mice when administered intraperitoneally as a single dose of as low as 2 mg/kg (Figure 2.3). In this respect, it was 5- to 10-fold more efficacious than PMEA. Furthermore, PMPDAP, like PMEDAP, showed marked anti-retroviral efficacy when administered orally to MSV-infected mice (26).

PHARMACOLOGICAL PROPERTIES OF PMEA

METABOLISM OF PMEA

Cellular uptake and metabolism of PMEA have been investigated in H9, MT-4, MRC-5 and CEM cells. Uptake by H9 cells did not occur via the nucleoside transport system, but through a different mechanism which may be compatible with an endocytosis-like process (28). Indeed, cellular uptake of PMEA (or HPMPA) was not affected by *S*-(paranitrobenzyl)-6-thioinosine (NBTI) or dipyridamole, whereas uptake of PMEA and HPMPA by the

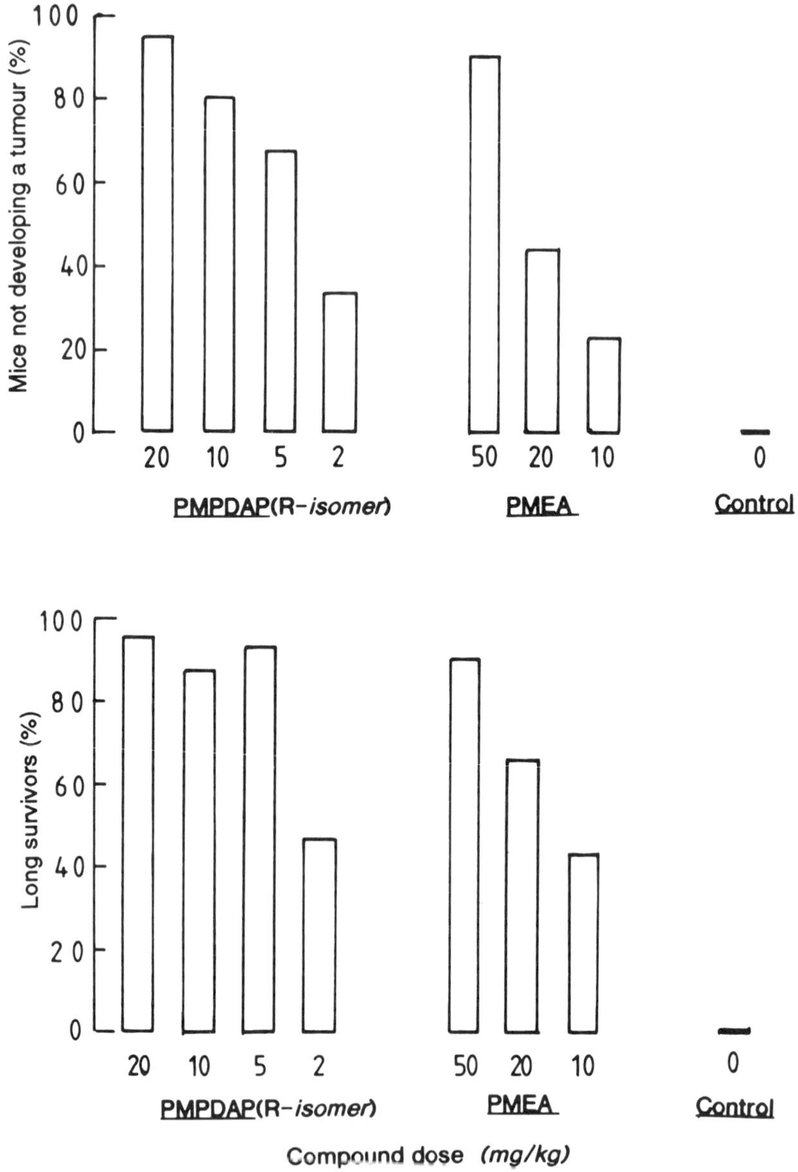

Figure 2.3. Anti-retroviral efficacy of PMEA and PMPDAP ((*R*)- enantiomer) in Moloney murine sarcoma virus (MSV)-infected NMRI mice. Two- to three-day-old NMRI mice were inoculated subcutaneously in the left hind leg with MSV and treated intraperitoneally with a single dose of test compound at 4 h prior to virus infection. Control mice receiving no test compound developed a tumour at four to five days post MSV infection and died from the infection at days 10–12 post infection

cells was virtually abolished at a temperature of 4 °C. Therefore, passive diffusion, as observed for AZT and a number of other 2′,3′-dideoxynucleosides (29,30), does not seem to occur with the acyclic nucleoside phosphonates. This is not surprising in view of the very polar nature of the test compounds. Also, extracellular DNA but not natural nucleosides compete with the uptake of PMEA, which again points to the possibility of an endocytosis-like uptake process (28). However, further studies are required to obtain clearer insight into the nature of cellular uptake of PMEA.

When the metabolism of PMEA in MT-4 cells was evaluated, only the parent compound and its mono- (PMEAp) and diphosphorylated (PMEApp) derivatives could be detected intracellularly (31). The appearance of PMEA and its metabolites in the MT-4 cells was concentration dependent and occurred proportionally with the initial extracellular PMEA concentrations. These observations strongly suggest that the enzymatic activity responsible for the anabolism of PMEA is not saturated for a PMEA concentration ranging from 0.5 to 300 μM. As a rule, at all concentrations tested, the phosphorylated derivatives of PMEA each represented approximately 10% of the parent compound in the intracellular compartment.

Relatively low amounts of PMEApp are formed intracellularly. At equimolar extracellular concentrations (e.g. 10 μM), AZT and D4T reach 5′-triphosphate levels that are at least 10-fold higher than those found for PMEApp under similar experimental conditions. Interestingly, when equivalent antivirally effective concentrations of AZT (0.006 μM), D4T (0.2 μM) and PMEA (5 μM) in MT-4 cells were compared, AZT-5′-triphosphate, D4T-5′-triphosphate and PMEApp levels after 24 h of incubation were 0.01, 0.06 and 0.07 nmol/10^9 cells, respectively (32,33).

No deaminated derivatives of PMEA (whether phosphorylated or not) could be detected intracellularly (31). These observations are in agreement with the findings that PMEA is not deaminated by adenylate deaminase even at enzyme concentrations that exceed by more than 1000-fold those that are sufficient to completely deaminate AMP within a few minutes (31). Since PMEHx, the deaminated product of PMEA, is inactive as an antiretroviral agent, resistance of PMEA to deamination by adenylate deaminase precludes the conversion of the antivirally active PMEA to its inactive congener PMEHx (Figure 2.4).

Studies on the intracellular retention of PMEA and its metabolites in MT-4 cells revealed an intracellular half-life for PMEApp of 16–18 h (31). This relatively long half-life may be due to the poor substrate properties of PMEApp for a number of catabolizing enzymes (e.g. ATPase, phosphodiesterase, nucleoside 5′-diphosphate (NDP) kinase) and may explain, at least in part, the long-lasting inhibitory effect of PMEA on retrovirus replication.

Bronson and co-workers investigated PMEA metabolism in human lymphocyte CEM and human fibroblast MRC-5 cells (34). They found that the uptake of PMEA by these cells was low (as had also been established for

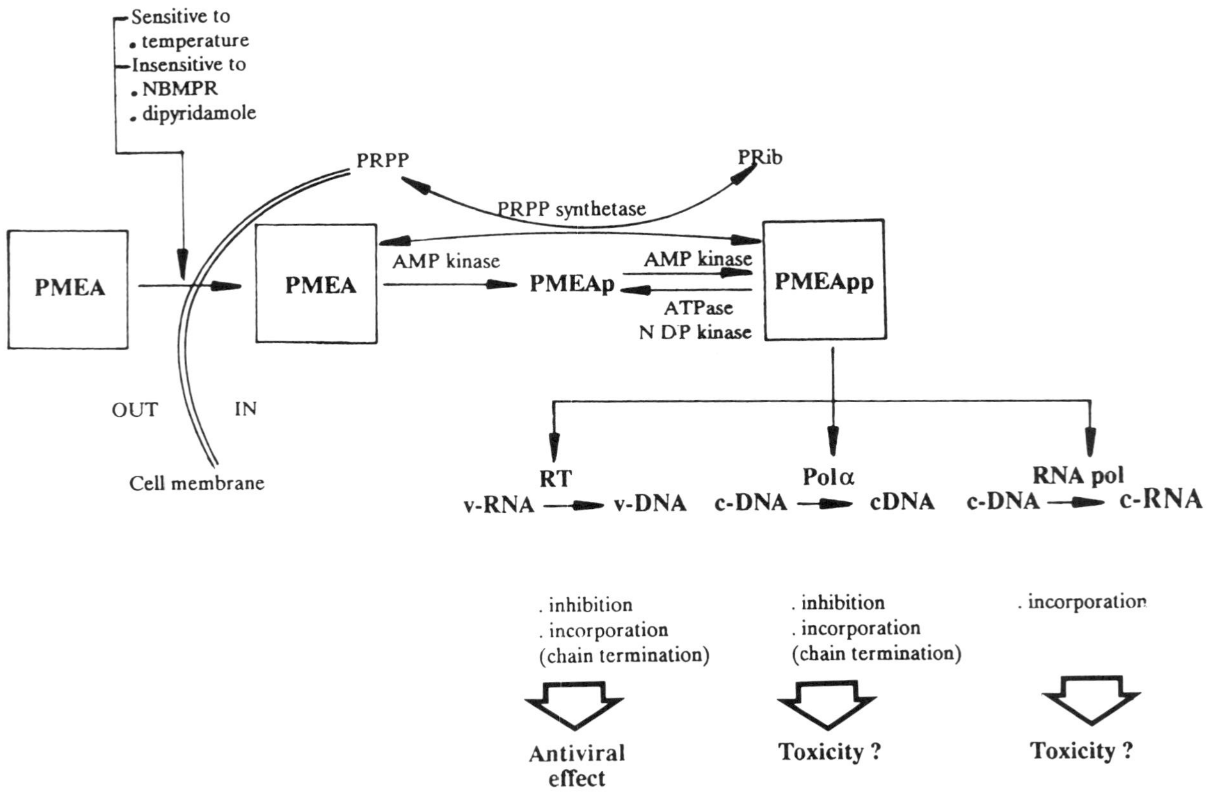

Figure 2.4. Proposed scheme of uptake and metabolism of PMEA

MT-4 cells). As metabolites, PMEAp and PMEApp could be detected in CEM cells. In MRC-5 cells, however, additional metabolites of PMEA were detected, but not characterized. Also Cerny and co-workers reported additional metabolites of PMEA in human cervix carcinoma HeLa cells, without being successful, however, in characterizing these metabolites (35).

CHARACTERIZATION OF ENZYMES THAT PHOSPHORYLATE PMEA

Role of AMP kinase in the conversion of PMEA to its phosphorylated metabolites

Which enzyme(s) are responsible for the phosphorylation of PMEA (and HPMPA)? AMP kinase from rabbit muscle and several other kinases (e.g. GMP kinase, nucleoside 5′-monophosphate kinase, NDP kinase) were found to be unable to catalyse the phosphorylation of PMEA (31,36). However, Merta and co-workers recently reported that an enzyme isolated from murine leukaemia L1210 cells was able to convert PMEA to its mono- and diphosphorylated form in the presence of ATP (37). AMP, dAMP and ADP were efficiently phosphorylated under the same experimental conditions. Phosphorylation of PMEA proceeded in two steps, PMEAp appearing first, followed by PMEApp. This phosphorylation pattern was also found for HPMPA and for the (*S*)- enantiomer of FPMPA, but not for the (*R*)- enantiomer of FPMPA. The latter compound was not phosphorylated at all by the isolated enzyme. This observation may explain the enantiospecificity of the antiviral effect of these compounds (i.e. HPMPA, FPMPA, PMPA), and points to a different metabolic behaviour of the (*S*)- and (*R*)- enantiomers. Thus, the enzyme responsible for the PMEA (HPMPA) phosphorylation is assumed to be AMP (dAMP) kinase (37). The purified enzyme has a molecular weight of 68 000 Da and is composed of two subunits of 40 000 and 29 000 Da, respectively. It seems to differ from the known AMP kinases (EC 2.7.4.3), which generally occur as monomers (molecular weight between 23 000 and 32 000 Da).

Role of 5-phosphoribosyl-1-pyrophosphate (PRPP) synthetase in the conversion of acyclic nucleoside phosphonate derivatives to their diphosphorylated derivatives

The acyclic purine nucleoside phosphonate derivatives can be considered as analogues of 2′-deoxyadenylate dAMP (viz. HPMPA) or 2′,3′-dideoxyadenylate (ddAMP) (viz. PMEA, FPMPA, PMPA). Their diphosphorylated derivatives could be considered as analogues of 2′-deoxyadenosine-5′-triphosphate (dATP) and 2′,3′-dideoxyadenosine-5′-triphosphate derivatives (ddATP). The structural analogy of HPMPA, PMEA, FPMPA and PMPA with AMP led us to an investigation of the susceptibility of the acyclic purine nucleoside derivatives as potential substrates for PRPP synthetase from *Escherichia coli* (31,38,39). PMEA, HPMPA and FPMPA were found to act as alternative substrates for PRPP synthetase. Their K_m was 2.5- to 8-fold higher, and their V_{max} 150- to 500-fold lower, than the K_m and V_{max} for AMP. Consequently, the phosphorylating capacity of PRPP synthetase for the acyclic nucleoside phosphonate derivatives (as evident from the K_m/V_{max} ratios) is 1000- to 2000-fold lower than for the natural substrate AMP.

PRPP synthetase is a key enzyme in purine and pyrimidine nucleotide synthesis and usually acts in the direction of the formation of 5-phosphoribose and ATP. When the diphosphorylated derivatives of PMEA, HPMPA and FPMPA were examined as substrates for the enzyme, the compounds had K_m values that were only 2- to 2.5-fold lower than that of ATP but, again, their V_{max} was 500- to 2000-fold lower than observed with ATP (38). Thus, not only the phosphorylation of PMEA to PMEApp but also the conversion of the diphosphorylated derivatives PMEApp, HPMPApp and FPMPApp to the unphosphorylated parent compounds occurred in a much less efficient manner than observed for ATP.

PMEA, HPMPA and FPMPA were not the only acyclic nucleoside phosphonates that showed an affinity for PRPP synthetase. Also the acyclic phosphonate analogues of 2,6-diaminopurine and the 6-hydrazino- and 6-hydroxylamino analogues of adenine were recognized as a substrate for PRPP synthetase (39) (Figure 2.5A). In contrast, substitution of the adenine base by a guanine, 2-aminopurine, hypoxanthine, 1,6-ethenoadenine, 6-thiopurine, 6-methylaminopurine or 6-dimethylaminopurine abrogated the affinity for the enzyme (Figure 2.5B). Thus, PRPP synthetase is very stringent with regard to the nature of the base moiety of the acyclic nucleoside phosphonates. On the other hand, PRPP synthetase is not very stringent with respect to the acyclic phosphonate moiety (Figure 2.5C). An increase in the number of methylene groups between the phosphonate moiety and the oxygen in the aliphatic chain, or between the oxygen and the base moiety, does not lead to a marked loss in substrate affinity for the enzyme (39). Also, several phosphonylalkyl derivatives of adenine were found to act as efficient substrates for PRPP synthetase, 5-phosphonylpentyladenine being the most efficient substrate (Figure 2.5C). Furthermore, translocation of the 2′-phosphonylmethoxy moiety to the 3′- position of the propyl chain in HPMPA, and substitution of the 3-OH group of HPMPA by a fluorine or hydrogen, is compatible with substrate affinity (Figure 2.5D).

In conclusion, PMEA, HPMPA, FPMPA, PMPA and their congeners are the first synthetic nucleoside analogues with an acyclic sugar moiety shown to act as substrates for PRPP synthetase. The above-mentioned studies were performed with purified *Escherichia coli* enzyme, but comparable data have recently been obtained with the PRPP synthetase from human erythrocytes or rat liver (our unpublished observations). The role of PRPP synthetase in the one-step conversion of the acyclic nucleoside phosphonates to their diphosphorylated derivatives in intact cells still needs to be demonstrated. It is possible that other cellular enzymes such as AMP kinase, as proposed by Merta and co-workers (37), play a more relevant physiological role than PRPP synthetase in the metabolic conversion of PMEA and related compounds to their active (phosphorylated) forms.

OTHER ENZYMES THAT MAY INTERACT WITH ACYCLIC NUCLEOSIDE PHOSPHONATES

PMEA and related analogues may interfere with a number of viral and cellular enzymes other than the viral reverse transcriptases, or cellular DNA polymerases, PRPP synthetase and AMP kinase. Holy and co-workers (36) demonstrated that the diphosphate derivatives of both the HPMP and PME congeners are able to inhibit HSV-1 ribonucleotide reductase (RR). The greatest inhibition was found for HPMPApp, PMEApp and PMEDAPpp against CDP reduction to dCDP. The conversion of ADP to dADP and of GDP to dGDP proved less sensitive to inhibition by these compounds. PMEGpp, PMEUpp, PMETpp and PMECpp did not show an appreciable inhibitory effect on HSV-1 RR at concentrations as high as 1 mM (36). The monophosphorylated derivatives of HPMPA, PMEA and PMEDAP were 500, 12 and > 50-fold less potent as inhibitors of HSV-1 RR than their diphosphorylated congeners. It remains to be demonstrated whether the diphosphorylated derivatives of PMEA and HPMPA also inhibit cellular RR to a significant extent.

Holy and co-workers also investigated the inhibitory effect of acyclic nucleoside phosphonate analogues on inosine (Ino) phosphorolysis by L1210 purine nucleoside phosphorylase (PNPase) (36,40). Several PME and HPMP derivatives were found to be potent inhibitors of PNPase. PMEA and HPMPA had K_i/K_m ratios equal to 0.012 and 0.046, respectively. Moreover, not only the parent compounds, but also the monophosphorylated derivatives (i.e. PMEAp, HPMPAp, PMEDAPp, PMEHxp and HPMPGp) proved exquisitely inhibitory to L1210 PNPase: K_i/K_m ratios ranged between 0.0005 and 0.017). However, these compounds may not affect PNPase activity in intact cells, since we found that PMEA and PMEDAP did not inhibit PNPase activity in intact L1210 or CEM cells (our unpublished observations). The assay to determine PNPase activity in intact cells was based upon a comparative measurement of tritium release from exogenously administered [2-^{3}H]inosine and [2-^{3}H]hypoxanthine (41). Tritium release occurs after inosine (via hypoxanthine) and hypoxanthine conversion by HGPRT (hypoxanthine guanine phosphoribosyl transferase) to inosinate (IMP) and subsequently by IMP dehydrogenase to xanthylate (XMP). A diminution in ^{3}H release from [2-^{3}H]Ino, as compared to ^{3}H release from

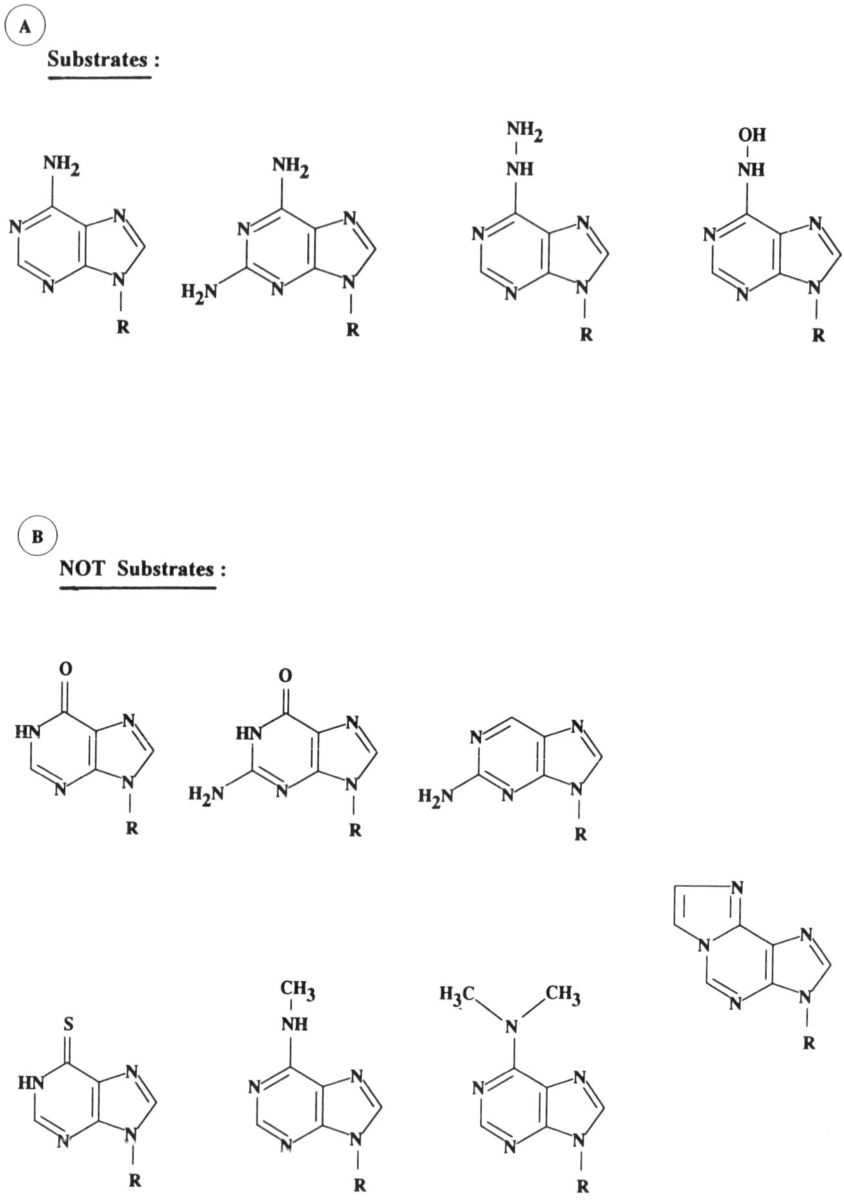

R = 2 - phosphonylmethoxyethyl

Figure 2.5. Structural features of acyclic nucleoside phosphonates that are required for recognition by *E. coli* PRPP synthetase

(C)

Substrates :

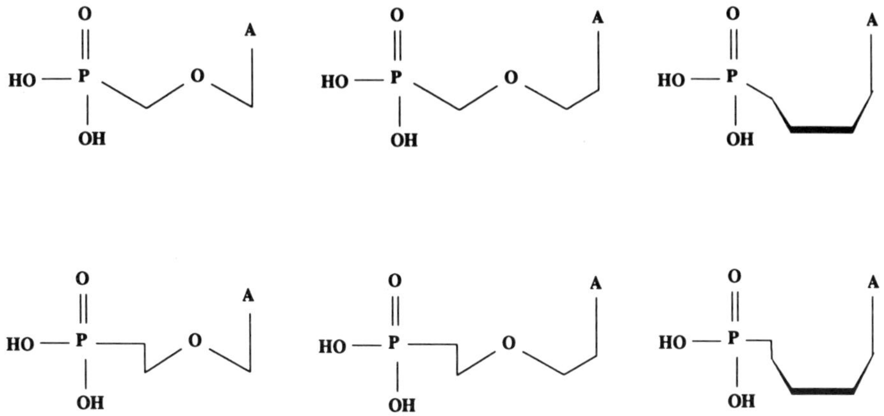

(D)

Substrates :

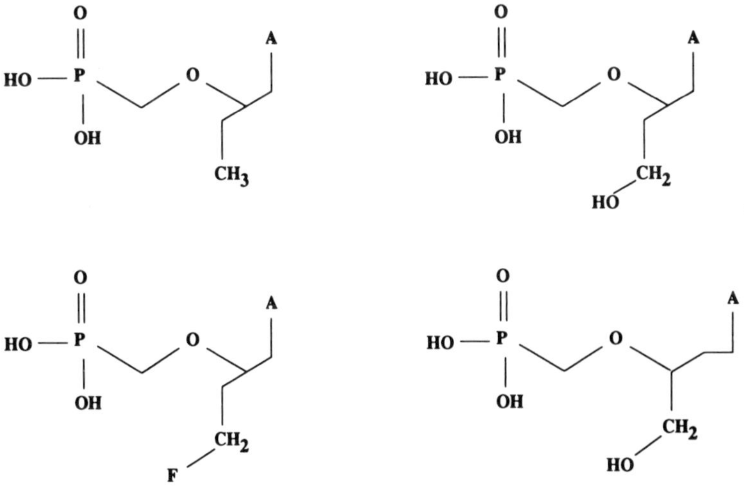

A = adenine

Figure 2.5. Continued

[2-^{3}H]Hx, must result from an inhibition of PNPase, the direct phosphorylation of Ino to IMP being undetectable and thus representing a minor metabolic pathway [41]. PMEA and PMEDAP (even after pre-incubation of the cells for 24 h) did not inhibit tritium release from either [2-^{3}H]Ino or [2-^{3}H]Hx, and this points to the failure of the test compounds to inhibit PNPase in intact cells (our unpublished data). These data also warn against extrapolation of data obtained from cell-free enzymatic systems to the intact cell situation.

PHARMACOKINETICS OF PMEA IN MICE

The pharmacokinetics of PMEA have been determined in mice and in rhesus monkeys (8,42). Upon intravenous (i.v.) bolus administration of PMEA at 25–500 mg/kg, PMEA was rapidly cleared from the murine plasma in a monoexponential and dose-independent manner (half-life ($T_{1/2}$): 7–12.5 min; distribution volume: 0.30–0.36 l/kg; total body clearance: 1.21–2.41 l/h per kilogram). The inter-animal pharmacokinetic parameters varied more extensively in rhesus monkeys than in mice and the plasma half-life proved also much higher in rhesus monkeys than mice (half-life: 1.09–3.07 h; distribution volume: 0.5–3.2 l/kg; total body clearance: 0.14–2.25 l/h per kilogram) (8). The PMEA clearance parameters in mice were similar to those reported for 2′,3′-dideoxynucleoside analogues such as AZT, AZddU, ddI and ddC (43–46). The linear and dose-independent pharmacokinetics of PMEA indicate that the process leading to elimination of PMEA is not saturated at therapeutically relevant doses.

As already mentioned, the oral bioavailability of PMEA is poor. An oral dose of PMEA at 100 mg/kg results in low plasma concentrations (0.4–7 μg/ml within 10–40 min after administration). These observations explain the poor anti-retrovirus activity of PMEA when administered orally (20,42).

PMEA was recovered as unchanged parent compound (67%) from the urine of mice within 24 h after i.v. administration. When given as an i.v. bolus injection, PMEA mainly accumulated in the kidney, liver and lungs. A similar tissue distribution has also been demonstrated in rhesus monkeys (8). Significant amounts of monophosphorylated, but not diphosphorylated, PMEA were detected in kidney and liver, but not in other tissues. Kidney and liver may possess high levels of an enzyme that converts PMEA to its monophosphorylated derivative (either directly from PMEA or indirectly from PMEApp). It seems advisable to extract, purify and characterize from these organs the enzyme that is responsible for the conversion of PMEA (or PMEApp) to PMEAp.

Low but significant levels of PMEA were obtained in the brain. In view of the neurological disorders associated with AIDS, penetration of PMEA into the central nervous system is an important property with regard to successful treatment of HIV infections. Although PMEA levels in the brain are relatively low, they may suffice to achieve a therapeutic effect since PMEA therapy has proved successful in the treatment of herpetic encephalitis and intracerebrally induced tumours in mice (7,21).

MECHANISM OF ANTI-RETROVIRAL ACTION

REVERSE TRANSCRIPTASE AS A TARGET ENZYME

The diphosphorylated derivatives of PMEA (e.g. PMEApp) and FPMPA (e.g. FPMPApp) are potent competitive inhibitors of HIV-1 reverse transcriptase (RT) with respect to the natural substrate dATP (27,31,34). The K_i values of HIV-1 RT for PMEApp and FPMPApp with poly(U)–oligo(dA) as template–primer and [^{3}H]dATP as the competing substrate are 0.09 and 0.03 μM, respectively (27,31). Under similar experimental conditions, the K_i value for ddATP was 0.166 μM. The K_i/K_m ratios for PMEApp, FPMPApp and ddATP were 0.01, 0.002 and 0.009, respectively. This means that these compounds have a much higher affinity for HIV-1 RT than the natural substrate dATP. The fact that PMEApp and FPMPApp are much weaker inhibitors of calf thymus DNA polymerase α (IC_{50}: 3.7 and 49 μM) than HIV-1 RT (IC_{50}: 0.08 and 0.02 μM) may account for the marked anti-retrovirus selectivity of PMEA and FPMPA (27,31). The ratio of IC_{50} of PMEA for HIV-1 RT to its IC_{50} for cellular DNA polymerase α is 46. Also, Votruba and co-workers (47) and Holy *et al.* (36) found a value of 37 for the ratio of the K_i/K_m of PMEApp for DNA polymerase α (from HeLa cells) to its K_i/K_m for the reverse transcriptase from avian myeloblastosis virus. As based on the ratio of the IC_{50} for DNA polymerase α to the IC_{50} for HIV-1 RT, FPMPApp proved even more selective than PMEApp (2900 versus 46), and this may account for the higher anti-retrovirus selectivity of FPMPA than PMEA.

In general, the retrovirus-associated reverse transcriptase can be inhibited by the acyclic nucleoside phosphonates by at least two different mechanisms which are not mutually exclusive and which may even complement each other. They can function as competitive inhibitors of RT with respect to the natural nucleoside 5′-triphosphates (as demonstrated with PMEApp and FPMPApp), and they can also serve as alternative substrates, be incorporated into the growing DNA chain and act as DNA chain terminators. In contrast to the natural substrates (dNTP) that contain a free 3′-hydroxyl which can be linked with the 5′-phosphate moiety of an incoming new nucleotide (Figure 2.6), the diphosphorylated acyclic nucleoside analogues do not allow further DNA chain elongation once they have been incorporated into the viral DNA. This is obviously due to the lack of a free 3′-OH group (Figure 2.1).

Pre-incubation studies of HIV-1 RT with PMEApp and FPMPApp for

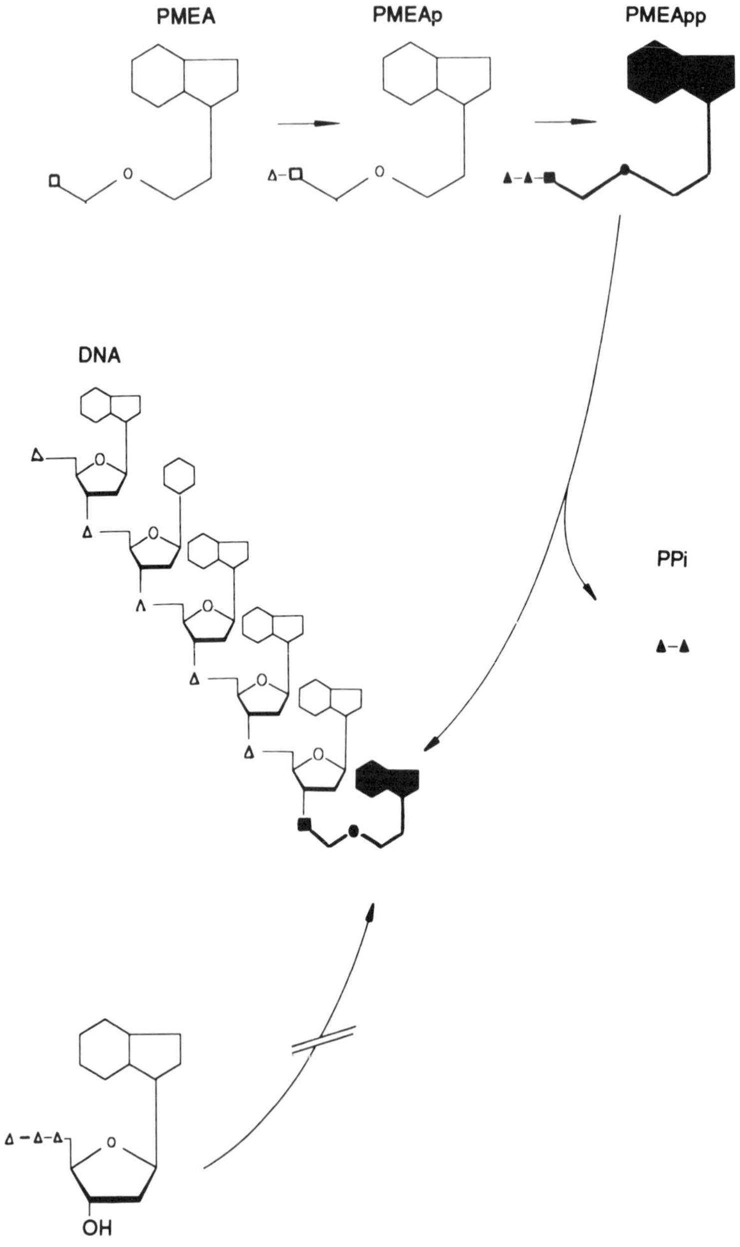

Figure 2.6. DNA chain termination by acyclic nucleoside phosphonates. △, ▲: phosphate; □, ■: phosphonate

different time periods in the presence of fixed concentrations of poly(U)–oligo(dA) as the template–primer but in the absence of dATP revealed a specific inactivation of the template–primer complex as a function of time (27,31). Progressive loss of RT activity was observed the longer the enzyme template–primer complex was pre-incubated with PMEApp and FPMPApp prior to starting the DNA polymerization reaction by the addition of [^{3}H]dATP. These findings are in agreement with those reported by Holy *et al.* (36), who found that PMEApp seems to be efficiently incorporated at the adenine sites but immediately causes DNA chain termination. Also, Balzarini *et al.* (27,31) found that both PMEApp and FPMPApp cause a dose-dependent and highly efficient DNA chain termination at the adenine sites in a Sanger sequencing reaction using HIV-1 RT and a phage N13 mp19 (+)-strand DNA: 17-base M13 template–primer.

Holy *et al.* (36) also found that HPMPApp is an alternative substrate for the *in vitro* DNA synthesis catalysed by HSV-1 DNA polymerase. HPMPApp is incorporated into the interior of the growing DNA chain of a denatured superhelical plasmid in the presence of Klenow polymerase and may eventually cause chain termination at distant A-rich sites in the DNA. These findings are also in agreement with our unpublished observations that HPMPApp is able to inhibit HIV-1 RT-catalysed DNA polymerization, but does not cause the virtually instant inactivation of the template–primer poly(U)–oligo(dA) that is achieved by PMEApp and FPMPApp under identical experimental conditions.

In conclusion, PMEApp, FPMPApp and HPMPApp inhibit the Klenow polymerase- and HIV-1 RT-catalysed DNA chain elongation. Yet, PMEA and FPMPA, but not HPMPA, are prominent anti-retrovirus agents. We might postulate, therefore, that DNA chain termination is a prerequisite for anti-retrovirus activity (viz. PMEA, FPMPA). In contrast, competitive inhibition of dATP incorporation in the HIV-1 RT-catalysed DNA polymerization reaction would not be sufficient *per se* to afford a selective inhibitory activity against retrovirus replication *in vitro* (viz. HPMPA).

IMMUNOMODULATORY PROPERTIES OF PMEA

The immunomodulatory properties of PMEA have been investigated in mice (48). In these studies, it was shown that PMEA administered intraperitoneally (i.p.) to C57Bl/6 mice at 25 mg/kg per day for five subsequent days significantly increased the levels of natural killer cell (NK) activity. The increase in NK activity achieved by PMEA was comparable to that observed for the murine spleen cells treated with 30 000 units of mouse interferon α/β (IFN-α/β) or 5 mg/kg of poly(I)–(C) at 24 h before performing the NK assay. Under identical experimental conditions, AZT was without any effect. PMEA was also found to induce IFN-α/β production in the plasma, i.e. following a single injection of PMEA at 25 mg/kg, or following daily injections for up to five consecutive days. The presence of IFN in the plasma could be detected at 24 h after PMEA injection; the highest IFN titres were noted at two to three days and IFN titres declined by the fifth day post injection. When administered i.p. at 30 mg/kg AZT failed to stimulate IFN-α/β production.

The enhancement of NK activity is a stepwise process controlled by a series of lymphokines released by lymphoid cells. The role of IFN and IL-2 is well defined in this process. IFN-α/β is known to be able to stimulate NK activity, while IL-2 is known to upregulate IFN-γ but not IFN-α/β. Thus, stimulation of IFN-α/β production found in PMEA-treated mice may well be the primary reason for the observed increase in NK activity. The molecular basis for the immunomodulatory potential of PMEA is unclear and should be further pursued. Also, it should be examined whether other acyclic nucleoside phosphonate derivatives also exhibit similar immunological properties to PMEA.

CONCLUSION

Since the discovery of the antiviral activity of the acyclic nucleoside phosphonates in 1986 by De Clercq, Holy and their co-workers, it has become clear that several members of this novel class of antiviral compounds represent promising candidate drugs for the treatment of retroviral infections. In particular, PMEA and PMEDAP (among the PME series), FPMPA (among the FPMP series), and PMPA and PMPDAP (among the PMP series) emerged as potent and selective retrovirus inhibitors. These compounds are all targeted at the retrovirus-associated reverse transcriptase. PMEA and its congeners have proved efficacious in various retrovirus models *in vivo* (e.g. mice, cats, monkeys) and, therefore, should be further pursued for their potential in the treatment of HIV infections.

REFERENCES

1. De Clercq, E., Holy, A., Rosenberg, I. *et al.* (1986). A novel selective broad-spectrum anti-DNA virus agent. *Nature*, **323**, 464–467.
2. De Clercq, E., Descamps, J., De Somer, P. and Holy, A. (1978). An aliphatic nucleoside analog with broad-spectrum antiviral activity. *Science*, **200**, 563–565.
3. Öberg, B. (1983). Antiviral effects of phosphonoformate (PFA, foscarnet sodium). *Pharmacol. Ther.*, **19**, 387–415.
4. De Clercq, E., Sakuma, T., Baba, M. *et al.* (1987). Antiviral activity of phosphonylmethoxyalkyl derivatives of purine and pyrimidines. *Antiviral Res.*, **8**, 261–272.
5. De Clercq, E. (1991). Broad-spectrum anti-DNA virus and anti-retrovirus activity of phosphonylmethoxyalkylpurines and -pyrimidines. *Biochem. Pharmacol.*, **42**, 963–972.
6. Pauwels, R., Balzarini, J., Schols, D. *et al.* (1988). Phosphonylmethoxyethylpurine

derivatives, a new class of anti-human immunodeficiency virus agents. *Antimicrob. Agents Chemother.*, **32**, 1025–1030.

7. De Clercq, E., Holy, A. and Rosenberg, I. (1989). Efficacy of phosphonylmethoxyalkyl derivatives of adenine in experimental herpes simplex virus and vaccinia virus infections *in vivo*. *Antimicrob. Agents Chemother.*, **33**, 185–191.
8. Balzarini, J., Naesens, L., Slachmuylders, J. *et al.* (1991). 9-(2-Phosphonylmethoxyethyl)adenine (PMEA) effectively inhibits retrovirus replication *in vitro* and simian immunodeficiency virus infection in rhesus monkeys. *AIDS*, **5**, 21–28.
9. Balzarini, J., Naesens, L., Herdewijn, P. *et al.* (1989). Marked *in vivo* antiretrovirus activity of 9-(2-phosphonylmethoxyethyl)adenine, a selective anti-human immunodeficiency virus agent. *Proc. Natl Acad. Sci. USA*, **86**, 332–336.
10. Naesens, L., Balzarini, J., Rosenberg, I. *et al.* (1989). 9-(2-Phosphonylmethoxyethyl)-2,6-diaminopurine (PMEDAP): a novel agent with anti-human immunodeficiency virus activity in vitro and potent anti-Moloney murine sarcoma virus activity in vivo. *Eur. J. Clin. Microbiol. Infect. Dis.*, **8**, 1043–1047.
11. Egberink, H., Borst, M., Niphuis, H. *et al.* (1990). Suppression of feline immunodeficiency virus infection *in vivo* by 9-(2-phosphonomethoxyethyl)adenine. *Proc. Natl Acad. Sci. USA*, **87**, 3087–3091.
12. Hartmann, K., Donath, A., Beer, B. *et al.* (1992). Use of two virustatica (AZT, PMEA) in the treatment of FIV and of FeLV seropositive cats with clinical symptoms. *Vet. Immunol. Immunopathol.*, **35**, 167–175.
13. Hartmann, K., Balzarini, J., Higgins, J. *et al.* (1994). *In vitro* activity of acyclic nucleoside phosphonate derivatives against feline immunodeficiency virus in Crandell feline kidney cells and feline peripheral blood lymphocytes. *Antiviral Chem. Chemother.*, **5**, 13–19.
14. Hoover, E. A., Ebner, J. P., Zeidner, N. S., and Mullins, J. I. (1991). Early therapy of feline leukemia virus infection (FeLV-FAIDS) with 9-(2-phosphonylmethoxyethyl)adenine (PMEA). *Antiviral Res.*, **16**, 77–92.
15. Gangemi, J. D., Cozens, R. M., De Clercq, E. *et al.* (1989). 9-(2-Phosphonylmethoxyethyl)adenine in the treatment of murine acquired immunodeficiency disease and opportunistic herpes simplex virus infections. *Antimicrob. Agents Chemother.*, **33**, 1864–1868.
16. Thormar, H., Balzarini, J., Holy, A. *et al.* (1993). Anti-Maedi/Visna virus activities of 2′,3′-dideoxynucleosides and acyclic nucleoside phosphonate analogues. *Antimicrob. Agents Chemother.*, **37**, 2540–2544.
17. Balzarini, J., Perno, C.-F., Schols, D. and De Clercq, E. (1991). Activity of acyclic nucleoside phosphonate analogues against human immunodeficiency virus in monocyte/macrophages and peripheral blood lymphocytes. *Biochem. Biophys. Res. Commun.*, **178**, 329–335.
18. Balzarini, J., Naesens, L. and De Clercq, E. (1990). Anti-retrovirus activity of 9-(2-phosphonylmethoxyethyl)adenine (PMEA) *in vivo* increases when it is less frequently administered. *Int. J. Cancer*, **46**, 337–340.
19. Naesens, L., Balzarini, J. and De Clercq, E. (1991). Single-dose administration of 9-(2-phosphonylmethoxyethyl)adenine (PMEA) and 9-(2-phosphonylmethoxyethyl)2,6-diaminopurine (PMEDAP) in the prophylaxis of retrovirus infection in vivo. *Antiviral Res.*, **16**, 53–64.
20. Naesens, L., Neyts, J., Balzarini, J. *et al.* (1993). Efficacy of oral 9-(2-phosphonylmethoxyethyl)-2,6-diaminopurine (PMEDAP) in the treatment of retrovirus and cytomegalovirus infections in mice. *J. Med. Virol.*, **39**, 167–172.
21. Balzarini, J., Sobis, L., Naesens, M. *et al.* (1990). Inhibitory effects of 9-(2-phosphonylmethoxyethyl)adenine and 3′-azido-2′,3′-dideoxythymidine on

tumor development in mice inoculated intracerebrally with Moloney murine sarcoma virus. *Int. J. Cancer*, **45**, 486–489.

22. Bron, J. J., Kim, C. U., Ghazzouli, I. *et al.* (1989). Synthesis and antiviral activity of phosphonylmethoxyethyl derivatives of purine and pyrimidine bases. In: *Nucleotide Analogues as Antiviral Agents*, J. C. Martin (ed.), American Chemical Society, Washington, DC, pp. 72–87.
23. Neyts, J., Sobis, H., Snoeck, R. *et al.* (1993). Efficacy of (*S*)-1-(3-hydroxy-2-phosphonylmethoxypropyl)cytosine and 9-(1,3-dihydroxy-2-propoxymethyl) guanine in the treatment of intracerebral murine cytomegalovirus infections in immunocompetent and immunodeficient mice. *Eur. J. Clin. Microbiol. Infect. Dis.*, **12**, 269–279.
24. Neyts, J., Stals, F., Bruggeman, C. and De Clercq, E. (1993). The anti-HIV agent 9-(2-phosphonylmethoxyethyl)-2,6-diaminopurine also exhibits marked efficacy against CMV infections *in vitro* and *in vivo*. *Eur. J. Clin. Microbiol. Infect. Dis.*, **12**, 437–446.
25. Neyts, J., Balzarini, J., Naesens, L. and De Clercq, E. (1992). Efficacy of (*S*)-1-(3-hydroxy-2-phosphonylmethoxypropyl)cytosine (HPMPC) and 9-(1,3-dihydroxy-2-propoxymethyl)guanine (DHPG) in the treatment of murine cytomegalovirus infections in severe combined immunodeficiency (SCID) mice. *J. Med. Virol.*, **37**, 67–71.
26. Balzarini, J., Holy, A., Jindrich, J. *et al.* (1993). Differential antiherpesvirus and antiretrovirus effects of the (*S*) and (*R*) enantiomers of acyclic nucleoside phosphonates: potent and selective *in vitro* and *in vivo* antiretrovirus activities of (*R*)-9-(2-phosphonomethoxypropyl)-2,6-diaminopurine. *Antimicrob. Agents. Chemother.*, **37**, 332–337.
27. Balzarini, J., Holy, A., Jindrich, J. *et al.* (1991). 9-[(2*RS*)-3-Fluoro-2-phosphonylmethoxypropyl] derivatives of purines: a class of highly selective antiretroviral agents *in vitro* and *in vivo*. *Proc. Natl Acad. Sci. USA*, **88**, 4961–4965.
28. Palú, G., Stefanelli, S., Rassu, M. *et al.* (1991). Cellular uptake of phosphonylmethoxyalkylpurine derivatives. *Antiviral Res.*, **16**, 115–119.
29. Zimmerman, T. P., Mahony, W. B. and Prus, K. L. (1987). 3′-Azido-3′-deoxythymidine: an unusual nucleoside analogue that permeates the membrane of human erythrocytes and lymphocytes by nonfacilitated diffusion. *J. Biol. Chem.*, **262**, 5748–5754.
30. Ahluwalia, G., Cooney, D. A., Mitsuya, H. *et al.* (1987). Initial studies on the cellular pharmacology of 2′,3′-dideoxyinosine, an inhibitor of HIV infectivity. *Biochem. Pharmacol.*, **36**, 3797–3800.
31. Balzarini, J., Hao, Z., Herdewijn, P. *et al.* (1991). Intracellular metabolism and mechanism of anti-retrovirus action of 9-(2-phosphonylmethoxyethyl)adenine, a potent anti-human immunodeficiency virus compound. *Proc. Natl Acad. Sci. USA*, **88**, 1499–1503.
32. Balzarini, J. (1993). Antiretrovirus and (anti)metabolic properties of acyclic phosphonylmethoxyalkyl purine derivatives: an overview. In: *Advances in Chemotherapy of AIDS*, R. B. Diasio and J.-P. Sommadossi (eds), in press.
33. Balzarini, J., Herdewijn, P. and De Clercq, E. (1989). Differential patterns of intracellular metabolism of 2′,3′-didehydro-2′,3′-dideoxythymidine and 3′-azido-2′,3′-dideoxythymidine, two potent anti-human immunodeficiency virus compounds. *J. Biol. Chem.*, **264**, 6127–6133.
34. Bronson, J. J., Ho, H.-T., De Boeck, H. *et al.* (1990). Biochemical pharmacology of acyclic nucleotide analogues. *Ann. NY Acad. Sci.*, **616**, 398–407.
35. Cerny, J., Foster, S. A. and Cheng, Y.-C. (1992). Cell-protective effect against

herpes simplex virus-1 and cellular metabolism of 9-(2-phosphonylmethoxyethyl)adenine in HeLa S3 cells. *Mol. Pharmacol.*, **42**, 537–544.
36. Holy, A., Votruba, I., Merta, A. *et al.* (1990). Acyclic nucleotide analogues: synthesis, antiviral activity and inhibitory effects on some cellular and virus-encoded enzymes in vitro. *Antiviral Res.*, **13**, 295–312.
37. Merta, A., Votruba, I., Jindrich, J. *et al.* (1992). Phosphorylation of 9-(2-phosphonomethoxyethyl)adenine and 9-(*S*)-(3-hydroxy-2-phosphonomethoxypropyl)adenine by AMP (dAMP) kinase from L1210 cells. *Biochem. Pharmacol.*, **44**, 2067–2077.
38. Balzarini, J. and De Clercq, E. (1991). 5-Phosphoribosyl 1-pyrophosphate synthetase converts the acyclic nucleoside phosphonates 9-(3-hydroxy-2-phosphonylmethoxypropyl)adenine and 9-(2-phosphonylmethoxyethyl)adenine directly to their antivirally active diphosphate derivatives. *J. Biol. Chem.*, **266**, 8686–8689.
39. Balzarini, J. and De Clercq, E. (1991). Conversion of acyclic nucleoside phosphonates to their diphosphate derivatives by 5-phosphoribosyl-1-pyrophosphate (PRPP) synthetase. In: *Purine and Pyrimidine Metabolism in Man VII*, Part A, R. A. Harkness, G. Elion and N. Zöllner (eds), Plenum Press, New York, pp. 29–32.
40. Šedivá, K., Ananiev, A. V., Votruba, I. *et al.* (1991). Inhibition of purine nucleoside phosphorylase by phosphonylmethoxyalkyl analogues of nucleotides. *Int. J. Purine Pyrimidine Res.*, **2**, 35–39.
41. Balzarini, J. and De Clercq, E. (1992). Assay method for monitoring the inhibitory effects of antimetabolites on the activity of inosinate dehydrogenase in intact human CEM lymphocytes. *Biochem. J.*, **287**, 785–790.
42. Naesens, L., Balzarini, J. and De Clercq, E. (1992). Pharmacokinetics in mice of the anti-retrovirus agent 9-(2-phosphonylmethoxyethyl)adenine. *Drug Metab. Dispos.*, **20**, 747–752.
43. Doshi, K. J., Gallo, J. M., Boudinot, F. D. *et al.* (1989). Comparative pharmacokinetics of 3′-azido-3′-deoxythymidine (AZT) and 3′-azido-2′,3′-dideoxyuridine (AZddU) in mice. *Drug Metab. Dispos.*, **17**, 590–594.
44. Eiseman, J. L., Bell, M. M., Billelo, J. A. *et al.* (1988). Pharmacokinetics of 3′-azido-3′-deoxythymidine (AZT) in retrovirus-infected mice. *FASEB J.*, **2**, A913.
45. Kalin, J. R. and Hill, D. L. (1988). Determination of 2′,3′-dideoxyadenosine, 2′,3′-dideoxyinosine and 2′,3′-dideoxycytidine in biological samples. *J. Chromatogr.*, **431**, 184–191.
46. Kelley, J. A., Litterst, C. L., Roth, J. S. *et al.* (1987). The disposition and metabolism of 2′,3′-dideoxycytidine, an *in vitro* inhibitor of human T-lymphotropic virus type III infectivity, in mice and monkeys. *Drug Metab. Dispos.*, **15**, 595–601.
47. Votruba, I., Trávnicek, M., Rosenberg, I. *et al.* (1990). Inhibition of avian myeloblastosis virus reverse transcriptase by diphosphates of acyclic phosphonylmethyl nucleotide analogues. *Antiviral Res.*, **13**, 287–294.
48. Del Gobbo, V., Foli, A., Balzarini, J. *et al.* (1991). Immunomodulatory activity of 9-(2-phosphonylmethoxyethyl)adenine (PMEA), a potent anti-HIV nucleotide analogue, on in vivo murine models. *Antiviral Res.*, **16**, 65–75.

3 Current Clinical Treatment of Retroviral Infections

E. F. BOWEN and M. ATKINS
Department of Thoracic Medicine, Royal Free Hospital, Pond Street, London

I. V. D. WELLER
Academic Department of Genitourinary Medicine, University College London Medical School and *Camden and Islington Community Health Services Trust, London*

M. A. JOHNSON
Department of Thoracic Medicine, Royal Free Hospital, Pond Street, London

In the 11 years since the identification of human immunodeficiency virus type 1 (HIV-1) and subsequently HIV-2 as the pathogens causing AIDS, the development of anti-retroviral agents has been incessant. Zidovudine was first made available for clinical use in 1986 and subsequently a large number of trials began. In 1989 the use of surrogate markers as trial endpoints was introduced. Although change in such markers may reflect some efficacy of a drug, to what extent this change may predict therapeutic outcome, as measured by clinical progression, is still not fully understood. Indeed, using clinical endpoints such as a new AIDS diagnosis is not without problems. A first AIDS event of oesophageal candidiasis compared with non-Hodgkin's lymphoma or cytomegalovirus (CMV) retinitis may carry equal weight as an endpoint in a study, yet each of these events has a very different prognostic implication. This suggests that future trials need to look more closely at virological and immunological endpoints in association with a more defined classification of clinical events. With greater understanding of the molecular biology of HIV-1 the development of new drugs has continued to expand. This knowledge has been used not only to develop new agents but also to understand the development of anti-retroviral resistance.

The clinically significant retroviruses known to infect man include HIV-1, HIV-2, HTLV-I and HTLV-II. This chapter will be limited to the treatment of HIV infection. The development of anti-retroviral agents hinges on the

Antiviral Chemotherapy. Edited by D.J. Jeffries and E. De Clercq

understanding of the HIV-1 replication cycle. This can be divided into two stages. In the first stage the HIV envelope protein gp120 binds to the cellular receptor CD4; fusion of the cell membrane and viral envelope follows, enabling the viral core to enter the cells. The core of the virus contains two identical strands of positive sense RNA. Once in the cells and uncoated, one strand of the RNA genome is converted to a DNA copy (proviral DNA) by viral reverse transcriptase (RT). The proviral DNA is then integrated into the host DNA at a random site by the action of a virally encoded integrase enzyme. Agents that block this first stage can prevent the infection of new cells but not the production of new virions by chronically infected cells.

Stage 2 concerns events following integration and involves transcription of the proviral DNA by host nuclear enzymes and viral regulating factors. The latter include the tat and rev proteins which promote transcription. The viral proteins are then processed and glycosylated in the cytoplasm by host cell enzymes. At the cell surface the core proteins are cleaved by a virally encoded proteinase, thus releasing virions that complete the cycle by budding from the cell surface. Therefore anti-retroviral agents focused at stage 2 may decrease or abate the production of infectious virus from chronically infected cells.

Figure 3.1 schematically shows the above stages and where various antivirals interfere with the cycle. Stage 1 anti-retrovirals include the dideoxy-

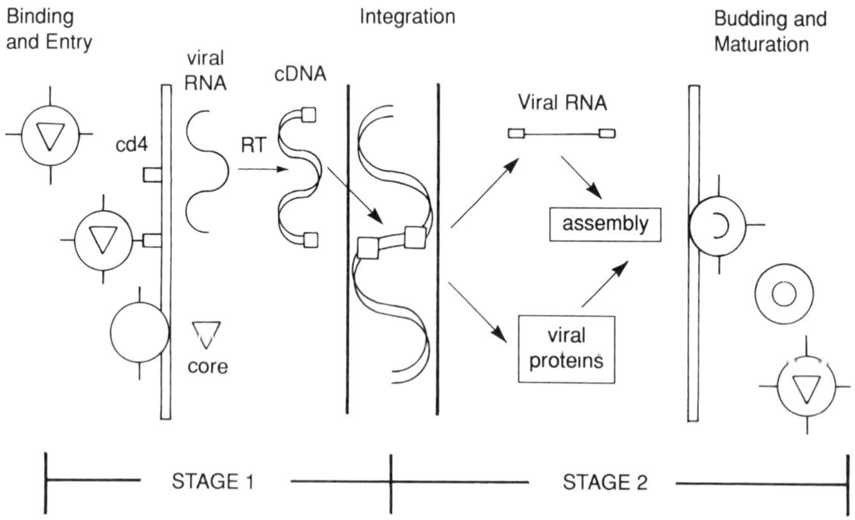

Figure 3.1. Schematic representation of HIV replication indicating possible target sites for antiviral drug intervention

nucleosides, potent *in vitro* RT inhibitors, and the non-nucleoside RT inhibitors (NNRTIs). Immunotherapy with agents such as soluble CD4 and chimeras to bind and kill gp120-expressing cells are not discussed in this chapter. Stage 2 agents include tat antagonists, glycosylation inhibitors and proteinase inhibitors.

This chapter aims to provide a review of anti-retrovirals either currently in clinical use or in clinical trials (phase I to phase III). Most of the early studies focused on zidovudine (ZDV) monotherapy but in the light of emerging viral resistance the trend has now moved to combination therapies and alternative agents.

NUCLEOSIDE MONOTHERAPY

The dideoxynucleosides remain the most studied and widely used anti-retrovirals. As triphosphates they compete with cellular deoxynucleoside-5′-triphosphates (essential substrates for RT) and also act as chain terminators in the synthesis of proviral DNA. ZDV, a thymidine analogue, was the first nucleoside RT inhibitor to be licensed for use in patients with HIV. It is of proven efficacy in patients with AIDS and is still the most commonly prescribed anti-retroviral agent for monotherapy. The licences for ZDV in Europe and the United States were granted with unprecedented speed even before the data from the first placebo-controlled trial of ZDV was published in July 1987 (1). This trial (BW002) compared 1500 mg of ZDV daily with placebo in 282 patients with a first episode of *Pneumocystis carinii* pneumonia (PCP) or AIDS-related complex (ARC). The study was terminated early, in accordance with the trial protocol, after an interim analysis by a Data and Safety Monitoring Board. The analysis revealed a significant reduction in mortality in the ZDV group with only one death out of 145 patients compared with 19 deaths out of 137 patients taking a placebo. There was also a reduction in the probability of developing an opportunistic infection, a modest increase in CD4 counts, a reduction in p24 antigenaemia, an improvement in the Karnofsky performance score and a significant increase in body weight in those patients taking ZDV. The trial highlighted the toxicity of ZDV. Nausea, myalgia, insomnia and headaches were reported more frequently by recipients of ZDV. Macrocytosis, as indicated by a raised mean corpuscular volume (MCV), developed within weeks in the majority of patients taking ZDV, which made it difficult to keep the trial truly blind to patients and physicians. Haematological toxicity was the most serious side effect. Anaemia with haemoglobin levels of less than 7.5 g/dl developed in 24% of ZDV recipients but only 4% of those on placebo ($p < 0.001$), and neutropenia (< 500 cells/mm^3) occurred in 16% of ZDV recipients compared with only 2% of those taking placebo.

The AIDS Clinical Trials Group (ACTG) 016 trial (2) compared 1200 mg of ZDV daily with placebo in 711 subjects with mildly symptomatic HIV infection as defined by either oral candidiasis, oral hairy leucoplakia, single dermatomal shingles, unintentional weight loss of > 10% of their body weight, intermittent diarrhoea or chronic fatigue. In August 1989, after a median follow-up period of only 11 months, the trial was terminated on the recommendation of an independent Data and Safety Monitoring Board because of the lower rate of disease progression among those taking ZDV. Twelve patients on ZDV with CD4 counts of > 200 but < 500 cells/mm^3 before treatment progressed to AIDS, ARC or death as a first critical event compared to 34 in the placebo group with the same CD4 count ($p = 0.0002$). Although serious anaemia and neutropenia were more common in the ZDV group, toxicity was less than that seen in the BW002 trial.

To evaluate the safety and efficacy of a lower daily dose of ZDV, the ACTG 002 trial (3) was conducted in 524 patients with AIDS. The trial compared 1500 mg daily with 600 mg daily. The median follow-up period was 25 months. The lower dose of ZDV used was at least as effective and significantly less toxic than the higher dose.

A more recently published study of a European cohort of AIDS patients looked at the use of ZDV at the time of AIDS diagnosis and the associated risk of death during a five-year follow-up (4). Patients receiving ZDV in the first year after an AIDS diagnosis had a lower death rate (relative risk of death 0.47). However, for patients on ZDV for longer than one year after AIDS the association with a reduction in mortality was decreased. Indeed for patients surviving more than two years, the differences between those treated and those not disappeared. This was not a randomized study but adjustment for other prognostic markers did not affect the mortality data. Observational studies such as this suggest that ZDV does have a beneficial effect in advanced disease but this effect may only be transient.

The ACTG 019 trial (5) was one of the earliest trials started in asymptomatic patients. A total of 1338 patients with CD4 counts < 500/mm^3 at entry were randomized to receive ZDV 500 mg or 1500 mg daily or placebo. The trial was stopped in August 1989 following an interim analysis when the median follow-up was 55 weeks. The data showed a reduction in the rate of progression to AIDS and ARC from 7.6 events per 100 patient years to 3.6 and 4.3 events per 100 patient years in the low- and high-dose groups respectively.

The higher dose of ZDV caused significantly more frequent severe anaemia (6.3%) and neutropenia (6.3%) compared with less than 2% in the lower dose and placebo groups. In 1990, on the basis of these early trial results, the National Institute of Allergy and Infectious Diseases recommended 500 mg per day of ZDV therapy for asymptomatic patients with CD4 counts of < 500/mm^3. Later the same year the ZDV product licence in Europe was extended to include asymptomatic patients with CD4 counts of < 200/mm^3

and those with counts between 200 and 500/mm^3 that were declining rapidly.

The European and Australian Collaborative Group Study (EACG 020), published in 1994 (6), was a placebo-controlled trial of 1000 mg per day of ZDV in 984 asymptomatic patients with CD4 > 400/mm^3. As there were so few progressions to ARC or AIDS other endpoints such as oral candidiasis, oral hairy leucoplakia and a decline of the CD4 count to < 350/mm^3 were used. The mean treatment period was 94 weeks. The study suggested that ZDV could delay the onset of clinical disease but the majority of endpoints were CD4 endpoints. The data were not analysed on an intention-to-treat basis and, therefore, a disproportionate number of patients with disease progression on ZDV might have been excluded from the analysis.

In addition, the European 017 trial (7) suggested that there was an early benefit from ZDV in asymptomatic patients, with CD4 counts of between 200 and 400/mm^3, versus placebo with a decreased rate of progression in the first two years only, but no difference in survival.

The largest and arguably most important trial to address the issue of immediate versus deferred ZDV monotherapy in asymptomatic patients is the Concorde study (8). The immediate arm (877 patients) received 1000 mg ZDV per day from the date of randomization, whereas the deferred group were to receive a placebo until AIDS or ARC developed. As a result of the preliminary announcement of the ACTG 019 trial the protocol was amended to allow participating physicians the discretion to start ZDV if patients had persistently low CD4 counts (below 500 cells/mm^3). The median follow-up time was 3.3 years. The number of clinical endpoints (347) in Concorde is greater than the total of those in all previously published trials in asymptomatic and early symptomatic disease. The results showed no significant difference in the three-year survival probabilities or in the three-year progression rates to symptomatic disease (ARC or AIDS). There was a small but significant increase in the CD4 counts in the immediate group compared with the deferred group. This difference persisted for up to three years but did not result in clinical benefit. This effect of ZDV explains why patients in the immediate group received prophylaxis for PCP later than the deferred group. ZDV was well tolerated, with a low frequency of severe adverse events. It may appear that there is an inconsistency between the Concorde results and those of ACTG 019 and EACG 020. However, if Concorde is re-analysed by the same entry criteria, endpoints and follow-up as these other trials then a difference is seen between the two groups in favour of early ZDV use, i.e. a small difference in progression of disease at one year and a significant difference between immediate and deferred therapy if a CD4 endpoint is used.

The results of Concorde discourage the use of ZDV monotherapy in asymptomatic adults and cast doubt on the uncritical use of CD4 cell counts as a surrogate endpoint for the assessment of clinical benefit. This has been reinforced by a recent follow-up analysis of the ACTG 019 trial. The initial increase in CD4 counts seen in patients on ZDV was not translated into slower progression to AIDS or survival benefit when the follow-up period was extended to a mean of 2.6 years (9).

Some treatment benefit with ZDV is seen in trials lasting less than 18 months. The lack of effect on mortality of early ZDV treatment is not inconsistent with the marked survival benefit seen by Fischl *et al.* (1). There the study groups were at a high risk of death and the median follow-up was only four months. Treatment was introduced late in the patients' clinical course and the benefit seen was to delay further late events, i.e. AIDS/death. With treatment early in a patient's clinical course the events that might be delayed transiently are less severe opportunistic events, not deaths. In this situation the risk/benefit equation is less clear. Indeed, a survival analysis adjusted for quality of life has been carried out on the ACTG 019 data, which also concluded that therapy with ZDV had little benefit (10). After 18 months patients treated with 500 mg of ZDV gained an average of 5 months without disease progression compared to the placebo group but had severe adverse events 6 months sooner. In this study the reduction in quality of life due to severe side effects equalled the increased quality of life associated with the delay in progression of disease. The authors concluded that in the absence of a demonstrated survival benefit a reasonable option for HIV infected asymptomatic patients may be to delay the initiation of antiretroviral therapy until there was clinical or laboratory evidence of disease progression.

In the light of the Concorde data many patients are also now reluctant to take ZDV monotherapy and instigation of such early treatment remains a personal choice of the physician and patient involved. However, there is one group of patients where early ZDV monotherapy may be very beneficial. A total of 463 pregnant women in America were randomly assigned to either 500 mg ZDV daily or placebo from 14 weeks gestation, a continuous intravenous infusion of ZDV (2 mg/kg loading dose followed by 6 mg/kg per hour) during labour and then ZDV/placebo syrup (2 mg/kg) to the baby for six weeks. Transmission to the baby occurred in 25.5% of the placebo arm but only 8.3% of the ZDV group. Obviously further long-term follow-up is important but these results are very encouraging (11). The US Food and Drug Administration (FDA) has recently approved the use of ZDV as therapy to prevent the transmission of HIV from the pregnant woman to her baby.

Two other nucleoside RT inhibitors have been investigated as monotherapeutic agents. Both didanosine (ddI) and zalcitabine (ddC) were made available to patients through expanded programmes during their formal evaluation in phase III clinical trials. DdI was evaluated in ACTG 116A (12) as monotherapy in ZDV naive patients with advanced disease and in 116B/117 (13) in patients with at least 16 weeks of previous ZDV exposure.

In 116A, in antiretroviral naive patients, ZDV appeared superior to ddI in preventing the occurrence of new AIDS-defining events or death at one year. However, in patients with 8–16 weeks previous ZDV exposure ddI was found to be superior in delaying disease progression. This is consistent with the findings in 116B/117 in which patients who had been on ZDV for a mean of 14 months switched to receive 500 mg of ddI and had a significantly slower progression to a new AIDS event than those who stayed on ZDV. This delayed progression was seen in patients who were asymptomatic or had ARC but was not seen in patients who already had an AIDS diagnosis nor was there a survival benefit. A further trial has examined the practice of switching to ddI when patients manifested signs of progressive disease on ZDV (14). The study population comprised 312 patients who had received at least six months of ZDV, had CD4 cell counts of 300/mm^3 or less and had shown clinical deterioration during the 12 weeks before study entry. Patients who continued to receive ZDV had a 50% greater risk for developing HIV-related events compared with those who had been switched to ddI. This benefit was consistent across subgroups of patients with either ARC or AIDS and was most apparent in patients with a CD4 count at entry of 100/mm^3 or greater. The Alpha trial (15) compared ddI at 200 mg per day versus 750 mg per day in patients with advanced disease and showed no difference between doses in terms of survival and disease progression in this population. By contrast there was a clear difference in adverse events, with 41 of the 908 patients in the high-dose group developing pancreatitis, from whom seven died, compared with only five out of 868 in the low-dose group. Peripheral neuropathy, a dry mouth and abnormal liver function tests were also more frequent in the high-dose group. Haematological abnormalities were uncommon. DdI at a dose of about 400 mg per day would appear to be an effective treatment for ZDV-experienced patients with signs of clinical or immunological decline. However, whether patients should be automatically switched to ddI after a finite period of ZDV exposure is still controversial. Further analysis of viral sensitivity to ZDV at entry to 116B/117 and further data on the virus phenotypes at entry may help to clarify if and when clinically stable patients should be electively switched to ddI monotherapy.

DdC is a more potent *in vitro* inhibitor of HIV RT than ddI or ZDV but there are less data available on its clinical efficacy. In ACTG 114 (16) patients with AIDS/ARC and CD4 counts less than 200/mm^3, with at least three months ZDV exposure, were randomized to continue on 600 mg ZDV or switched to ddC 2.25 mg per day. In the latter group there were significantly more clinical events and deaths. In ACTG 119, AIDS patients who switched to ddC after at least 48 weeks of ZDV, showed no difference in clinical endpoints or survival compared to those who continued on ZDV (17). There was a slower rate of decline both in CD4 and weight loss in the ddC arm but a small sample size (59 in the ZDV arm and 52 in the ddC arm) and the longer period of prior ZDV use makes the significance of these results difficult to interpret. The most recent trial (Community Programs for Clinical Research on AIDS 002) comparing ddI (500 mg per day) or ddC (2.25 mg per day) monotherapy after ZDV by Abrams *et al.* (18) found that ddC was at least as efficacious as ddI in delaying disease progression and death in patients with AIDS or a CD4 count $< 300/mm^3$. It appeared that ddC might provide a slight survival advantage. The rates of adverse events were similar in both groups but the nature of the events were different. Peripheral neuropathy and stomatitis were significantly more frequent in the ddC group. Pancreatitis only occurred in patients on ddI. At present ddC is licensed for combination therapy with ZDV on the basis of surrogate marker data and second-line monotherapy in ZDV-experienced patients with intolerance to ZDV or ddI. Peripheral neuropathy is a contraindication to its use.

Other nucleoside RT inhibitors considered for monotherapy include Stavudine (d4T) and 3TC. D4T is a thymidine analogue with potent *in vitro* activity against HIV. Results from phase I/II studies showed a decline in p24 antigenaemia and a rise in CD4 cell counts sustained for more than a year at doses above 1 mg/kg per day (19). However, toxicity, predominantly a peripheral neuropathy, was common (20% cases) particularly at doses of 2 mg/kg per day and was dose limited. Current II/III studies in the USA are comparing d4T as monotherapy to ZDV in patients with CD4 counts $< 300/mm^3$. As of June 1994 d4T is licensed in the USA as monotherapy in patients who have either failed or are intolerant of ZDV or ddI. In the UK d4T is only available in a study for patients who have failed on therapy with ZDV and ddI.

3TC (2′-deoxy-3′-thiacytidine) exhibits synergistic activity with ZDV against HIV *in vitro* and is active against ZDV-resistant strains. Preliminary results from phase I/II studies show the drug to be well tolerated and relatively non-toxic (20). Although 3TC's own antiviral activity is relatively modest, it is an attractive option for combination therapy. Phase II/III trials underway are examining 3TC in combination with ZDV both in ZDV-naive (NUCB 3001) and experienced patients (NUCB 3002). It also has activity against hepatitis B virus both *in vivo* and *in vitro*.

Foscarnet is a phosphonoformate derivative that has been shown to have an anti-HIV effect *in vitro* and to be synergistic with ZDV. An additive effect has also been demonstrated *in vivo* with beneficial changes in surrogate markers in patients on combined ZDV and foscarnet (21). In the SOCA study foscarnet was used as monotherapy for patients with CMV retinitis (22). There was no difference in the two treatment groups in the rate of retinitis progression. However, there was a survival advantage in the foscarnet treatment group and an increase in median CD4 count suggesting an anti-retroviral effect. Trials of foscarnet as an anti-retroviral agent as monotherapy and in combination with ZDV continue.

NON-NUCLEOSIDE RT INHIBITORS

Several selective NNRTIs have been identified. They are active against HIV-1 only and not HIV-2 RT or other viral polymerases. Although the structures of the drugs are very different they all seem to bind to a similar region of RT distant from the active site. This has been their major problem in that single point mutations may develop within days or weeks of instigating therapy which can confer cross-resistance to the other NNRTIs without noticeable effect on the enzyme activity. The benzodiazipine-like drug TIBO was the first NNRTI to be identified. Early trials showed a large but transient reduction in viral load; oral bioavailability is poor but the drug is of relatively low toxicity (23). The next-generation TIBOL, loviride, showed a sustained elevation in CD4 in asymptomatic patients with counts $> 400/\text{mm}^3$ compared with placebo (24). The side effects were rash and itching but there was no evidence of the development of resistant virus. Continuing studies are comparing loviride to ZDV as monotherapy and both agents in combination.

Nevirapine is a non-competitive inhibitor of RT that interacts with tyrosine residues at positions 181 and 188. It is synergistic with ZDV, active against ZDV-resistant HIV-1 but inactive against TIBO-resistant virus (25). In nucleoside-experienced p24 antigen-positive patients the addition of nevirapine cause a rapid decline in viral load, fall in p24 antigenaemia and increase in CD4 cells. The decreased antigenaemia was sustained at 16 weeks. As monotherapy in ZDV-naive patients similar results were obtained but the increase in CD4 count and fall in viral load returned to baseline. Rashes were the main side effect. Despite the rapid development of resistance NNRTIs may be useful in situations where only a limited duration of therapy is required but where a lack of toxicity is of particular importance such as during pregnancy or following a needlestick injury from an HIV-infected patient.

TAT ANTAGONISTS

In recent early Phase I and II trials, tat antagonists have been disappointing. Despite seemingly good molecular design and good *in vitro* results preliminary data showed RO-24-7429 not to be active *in vivo* and studies have now been discontinued.

PROTEINASE INHIBITORS

Recently there has been much interest in drugs that inhibit chronically infected cells by targeting enzymes required for stage 2 of the replication cycle. Viral proteinase is required for the specific cleavage of HIV protein precursors both in virus particles undergoing maturation and in the infected cell. There is no known host enzyme with the same specificity as this viral proteinase. Proteinase inhibitors have been designed by cloning and expressing the protease and with the aid of data obtained from the high-resolution crystal structure of the enzyme (26). The currently most studied and most advanced inhibitor is Saquinavir (Ro 31-8959). Early phase I/II studies using three different doses as monotherapy showed Sequinavir to be relatively non-toxic but early improvements in surrogate markers were not sustained at 16 weeks (27). ACTG 229 compared the three-drug combination of Saquinavir, ddC and ZDV versus Saquinavir and ZDV versus ddC and ZDV in 302 patients with CD4 counts of 50 to $300/mm^3$ and at least four months previous ZDV therapy (28). There were no major differences in toxicities in the three regimens. At 24 weeks 31% of patients on the triple therapy arm had CD4 counts that had returned to baseline compared with 37% for Saquinavir/ZDV and 55% on ddC/ZDV. There was also a greater decrease in viral burden in patients receiving triple therapy. Of the 11 patients who had a major clinical event in the 24-week study one was on the triple combination, four on ZDV/ddC and six on Saquinavir/ZDV. Further larger studies on combination therapy with Saquinavir are underway and results eagerly awaited. Work on proteinase inhibitors has been limited, in part, by their complexity of synthesis and their relatively poor bioavailability. Promising and potent agents under development such as the non-peptidic compounds AG1343 (29) and VX-478 (30), and the cyclic urea inhibitors (31) may overcome these problems.

COMBINATION THERAPY

Combination chemotherapy looks at present to be the most promising strategy to control HIV infection. Two modes of combination have been studied: convergent therapy, when the drugs used are in the same class, i.e. nucleoside RT inhibitors ddI/ddC and ZDV; and divergent therapy, when the drugs used have different targets, i.e. a protease inhibitor and an RT inhibitor. Apart from slowing the progress of disease and decreasing mortality, one of the aims of combination therapy is to slow down the development of antiviral resistance. Despite good preliminary results showing an improvement in surrogate markers with combination therapy, data showing a reduction in the emergence of antiviral resistance *in vivo* are lacking at present.

One exciting prospect of convergent therapy is the potential to produce multiple point mutations in resistant strains that actually render the virus non-viable. Chow *et al.* isolated and sequenced a mutant virus with substitutions conferring resistance to ZDV and ddI that became non-viable when cultured with an NNRTI after a mutation to the latter drug had arisen (32). Several groups have since attempted to repeat this work and select such a non-viable mutant. Larder *et al.* cultured virus with dual resistance to ZDV and ddI in increasing concentrations of nevirapine (33). In just three passages virus appeared that was nevirapine resistant but also had enhanced resistance to ZDV. Subsequently Chow, on more extended sequencing of his non-viable mutant, found further unintentional lethal mutations in the RT coding region that were irrelevant to drug resistance (34). Therefore at present the rationale behind convergent chemotherapy is still theoretical but remains an exciting prospect.

CONVERGENT CHEMOTHERAPY

ZDV and ddC have been evaluated in combination in ACTG 106 in patients with advanced HIV disease (35). Fifty-six patients were assigned to one of six regimens of ZDV/ddC at different doses with a ZDV alone control arm. No unexpected toxicities or pharmacokinetic interactions were observed. No group showed a clinical advantage but over a median follow-up of 40 weeks fewer clinical endpoints were reached compared with historical monotherapy studies. The combination of ddC with doses of ZDV greater than 150 mg per day produced the largest and most persistent effect on both CD4 counts and p24 antigenaemia. The enhanced anti-retroviral effect may be due to direct synergism or the delayed emergence of resistant strains. The latter was looked for in a small subgroup of patients on ddC/ZDV combination therapy (36). The more sustained CD4 cell responses conferred by the addition of ddC to ZDV could not be ascribed to the delayed emergence of ZDV resistance.

ACTG 143 was a phase I/II study looking at the combination of ddI and ZDV versus monotherapy (37). Asymptomatic patients with CD4 counts of 200 to 500/mm^3, stratified according to previous ZDV exposure, were randomized to receive either low- or high-dose ZDV and ddI or ddI monotherapy. Results showed an increase in median CD4 counts in the combination groups compared to the monotherapy arms but no significant clinical benefit.

These studies illustrate the need to assess drug efficacy with clinical endpoints to examine whether promising changes in surrogate markers are translated into a medium- to long-term clinical benefit. Hopefully this question will be answered by the Delta Trial. Over 2000 patients, with CD4 counts less than 350/mm^3 have been randomized to either ZDV monotherapy or ZDV and ddI or ZDV and ddC. The ACTG 155 trial (38) was a randomized, double-blind study comparing the safety and efficacy of ZDV and ddC in combination, with ZDV alone or ddC alone in 991 patients who were ZDV experienced for at least 6 months. A combination of ddC 2.25 mg per day and ZDV 600 mg per day was given to 423 patients; 285 received ddC 2.25 mg per day only and 283 continued ZDV 600 mg per day. The median duration of follow-up was 17.7 months. There was no significant difference in the rate of progression to AIDS or death between the groups overall. However, in a subset analysis, patients with a CD4 count of $> 150/mm^3$ at entry given the combination had a significantly lower rate of progression, with only a small increase in toxicity.

Other convergent combination trials including three and four drug combinations are on-going or about to start.

ANTI-RETROVIRAL RESISTANCE

It is widely believed that anti-retroviral resistance is likely to be a major factor in limiting the effectiveness of current and future therapies. Since the first report of ZDV resistance in 1989 much more is now understood about the development of resistance. ZDV resistant virus can be cultured from patients after about six months to one year of treatment. Resistance appears to become more frequent and arise more rapidly in patients with advanced disease (39). The five point mutations in the viral RT that most commonly confer ZDV resistance arise in a temporally defined sequence at amino acid positions 41, 67, 70, 215 and 219 (40). The mutations at positions 41, 70 and 215 seem to be the most important. Resistance has also been described for the other widely used nucleoside and non-nucleoside RT inhibitors. Isolates with reduced sensitivity to ddI and ddC have been described although the decrease in susceptibility is more modest. The specific point mutations associated with resistance are at positions 74 for ddI and 69 for ddC (24). Interestingly the 74-point mutation in ddI confers decreased sensitivity to ddC but increased susceptibility to ZDV.

Mutations to the NNRTIs such as TIBO and Nevirapine emerge rapidly both *in vitro* and *in vivo*, conferring cross-resistance of HIV-1 to other NNRTIs. The point mutations involve the substitution of tyrosine at positions 181 and 188 for cysteine and asparagine respectively (36). These tyrosine residues are critical for NNRTI binding to the RT; therefore single point mutations at these sites render the virus resistant to those drugs.

Although correlations have been suggested, the true relationship between the emergence of *in vitro* resistance virus and clinical deterioration has yet to be proved (41). Factors which make such a correlation difficult include whether the increasing viral load is a cause or effect of developing ZDV resistance, whether *in vitro* culture may select different subspecies through selective amplification in the laboratory, and finally the importance of the presence of syncytia (SI)- or non-syncytia (NSI)-inducing isolates. The isolation of an SI phenotype has been associated with a rapid CD4 decline. A small cohort of 32 asymptomatic patients with detectable p24 Ag was followed for clinical disease progression. Eight of the 12 patients harbouring

SI variants for a total of 223 months progressed to AIDS, compared with only one of 20 patients having NSI isolates for a total of 559 months (41). More importantly, there was no difference between the frequency of ZDV-resistant mutations in the SI or NSI isolates.

CONCLUSION

Antiviral therapy of HIV-infected patients should be influenced predominantly by the clinical status of the patient and not the CD4 count. Although the CD4 count is a useful aid to management, it is not a test of antiviral efficacy. On the basis of the evidence available it is difficult to justify treating asymptomatic patients who have stable CD4 counts of $> 200/mm^3$ with anti-retrovirals. Benefit, if any, is transient, not without toxicity in the short term, of unknown long-term safety and is very expensive. ZDV monotherapy should be reserved for when the first symptoms of HIV disease appear or if the CD4 count trend suggests that this is imminent. This, along with regular clinical assessments and adequate PCP prophylaxis, should form the mainstay of treatment. If ZDV monotherapy fails due to continuing disease progression or toxicity then changing to another agent should be considered. Most experience has been gained with ddI and ddC. No drug combination has yet been shown to offer a clinical benefit and be as, or less, toxic than monotherapy. The use of other agents such as d4T, 3TC or Nevirapine should be reserved for clinical trials until their effectiveness has been established.

REFERENCES

1. Fischl, M., Richman, D., Grieco, M. *et al.* (1987). The efficacy of AZT in the treatment of patients with AIDS and ARC. *N. Engl. J. Med.*, **317**, 185–191.
2. Fischl, M., Richman, D., Hanson, N. *et al.* (1990). The safety and efficacy of AZT in the treatment of patients with mildly symptomatic HIV infection. *Ann. Intern. Med.*, **112**, 727–737.
3. Fishl, M., Parker, C., Pertinelli, C. *et al.* (1990). A randomised controlled trial of a reduced daily dose of zidovudine in patients with AIDS. *N. Engl. J. Med.*, **323**, 1009–1014.
4. Lundgren, J., Phillips, A., Pedersen, C. *et al.* (1994). Comparison of the long term prognosis of patients with AIDS treated and not treated with zidovudine. *JAMA*, **271**, 1088–1092.
5. Volberding, P., Lagakos, W., Koch, M. *et al.* (1990). Zidovudine in asymptomatic HIV infection: a controlled trial in patients with fewer than 500 CD4 cells. *N. Engl. J. Med.*, **322**, 941–949.
6. Cooper, D., Gatell, J., Kroon, S. *et al.* (1993). Zidovudine in persons with asymptomatic HIV infection and CD4+ cell counts greater than 400 per cubic millimetre. *N. Engl. J. Med.*, **329**, 297–303.
7. Mulder, J., Cooper, D., Mathieson, L. *et al.* (1994). Zidovudine twice daily in

asymptomatic subjects with HIV infection and a high risk of progression to AIDS. *AIDS*, **8**, 313–321.
8. Concorde Coordinating Committee. MRC/ANRS (1994). A randomised double-blind controlled trial of immediate versus deferred zidovudine in symptom free HIV infection. *Lancet*, **343**, 871–881.
9. Volberding, P., Lagakos, S., Grimes, J. M. *et al.* (1994). Zidovudine in early asymptomatic HIV disease: a controlled trial in subjects with greater than 500 CD4+ cells/μl (Abstract). *Xth International Conference on AIDS*, Yokohama, Japan.
10. Lenderking, W.R., Gelber, R.D., Cotton, D.J. *et al.* (1994). Evaluation of the quality of life associated with zidovudine treatment in asymptomatic human immunodeficiency virus infection. *N. Eng. J. Med.*, **330**, 738–743.
11. Executive summary: AZT and vertical transmission of HIV infection (1994). *Royal College of Obstetrics and Gynaecology Newsletter*, **19** (June), 2.
12. Editorial (1993). Didanosine and ACTG 116A. *Lancet*, **341**, 109.
13. Kahn, J., Lagakos, S., Richman, D. *et al.* (1992). A controlled trial comparing continued zidovudine with ddI in HIV infection. *N. Engl. J. Med.*, **327**, 581–587.
14. Spruance, S., Pavia, A., Peterson, D. *et al.* (1994). DDI compared with continuation of zidovudine in HIV infected patients with signs of clinical deterioration while receiving zidovudine. *Ann. Intern. Med.*, **120**, 360–368.
15. Abouker, J.-P. and the MRC/ANRS International Alpha Trial Coordinating Committee (1992). Didanosine for zidovudine intolerant patients with HIV disease. *Lancet*, **340**, 1346–1347.
16. Collier, A., Henry, K., Japour, A. *et al.* (1993). Switching and combining antiretroviral therapies. *AIDS Clin. Care*, **5**, 33–37.
17. Fischl, M., Olsen, R., Follensbee, S. *et al.* (1993). Zalcitabine compared with zidovudine in patients with advanced HIV-1 infection who received previous zidovudine therapy. *Ann. Intern. Med.*, **188**, 762–769.
18. Abrams, D., Goldman, A., Lainer, C. *et al.* (1994). A comparative trial of ddI or zalcitabine after treatment with zidovudine in patients with HIV-1 infection. *N. Engl. J. Med.*, **330**, 657–662.
19. Browne, M., Mayer, K., Chafee, S. *et al.* (1993). D4T in patients with AIDS or ARC: a phase I trial. *J. Infect. Dis.*, **167**, 21–29.
20. Kitchen, V., Danner, S., Katlaria, C. *et al.* (1992). A phase I/II trial of the efficacy of 3TC in asymptomatic or oligosymptomatic subjects with HIV infection. *AIDS*, **6** (suppl.), s89–s94.
21. Jacobson, M., van der Hurst, C., Causey, D. *et al.* (1991). In vivo additive antiretroviral effect of combined zidovudine and foscarnet for HIV infection. *J. Infect. Dis.*, **163**, 1219–1222.
22. SOCA Trials Group (1992). Mortality in patients with AIDS treated with either foscarnet or ganciclovir for CMV retinitis. *N. Engl. J. Med.*, **326**, 213–220.
23. Sandstrum, E. and Oberg, B. (1993). Antiviral therapy in HIV infection. Current status (part 2). *Drugs*, **45** (5), 637–653.
24. AIDS Treatment Update, June 1994.
25. Yeni, P., Schooley, R., Harver, S. *et al.* (1993). Antiretroviral and immune based therapies: update. *AIDS*, **7** (suppl.), S173–S184.
26. Weber, J. (1993). The molecular basis of antiretroviral therapy. *J. Antimicrob. Chemother.*, **32**, 789–792.
27. Collier, A., Coombs, R., Timpone, J. *et al.* (1994). Comparative study of Ro 31-8959 and zidovudine (ZDV) vs. ZDV and zalcitabine (ddC) vs. Ro 31-8959, ZDV and ddC. *Xth International Conference on AIDS*, Yokohama, Japan.
28. Bassett, R., Schoerfeld, D. and Collier, A. ACTG Executive Summary, May 1994.

29. Shetty, B., Kaldor, S., Reich, S. *et al.* (1994). AG1343, an orally available non-peptidic HIV-1 protease inhibitor (Abstract). *Xth International Conference on AIDS*, Yokohama, Japan.
30. Kim, E., Rao, B., Deininger, D. *et al.* (1994). Structural comparison of the clinically relevant inhibitors of the HIV-1 protease (Abstract). *Xth International Conference on AIDS*, Yokohama, Japan.
31. Otto, M., Aldrich, P., Grubb, M. *et al.* (1994). XM412, an improved cyclic urea inhibitor of HIV protease for oral administration (Abstract). *Xth International Conference on AIDS*, Yokohama, Japan.
32. Chow, Y., Hirsch, M., Mensll, D. *et al.* (1993). Use of evolutionary limitations of HIV-1 multi-drug resistance to optimize therapy. *Nature*, **361**, 650–654.
33. Larder, B. (1994). Interactions between drug resistance mutations in HIV-1 reverse transcriptase. *J. Gen. Virol.*, **75**, 951–957.
34. Chow, Y., Hirsch, M., Kaplan, J. *et al.* (1993). HIV-1 error revealed. *Nature*, **362**, 678.
35. Meng, T., Fischl, M., Boota, A. *et al.* (1992). Combination therapy with ZDV and ddC in patients with advanced HIV infection. *Ann. Intern. Med.*, **116**, 13–20.
36. Richman, D., Meng, T., Specter, S. *et al.* (1994). Resistance to AZT and ddC during long term combination therapy in patients with advanced HIV. *J. AIDS*, **7**, 135–138.
37. Collier, A., Coombs, R., Fischl, M. *et al.* (1993). Combination therapy with zidovudine and ddI compared to zidovudine alone in HIV-1 infection. *Ann. Intern. Med.*, **119**, 786–793.
38. ACTG 155 Trial (1994). Executive Summary. Roche, Strasbourg.
39. Larder, B., Darby, C., Richman, D. *et al.* (1989). HIV with reduced sensitivity to AZT isolated during prolonged therapy. *Science*, **243**, 1731–1734.
40. Kellam, P., Boucher, C. and Tifnagel, J. (1994). Zidovudine treatment results in the selection of HIV-1 variants whose genotypes confer increasing levels of drug resistance. *J. Gen. Virol.*, **75**, 341–351.
41. Tudor-Williams, G., St Claire, M., McKinney, R. *et al.* (1992). HIV-1 sensitivity to zidovudine and clinical outcome in children. *Lancet*, **339**, 15–19.
42. Boucher, C., Lange, J., Miedema, F. *et al.* (1992). HIV-1 biological phenotype and the development of zidovudine resistance in relation to disease progression in asymptomatic individuals during treatment. *AIDS*, **6**, 1259–1264.

Part B

HERPESVIRUSES

Basic Research

Clinical Treatment

4 Selective Inhibition of Cytomegalovirus Replication

MARY L. HAFFEY
Bristol-Myers Squibb Pharmaceutical Group, Princeton, New Jersey, USA

A. KIRK FIELD
Hybridon, Inc., Worcester, Massachusetts, USA

INTRODUCTION

Human cytomegalovirus (HCMV) has been described since the early 1900s, but during the last decade several factors have contributed to a blossoming of literature and heightened interest in HCMV. In the laboratory, the use of molecular techniques, monoclonal antibodies and advances in cell culture technology have facilitated the study of HCMV replication at the molecular level. The expansion of immunosuppressed populations and the habits of modern Western civilization have contributed to an increased incidence of HCMV disease. In the past, HCMV was a clinically important pathogen primarily for the fetus and neonate. Now, increasing numbers of immunosuppressed children and adults are also susceptible to debilitating and life-threatening HCMV disease. Finally, the ever-increasing use of antiviral chemotherapy has clearly demonstrated that viral diseases are amenable to treatment, fostering a search for safe and effective agents to combat HCMV infections.

The possibility of antiviral chemotherapy for serious HCMV infections began with the approval in the late 1980s of the intravenous (i.v.) form of ganciclovir (GCV) and continues in the 1990s with the approval of i.v. sodium phosphonoformate (PFA, foscarnet) for the treatment of HCMV retinitis. The successful use of these agents and the expanding knowledge of essential viral targets have extended the hope that more effective and acceptable therapies are possible.

In this chapter, we will analyse the present knowledge of HCMV structure, replication and pathogenesis, and the existing armamentarium of antivirals in clinical use and in development. This discussion will highlight both the benefits and deficiencies of present therapy and the opportunities for future therapies against new HCMV targets. By design, we have focused on the chemotherapeutic approaches to the management of HCMV disease

Antiviral Chemotherapy. Edited by D.J. Jeffries and E. De Clercq

and have not discussed vaccines. An excellent review of HCMV vaccine development is presented by Gonczol and Plotkin (1).

DISCOVERY AND EMERGING ROLE AS A HUMAN PATHOGEN

HCMV was named after the enlarged, inclusion body-containing cells found in infected patients (reviewed in reference 2). These inclusion-bearing cells were first noted in 1904 (3,4) in histological examinations of tissues from newborn infants at autopsy, but the viral aetiology of the inclusions was not postulated until 1921 (5). In 1926, Cole and Kuttner (6) showed that inclusion-bearing, guinea-pig salivary glands could transmit infection after filtration, leading to the generic designation of HCMV as the 'salivary gland virus'. Fifty years after the first reports, researchers (7–9) successfully propagated HCMV in cell culture. The AD 169 strain of HCMV, which is frequently studied today, was recovered from the adenoids of a young girl in one of these early studies (7). After propagation in cell culture was accomplished, serological methodology developed rapidly, demonstrating the antigenic variation of the virus and confirming its widespread epidemiology in the human population (10,11). Later biochemical analysis and electron microscopy revealed that HCMV is a DNA virus, and a member of the herpesvirus family (reviewed in references 12 and 13). The term 'cytomegalovirus' was coined by Weller in 1960 to describe the 'salivary gland virus' which caused 'cytomegalic inclusion disease' (11).

HCMV is ubiquitous, with seropositivity in developed countries averaging about 75% and in developing countries close to 100% of the population (2,14). In the otherwise normal host, HCMV usually establishes a latent asymptomatic infection. However, in populations where cell-mediated immunity is suppressed, HCMV is a major pathogen. The developing fetus, neonate, allograft recipients, cancer patients and AIDS patients are all at risk of serious disease caused by HCMV (2). Host immune function, the route of infection and the size of inoculum all contribute to the extent and severity of HCMV disease (13).

Primary infection in immunocompetent hosts, while usually asymptomatic, can manifest itself as a mononucleosis-like syndrome with fever, hepatitis and/or fatigue, characterized by atypical circulating lymphocytes. Seven per cent of all infectious mononucleosis may be due to HCMV infection (15). Following primary infection there is often a prolonged interval where no apparent tissue damage or illness occurs, but the virus remains 'latent' in many tissues.

As mentioned above, some of the increasing morbidity and mortality seen with HCMV infection in recent decades is a function of the changes in habits of modern Western societies (17). People are less frequently exposed to the virus in childhood due to reduced breast feeding and less crowded living conditions. As a result, primary HCMV infection occurs with increasing frequency in adults, and is more likely to result in clinical manifestations. In women, infection during pregnancy can have devastating consequences. Maternal/fetal transfer results in congenital infection, leading to fetal hepatosplenomegaly, jaundice, thrombocytopenic purpura, microcephaly, low birth weight and, in the most severe cases, irreversible central nervous system (CNS) damage. HCMV is the major infectious cause of mental retardation in children (17).

Organ transplantation, cancer chemotherapy and acquired immune deficiency syndrome (AIDS) have also expanded the population susceptible to HCMV infection and disease. Interstitial pneumonia due to HCMV kills at least 15% of bone marrow transplant patients; in renal transplants, HCMV results in 20% of graft rejection and accounts for 25% of all mortality (15). In addition, approximately 20% of AIDS patients develop HCMV retinitis which, if untreated, is a progressive infection resulting in blindness (16).

STRUCTURE AND REPLICATION OF HCMV

In general, cytomegaloviruses are species specific for replication and pathogenesis. Their classification as beta herpesviruses is based on biological features of replication and the proposed, non-neuronal site for latency. HCMV replicates slowly compared to other herpesviruses both in cell culture and in man (reviewed in references 12 and 13).

VIRION AND GENOME STRUCTURE

The HCMV virion consists of an electron-dense, nucleic acid-containing core enclosed in an icosahedral capsid which is surrounded by a lipid envelope (Figure 4.1). The tegument is a fibrillar/granular layer containing matrix proteins which anchors the envelope to the capsid. Virions are pleomorphic, and range in diameter from 150 to 300 nm. Details of the HCMV virion proteins have recently been reviewed by Stinski (13) and Gibson (18).

Among the human herpesviruses studied to date, the genome of HCMV and HHV-6 are most closely related (19). A comparison of the prototypical organization of the various herpesvirus genomes is shown in Figure 4.2. HCMV is the largest of the human herpesvirus genomes (20); it is composed of double-stranded DNA, about 150×10^6 Da in molecular weight and exhibits a buoyant density of 1.716–1.717 g/cm^3 (20,21). As is true of many viruses, high-multiplicity passage of viral stocks in culture can result in the generation of defective genomes (smaller than wild type: 100×10^6 Da) which are packaged into virions, thus increasing the number of non-infec-

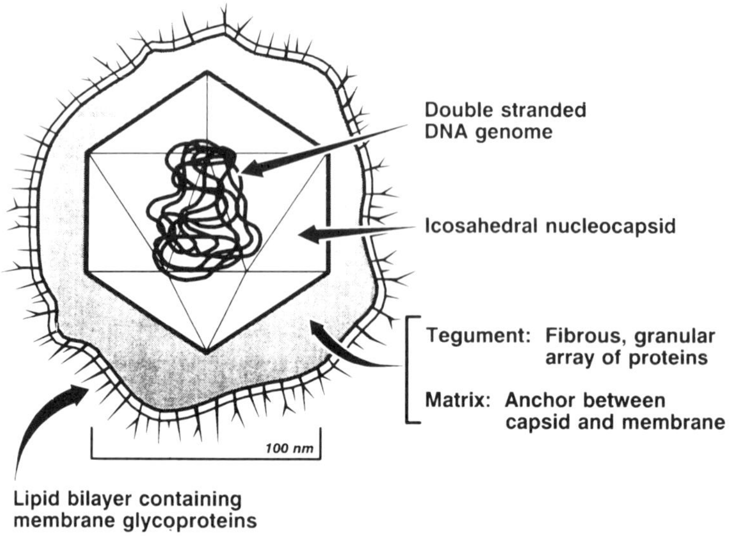

Figure 4.1. Generalized structure of HCMV virion

tious particles in such stocks. These defective particles have not yet been observed in infected hosts (13).

As reviewed in Stinski (13), HCMV isolates generally have at least 50% greater DNA sequence complexity than do HSV isolates, due to gene acquisitions and duplications. Like HSV strains, HCMV genomes found in infectious virion preparations contain nicks and gaps, and can exist in four isomeric configurations. Long (L) and short (S) segments each have inverted (internal and terminal) repeats (refer to Figure 4.2). In the isomerizing genome represented in the Towne strain, the unique L region (UL) is 175 kilobase pairs (kb) in length bounded by repeats of 11 kb and the unique S (US) region is 38 kb with 2 kb repeat. HCMV 'a' sequence amplification causes L–S junction variations which result in sequence divergence between strains.

The complete DNA sequence of strain AD 169 was recently reported, and is described as 229 354 base pairs long, with a guanine + cytosine content of 57.2% (21). Because this DNA sequence was obtained from a high-passage strain of HCMV (AD 169) which is poorly pathogenic, some care should be taken in extrapolating directly to clinical strains.

Sequencing of the AD 169 strain revealed 208 open reading frames (22); however, very little of the genome has been mapped with respect to transcription or protein expression. Of the roughly 200 presumed genes identified, about 30–40 have homologues in the HSV genome based upon predicted protein sequence similarities, and most of those (30–35 genes) appear to be 'herpesvirus common'. A summary of the proposed homologues for which functions have been assigned is listed in Table 4.1. As described in more detail by Mocarski (27,28), these genes are involved in DNA replication, genome packaging and virion structure. Certain types of DNA elements are also common to the herpesvirus family, but those found in HCMV do not have close sequence homology to the other herpesvirus sequences. These DNA elements include DNA packaging signals at the ends of the viral genome and inverted terminal and internal repeats. Recently, additional herpesvirus common genes have been described. The proteinase genes of CMV (29) and HSV-1 (30) are reported to share sequence homology, and the enzyme responsible for the phosphorylation of ganciclovir in HCMV-infected cells (UL97) has been shown to have a homologue in other herpesviruses (34).

Curiously, potential homologues of cellular genes have also been identified in the HCMV genome. These include (i) an HLA homologue (UL18 gene) capable of binding β_2-microglobulin (β_2m) (36), (ii) a T cell receptor, γ-chain (UL20 gene), and (iii) G-protein coupled receptors (GCRs) (UL33, US27, US28 genes). HCMV can activate second messengers in a manner analogous to other GCRs, some of which are potential oncogenes. This activation process may be related to pathogenesis (37). If HCMV GCR homologues contain ligand binding sites, a novel class of antivirals could be envisioned by analogy with the β-adrenergic receptors where ligand mimics could potentially be designed which would interfere with signal transduction (21). In light of these protein sequence homologies, it is not surprising that cross-hybridization with human cellular genes and 28 S ribosomal RNA sequences has also been reported (38).

One challenge open for the future is to explain the function of all the genes catalogued from the sequence analysis. We have discussed how protein sequence homologies can be used to derive clues to gene function. Another approach used in the past is heterologous expression of viral proteins, and such studies in the future with HCMV will also be facilitated by the AD 169 sequence analysis.

Restriction endonuclease length polymorphisms (RLPs) exist between various HCMV isolates, indicating that different HCMV strains have some sequence variations. RLPs between strains are not the result of major sequence changes, nor do they appear to affect biology of the viruses, as reflected in 80% general homology and colinearity between isolates studied to date. (Refer to reference 13 or 39 for restriction maps).

In much the same way as has been described for HSV (40,41), the HCMV RLPs can be used to trace viral transmission in correlation to the clinical consequences of infections and reactivations. In renal transplant patients, disease has been traced primarily to HCMV strains present in the donor kidney (42). By contrast, reactivation of endogenous latent strains appears to cause disease more often in bone marrow transplant (BMT) patients (43). Seropositive HCMV donor marrow can in fact be protective in BMT recipi-

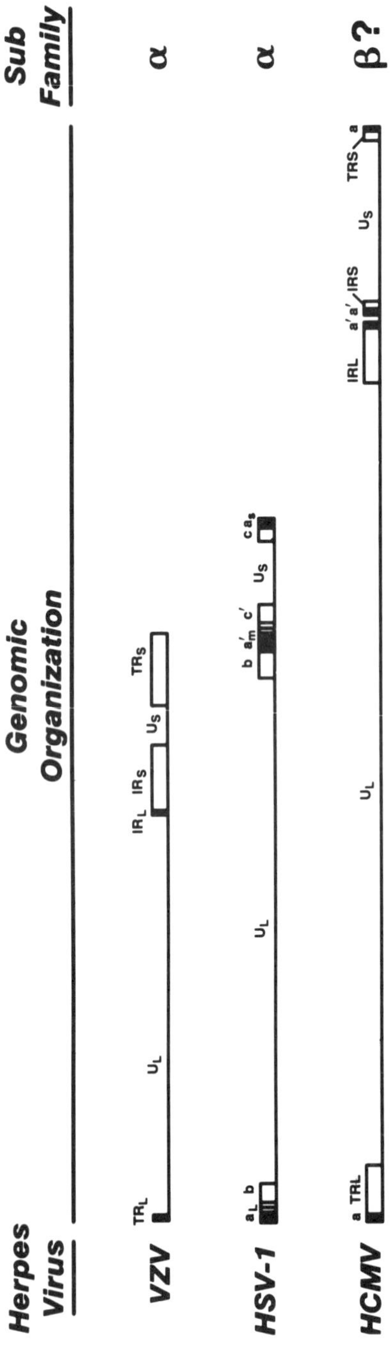
Herpes Virus
Genomic Organization
Sub Family
VZV
TRL UL IRL IRS US TRS
α
HSV-1
aL b UL b a'm c' US c aS
α
HCMV
a TRL UL IRL a' a' IRS US TRS a
β?

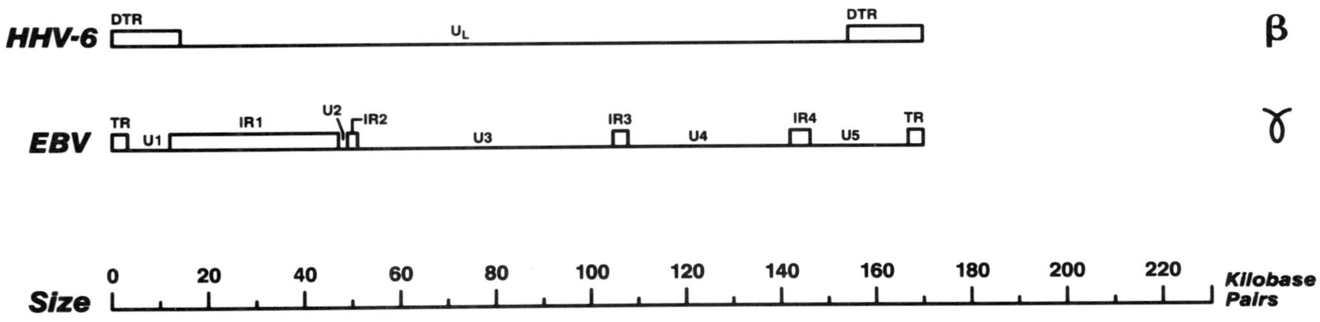

Figure 4.2. Genomic organization of human herpesviruses: varicella zoster virus (VZV), herpes simplex virus type 1 (HSV-1), human cytomegalovirus (HCMV), human herpesvirus 6 (HHV-6) and Epstein–Barr virus (EBV). The details of each scheme are found in references 185, 186, 13, 187 and 188, respectively. Terminal repeats (TR), internal repeats (IR), direct terminal repeats (DTR), unique (U), long (L) and short (S) designations are noted

Table 4.1. Homologous genes

Gene	HCMV	HSV	VZV	EBV
Pol accessory	UL44	UL42		BMRF1
Ribonucleotide reductase?	UL45	UL39	VZV19	BORF2
Capsid/assembly?	UL46	UL38?	VZV20?	BORFI?
Virion protein?	UL48	UL36	VZV22	BPLF1
DNA polymerase	UL54	UL30	VZV28	BALF5
Glycoprotein B	UL55	UL27	VZV31	BALF4
Major DNA binding protein	UL57	UL29	VZV29	BALF2
Transactivator?	UL69	UL54	VZV4	BMFL1
DNA replication	UL70	UL52	VZV6	BSLF1
dUTPase	UL72	UL50	VZV8	BLLF1
Glycoprotein H	UL75	UL22	VZV37	BXLF1
Virion protein?	UL77	UL25	VZV34	BVRF1
Assembly protein	UL80	UL26	VZV33	BVRF2
Major capsid protein	UL86	UL19	VZV40	BCLF1
Protein kinase	UL97	UL13	VZV47	BGLF4
Deoxyribonuclease	UL98	UL12	VZV48	BGLF5
DNA replication?	UL101	UL9?	VZV51?	BBLF2?
DNA replication?	UL102	UL8?	VZV52?	BBLF3?
Virion protein?	UL104	UL6	VZV54	BBRF1
Helicase	UL105	UL5	VZV55	BBLF4
Uracil-DNA glycosylase	UL114	UL2	VZV59	BKRF3

Information contained in this table is derived from references 22 and 23. A question mark (?) refers to designations of gene function or homology for which some uncertainty still exists.

ents (44). These RLP variations have also revealed that an individual can be co-infected by more than one HCMV strain.

Heterogeneity in HCMV strains may also be evidenced from the varied molecular sizes reported for specific viral proteins (15). Whether this is due to different analytical systems or intrinsic strain differences is not always clear.

RECEPTORS AND CELL ENTRY

It is assumed that the early stages of HCMV replication are similar to those described for HSV (12,45), involving an interaction between the virion envelope and the host cell membrane. As noted in Table 4.1, several virion proteins and glycoproteins are conserved among the herpesvirus family.

At least three virion proteins are implicated in the HCMV attachment/penetration process: gB (UL55 gene), gH (UL75 gene) and the HLA homologue (UL18 gene) (18). Among these, the HCMV UL18 gene is unique in that it is not conserved in the herpesvirus family.

The HCMV glycoproteins have been described by various titles in the literature, including three complexes: gcI, II and III (13). The gcI complex contains gB and related glycoproteins; the gcII complex is equivalent to a repetitive gene family (US6), and the gcIII complex contains the gH glycoprotein, among others. The genome of HCMV contains 30 reading frames for proteins with characteristics of glycoproteins (21) but all of their gene products have not yet been assigned.

The gcI complex contains proteins of 160–300 kDa which dissociate upon reduction for electrophoretic analysis (46). Of these, the conserved viral glycoprotein, gB (UL55, gp58/116), begins as a precursor of more than 900 amino acids which is glycosylated to form a 150–160 kDa molecule and subsequently endoproteolysed into gp116 and gp58. The antigenic domain of gp58 (AD-1) has been recently characterized (47).

In contrast, the conserved gH glycoprotein shifts modestly in apparent molecular weight from 80–85 kDa to 86 kDa (gp86) as it is processed from precursor to product, respectively. Recently, Keay and Baldwin demonstrated that the human fibroblast receptor of gp86 is a phosphorylated glycoprotein (48).

A monoclonal antibody (1G6), directed at the gH glycoprotein, has been described which can neutralize HCMV in the absence of complement (49). Antibodies to gB can also neutralize viral infectivity (49). These results suggest that the gH and gB glycoproteins are directly involved in virion infectivity, as has been described for their HSV homologues (45). A recent study compared the complete coding sequences of 10 clinical strains of HCMV and determined that, compared to glycoprotein gB, gH is more highly conserved among strains and may be expected to have more limited immunological diversity (51). One anti-gH monoclonal antibody (MSL106) is reportedly in phase I clinical trials for HCMV infection in bone marrow transplant recipients (50).

The HCMV glycoproteins have been reviewed in greater detail by Stinski (13), Landini and Michelson (15), Chee *et al.* (21), Mach *et al.* (39) and Gibson (18). From the perspective of antiviral drug targeting, several possibilities exist in addition to the monoclonal antibodies approach. Glycosylation inhibitors which prevent precursor processing of essential glycoproteins may block HCMV replication, as has been shown for other viruses (52). Identification of small molecules capable of blocking cellular receptors is another antiviral approach, and attempts to define the cellular receptor(s) involved in virion attachment have also been initiated. Recent studies by Cooper *et al.* (53), using ^{35}S-labelled HCMV, demonstrated that virions bind to numerous cell types in culture, including human lymphocytes and monocytes. However, human fibroblasts and umbilical vein endothelial cells have been reported to bind 10-fold greater numbers of virions compared to other cell types. Cooper *et al.* have further demonstrated that the binding to monocytes is mediated by a cell membrane glycoprotein which has a molecular weight of about 30 kDa and which appears to bind HCMV glycoprotein gB (54). In contrast, gH has been shown to bind to a 92 kDa protein which is expressed on the surface of cells susceptible to HCMV infection. The structure and cellular functions of these putative 30 kDa and 92 kDa HCMV receptors have not yet been described. Initiation of HCMV infection also requires interaction with the cell surface heparin sulphate (55). Furthermore, sulphated polymers inhibit this interaction (56) as was previously described for HSV (57).

An additional, interesting hypothesis has been raised to explain HCMV entry into cells. HCMV virions have been shown to bind β_2m, and it has been postulated that β_2m on the cell surface binds to the UL18 gene product (the homologue of the HLA α-chain) to facilitate cell attachment and/or virion penetration (reviewed by Stinski, reference 13). Based upon this scenario, it may be possible to envision antivirals directed at specific disruption of the UL18/β_2m interaction resulting in the loss of virion infectivity.

The studies mentioned above have only begun to unravel the process of virion/cell receptor interaction at the molecular level. Further detailed understanding could be an important start in defining a new antiviral strategy, as has been described for the rhinoviruses (ICAM) and HIV (CD4) receptors (reviewed by Lentz, reference 58).

REGULATION OF GENE EXPRESSION

HCMV requires differentiated cells for growth in cell culture and, unlike HSV, HCMV only arrests host cell protein synthesis briefly at the initial stage of infection. In infected cells, 30% and 60% of the observed protein synthesis is HCMV specific at early and late times in infection, respectively (15). This overlapping pattern of gene expression makes it difficult to distinguish host proteins from viral proteins. Additionally, synthesis of the following cellular proteins is stimulated after infection: cellular DNA polymerases α and γ (mitochondrial DNA synthesis increases), poly ADP ribose synthetase, RNA polymerases I, II and III, cytosolic and mitochondrial thymidine kinases, ornithine decarboxylase, plasminogen activator and DNases (15). The reason for this stimulation of host protein synthesis in HCMV infection is unclear, but one could imagine a requirement for at least some of these cellular enzymes in the viral replication process. Perhaps because of the stimulation of host cell protein synthesis, and in order to compete for cellular RNA polymerase (pol), several HCMV mRNAs have strong upstream regulatory and enhancer elements containing consensus binding sites for a variety of cellular transcription factors. This may also explain why expression from these promoters is high in many cell types.

The overall scheme for HCMV replication partially resembles the other herpesviruses studied to date. The temporal cascade, which was originally described by Honess and Roizman (59) for HSV replication, consisted of sequential expression of immediate–early (IE or α); early (E or β); and late (L or γ) transcripts and/or proteins. Strictly speaking, IE gene expression requires no prior viral protein synthesis, while E genes require IE viral gene expression and L genes are expressed after viral DNA synthesis has occurred. The original HSV cascade scheme has since been modified to account for new findings and the exceptions to this rule (12), but overall the pattern serves as a framework for discussion of the sequential waves of viral protein synthesis in infected cells. During productive HCMV infection, IE, E and L gene expression occur to varying degrees, simultaneously.

IE gene expression which occurs within 3–4 h post infection (pi) is sensitive to α-amanitin in cell-free translation assays, indicating that it is likely to be dependent upon cellular RNA pol II.

Four major IE transcription units (IE1–4) have been mapped on the HCMV genome to map units (mu) .66–.76 (refer to Figure 4.3). About 88% of IE transcription occurs in this distinct region of UL. Low levels of IE transcription are seen from two other regions, between .21 and .24 mu in UL and .8–.86 mu in US. In the major transcription unit (Figure 4.3) a complex pattern of the IE1 and IE2 transcripts is generated from a single promoter region by differential splicing. Details of the features of the HCMV IE promoter have been reviewed by Stinski (13) and Mocarski (27,28).

IE gene products are involved in stimulating both viral and host gene expression, as viral and cellular transcription increases dramatically pi. IE1 induces the cellular nuclear factor, NF-κB, which induces several genes including IE1 itself. IE2, although less abundant than IE1, was also recently shown to upregulate the expression of cellular genes, e.g. interleukin (IL)-2 and the IL-2 receptor (60). Thus, the expression of IE2 may be involved in modulation of immune responses to HCMV infection. IE2 also represses IE gene expression through a signal found upstream of the IE1–2 transcription unit. Phosphorylated IE1 migrates to the nucleus and it appears to autoregulate, transiently shutting down by 8 h pi but then accumulating to high levels at late times pi. The IE2 protein is produced throughout the replication cycle, and its synthesis increases with time. IE2 can act alone or be stimulated by IE1 protein. Recently, it has been shown that the DNA binding domain of IE2 spans a large region in the carboxy-terminal half of the protein and that IE2 can contribute to transactivation, but may require additional transcription factors (62,63). At late times pi only the C-terminal portion of IE2 may be transcribed (61).

This complex control of IE gene expression is a potential target for antiviral intervention. Since this control is essential to the viral replicative cycle, inhibition of an IE gene function by an antiviral agent could truncate the replicative cycle prematurely.

The E phase, initiated prior to HCMV DNA replication, lasts 24 h or more. Little functional distinction can be made between E and L genes because most, but not all, L genes are made in the absence of DNA synthesis and are proportional to the overall levels of transcription. One late gene is transcribed but not fully processed into a functional cytoplasmic mRNA

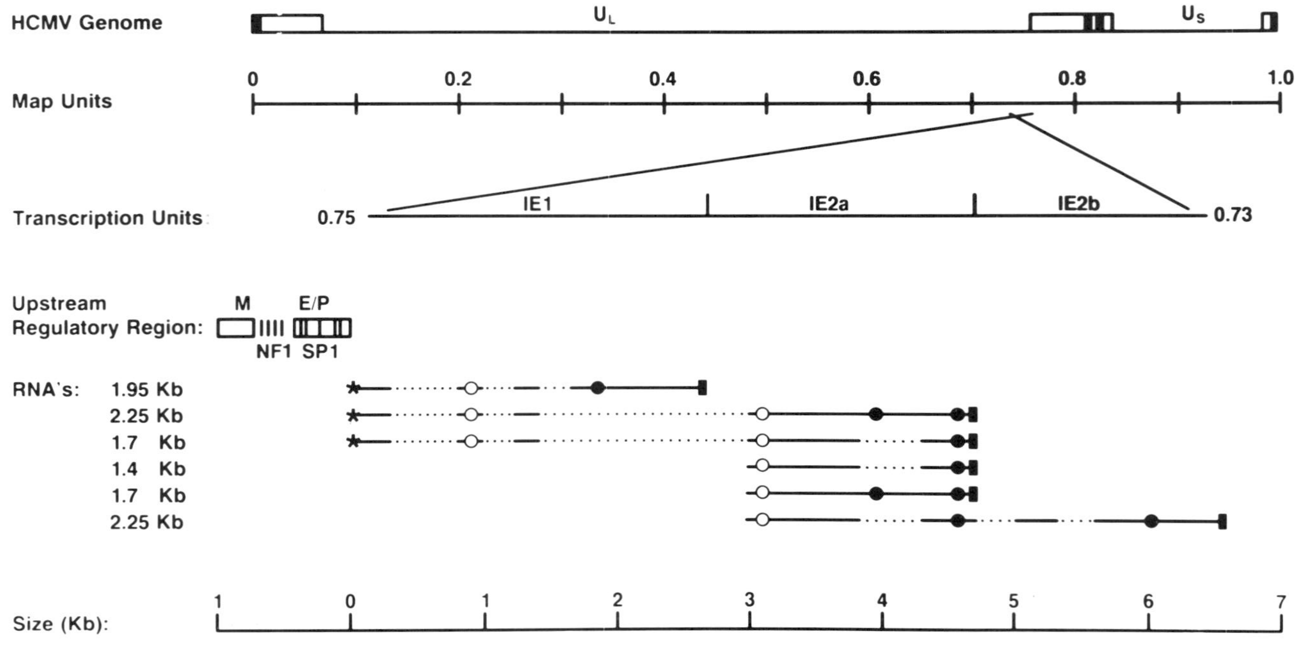

Figure 4.3. Organization of the HCMV major immediate early transcription unit. A region between 0.73 and 0.75 map units containing the IE1 and IE2 transcripts is shown. Upstream regulatory elements include enhancer/promoter (E/P) and modulator (M) regions as well as binding sites for nuclear factors NF1 and SP1. Sizes are shown in kilobase pairs (Kb). Location of cap site (*), initiation codons (○), termination codons (●) and poly-A signals (■) are indicated on RNAs. Solid black lines indicate exons and dotted lines introns of RNA. Information is from references 2, 13 and 39

until DNA synthesis is complete (64); such post-transcriptional regulation may involve a viral or cellular gene which is stimulated by DNA synthesis and whose gene product interacts with *cis*-acting elements in 5′ or 3′ ends of precursor RNAs. One 'true' late promoter has been described within the IE2 gene (61), which is apparently not active when DNA synthesis is inhibited. Overall, the level of viral transcription increases with time after infection.

DNA REPLICATION

The time required for initiation of HCMV DNA synthesis in cultured cells is slower than for the alpha herpesviruses; and two peaks of HCMV DNA replication may occur, at one and three days pi, respectively. At high multiplicities of infection, DNA synthesis starts at 12 h pi and reaches a maximum rate at 72–96 h pi. In contrast, alpha herpesvirus DNA replication occurs at 4–6 h pi. The reason for this disparity is unknown, but the relatively low levels of HCMV protein expression (e.g. viral E proteins essential for DNA replication) and/or competition for essential cellular factors could account for the length of time. Consistent with this time difference, HCMV plaques in cell culture appear in 7–14 days, about a week later than for HSV plaque development (one to two days) (13).

The details of HCMV DNA replication have not been established (65), and much of what is known is inferred from the studies of HSV. By analogy with the HSV DNA replication genes identified by Challberg (66), one might have expected to identify seven HCMV gene products essential for viral DNA replication. For HSV these would include the DNA polymerase (HSV UL30 gene), an accessory protein (HSV UL42 gene) which increases processivity of DNA replication, a single-stranded DNA binding protein (HSV UL29 gene, also known as ICP8), a DNA origin-of-replication binding protein (HSV UL9 gene), and a three-protein complex (HSV UL5, 8 and 52 genes) which provide helicase and primase activities. Many of these HSV proteins have HCMV homologues (Table 4.1). Pari and Anders (23) demonstrated that eleven loci encode trans-acting factors are required for origin dependent HCMV DNA replication, using a co-transfection method similar to that described by Challberg (66). Of the eleven, six genes are homologues of the required HSV genes. (HCMV UL44 = HZV UL42; HCMV UL54 = HSV UL30; HCMV UL57 = HSV UL29; HCMV UL70 = HSV UL52; HCMV UL105 = HSV UL5; HCMV UL101-102 = HSV UL8). In addition, five other HCMV reading frames appear to be unique (UL36-38, UL112-113, IE1/IE2, IRS1, and UL84). These essential genes and gene products are each potential key targets for antiviral intervention. To date, inhibitors of the viral DNA polymerase have been used successfully in the clinic, but intense efforts are underway to identify novel inhibitors of other viral replication targets.

The HCMV DNA polymerase (UL54 gene) is a 140 kDa protein which bears only 24% amino acid sequence homology to the HSV polymerase (22). Like HSV, the HCMV polymerase also has a 3′–5′ exonuclease activity and is active in high salt. HCMV DNA polymerase is found associated with a 51–58 kDa protein, referred to as ICP36 (UL44 gene product). ICP36 binds DNA and may play a role in DNA replication (like the HSV UL42 gene product (68)). ICP36 was recently shown to bind to HCMV DNA polymerase and stimulate enzymatic activity (26). One HCMV protein (UL57 gene, also known as DB140) has been described which has apparent homology to HSV ICP8 (69). It is found in low abundance in the nucleus. The HCMV UL57 gene has been mapped adjacent to the origin of lytic DNA replication, like HSV ICP8 (70). Four other HCMV nuclear E proteins have been identified, and their functions are being clarified (18). The functions of the unique HCMV genes required for replication include both immediate and early expressed genes. The UL36-38 region is complex and is expressed at immediate early times (24). Recently, potent and selective antisense inhibitors of this region have been found which inhibit virus replication, indicating the essential nature of UL36-38 (personal communication). Similarly, antisense inhibitors of the IE2 region are also potent inhibitors of HCMV replication (25).

HCMV and HSV have similar genome arrangements (Figure 4.2); UL and US regions with repetitive 'a' sequences at each end and an internal 'a' sequence to permit rearrangement. Like HSV, replication may involve a circular intermediate which can be formed by hybridization of direct repeat sequences at the ends of the HCMV genome (41,65). The HCMV 'a' sequences are partially homologous with HSV 'a' sequences, and experiments with recombinant viruses have shown that HSV can functionally use the HCMV 'a' sequence. Cleavage of unit length genomes occurs within 30–35 bases of the homology sequence. Because evidence exists for concatemers, loops, forks and four isomers, a mechanism similar to that described for HSV replication is envisioned for HCMV (67). Thus, it appears that DNA maturation may be similar for several members of the herpesvirus family. Further characterization of this DNA maturation process could result in identification of 'herpesvirus common' targets for antiviral intervention.

ASSEMBLY

Virion assembly in the infected cell is a complex and incompletely understood process. The most immature particles, referred to as B-capsids, contain essentially no DNA or envelope. B-capsids do contain the major capsid protein (UL86), other less abundant capsid proteins and an assembly protein (UL80). The assembly protein is present in immature particles, is phosphorylated, undergoes maturational cleavage, and is absent from the mature virions (18). Gibson (18) has disclosed that the maturation of assembly protein is the result of proteinase activity (referred to as *assemblin*) associated with the UL80 gene product(s). Detailed characterization of the assemblin and essential substrate cleavage site(s) necessary for maturation of the virion are ongoing for both this proteinase (29,31,32,33) and the HSV-1 protease (UL26 gene product) recently identified by Liu and Roizman (30). Success in this characterization should identify herpesvirus targets and a new avenue for antiviral intervention, as has been the case for inhibition of the human immunodeficiency virus (HIV) proteinase.

Continued maturation of the B-capsids into infectious virions requires elimination of the assembly protein, acquisition of unit-length DNA, tegument/matrix proteins and finally envelopment. A variety of phosphoproteins have been reported to be part of the HCMV tegument/matrix. These include: pp28—a hydrophilic, immunogenic phosphoprotein; pp64—a putative protein kinase; pp65—another putative protein kinase also referred to as the 'lower matrix protein'; pp71—the 'upper matrix protein'; and pp150—a large, basic, immunogenic, glycosylated phosphoprotein. The role of each phosphoprotein is yet to be determined. The complex process of virion maturation has been summarized recently by Gibson (18) and may be considered as a general target for antiviral chemotherapy. Elucidation of the functional requirements for the putative protein kinases could also yield specific new targets for antiviral intervention.

PATHOGENESIS AND THE AVAILABILITY OF ANTIVIRAL TARGETS

To appreciate more fully the challenge of selective inhibition of HCMV by an antiviral agent, we should also examine the nature of HCMV infections, latency and disease. Unfortunately, just as our understanding of the details of replication and the functions of the 200 genes of HCMV is relatively rudimentary, our knowledge of the details of pathogenesis is also only fragmentary. In this section, we will highlight those aspects of the infection and disease process which are important to antiviral strategies. More detailed descriptions of infection and disease in the normal and immunocompromised host have been provided by Alford and Britt (2) and Falloon and Masur (71).

HCMV may enter the host via saliva, urine, cervical and vaginal secretions, semen, breast milk, tears, faeces and blood. On average, 1% of infants are infected *in utero*, and up to 60% become infected by age six months. The natural progression of the infection is subclinical in the immunocompetent host, often initiated by infection of ductal epithelial cells, which in infants and children results in salivary gland infection and pharyngeal shedding, thus providing the main routes of viral spread to other children and caregivers. Blood transfusions and organ transplants are also a source of virus transmission which can result in either primary infection or reactivation. As a result, the clinical incidence of HCMV infection in graft recipients, AIDS patients and other immunosuppressed populations varies from 40% to 100% .

After infection, virus spreads to a variety of organs by viraemia which may persist for weeks or months. Neutrophils and mononuclear cells are the apparent main source of HCMV in the blood. Other organs which potentially may be infected include the kidneys (prolonged infection can result in viruria, but generally not renal dysfunction, except in renal transplant patients), liver, lungs (especially in immunocompromised bone marrow transplant recipients), gastrointestinal tissue including oesophagus, small bowel, colon and rectum (usually secondary to HIV infection), myocardium and the CNS (in the newborn and in adults as a complication of AIDS).

Although relatively little work has been done to define the cells which are involved in virus replication *in vivo*, studies of primary cell cultures have shown that different cell types are not equally susceptible to HCMV infection (13,72). HCMV replicates to varying degrees in mesangial cells, glomerular visceral epithelial cells and renal tubular epithelial cells. T lymphocyte populations, stimulated in an allogeneic mixed lymphocyte reaction, also support HCMV replication (73). Human fetal thymic tissue engrafted into SCID-Hu mice will support HCMV replication (108). Epithelial cells in the thymic medulla are the primary host cells. Fibroblasts support viral replication more readily than do epithelial or transformed cells (13), and the ability of HCMV to replicate in peripheral leucocytes is reduced after passage of the virus in fibroblasts in cell culture. Cells non-permissive for HCMV replication exhibit limited viral gene expression and no viral DNA replication, but they may become permissive after exposure to certain inducing agents. For example, restriction of HCMV gene expression in undifferentiated human teratocarcinoma cells is lifted when cells are induced to differentiate by the addition of retinoic acid. This is accompanied by changes in chromatin structure (DNase 1 hypersensitivity) and in the regulatory region, IE1 (74). It has been suggested that activation of nuclear factor NF1/CBP sites may play a role in the switch to productive HCMV replication (13). T lymphocyte subsets $CD4^+$ and $CD8^+$ routinely support the replication of HCMV, following stimulation by cultivation in IL-2 (73), suggesting that T cell permissiveness *in vivo* may be enhanced by T cell activation. Recently Lathey and Spector (75) demonstrated that HCMV replicates poorly in monocytes in the presence of phytohaemagglutinin-P-stimulated T cells, but addition of therapeutic concentrations of hydrocortisone (HC) gave a 10–100-fold stimulation of virus production without cell lysis. HC treatment of macrophage can increase infectious virus production *in vitro* (77). This finding may have implications *in vivo* since HC is used in immunosuppression regimens post transplantation.

These various observations suggest that differential transcriptional activation may explain differences in HCMV permissiveness in various cells. In addition, the observations indicate that a variety of cells, including monocytes, may shed infectious HCMV under physiological conditions and participate in virus dissemination (75). A recent study to localize HCMV precisely in different leucocyte populations obtained from 14 immunocompromised patients found that 45% of polymorphonuclear leucocytes were positive for infectious virus, while only 17% of monocyte/macrophages were positive. Viral DNA was found in T and B cells, but virus could not be isolated, suggesting that these populations may be latent reservoirs for virus (76).

In subclinical infections, humoral and cell-mediated responses are activated and infection is resolved as a result of the specific immune response; cell-mediated immunity (cytotoxic T lymphocytes, CD4 helper/inducer T lymphocytes and NK cells) plays a dominant role in halting the progression to clinical disease (2). However, as described by others (78,79), the details of infection and resolution of that infection are complex. Grundy (79) has observed that 'HCMV has evolved mechanisms to utilize host cell molecules or to alter their expression so as to evade both humoral and cell-mediated immune responses'.

As mentioned previously, HCMV binds to β_2m, which enhances virion infectivity and may allow virus to bind to other cellular receptors (79). The binding of β_2m can impose two additional consequences on infection: protection of the virion from neutralization by antibody in extracellular fluids, and alteration of the transport of class I HLA molecules within the infected cell. β_2m is involved in the transport of class I HLA heavy chains to the cell surface. Sequestration of β_2m in the cytoplasm of HCMV-infected cells may account for the observed progressive decrease of class I HLA on the cell surface, resulting in a decreased presentation of viral antigens to cytotoxic T cells late in infection (79,80,81). In addition, HCMV also induces a protein which binds the Fc portion of immunoglobulins and is found on the surface of infected cells. This provides the potential for non-specific IgG binding to infected cells and further protection from specific immune attack (2).

HCMV can cause immunosuppression (71), with a reduction in helper/suppressor ($CD4^+/CD8^+$) ratio (82). This may be the direct effect of infection of cells of the immune system. Rice *et al.* (83) demonstrated that HCMV sometimes abortively infects human monocytes and lymphocytes.

Kapasi and Rice further demonstrated that HCMV infection suppresses monocyte phagocytic activity (84). Transient neutropenia and thrombocytopenia, which occur during acute infection, may be the result of infection of the haematopoietic cells. Inhibition of the formation of haematopoietic colonies by HCMV infection has been demonstrated *in vitro* (85).

HCMV-induced immunosuppression may also be the indirect result of infection. Monocytes and macrophages produce interleukin 1 (IL-1), which activates T cells. HCMV infection of monocytes appears to nullify IL-1 activity by the release of a protein which inhibits IL-1 activity (86). In addition, the HCMV UL18 gene has apparent homology to the HLA DR, class II transplantation antigen, and it may be that antibodies to HCMV UL18 gene product, cross-reacting with class II HLA, contribute to the increased graft rejection seen in HCMV-infected transplant patients (87).

Thus, when HCMV-induced disease occurs in immunodeficient hosts, HCMV may exacerbate the immunosuppression by directly and indirectly destroying elements of the immune system. From the viewpoint of antiviral therapy, approaches which inhibit viral replication, together with those which alter immune function (enhance or suppress, depending on the situation as described below), may be most appropriate.

It is quite clear that following primary infection of the immunocompetent host HCMV persists in a latent state, with periodic reactivation and virus production. McVoy and Adler (88) surveyed for the presence of IgM to HCMV as a measure of primary immune response in seropositive individuals, and found that the rate of IgM positivity increased with age. This suggested that in immunocompetent individuals HCMV reactivation occurs with a frequency which increases with age. Reactivations and reinfections occur in individuals already displaying IgG antibodies to HCMV, indicating that reactivation or reinfection occurs in the immune host and usually remains a subclinical infection. Unfortunately, we know very little about the nature of latency and the reactivation process for HCMV.

In immunocompetent HCMV-seropositive individuals, expression of immediate–early proteins occurs in cells of the brain, kidney, spleen, lung and liver, without detection of productive infection (89). This observation may indicate that an array of cells in many organs are latently infected, and explain the very high frequency of transmission of HCMV from seropositive organ donors to seronegative recipients (90). However, to date no evidence for integration of the HCMV genome into host cells has been reported (13). As mentioned above, human monocytes support only low-level productive infection, and resting lymphocytes are considered non-permissive, with no HCMV DNA replication occurring in these cells (13,72,91). Thus, under conditions in the normal host, these lymphocytes are likely candidates for latent infection.

In the immunocompromised host, reactivation may be manifest as clinical disease. Some 20% of AIDS patients develop HCMV retinitis; solid organ and bone marrow transplant patients have a high probability of developing serious HCMV disease, generally as a result of reactivation of virus from the donor organ (92–94). Thus, the host immune response appears to be a main factor in controlling both virulence and reactivation from latency. Most AIDS patients have active HCMV infections and may shed multiple strains of virus (94). Since HCMV infection is immunosuppressive, as described above, this may lower the immunocompetence of the host and enhance the spread of HIV. HCMV has been reported to induce class I HLA antigens on certain cells, which may result in enhanced spread of HIV, using HLA antigens as receptors (95). Furthermore, HCMV and HIV can co-infect cells, as shown both in AIDS patients (96,97) and in cell culture (98). In co-infected cells in culture, HCMV and HIV cause reciprocal enhancement of virus replication compared with single virus-infected cells (98). In doubly infected T cells, mitogen stimulation results in enhanced HIV gene expression compared to that observed in cells not infected by HCMV (99). Since HCMV immediate–early proteins are capable of trans-activating HIV transcription, and since T cell activation appears to have a synergistic effect on HIV gene expression in HCMV-infected cells (99), it may be that HCMV plays a direct role in enhancing HIV replication and exacerbating the spread of HIV infection (96,97) and the progression of AIDS.

The presence of HIV may result in enhanced spread of acute HCMV infection as well. Infection of T lymphocytes by HIV removes the block of HCMV replication in these cells, resulting in an expanded susceptible population for productive HCMV infection (100). Recently, Webster (101) observed that in HIV-infected haemophiliacs the risk of developing AIDS was 2.5-fold higher in CMV seropositive patients than in seronegative patients. These observations do not prove a synergistic relationship between HCMV and HIV in the progression of AIDS, but they do emphasize the importance of understanding the role of dual pathogenesis of HCMV and HIV in the immunocompromised host. This understanding is essential in designing optimal antiviral strategies for the AIDS patient.

ANTIVIRAL STRATEGIES

The development of antiviral agents has been an evolving process. In general, when little is known about the details of virus replication and antiviral targets, the identified antiviral agents can be poorly selective and quite cytotoxic. As details of the proteins of virion structure and replication become available, the ability to identify antivirals which are more precisely targeted and potentially less cytotoxic is improved. We are now entering an era in which the architecture of protein active sites and drug/target interaction is being defined at the molecular level through the analysis of X-ray crystal structures. We should expect this work to result in a more rational design of antiviral drugs. This is the case for design of HIV proteinase inhibitors where the tertiary structure of the active site of the proteinase dimer is well defined and the cleavage sites of the natural substrates are known. This knowledge has led to the synthesis of potent and selective HIV proteinase inhibitors which are presently in development (102,103). X-ray crystal structures have also been of value for developing agents directed towards the picornaviruses (104) and the influenza viruses. The goal of structurally based, rational drug design appears more distant, but eventually attainable, for the herpesviruses, including HCMV. Nonetheless, current strategies which take advantage of inhibition of key HCMV target proteins or modulate viral immunosuppression have shown promise and, where monotherapy fails, the use of combination therapy is attractive. These strategies and future approaches are outlined below.

The usual progression in the development of an anti-infective agent is to establish the efficacy and therapeutic index of a drug in cell culture; proceed to animal protection studies, pharmacokinetic and toxicity profiles in multiple species; stability studies and formulation for human use, and entry into phase I clinical evaluation. For many viruses, the human pathogen can cause a disease in animals comparable to the human infection. However, HCMV is very host specific and does not generally infect other animal species (105). Recently, an HCMV model of induced retinitis has been described for the rabbit eye (106) and a novel method for evaluation of antiviral drugs against HCMV-infected cells entrapped in agarose plugs implanted in mice has been described (107). Neither of these models is sufficiently validated to be a predictive model for anti-HCMV drug efficacy in humans at this time. Two models which employ engraftment of human tissue into immunodeficient (SCID) mice may prove useful. Del Cerra has described HCMV infection of human retinal tissue implanted into the anterior eye chambers of SCID mice (108). A SCID-hu mouse/HCMV infection model has also been characterized and may eventually be very useful for evaluation of new HCMV drugs (109). Until such HCMV animal infection models are validated further, surrogate models using mice, guinea-pigs and rats infected with the respective endogenous CMV have been employed to evaluate antiviral drugs (110,111) and study the pathogenesis of CMV infections. The murine CMV (MCMV) model has been particularly useful in this regard (111,112). As in the human infection, latent MCMV can be transferred by organ transplantation. Latently infected mice can be immunosuppressed, resulting in MCMV reactivation, severe disease in a variety of organs, and failure of haematopoiesis. Latent virus can be recovered from the spleen, kidney, heart and peripheral blood cells in the infected mice and appears to be associated with stromal cells (112). Unfortunately, the precise identity of the cell type(s) which harbour latent virus and the status of the viral genome during the latent phase remain unclear. The recently described murine acquired immunodeficiency syndrome (MAIDS) model susceptible to MCMV as an opportunistic infection is a useful surrogate for HCMV infections of immunocompromised patients (113). Evaluation of

GCV in the murine models correctly predicted the potential for clinical utility (111,114) of this drug and supports the value of these models in identifying drugs for future clinical development.

In general, the strategy which has dominated the quest for inhibitors of herpesvirus replication has focused on defining agents which are DNA polymerase substrate analogues and interfere with DNA synthesis. These are most notably represented by acyclovir (ACV) (Zovirax), the triphosphate of which is an analogue of dGTP (115), and foscarnet (PFA) (Foscavir), a pyrophosphate analogue (116). The early work on substrate analogues was often targeted towards cancer chemotherapy (117), and resulted in a variety of nucleoside analogues that presented a narrow therapeutic index. These drugs were either unacceptable for controlled antiviral investigations (ara-C), or could only be used in a limited antiviral setting (IUdR for HSV keratitis). Adenine arabinoside (ara-A, vidarabine, Vira A) has an acceptable therapeutic index against HSV in cell culture, and was the first antiviral drug approved for parenteral administration. Vira A has been a useful drug in the treatment of HSV encephalitis, neonatal HSV infections and varicella zoster infection in immunocompromised patients (118,119), but the potency against HCMV is insufficient to result in an effective anti-HCMV drug.

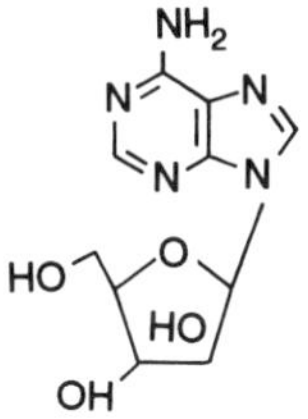

Ara A

The discovery of ACV as an orally active, potent and selective inhibitor of HSV replication demonstrated that an antiviral agent can be presented to the host as a prodrug and specifically activated in virus-infected cells to become a selective inhibitor of viral DNA polymerase (ACV triphosphate) (120). ACV triphosphate is an analogue of dGTP and inhibits viral DNA replication by incorporation into HSV DNA as a chain terminator (120,121). ACV inhibits HCMV replication only at high concentrations ($ED_{50} = 20$–$40\ \mu M$), a reflection of the fact that HCMV does not encode a kinase capable of efficiently phosphorylating ACV (122). However, the success with ACV stimulated efforts to discover new nucleoside and nucleotide analogues which are also potent inhibitors of HCMV (see summary in Table 4.2). ACV has been approved for a wide variety of HSV and VZV infections and an ACV prodrug (BW 256U87, valaciclovir) has recently been reported to be

Table 4.2. Summary of HCMV antiviral drugs

Drug	Chemical class	HCMV ED_{50} (μM)	Proposed antiviral mechanism	Potential advantages	Potential disadvantages	Development status	Reference
Ganciclovir (GCV)	Acyclic nucleoside analogue (NA)	1–10	Phosphorylation-dependent DNA polymerase inhibitor	Efficacy against HCMV retinitis	Poor oral bioavailability Haematotoxicity	Approved (i.v.) for retinitis in AIDS patients	111, 124, 134
Foscarnet (PFA)	Pyrophosphate analogue	20–40	DNA polymerase inhibitor; blocks pyrophosphate binding site	Efficacy against HCMV retinitis Active against GCV-resistant HCMV and HIV	Renal toxicity Seizures	Approved (i.v.) for retinitis in AIDS patients	168
Acyclovir	Acyclic NA	20–40	Phosphorylation-dependent DNA polymerase inhibitor	Proven safety	Poor efficacy	Approved for HSV, not HCMV	120, 121
DHPC (BW 1117U81)	Acyclic NA	1–14	Probable phosphorylation-dependent DNA polymerase inhibitor	Favourable therapeutic index in cell culture	Toxicities and bioavailability unknown	Pre-clinical	136, 137
Pyrrolo-(2,3-*d*)-pyrimidine	Acyclic NA	1–10	Uncertain	Antiviral potency in cell culture	Toxicities and bioavailability unknown	Pre-clinical	138, 140, 141

2′-nor-cGMP	NA cyclophosphate	1–2	Probable DNA polymerase inhibitor	Possible activity Active against GCV-resistant HCMV	Toxicities and bioavailability unknown	Pre-clinical	142–144
HPMPC (GS 504)	NA phosphonate	0.1	DNA polymerase inhibitor	Infrequent dosing Active against GCV-resistant HCMV	Low oral bioavailability Nephrotoxicity	Phase II/III Clinical	113, 132, 149, 150, 152
FIAC/FIAU	Halogenated NA	1–10	Probable DNA polymerase inhibitor	Oral bioavailability Active against GCV-resistant HCMV	Gastrointestinal, bone, marrow and liver toxicities	Discontinued	132, 162, 163
BHCG (lobucavir)	Cyclobutyl NA	1–10	Phosphorylation-dependent DNA polymerase inhibitor	Possible oral bioavailability Active against GCV-resistant HCMV	Toxicities and bioavailability unknown	Phase I Clinical	157, 159–161, 163
Immune modulators (interferons, growth-stimulating factors)	Proteins Peptides	–	Inhibit virus replication; alter immune response	Immune stimulation Potential for combination therapy	Wide array of side-effects	Experimental and clinical, CMV-Ig approved for prophylaxis in kidney Tx	176–180

in clinical development for a variety of herpesvirus infections, including HCMV (123).

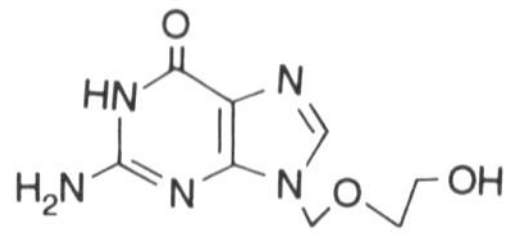

ACV

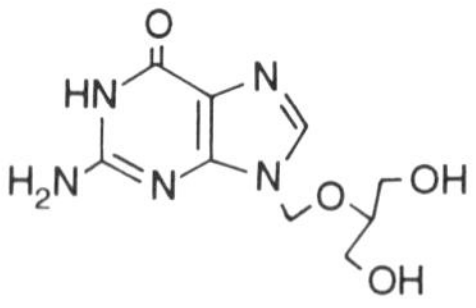

GCV

GANCICLOVIR

Ganciclovir (GCV, DHPG, 2′NDG, Cytovene) has an acyclic structure similar to that of ACV. Like ACV, it is an excellent substrate for HSV thymidine kinase (TK) and is converted to the triphosphate, which inhibits viral DNA synthesis. However, unlike ACV, GCV is an inhibitor of HCMV at 1–10 μM. The antiviral activities, mechanism of action and pharmacokinetic properties of GCV have been reviewed in more detail by Matthews and Boehme (124) and Fauld and Hee (128). Briefly, GCV is phosphorylated in HCMV-infected cells, and GCV triphosphate selectively inhibits the viral DNA polymerase (124,129,130). These observations imply that GCV inhibits HCMV replication in a manner similar to the ACV inhibition of HSV replication.

Since HCMV does not encode a TK equivalent to that of HSV, but does stimulate cellular kinases (122,131), it was originally proposed that phosphorylation of GCV may be the indirect effect of HCMV infection. This mechanism of action was supported by the isolation of GCV-resistant HCMV mutants which neither stimulate the phosphorylation of GCV nor have altered DNA polymerases (132,133). Recently, however, the HCMV gene responsible for GCV phosphorylation has been reported (34,35). As described earlier, this gene is encoded by the UL97 reading frame and is believed to be a protein kinase which has homologues in other herpesviruses.

As mentioned above, the efficacy of GCV was also confirmed in animal protection studies (111,124); however, two deficiencies were suggested from the results. The oral bioavailability of GCV was poor in some species. In the treatment of MCMV interstitial pneumonia in mice, GCV reduced virus replication in the lungs, but did not block the development of pneumonia (124).

In man, GCV has only marginal oral bioavailability, but is approved for i.v. administration and is currently being studied at high oral doses as well. The clinical efficacy, pharmacology and toxicity of GCV have been reviewed (125–7,134). Since neutropenia has been a major complication associated with GCV therapy, GCV has also been administered experimentally by intravitreal injection for treatment of HCMV retinitis in patients with significant pre-existing bone marrow suppression. GCV has been poorly effective against HCMV pneumonitis in humans, except when used in combination with immunotherapy (see discussion below). Thus, the animal studies have been reasonably predictive of the eventual clinical experiences with GCV.

OTHER ACYCLIC NUCLEOSIDES

The carba analogues of GCV and ACV (DHBG and HBG) were described by Wahren *et al.* (135). Both compounds are only poorly active against HCMV, with ED_{50} values comparable to those of ACV.

The K_i values for inhibition of HCMV DNA polymerase by the respective triphosphates are at least 100-fold lower than that for ACV triphosphate, suggesting that the poor ED_{50} values may have resulted from inefficient cellular pharmacokinetics or anabolism.

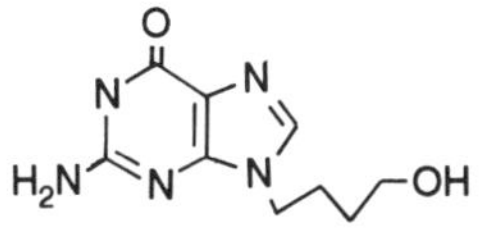

HBG

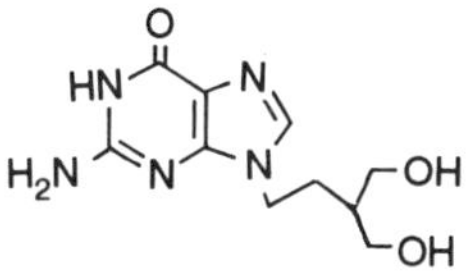

DHBG

The cytosine analogue of GCV, 1-[2-hydroxy-1-(hydroxy-methyl)ethoxymethyl]cytosine (DHPC or BW 1117U81), has anti-HCMV activity in human fibroblast cell cultures, with an ED_{50} value of 1.9–14 μM depending on the cells used (136). The IC_{50} for cell growth inhibition is greater than 1 mM, resulting in a favourable therapeutic index. DHPC is phosphorylated by deoxycytidine kinase, but is only poorly anabolized in either HCMV-infected or uninfected cells. HCMV mutants selected for resistance to DHPC are also resistant to HPMPC and foscarnet, suggesting that HCMV DNA polymerase is the antiviral target (137).

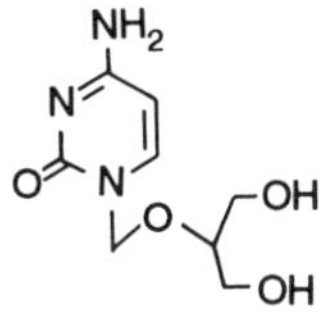

DHPC

Pyrrolo[2,3-*d*]pyrimidine nucleosides have been investigated for antitumour and antiviral activities for some years (recently reviewed by Townsend *et al.* in reference 138). As a result of these investigations, halogenated tubercidin nucleoside analogues, in which the sugar moiety is replaced with either 7-hydroxyethoxymethyl (HEM) or 7-dihydroxypropoxymethyl (DHPM), were prepared.

Two compounds have been identified which inhibit HCMV in cell culture at less than 10 μM. These are HEM bromo-tubercidin and DHPM bromo-tubercidin (139,140).

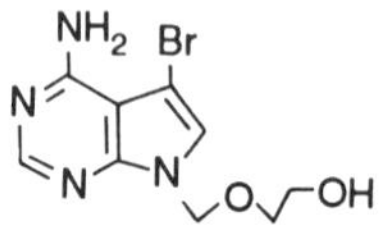

HEM Br-TUBERCIDIN

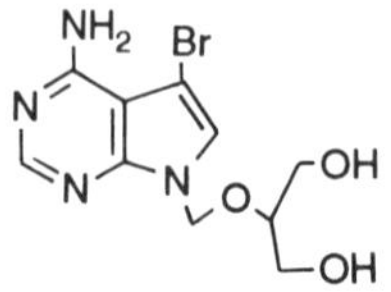

DHPM Br-TUBERCIDIN

Both compounds cause no changes in cell morphology, but do cause cell growth inhibition near the antiviral concentrations (141). Although HEM bromo-tubercidin did not protect mice against fatal MCMV infection, DHPM bromo-tubercidin administered at 5.6 mg/kg per day i.p. for five days resulted in a significant increase in murine survival with minimal toxicity (140). Details of the mechanism of action, pharmacokinetics and toxicity profile for DHPM bromo-tubercidin are not yet available.

NUCLEOSIDE PHOSPHATES AND PHOSPHONATES

In attempts to derive nucleosides with a broader spectrum of antiviral activities, several laboratories have synthesized stable phosphate or phosphonate derivatives. These derivatives would be expected to have activity against TK^- viruses such as HCMV, and ACV or GCV mutants of HSV which are drug resistant due to TK deficiency. Since these compounds circumvent viral-induced phosphorylation, one of the selective steps which occurs only in infected cells—the potential for greater toxicity—is also increased.

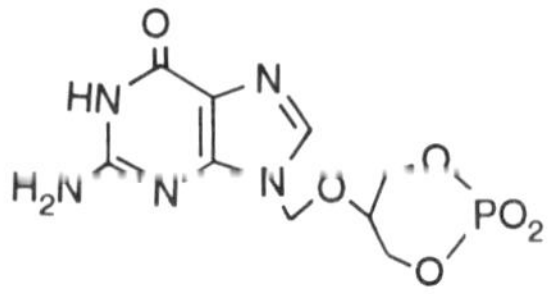

2'-nor-cGMP

The cyclic phosphate derivative of GCV, 2′-nor-cGMP, has broad-spectrum activity against DNA viruses, including HCMV (142). The antiviral activity against HSV in cell culture or in animal protection studies is equivalent for TK^+ and TK^- strains (143,144), suggesting that the anti-HCMV activity is independent of virus-induced phosphorylation, and that 2′-nor-dGMP is not dephosphorylated to yield GCV. 2′-nor-dGMP is also more toxic than GCV to uninfected cells (144). 2′-nor-dGMP is 15–20-fold more potent than GCV against guinea-pig CMV (GPCMV) in cell culture, and effective in clearing infection in infected guinea-pigs (145). At the effective doses administered subcutaneously, the drug was well tolerated in animals. At higher doses the drug was toxic to the kidney and bone marrow in animals.

A number of nucleoside phosphonates have been synthesized and evaluated for anti-HCMV efficacy. Phosphonates could provide an added advantage over phosphates by eliminating the labile P—O bond and replacing it with the P—C bond, which is more resistant to enzymatic hydrolysis. Prisbe *et al.* (144) synthesized a phosphonate derivative of GCV which has reduced antiviral activity against HSV types 1 and 2, reduced toxicity in Vero cells, but retains anti-HCMV activity (ED_{50} = 10 μM). Similarly, Sidwell *et al.* (146) have reported that the phosphonate monoethyl ester of GCV (SR 3727) is active against HCMV (ED_{50} = 2.5–5.4 μg/ml) in cell culture and protects mice against MCMV at 125 mg/kg per day (i.p.).

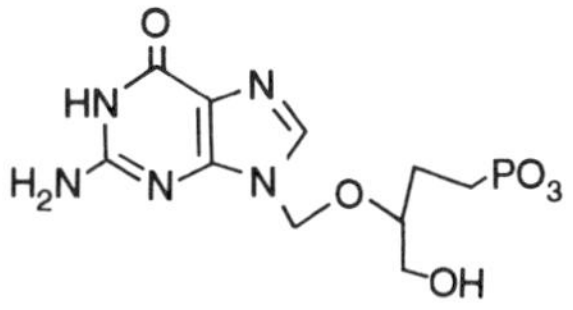

GCV PHOSPHONATE

A novel series of phosphonylmethoxyalkyl derivatives of purines and pyrimidines was first disclosed in 1986 with the description of (*S*)-HPMPA (147). As expected, (*S*)-HPMPA and other base analogues (e.g. (*S*)-HPMPG, (*S*)-HPMPC) have activity against a broad spectrum of DNA viruses, and are not viral TK dependent (147–149).

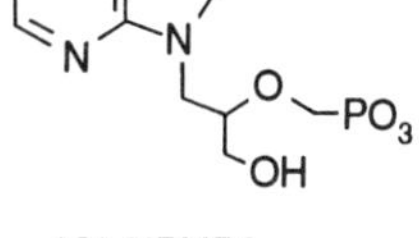

(*S*)-HPMPA

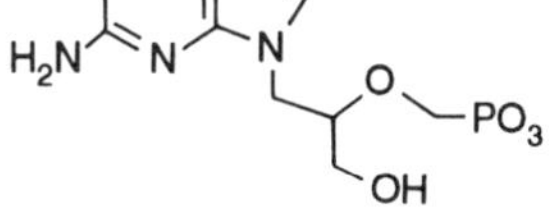

(*S*)-HPMPG

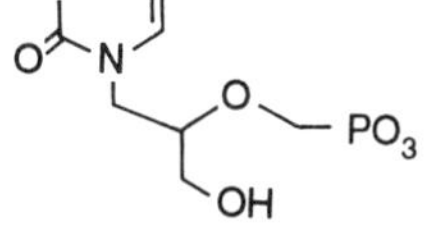

(*S*)-HPMPC

Among these, (*S*)-HPMPC (GS 504) has the most attractive antiviral activity profile in cell culture, with an ED_{50} of about 0.1 μg/ml for HCMV, more potent than GCV, and with a therapeutic index of 1500 (149). Unlike GCV, (*S*)-HPMPC is metabolized to the mono- and diphosphate (the triphosphate equivalent) in both virus-infected and uninfected cells. The diphosphate is a competitive inhibitor (*vis-à-vis* dCTP) of viral DNA polymerase, with a 25–50-fold selectivity relative to cellular DNA polymerase α (150). One proposed consequence of metabolism in uninfected cells is that exposure of cells to HPMPC prior to infection may block subsequent HCMV infection more effectively (151). GCV-resistant HCMV clinical isolates which are incapable of inducing phosphorylation of GCV in infected cells may retain susceptibility to (*S*)-HPMPC (132).

Importantly, (*S*)-HPMPC diphosphate has an extended half-life of 17 h in human cells (150). The long intracellular half-life suggests that infrequent dosing with (*S*)-HPMPC *in vivo* may be possible. Stals *et al.* (152) recently demonstrated that (*S*)-HPMPC is effective in preventing rat CMV replication when added four days prior to cell culture infection, or seven days prior to rat infection. GCV was ineffective in the same experimental regimen. In addition, HPMPC was highly efficacious in the MAIDS mouse infected with MCMV, a disease syndrome similar to that of HCMV infection of AIDS patients (113). Thus, (*S*)-HPMPC is a highly potent inhibitor of CMV. Its metabolism in uninfected cells and extended half-life for the diphosphate may provide the opportunity for infrequent dosing in the treatment of HCMV disease. However, (*S*)-HPMPC also causes nephrotoxicity, which varies in severity from species to species, being most pronounced in the guinea-pig (153). The key to the success of (*S*)-HPMPC for the treatment of HCMV disease will be the attraction of an infrequent treatment regimen which maintains efficacy and minimizes potential toxicities. HPMPC has recently entered into phase I clinical trials.

HALOGENATED PYRIMIDINES

Colacino and Lopez (154) demonstrated that FIAC (2′-deoxy-2′-fluoro-β-D-arabinofuranosyl-5-iodocytosine) is a potent anti-HCMV compound ($ED_{50} = 0.6\ \mu M$), with a selectivity index of 13. The closely related fluoriodoarabinouracil analogue (FIAU) has similar anti-HCMV activity, and FIAC is a prodrug for FIAU following deamination.

Although the antiviral activity and selectivity indices are not outstanding,

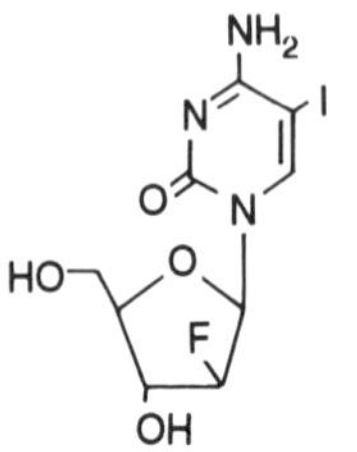

FIAC

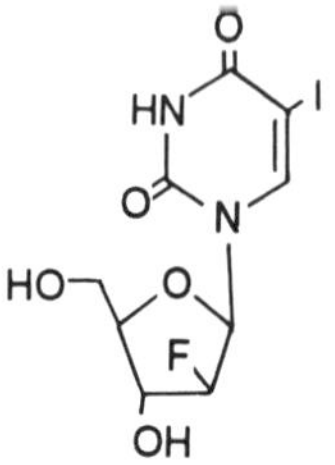

FIAU

there had been renewed interest in the development of these nucleoside analogues. They have excellent oral bioavailability (155), are more active than GCV in cell culture, and show antiviral activity against GCV-resistant isolates of HCMV (132,155). However, FIAC is incorporated into DNA of both infected and uninfected cells (154), and in clinical studies oral or i.v. administration of FIAC results in gastrointestinal and haematological toxicity (155). The clinical development of FIAU was recently discontinued due to severe delayed liver toxicity in a hepatitis B virus treatment study.

CYCLOBUTYL NUCLEOSIDE ANALOGUES

Within the past few years several laboratories have focused attention on a series of nucleoside analogues in which the sugar moiety is replaced by a cyclobutyl ring. Particular interest was first focused on the racemic guanosine analogues ((±)-BHCG (also referred to as SQ 33,054, cyclobut-G (CBG)), and (±)-HHCG), and the adenine analogue ((±)-BHCA, also referred to as cyclobut-A (CBA)) (156–160).

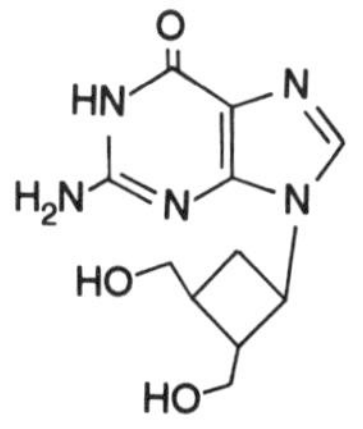

BHCG

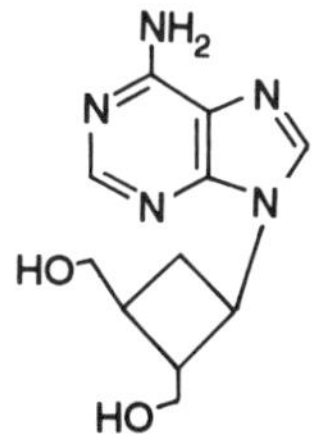

BHCA

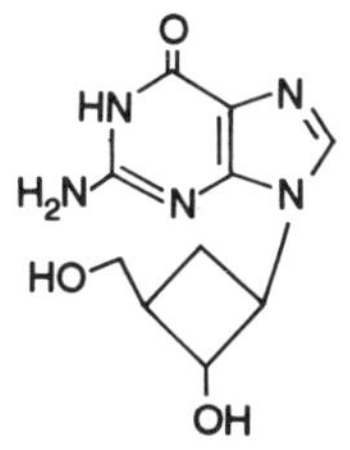

HHCG

BHCG is potently active against HSV (types 1 and 2), and shows a 25–50-fold decrease in antiviral activity against TK^- strains. By contrast, BHCA has similar broad anti-herpesvirus activities, but no dependence on virus-induced TK. Both BHCG and BHCA have anti-HIV activity. Although the anti-HIV activity in T cell cultures is at concentrations approaching cytotoxic levels, in monocyte/macrophage cultures both compounds inhibit HIV replication at nanomolar concentrations, well below the cytotoxic levels. In addition, BHCG, BHCA and HHCG each have ED_{50} values of 1–4 μM against HCMV.

The activities of racemic BHCG and BHCA have prompted further characterization of the active enantiomers (161–163). The antiviral activities are associated with the (*R*)-enantiomer. *R*-BHCG (lobucavir) has oral efficacy comparable to that of GCV in mice infected with MCMV. Detailed pharmacokinetic profiles in mice and rats indicate that *R*-BHCG is excreted mainly in the urine, with a calculated bioavailability in excess of 50%.

The mechanism of antiviral action of *R*-BHCG has been elucidated primarily for HSV. Although *R*-BHCG is a relatively poor substrate for HSV-1 TK compared to the (*S*)-isomer (164,165), in HSV-1-infected cells *R*-BHCG rapidly accumulates as the triphosphate (TP), which has a half-life of about 10 h (165). *R*-BHCG-TP competitively inhibits HSV-1 DNA polymerase with respect to dGTP (166). The inhibition constant for HSV-1 DNA polymerase (K_i = 17 nM) is about 30-fold lower than for HeLa DNA polymerase α (166). In HCMV-infected cells, *R*-BHCG is phosphorylated only to a small degree (less than 0.5 pmol/10^6 cells compared to greater than 50 pmol/10^6 cells for GCV using 25 μM ^{3}H-labelled nucleoside analogue) (167). Thus, it appears that although the anti-HCMV activities are similar for *R*-BHCG and GCV, *R*-BHCG is a poorer substrate for the HCMV-induced kinase. *R*-BHCG also retains its antiviral activity against GCV-resistant HCMV, which is incapable of phosphorylating GCV (discussed below). Taken together, these observations suggest that the mechanism of action of *R*-BHCG against HCMV may be somewhat different from its mechanism of action against HSV, and that additional effort to clarify that mechanism is needed. *R*-BHCG has recently entered phase I clinical trials.

R-BHCA is the antiviral enantiomer of racemic BHCA. Unlike *R*-BHCG, *R*-BHCA is neither a substrate for HSV-1 TK, nor is its phosphorylation enhanced in HSV-1-infected cells. However, in HCMV-infected cells *R*-BHCA is phosphorylated as efficiently as is GCV. Furthermore, *R*-BCHA retains antiviral activity, and is phosphorylated in cells infected with a GCV-resistant HCM unable to phosphorylate GCV (167).

FOSCARNET

Foscarnet (Foscavir, the trisodium salt of phosphonoformic acid, PFA) is a pyrophosphate analogue which selectively inhibits herpesvirus DNA polymerases and the reverse transcriptase of HIV.

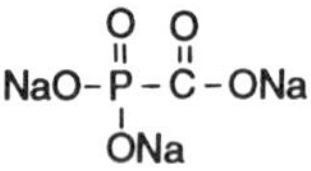

PFA (FOSCARNET)

A recent detailed review of the biology, biochemistry and clinical use in patients with HCMV retinitis has been prepared by Chrisp and Clissold (168). Thus, we will only briefly summarize a few important features of foscarnet. Unlike the aforementioned drugs which are prodrugs until phosphorylated to the respective triphosphates, foscarnet is a direct DNA polymerase inhibitor by competitive blockade of the pyrophosphate binding site. As suggested by this difference in mechanism of action, virus mutants resistant to GCV may remain sensitive to foscarnet (132). However, recently

Sullivan and Coen isolated foscarnet-resistant HCMV mutants by serial passage at progressively higher drug concentrations in cell culture (169). Two independent mutants were cross-resistant to phosphonoacetic acid (PAA, a related pyrophosphate analogue) and ACV. They remained sensitive to GCV, ara-A, FIAC and HPMPC, and were hypersensitive to aphidicolin and HPMPA. Since PAA resistance for HCMV is due to mutation in the DNA polymerase (170), these foscarnet-resistant mutants may also contain polymerase mutations. These observations also suggest that foscarnet-resistant HCMV mutants might arise in the clinic.

Foscarnet (i.v.) has been approved for treatment of HCMV retinitis in AIDS patients. Its potential for inhibition of HCMV, GCV-resistant HCMV and HIV may make it an attractive alternative therapy to GCV. Foscarnet has the potential to cause acute renal failure and seizures—a substantial disadvantage; however, it does not contribute to bone marrow suppression.

COMBINATION THERAPY

It is apparent that although new therapeutic agents with improved efficacy are being described, many may be burdened with toxicity and/or bioavailability profiles which may limit their clinical use. In addition, since the first observation of clinical resistance of HCMV to antiviral treatment (171), several reports of resistance to ganciclovir (UL 97 kinase mutation) and foscarnet (UL 54 DNA polymerase) have emerged. Resistance development for HCMV was recently reviewed by Field and Biron (172). Another approach which is increasing in favour is combination therapy, which offers potential significant improvements over monotherapies. Schinazi recently reviewed this approach (173). Among his rationale for combination drug therapy are: (i) the possible reduction of toxicity while maintaining high efficacy by using reduced doses of each of two antiviral drugs having different toxicity profiles and additive or synergistic antiviral effects; (ii) the reduction in the emergence of resistant virus mutants by using two drugs with different mechanisms of action (a proposal which is yet to be proven); and (iii) a possible decrease in the incidence of non-responsiveness by combining antiviral drug therapy with immunotherapy.

For HCMV infections, the strategies attempted to date include combining antiviral compounds which have different mechanisms of action, in the hope of achieving synergistic efficacy; combining an antiviral compound with an immune modulator either to achieve antiviral synergy or to reverse immunosuppression; or combining an antiviral compound with immunoglobulin to achieve antiviral synergy and perhaps modulation of pathological immune responses to HCMV infection.

GCV and foscarnet

Although the antiviral target of both GCV and foscarnet is the viral DNA polymerase, GCV-resistant HCMV do not necessarily show cross-resistance to foscarnet (132,174), and in cell culture protection studies GCV and foscarnet have synergistic anti-HCMV effects (175). If the synergistic effect is achievable in the clinic, then efficacy at drug combinations well below toxic thresholds may also be achievable.

GCV and immune modulators

The use of human leucocyte interferon (IFN-α) alone for the treatment of HCMV in organ transplant recipients has had mixed results. Hirsch *et al.* found that prophylaxis in renal transplant recipients protected against serious infections (176), whereas Meyers *et al.* (177) found no effect of similar doses in allogeneic bone marrow recipients. Since interferons and GCV have different mechanisms of action, a synergistic antiviral effect might be expected. Rasmussen *et al.* evaluated combinations of GCV and recombinant interferons in cell culture studies and observed that whereas with IFN-α only additive effects were observed, with IFN-β there was synergy with GCV over a narrow range of dose combinations (178).

The major toxicity associated with GCV therapy is dose-related neutropenia; this in a patient population which may be experiencing neutropenia as a result of HCMV infection (179). Granulocyte–macrophage colony-stimulating factor (GM-CSF) regulates the proliferation and maturation of haematopoietic stem cells, and in AIDS patients has been used to increase the number of circulating leucocytes (179). GM-CSF has been administered during GCV therapy in the hope of reducing the GCV-associated bone marrow suppression while preventing the progression of HCMV retinitis in AIDS patients. Preliminary results have indicated that the therapeutic efficacy of GCV can be maintained with a reduction in the episodes of neutropenia (179,180). This approach to dual therapy may be promising for allowing increased dosing and length of GCV treatment.

GCV and immunoglobulin

As briefly discussed previously, GCV therapy of HCMV pneumonitis in bone marrow transplant patients can successfully reduce virus titres in the lungs, but fails to alter disease significantly. In addition, hyperimmune globulin can effectively treat HCMV pneumonitis, but not neutralize virus. Thus, the effectiveness of antisera appears to be through a mechanism other than by neutralization (181). Grundy *et al.* have proposed that HCMV pneumonitis in transplant recipients is an immunopathological T cell response to viral antigens on cells of the lung (181). An explanation for the protective role of immunoglobulin could be its combination with and masking of viral antigens on infected cells, minimizing the T cell response. Their hypothesis is further supported by observations that the induction of pneumonitis by MCMV involves a T cell response and not virus replication alone (182). Recently Rubin *et al.* demonstrated that in the MCMV infection model GCV in combination with hyperimmune antibody was more effective than either therapy alone (183), consistent with the clinical observations (184). HCMV immune globulin (CMV-Ig (MedImmune)) has also been successfully used and has been approved for prevention of CMV disease in kidney transplant patients.

Antisense oligonucleotides

As indicated earlier, most of the antiviral drugs in clinical use or under development are inhibitors of HCMV DNA polymerase; with the anticipation that a new class of HCMV proteinase inhibitors will also soon emerge. Yet HCMV encodes for more than 200 open reading frames, all of which are potential targets for antiviral intervention. The problem has traditionally been one of not having a clear research path to identify inhibitors of these potential targets. That limitation may be circumvented by a new approach; the design of antisense oligonucleotide inhibitors. Since the HCMV genome has been sequenced, the theoretical opportunity exists to synthesize antisense oligonucleotide inhibitors targeted to any of the open reading frames or their predicted mRNA sequence and function configurations such as splice sites or translation start sites. With alterations in the phosphate backbone chemistry of the antisense oligonucleotides, stable compounds with potent antiviral activities can be synthesized.

This opportunity was seized by Azad *et al.* (26) in the design and characterization of ISIS 2922, a 21-mer phosphorothioate oligonucleotide which is antisense to a sequence in the coding region of IE2. ISIS 2922 shows sequence specificity and an ED_{50} value of about 0.3 μM. This compound has now entered clinical trial for intravitreal delivery in the treatment of HCMV retinitis in AIDS patients.

A second and more potent inhibitor has been by Pari *et al.* (personal communication). This antisense oligonucleotide is complementary to a UL 36 sequence, shows excellent target specificity, selectivity index, an ED_{50} value of about 0.06μM, and activity against ganciclovir-resistant, HPMPC-resistant and foscarnet-resistant HCMV strains. Preclinical studies are currently in progress.

CHALLENGES FOR THE FUTURE

It should be apparent from the foregoing discussion that while HCMV-associated disease is fast becoming a major health problem due to increased numbers of immunocompromised hosts, development of effective therapies has not kept pace. The current armamentarium of anti-HCMV therapeutics has, by and large, emerged as a secondary interest to identifying antiviral agents against other herpesviruses. The need for a safe, orally active, selective HCMV inhibitor is evident. The ideal agent would irreversibly block HCMV infection without interfering with the ability of the immune system to resist overt infection.

Our hope for future effective and substantially less toxic therapy can come from a much more in-depth understanding of HCMV at the molecular level, enabling the identification of unique features of viral proteins as targets for selective antiviral intervention. The HCMV genome encodes for some 200 proteins and probably includes enzyme targets yet to be identified. Elucidation of the virion and cellular receptors, the IE gene products and the HCMV proteinase could all lead to novel antiviral strategies. These and other antiviral approaches should emerge as an indirect product of the more detailed understanding of HCMV structure and replication.

REFERENCES

1. Gonczol, E. and Plotkin, S. (1990). Progress in vaccine development for prevention of human CMV infection. In *Current Topics in Microbiology and Immunology*, J. K. McDougall (ed.), Springer-Verlag, Berlin, pp. 255–274.
2. Alford, C. A. and Britt, W. J. (1990). Cytomegalovirus. In *Virology*, B. N. Fields and D. M. Knipe (eds), Raven Press, New York, pp. 1981–2010.
3. Jesionek, A. and Kiolemenoglou, B. (1904). Ueber einen befund von protozoenartigen gebilden in den organen eines heriditar-leutischen Fotus. *Munch. Med. Wochenschr.*, **15**, 1905–1907.
4. Ribbert, D. (1904). Über protozoenartige zellen in der niere eines syphilitischen neugoborenen und in der parotis von kindern. *Centralbl. Allg. Pathol. Anat.*, **15**, 945–948.
5. Lipschutz, B. (1921). Untersuchengen über die ätiologie der krankheiten der herpesgruppe (herpes zoster, herpes genitalis, herpes febrilis). *Arch. Derm. Syph. (Berl.)*, **136**, 428–482.
6. Cole, R. and Kuttner, A. G. (1926). A filterable virus present in the submaxillary glands of guinea pigs. *J. Exp. Med.*, **44**, 855–873.
7. Rowe, W. P., Hartley, J. W., Waterman, S. *et al.* (1956). Cytopathogenic agents resembling human salivary gland virus recovered from tissue of human adenoids. *Proc. Soc. Exp. Biol.*, **92**, 118 424.
8. Smith, M. G. (1956). Propagation in tissue cultures of a cytopathogenic virus from human salivary gland disease. *Proc. Soc. Exp. Biol.* , **92**, 424–430.
9. Weller, T. H., Macauley, J. C., Craig, J. M. and Wirth, P. (1956). Isolation of intranuclear inclusion producing agents from infant illnesses resembling cytomegalic inclusion disease. *Proc. Soc. Exp. Biol.*, **94**, 4–12.
10. Farber, S. and Wolbach, S. B. (1932). Intranuclear and cytoplasmic inclusions ('protozoan-like bodies') in the salivary glands and other organs of infants. *Am. J. Pathol.*, **8**, 123–126.
11. Weller, T. H., Hanshaw, J. B. and Scott, D. E. (1960). Serologic differentiation of viruses responsible for cytomegalic inclusion disease. *Virology*, **12**, 130–132.

12. Roizman, B. (1990). Herpesviridae: a brief introduction. In *Virology*, B. N. Fields and D. M. Knipe (eds), Raven Press, New York, pp. 1787–1794.
13. Stinski, M. F. (1990). Cytomegalovirus and its replication. In *Virology*, B. N. Fields and D. M. Knipe (eds), Raven Press, New York, pp. 1959–1980.
14. Emery, V. C. and Griffiths, P. D. (1990). Current status review: molecular biology of cytomegalovirus. *Int. J. Exp. Pathol.*, **71**, 905–918.
15. Landini, M.-P. and Michelson, S. (1988). Human cytomegalovirus proteins. *Prog. Med. Virol.*, **35**, 152–185.
16. Studies of the ocular complications of AIDS in collaboration with the AIDS Clinical Trials Group (1992). Mortality in patients with the acquired immunodeficiency syndrome treated with either foscarnet or ganciclovir for cytomegalovirus retinitis. *N. Engl. J. Med.*, **326**, 213–220.
17. Adler, S. P. (1990). New insights into human cytomegaloviral infections. *Prog. Med. Virol.*, **37**, 136–155.
18. Gibson, W. (1991). Cytomegalovirus protein structure and function. In *Progress in Cytomegalovirus Research*, M. P. Landini (ed.), Elsevier, Amsterdam, pp. 357–370.
19. Lawrence, G. L., Chee, M. S., Craxton, M. A. *et al.* (1990). Human herpesvirus 6 is closely related to human cytomegalovirus. *J. Virol.*, **64**, 287–299.
20. McDougall, J. K. (ed.) (1990). *Current Topics in Microbiology and Immunology*, Springer-Verlag, Berlin, preface.
21. Chee, M. S., Bankier, A. T., Beck, S. *et al.* (1990). Analysis of the protein-coding content of the sequence of human cytomegalovirus strain AD 169. In *Current Topics in Microbiology and Immunology*, J. K. McDougall (ed.), Springer-Verlag, Berlin, pp. 125–170.
22. Chee, M. S. (1991). The HCMV genome project: what has been learned and what can be expected in the future. *Transplant Proc.*, **23**, 174–180.
23. Pari, G. S. and Anders, D. G. (1993). Eleven loci encoding trans-acting factors are required for transient complementation of human cytomegalovirus 0riLyt-dependent DNA replication. *J. Virol.*, **67**, 6979–6988.
24. Tenney, D. J. and Colberg-Poley, A. M. (1991). Expression of the human cytomegalovirus UL 36–38 immediate early region during permissive infection. *Virol.*, **182**, 199–210.
25. Azad, R. F., Driver, V. B., Tanaka, K. *et al.* (1993). Antiviral activity of a phosphorothioate oligonucleotide complementary to RNA of the human cytomegalovirus major immediate-early region. *Antimicrob. Agents Chemother.*, **37**, 1945–1954.
26. Ertl, P. F. and Powell, K. L. (1992). Physical and functional interaction of human cytomegalovirus DNA polymerase and its accessory protein (ICP36) expressed in insect cells. *J. Virol.*, **66**, 4126–4133.
27. Mocarski, E. S., Jr (1991). Initial events involved in cytomegalovirus–cell interactions. *Transplant. Proc.*, **23**, 43–47.
28. Mocarski, E. S., Jr, Abenes, G. B., Manning, W. C. *et al.* (1990). Molecular genetic analysis of cytomegalovirus and gene regulation in growth, persistence and latency. In *Current Topics in Microbiology and Immunology*, J. K. McDougall (ed.), Springer-Verlag, Berlin, pp. 47–74.
29. Welch, A. R., Woods, A. S., McNally, L. M. *et al.* (1991). A herpesvirus maturational proteinase, assemblin: identification of its gene, putative active site domain, and cleavage site. *Proc. Natl Acad. Sci. USA*, **88**, 10792–10796.
30. Liu, F. and Roizman, B. (1991). The herpes simplex virus 1 gene encoding a protease also contains within its coding domain the gene encoding the more abundant substrate. *J. Virol.*, **65**, 5149–5156.

31. Baum, E. Z., Bebernitz, G. Z., Hulmes, J. D. *et al.* (1993). Expression and analysis of the human cytomegalovirus UL80-encoded protease: Identification of autoproteolytic sites. *J. Virol.* **67**: 497–506.
32. Jones, T. R., Sun, L., Bebernitz, G. A. *et al.* (1994). Proteolytic activity of human cytomegalovirus UL80 protease cleavage site mutants. *J. Virol.*, **68**, 3742–3752.
33. Jones, T. R., Muzithras, V. P., Sun, L. *et al.* (1993). Expression and localization of the HCMV UL80-encoded protease in mammalian cells. (Michelson and Plotkin, ed.) *Fourth Internat. Cytomegalovirus Workshop*, Excerpta Medica. Amsterdam.
34. Sullivan, V., Talarico, C. L., Stanat, S. C. *et al.* (1992). A protein kinase homologue controls phosphorylation of ganciclovir in human cytomegalovirus-infected cells. *Nature*, **358**, 162–164.
35. Littler, E., Stuart, A. D. and Chee, M. S. (1992). Human cytomegalovirus UL97 open reading frame encodes a protein that phosphorylates the antiviral nucleoside analog ganciclovir. *Nature (London)*, **358**. 160–162.
36. Beck, S. and Barrell, G. B. (1988). Human cytomegalovirus encodes a glycoprotein homologous to MHC class 1 antigens. *Nature*, **331**, 269–272.
37. Albrecht, T., Fons, M. P., Boldogh, I. *et al.* (1991). Metabolic and cellular effects of human cytomegalovirus infection. *Transplant. Proc.*, **23**, 48–55.
38. Shaw, S. B., Rasmussen, R. D., McDonough, S. H. *et al.* (1985). Cell-related sequences in the DNA genome of human cytomegalovirus strain AD169. *J. Virol.*, **55**, 843–848.
39. Mach, M., Stamminger, T. and Jahn, G. (1989). Review article. Human cytomegalovirus: recent aspects from molecular biology. *J. Gen. Virol.*, **70**, 3117–3146.
40. Buchman, T. G., Roizman, B., Adams, G. and Stover, B. H. (1978). Restriction endonuclease fingerprinting of herpes simplex DNA: a novel epidemiological tool applied to a nosocomial outbreak. *J. Infect. Dis.*, **138**, 488–498.
41. Roizman, B. (1979). The structure and isomerization of herpes simplex virus genomes. *Cell*, **16**, 481–494.
42. Grundy, J. E., Lui, S. F., Super, M. *et al.* (1988). Symptomatic cytomegalovirus infection in seropositive kidney recipients: reinfection with donor virus rather than reactivation with recipient virus. *Lancet*, **ii**, 132–135.
43. Winston, D. J., Huang, E.-S., Miller, M. J. *et al.* (1985). Molecular epidemiology of cytomegalovirus infections associated with bone marrow transplantation. *Ann. Intern. Med.*, **102**, 16–20.
44. Grob, J. P., Grundy, J. E., Prentice, H. G. *et al.* (1987). Immune donors can protect marrow-transplant recipients from severe cytomegalovirus infections. *Lancet*, **i**, 774–776.
45. Spear, P. G. (1984). Glycoproteins specified by herpes simplex viruses. In *The herpesviruses*, B. Roizman (ed.), Plenum Press, New York, pp. 315–356.
46. Britt, W. J. and Vulger, L. G. (1989). Processing of the gp55–116 envelope glycoprotein complex (gB) of human cytomegalovirus. *J. Virol.*, **63**, 403–410.
47. Wagner, B., Kropff, B., Kalbacher, H. *et al.* (1992). A continuous sequence of more than 70 amino acids is essential for antibody binding to the dominant antigenic site of glycoprotein gp58 of human cytomegalovirus. *J. Virol.*, **66**, 5290–5297.
48. Keay, D. and Baldwin, B. (1992). The human fibroblast receptor for gp86 of human cytomegalovirus is a phosphorylated glycoprotein. *J. Virol.*, **66**, 4834–4838.
49. Rasmussen, L., Nelson, M., Neff, M. and Merigan, T. C., Jr (1988). Characterization of two different human cytomegalovirus glycoproteins which are targets for neutralizing antibody. *Virology*, **163**, 308–318.

50. Drobyski, W. R., Gottlieb, M., Carrigan, D. *et al.* (1991). Phase 1 study of safety and pharmacokinetics of a human anticytomegalovirus monoclonal antibody in allogeneic bone marrow transplant recipients. *Transplantation*, **51**, 1190–1196.
51. Chou, S. (1992). Molecular epidemiology of envelope glycoprotein H of human cytomegalovirus. *J. Infect. Dis.*, **166**, 604–607.
52. Klenk, H-D. and Schwarz, R. T. (1982). Viral glycoprotein metabolism as a target for antiviral substances. *Antiviral Res.*, **2**, 177–190.
53. Cooper, N. R., Nowlin, D., Taylor, H. P. and Compton, T. (1991). Cellular receptor for human cytomegalovirus. *Transplant. Proc.*, **23**, 56–59.
54. Rasmussen, L., Resta, S. and Merigan, T. (1991). Human cytomegalovirus glycoprotein–receptor interactions. *Transplant. Proc.*, **23**, 60–63.
55. Compton, T., Nowlin, D. M. and Cooper, N. R. (1993). Initiation of human cytomegalovirus infection requires initial interaction with cell surface heparan sulfate. *Virol.*, **193**, 834–841.
56. Neyts, J., Snoeck, R., Schols, D. *et al.* (1992). Sulfated polymers inhibit the interaction of human cytomegalovirus with cell surface heparan sulfate. *Virol.*, **189**, 48–58.
57. Shieh, M. T., WuDunn, D., Montgomery, R. I., Esko, J. D. and Spear, P. G. (1992). Cell surface receptors for herpes simplex virus are heparin sulfate proteoglycans. *J. Cell Biol.*, **116**, 1273–1281.
58. Lentz, T. L. (1990). Review article. The recognition event between virus and host cell receptor: a target for antivirals. *J. Gen. Virol.*, **71**, 751–766.
59. Honess, R. W. and Roizman, B. (1974). Regulation of herpesvirus macro-molecular synthesis. *J. Virol.*, **14**, 8–19.
60. Geist, L. J., Monick, M. M., Stinski, M. F. and Hunninghake, G. W. (1991). The immediate early genes of human cytomegalovirus upregulate expression of the interleukin-2 and interleukin-2 receptor genes. *Am. J. Respir. Cell Mol. Biol.*, **5**, 292–296.
61. Puchtler, E. and Stamminger, T. (1991). An inducible promoter mediates abundant expression from the immediate–early 2 gene region of human cytomegalovirus at late times after infection. *J. Virol.*, **65**, 6301–6306.
62. Schwartz, R., Sommer, M. H., Scully, A. and Spector, D. H. (1994). Site-specific binding of the human cytomegalovirus IE2 86-kilodalton protein to an early gene promoter. *J. Virol.*, **68**, 5613–5622.
63. Arlt, H., Lang, D., Gebert, S. and Stamminger, T. (1994). Identification of binding sites for the 85-kilodalton IE2 protein of human cytomegalovirus within an IE-2 responsive viral early promoter. *J. Virol.*, **68**, 4117–4125.
64. Goins, W. F. and Stinski, M. F. (1986). Expression of a human cytomegalovirus late gene is posttranscriptionally regulated by a 3′-end-processing event occurring exclusively late after infection. *Mol. Cell. Biol.*, **6**, 4202–4213.
65. McVoy, M. A. and Adler, S. P. (1991). Analysis of human cytomegalovirus (HCMV) DNA replicative intermediates: DNA forms not predicted by the rolling circle model. In *Progress in Cytomegalovirus Research*, M. P. Landini (ed.), Elsevier, Amsterdam, pp. 53–56.
66. Challberg, M. D. (1986). A method for identifying the viral genes required for herpesvirus DNA replication. *Proc. Natl Acad. Sci. USA*, **83**, 9094–9098.
67. McVoy, M. A. and Adler, S. P. (1994). Human cytomegalovirus DNA replicates after early circularization by concatemer formation, and inversion occurs within the concatemer. *J. Virol.*, **68**, 1040–1051.
68. Parris, D. S., Cross, A., Haarr, L. *et al.* (1988). Identification of the gene encoding the 65-kilodalton DNA-binding protein of herpes simplex virus type 1. *J. Virol.*, **62**, 818–825.

69. Kemble, G. W., McCormick, A. L., Pereira, L. and Mocarski, E. S. (1987). A cytomegalovirus protein with properties of herpes simplex virus ICP8: partial purification of the polypeptide and map position of the gene. *J. Virol.*, **61**, 3143–3151.
70. Hamzeh, F. M., Leitman, P. S., Gibson, W. and Hayward, G. S. (1990). Identification of the lytic origin of replication in human cytomegalovirus by a novel approach utilizing ganciclovir-induced chain termination. *J. Virol.*, **64**, 6184–6195.
71. Falloon, J. and Masur, H. (1990). Cytomegalovirus and the immunosuppressed patient. In *Antiviral Agents and Viral Diseases of Man*, G. J. Galasso, R. J. Whitley and T. C. Merigan (eds), Raven Press, New York.
72. Nelson, J. A., Gwann, J. W., Jr and Ghazal, P. (1990). Regulation and tissue-specific expression of human cytomegalovirus. In *Curr. Top. Microbiol. Immunol.*, **154**, 75–100.
73. Braun, R. W. and Reiser, H. C. (1986). Replication of human cytomegalovirus in human peripheral blood T cells. *J. Virol.*, **60**, 29–36.
74. Nelson, J. A. and Groudine, M. (1986). Transcriptional regulation of human cytomegalovirus major immediate–early gene is associated with induction of DNase-I hypersensitivity sites. *Mol. Cell. Biol.*, **6**, 452–461.
75. Lathey, J. L. and Spector, S. A. (1991). Unrestricted replication of human cytomegalovirus in hydrocortisone-treated macrophages. *J. Virol.*, **65**, 6371–6375.
76. Gerna, G., Zipeto, D., Percivalle, E. *et al.* (1992). Human cytomegalovirus infection of the major leukocyte subpopulations and evidence for initial viral replication in polymorphonuclear leukocytes from viremic patients. *J. Infect. Dis.*, **166**, 1236–1244.
77. Lathey, J. L. and Spector, S. A. (1991). Unrestricted replication of human cytomegalovirus in hydrocortisone-treated macrophages. *J. Virol.*, **65**, 6371–6375.
78. Zalia, J. A. (1991). Pathogenesis of CMV-associated diseases in 1990. *Transplant. Proc.*, **23**, 1–4.
79. Grundy, J. E. (1991). Alterations of cellular proteins in human cytomegalovirus infection: potential for disease pathogenesis. *Transplant. Proc.*, **23**, 38–42.
80. Browne, H., Smith, G., Beck, S. and Minson, T. (1990). A complex between the MHC class 1 homologue encoded by human cytomegalovirus and B_2 microglobulin. *Nature*, **347**, 770–772.
81. Barnes, P. D. and Grundy, J. E. (1992). Down-regulation of the class 1 HLA heterodimer and beta 2-microglobulin on the surface of cells infected with cytomegalovirus. *J. Gen. Virol.* **73**, 2395–2403.
82. Carney, W. P., Rubin, R. H., Hoffman, R. A. *et al.* (1981). Analysis of T lymphocyte subsets in cytomegalovirus mononucleosis. *J. Immunol.*, **126**, 2114–2116.
83. Rice, G. P. A., Schrier, R. D. and Oldstone, M. B. A. (1984). Cytomegalovirus infects human lymphocytes and monocytes: virus expression is restricted to immediate–early gene products. *Proc. Natl Acad. Sci. USA*, **81**, 6134–6138.
84. Kapasi, K. and Rice, G. P. A. (1986). Role of the monocyte in cytomegalovirus-mediated immunosuppression *in vitro*. *J. Infect. Dis.*, **154**, 881–884
85. Rakusan, T. A., Juneja, H. S. and Fleischmann, W. R. (1989). Inhibition of hemopoietic colony formation by human cytomegalovirus *in vitro*. *J. Infect. Dis.*, **159**, 127–130.
86. Rodgers, B. C., Scott, D. M., Mundin, J. and Sissons, J. G. P. (1985). Monocyte-derived inhibitor of interleukin 1 induced by human cytomegalovirus. *J. Virol.*, **55**, 527–532.
87. Fujinami, R. S., Nelson, J. A., Walker, L. and Oldstone, M. B. A. (1988). Sequence homology and immunologic cross-reactivity of human cytomegalovirus with

HLA-DR beta chain: a means for graft rejection and immunosuppression. *J. Virol.*, **62**, 100–105.

88. McVoy, M. A. and Adler, S. P. (1989). Immunologic evidence for frequent age-related cytomegalovirus reactivation in seropositive immunocompetent individuals. *J. Infect. Dis.*, **160**, 1–10.
89. Toorkey, C. B. and Carrigan, D. R. (1989). Immunohistochemical detection of an immediate early antigen of human cytomegalovirus in normal tissues. *J. Infect. Dis.*, **160**, 741–751.
90. Ho, M. (1991). Hepatitis C virus, another agent transmitted by transplanted organs. *N. Engl. J. Med.*, **325**, 507–509.
91. Rice, G. P. A., Schrier, R. D. and Oldstone, M. B. A. (1984). Cytomegalovirus infects human lymphocytes and monocytes: virus expression is restricted to immediate–early gene products. *Proc. Natl Acad. Sci. USA*, **81**, 6134–6138.
92. Chou, S. (1989). Neutralizing antibody responses to reinfecting strains of cytomegalovirus in transplant recipients. *J. Infect. Dis.*, **160**, 16–21.
93. Grundy, J. E., Super, M., Sweny, P. *et al.* (1988). Symptomatic cytomegalovirus infection in seropositive kidney recipients: reinfection with donor virus rather than reactivation of recipient virus. *Lancet*, **ii**, 132–135.
94. Spector, S. A., Hirata, K. K. and Neuman, T. R. (1984). Identification of multiple cytomegalovirus strains in homosexual men with acquired immunodeficiency syndrome. *J. Infect. Dis.*, **150**, 953–955.
95. Grundy, J. E., Ayles, H. M. and McKeating, J. A. (1988). Enhancement of class 1 HLA antigen expression by cytomegalovirus: role in amplification of viral infection. *J. Med. Virol.*, **25**, 483–495.
96. Nelson, J. A., Reynolds-Kohler, C., Oldstone, M. B. A. and Wiley, C. A. (1988). HIV and HCMV coinfect brain cells in patients with AIDS. *Virology*, **165**, 286–290.
97. Finkle, C., Tapper, M. A., Knox, K. K. and Carrigan, D. R. (1991). Coinfection of cells with the human immunodeficiency virus and cytomegalovirus in lung tissues of patients with AIDS. *J. AIDS*, **4**, 735–736.
98. Ho, W.-Z., Harouse, J. M., Rando, R. F., Gonczol, E. *et al.* (1990). Reciprocal enhancement of gene expression and viral replication between human cytomegalovirus and human immunodeficiency virus type 1. *J. Gen. Virol.*, **71**, 97–103.
99. Paya, C. V., Virelizier, J.-L. and Michelson, S. (1991). Modulation of T-cell activation through protein kinase C- or A-dependent signalling pathways synergistically increases human immunodeficiency virus long terminal repeat induction by cytomegalovirus immediate–early proteins. *J. Virol.*, **65**, 5477–5484.
100. Skolnik, P. R., Kosloff, B. R. and Hirsch, M. S. (1988). Bidirectional interactions between human immunodeficiency virus type 1 and cytomegalovirus. *J. Infect. Dis.*, **157**, 508–514.
101. Webster, A. (1991). Cytomegalovirus as possible cofactor in HIV disease progression. *J. AIDS*, **4**, S47–S52.
102. Kempf, D. J., Marsh, K. C., Paul, D. A. *et al.* (1991). Antiviral and pharmacokinetic properties of C_2 symmetric inhibitors of the human immunodeficiency virus type 1 protease. *Antimicrob. Agents Chemother.*, **35**, 2209–2214.
103. Debouck, C. and Metcalf, B. W. (1990). Human immunodeficiency virus protease: a target for AIDS therapy. *Drug. Dev. Res.*, **21**, 1–17.
104. Chapman, M. S., Minor, I., Rossman, M. G. *et al.* (1991). Human rhinovirus 14 complexed with antiviral compound R61837. *J. Mol. Biol.*, **217**, 455–463.
105. Kern, E. R. (1991). Value of animal models to evaluate agents with potential activity against human cytomegalovirus. *Transplant. Proc.*, **23**, 152–155.

106. Dunkel, E. C. (1991). HCMV-induced chorioretinitis in the rabbit. *Transplant. Proc.*, **23**, 25–28.
107. Allen, L. B., Li, S., Arnett, G. *et al.* (1992). Novel method for evaluating antiviral drugs against human cytomegalovirus in mice. *J. Virol.*, **36**, 206–208.
108. DiLorato, D., Epstein, L. G., Lazar, E. S., Britt, W. J. and del Cerro, M. (1994). Cytomegalovirus infection of human retinal tissue: An in vivo model. *Lab. Investigations*, **71**, 141–148.
109. Mocarski, E. S., Bonyhadi, M., Salimi, S., *et al.* (1993). Human cytomegalovirus in SCID-HU mouse thymic epithelial cells are prominent targets of replication. *Proc. Natl. Acad. Sci. USA*, **90**, 104–108.
110. Stals, F. S., Bosman, F., Van Boven, C. P. A. and Bruggeman, C. A. (1990). An animal model for therapeutic intervention studies of CMV infection in the immunocompromised host. *Arch. Virol.*, **114**, 91–108.
111. Kern, E. R. (1990). Preclinical evaluation of antiviral agents: *in vitro* and animal model testing. In *Antiviral Agents and Viral Diseases of Man*, G. J. Galasso, R. J. Whitley and T. C. Merigan (eds), Raven Press, New York.
112. Jordan, M. C. and Pomeroy, C. (1991). Latent CMV infection in the mouse. *Transplant Proc.*, **23**, 17–21.
113. De Castro, L. M., Kern, E. R., De Clercq, E. *et al.* (1991). Phosphonylmethoxyalkyl purine and pyrimidine derivatives for treatment of opportunistic cytomegalovirus and herpes simplex virus infections in murine AIDS. *Antiviral Res.*, **16**, 101–114.
114. Smee, D. F., Burger, R. A., Coombs, J. *et al.* (1991). Progressive murine cytomegalovirus disease after termination of ganciclovir therapy in mice immunosuppressed by cyclophosphamide treatment. *J. Infect. Dis.*, **164**, 958–961.
115. Elion, G. B. (1986). History, mechanism of action, spectrum and selectivity of nucleoside analogues. In *Antiviral Chemotherapy: New Directions for Clinical Applications and Research*, J. Mills and L. Corey (eds), Elsevier, New York.
116. Oberg, B. (1989). Antiviral effects of phosphonoformate (PFA, foscarnet sodium). *Pharmacol. Ther.*, **40**, 213–285.
117. Elion, G. B. (1989). The purine path to chemotherapy. *Science*, **244**, 41–47.
118. Whitley, R. J., Nahmias, A. J., Soong, S.-J. *et al.* (1980). Vidarabine therapy of neonatal herpes simplex virus infection. *Pediatrics*, **66**, 495–501.
119. Whitley, R. J., Alford, C. A., Hirsch, M. S. *et al.* (1986). Vidarabine versus acyclovir therapy in herpes simplex encephalitis. *N. Engl. J. Med.*, **314**, 144–149.
120. Derse, D., Cheng, Y.-C., Furman, P. A. *et al.* (1981). Inhibition of purified human and herpes simplex virus-induced DNA polymerases by 9-(2-hydroxyethoxymethyl)guanine triphosphate. *J. Biol. Chem.*, **256**, 11447–11451.
121. Reardon, J. E. and Spector, T. (1989). Herpes simplex virus type 1 DNA polymerase. *J. Biol. Chem.*, **264**, 7405–7411.
122. Estes, J. E. and Huang, E. S. (1977). Stimulation of cellular thymidine kinases by human cytomegalovirus. *J. Virol.*, **24**, 13–21.
123. Beauchamp, L. M., Orr, G. F., deMiranda, P. *et al.* (1992). Amino acid ester prodrugs of acyclovir. *Antiviral Chem. Chemother.*, **3**, 157–164.
124. Matthews, T. and Boehme, R. (1988). Antiviral activity and mechanism of action of ganciclovir. *Rev. Infect. Dis.*, **10**, S490–S494.
125. Levinson, M. L. and Jacobson, P. A. (1992). Treatment and prophylaxis of cytomegalovirus disease. *Pharmacotherapy*, **12**, 300–318.
126. Paul, S. and Dummer, S. (1992). Topics in clinical pharmacology: ganciclovir. *Am. J. Med. Sci.*, **304**, 272–277.
127. Nevins, T. E. and Dunn, D. L. (1992). Use of ganciclovir for cytomegalovirus infection. *J. Am. Soc. Nephrol.*, **2**, S270–S273.

128. Fauld, D. and Hee, R. C. (1990). Ganciclovir. *Drugs*, **39**, 597–638.
129. Biron, K. K., Fyfe, J. A., Stanat, S. C. *et al.* (1986). A human cytomegalovirus mutant resistant to the nucleoside analog 9-{[2-hydroxy-1-(hydroxymethyl) ethoxy]methyl} guanine (BW B759U) induces reduced levels of BW B759U triphosphate. *Proc. Natl Acad. Sci. USA*, **83**, 8769–8773.
130. Mar, E.-C., Chiou, J. F., Cheng, Y. C. and Huang, E. S. (1985). Inhibition of cellular DNA polymerase a and human cytomegalovirus-induced DNA polymerase by the triphosphates of 9-(2-hydroxyethoxymethyl)guanine and 9-(1,3-dihydroxy-2-propoxymethyl)guanine. *J. Virol.*, **53**, 776–780.
131. Lewis, R. A., Watkins, L. and St Jeor, S. (1985). *Mol. Cell. Biochem.*, **65**, 67–71.
132. Stanat, S. C., Reardon, J. E., Erice, A. *et al.* (1991). Ganciclovir-resistant cytomegalovirus clinical isolates: mode of resistance to ganciclovir. *Antimicrob. Agents Chemother.*, **35**, 2191–2197.
133. Coen, D. M. (1991). Drug resistance and drug targets in HSV and CMV, *16th International Herpesvirus Workshop*, Abstr. SA-17.
134. Fan-Havard, P., Nahata, M. C. and Brady, M. T. (1989). Ganciclovir: a review of pharmacology, therapeutic efficacy and potential use for treatment of congenital cytomegalovirus infections. *J. Clin. Pharm. Ther.*, **14**, 329–340.
135. Wahren, B., Larsson, A., Ruden, U. *et al.* (1987). Acyclic guanosine analogs as inhibitors of human cytomegalovirus. *Antimicrob. Agents Chemother.*, **31**, 317–320.
136. Beauchamp, L. M., Serling, B. L., Kelsey, J. E. *et al.* (1988). Effect of acyclic pyrimidines related to [(dihydroxy-2-propoxy)methyl]guanine on herpesviruses, *J. Med. Chem.*, **31**, 144–149.
137. Talarico, C., Stanat, S., Lambe, C. *et al.* (1990). Mode of action studies on the anti-cytomegalovirus nucleoside analog [1-(2-hydroxy-1-(hydroxymethyl) ethoxymethyl)-cytosine]. *Antiviral Res.* (Suppl. 1), abstr. 92, 87.
138. Townsend, L. B., Drach, J. C., Wotring, L. L. *et al.* (1991). Design, synthesis, and studies on the activity relationships of certain pyrrolo[2,3-*d*]pyrimidine nucleosides and structurally related analogs as potential antiveoplastic and antiviral agents. *Il Farmaco*, **46**, 113–139.
139. Pudlo, J. S., Saxena, N. K., Nasiri, M. R. *et al.* (1988). Synthesis and antiviral activity of certain 4- and 4,5-disubstituted 7-[(2-hydroxyethoxy)methyl]pyrrolo[2,3-*d*]pyrimidines. *J. Med. Chem.*, **31**, 2086–2092.
140. Pudlo, J. S., Nassiri, M. R., Kern, E. R. *et al.* (1990). Synthesis, antiproliferative, and antiviral activity of certain 4-substituted and 4,5 disubstituted 7-[(1,3-dihydroxy-2-propoxy)-methyl]pyrrolo[2,3-*d*]pyrimidines. *J. Med. Chem.*, **33**, 1984–1992.
141. Nassiri, M. R., Hudson, J. L., Pudlo, J. S. *et al.* (1990). Flow cytometric evaluation of the cytotoxicity of novel antiviral compounds. *Cytometry*, **11**, 411–417.
142. Tolman, R. L., Field, A. K., Karkas, J. D. *et al.* (1985). 2′-Nor-cGMP: a seco-cyclic nucleotide with powerful anti-DNA-viral activity. *Biochem. Biophys. Res. Commun.*, **128**, 1329–1335.
143. Field, A. K., Davies, M. E. M., De Witt, C. M. *et al.* (1986). Efficacy of 2′-nor-cyclic GMP in treatment of experimental herpes virus infections. *Antiviral Res.*, **6**, 329–341.
144. Prisbe, E. J., Martin, J. C., McGee, P. C. *et al.* (1986). Synthesis and antiherpes virus activity of phosphate and phosphonate derivatives of 9-[(1,3-dihydroxy-2-propoxy)methyl] guanine, *J. Med. Chem.*, **29**, 671–675.
145. Yang, Z. H., Lucia, H. L., Tolman, R. L. *et al.* (1989). Effect of 2′-nor-cyclic GMP against guinea pig cytomegalovirus infection. *Antimicrob. Agents Chemother.*, **33**, 1563–1568.

146. Sidwell, R. W., Huffman, J. H., Barnard, D. L. *et al.* (1992). In vitro and in vivo cytomegalovirus-inhibitory effects of 9-[3-ethylphosphono-1-hydroxymethyl-propyloxy methyl]guanine (SR3727): Interscience Conf. *Antimicrob. Agents Chemother.*, Abstr. 1318.
147. De Clercq, E., Holy, A., Rosenbery, I. *et al.* (1986). A novel selective broad-spectrum anti-DNA virus agent. *Nature (London)*, **323**, 464–467.
148. Terry, B. J., Mazina, K. E., Tuomari, A.V. *et al.* (1988). Broad-spectrum antiviral activity of the acyclic guanosine phosphonate (*R,S*)-HPMPG. *Antiviral Res.*, **10**, 235–252.
149. Snoeck, R., Sakuma, T., De Clercq, E. *et al.* (1988). (*S*)-1-(3-Hydroxy-2-phosphonylmethoxypropyl)cytosine, a potent and selective inhibitor of human cytomegalovirus replication. *Antimicrob. Agents Chemother.*, **32**, 1839–1844.
150. Ho, H.-T., Woods, K. L., Bronson, J. J., De Boeck, H. *et al.* (1992). Intracellular metabolism of the antiherpes agent (*S*)-1[3-hydroxy-2-(phosphonyl-methoxy)propyl]cytosine on lymphocyte transformation and delayed-type hypersensitivity responses. *Mol. Pharmacol.*, **41**, 197–202.
151. Neyts, J., Snoeck, R., Balzarini, J. and De Clercq, E. (1991). Particular characteristics of the anti-human cytomegalovirus activity of (*S*)-1-(3-hydroxy-2-phosphonylmethoxypropyl)cytosine (HPMPC) *in vitro*. *Antiviral Res.*, **16**, 41–52.
152. Stals, F. S., De Clercq, E. and Bruggeman, C. A. (1991). Comparative activity of (*S*)-1-(3-hydroxy-2-phosphonylmethoxypropyl)cytosine [HPMPC] and 9-(1,3-dihydroxy-2-propoxymethyl)guanine [DHPG] against rat cytomegalovirus infection *in vitro* and *in vivo*. *Antimicrob. Agents Chemother.*, **35**, 2262–2266.
153. Li, S. B., Yang, Z. H., Feng, J. S. *et al.* (1990). Activity of (*S*)-1-(3-hydroxy-2-phosphonylmethoxypropyl)cytosine (HPMPC) against guinea pig cytomegalovirus infection in cultured cells and in guinea pigs. *Antiviral Res.*, **13**, 237–252.
154. Colacino, J. M. and Lopez, C. (1985). Antiviral activity of 2′-deoxy-2′-fluoro-β-D-arabinofuranosyl-5-iodocytosine against human cytomegalovirus in human skin fibroblasts. *Antimicrob. Agents Chemother.*, **28**, 252–258.
155. King, D. H. (1991). Fluorinated pyrimidines: a new change for old drugs. *Transplant. Proc.*, **23**, 168–170.
156. Slusarchyk, W. A., Young, M. G., Bisacchi, G. S. *et al.* (1989). Synthesis of SQ-33,054, a novel cyclobutane nucleoside with potent antiviral activity. *Tetrahedron Lett.*, **30**, 6453–6456.
157. Field, A. K., Tuomari, A. V., McGeever-Rubin, B. *et al.* (1990). (±)-(1α, 2β, 3α)-9-[2,3-bishydroxymethyl)-cyclobutyl]guanine [(±)-BHCG or SQ 33054]: a potent and selective inhibitor of herpesviruses. *Antiviral Res.*, **13**, 41–52.
158. Terry, B. J., Mazina, K. E., Tuomari, A. V. *et al.* (1990). Anti-herpetic activity of (±)-(1α,2β,3α)-9-[2-hydroxy-3-(hydroxymethyl)cyclobutyl]guanine and inhibition of HSV-1 DNA polymerase. *Antiviral Chem. Chemother.*, **1**, 263–268.
159. Hayashi, S., Norbeck, D. W., Rosenbrook, W. *et al.* (1990). Cyclobut-A and cyclobut-G, carbocyclic oxetanocin analogs that inhibit the replication of human immunodeficiency virus in T cells and monocytes and macrophages *in vitro*. *Antimicrob. Agents Chemother.*, **34**, 287–294.
160. Norbeck, D. W., Kern, E., Hayashi, S. *et al.* (1990). Cyclobut-A and cyclobut-G: broad-spectrum antiviral agents with potential utility for the therapy of AIDS. *J. Med. Chem.*, **33**, 1281–1285.
161. Ichikawa, Y., Narita, A., Shiozawa, A. *et al.* (1989). Enantio- and diastereo-selective synthesis of carbocyclic oxetanocin analogues. *J. Chem. Soc. Chem. Commun.*, 1919–1921.
162. Bisacchi, G. S., Braitman, A., Cianci, C. W. *et al.* (1991). *J. Med. Chem.*, **34**, 1415–1421.

163. Braitman, A., Swerdel, M. R., Olsen, S. J. *et al.* (1991). Evaluation of SQ 34,514: pharmacokinetics and efficacy in experimental herpesvirus infections in mice. *Antimicrob. Agents Chemother.*, **35**, 1464–1468.
164. Kohlbrenner, W. E., Carter, C. D., Fesik, S. W. *et al.* (1990). Efficiency of phosphorylation of the cyclobut-G (A-69992) enantiomers by HSV-1 thymidine kinase does not correlate with their anti-herpesvirus activity. *Biochem. Pharmacol.*, **40**, R5–R10.
165. Yamanaka, G., Tuomari, A. V., Hagen, M. M. *et al.* (1991). Selective activity and cellular pharmacology of (1*R*-1α,2β,3α)-9-[2,3-bis(hydroxymethyl)cyclobutyl]-guanine in herpesvirus infected cells. *Mol. Pharmacol.*, **40**, 446–453.
166. Terry, B. J., Cianci, C. W. and Hagen, M. E. (1991). Inhibition of HSV-1 DNA polymerase by [1*R*(1α,2β,3α)]-9-(2,3-bis(hydroxymethyl)cyclobutyl]guanine. *Mol. Pharmacol.*, **40**, 591–596.
167. Yamanaka, G., Tuomari, A. V., Christodoulides, M. *et al.* (1991). (*R*)-BHCA(SQ 34,990): a dihydroxymethylcyclobutyl deoxyadenosine analog active against ganciclovir-resistant HCMV. In *Progress in Cytomegalovirus Research*, M. P. Landini (ed.), Elsevier, Amsterdam, pp. 341–344.
168. Chrisp, P. L. and Clissold, S. P. (1991). Foscarnet. *Drugs*, **41**, 104–129.
169. Sullivan, V. and Coen, D. M. (1991). Isolation of foscarnet-resistant human cytomegalovirus patterns of resistance and sensitivity to other antiviral drugs. *J. Infect. Dis.*, **164**, 781–784.
170. D'Aquila, R. T., Hayward, G. S. and Summers, W. C. (1989). Physical mapping of the human cytomegalovirus (HCMV) (Towne) DNA polymerase gene: DNA-mediated transfer of a genetic marker for an HCMV gene. *Virology*, **171**, 312–316.
171. Erice, A., Chou, S., Biron, K. K. *et al.* (1989). Progressive disease due to ganciclovir-resistant cytomegalovirus in immunocompromised patients. *N. Engl. J. Med.*, **320**, 289–293.
172. Field, A. K. and Biron, K. K. (1994). 'The end of innocence' revisited: resistance of herpesviruses to antiviral drugs. *Clin. Microbiol. Rev.*, **7**, 1–13.
173. Schinazi, R. F. (1991). Combined chemotherapeutic modalities for viral infections: rationale and clinical potential. In *Synergism and Antagonism in Chemotherapy*, Academic Press, New York, Ch. 4.
174. Crumpacker, C. S. and Heath-Chiozzi, M. (1991). Overview of cytomegalovirus infections in HIV-infected patients: current therapies and future strategies. *J. AIDS*, **4**, S1–S5.
175. Manischewitz, J. F., Quinnan, G. V., Lane, H. C. and Wittek, A. E. (1990). Synergistic effect of ganciclovir and foscarnet on cytomegalovirus replication *in vitro*. *Antimicrob. Agents Chemother.*, **34**, 373–375.
176. Hirsch, M. S., Schooley, R. T., Cosimi, A. B. *et al.* (1983). Effects of interferon-alpha on cytomegalovirus reactivation syndromes in renal-transplant recipients. *N. Engl. J. Med.*, **308**, 1489–1493.
177. Meyers, J. D., Flournoy, N., Sanders, J. E. *et al.* (1987). Prophylactic use of human leukocyte interferon after allogeneic marrow transplantation. *Ann. Intern. Med.*, **107**, 809–816.
178. Rasmussen, L., Chen, P. T., Mullenax, J. G. and Merigan, T. C. (1984). Inhibition of human cytomegalovirus replication by 9-(1,3-dihydroxy-2-propoxymethyl)guanine alone and in combination with human interferons. *Antimicrob. Agents Chemother.*, **26**, 441–445.
179. Grossberg, H. S., Bonnem, E. M. and Buhles, W. C. (1989). GM-CSF with ganciclovir for the treatment of CMV retinitis in AIDS. *N. Engl. J. Med.*, **320**, 1560.
180. Hardy, W. D. (1991). Combined ganciclovir and recombinant human granulo-

cyte–macrophage colony-stimulating factor in the treatment of cytomegalovirus retinitis in AIDS patients. *J. AIDS*, **4**, S22–S28.
181. Grundy, J. E., Shanley, J. D. and Griffiths, P. D. (1987). Is cytomegalovirus interstitial pneumonitis in transplant recipients an immunopathological condition? *Lancet*, **ii**, 996–999.
182. Shanley, J. D. (1991). Murine models of cytomegalovirus-associated pneumonitis. *Transplant. Proc.*, **23**, 12–16.
183. Rubin, R. H., Lynch, P., Pasternack, M. S. *et al.* (1989). Combined antibody and ganciclovir treatment of murine cytomegalovirus-infected normal and immunosuppressed BALB/c mice. *Antimicrob. Agents Chemother.*, **33**, 1975–1979.
184. Schmidt, G. M. (1991). Treatment of CMV infections and disease in transplantation. *Transplant Proc.*, **23**, 126–130.
185. Gelb, L. W. (1990). Varicella–zoster virus. In *Virology*, B. N. Fields and D. M. Knipe (eds), Raven Press, New York, pp. 2011–2054.
186. Roizman, B. and Sears, A. E. (1990). Herpes simplex viruses and their replication. In *Virology*, B. N. Fields and D. M. Knipe (eds), Raven Press, New York, pp. 1795–1842.
187. Kieff, E. and Liebowitz, D. (1990). Epstein–Barr virus and its replication. In *Virology*, B. N. Fields and D. M. Knipe (eds), Raven Press, New York, pp. 1889–1920.
188. Lopez, C. and Honess, R. W. (1990). Human herpesvirus. In *Virology*, B. N. Fields and D. M. Knipe (eds), Raven Press, New York, pp. 2055–2062.

5 Chemotherapy of Herpes Simplex Virus Infections: A Laboratory Perspective

HUGH J. FIELD and SIÂN E. GOLDTHORPE
Cambridge University Department of Veterinary Medicine, Cambridge, UK

HERPES SIMPLEX VIRUS AND ITS REPLICATION CYCLE

HERPES SIMPLEX VIRUS AS A TARGET OF CHEMOTHERAPY

The chemotherapy of herpes simplex virus (HSV) has enjoyed singular success: several very effective drugs have been discovered and their development widely reported. More data have been accumulated on inhibitors of HSV, *in vivo* and *in vitro*, than perhaps of any other virus to date. Notwithstanding the hundreds of laboratories working with this virus, there remain features of HSV infection that are not fully elucidated. Furthermore, there are many aspects of the interactions between HSV and chemotherapeutic agents which have still to be thoroughly investigated.

For some commentators, the mere demonstration of clinical efficacy may seem to be the end of the investigative study of a particular anti-herpes drug. Such an attitude is undoubtedly simplistic, given the complexity of the interactions between HSV and the human host. Continued study of the molecular mechanisms of virus replication and pathogenesis in the presence of inhibitors is required, in order that antiviral agents may realize their full potential. In this way, the limitations of current compounds may be determined and overcome by the design of novel therapeutic strategies.

Of all virus diseases, those caused by HSV have so far proved most amenable to chemotherapy. The reasons for this relative success include the following.

1. The virus has a relatively large DNA genome which encodes at least 70 gene products and hence numerous potential targets for inhibition.
2. Several virus-specific enzymes involved with DNA metabolism are induced in infected cells which are then suitable targets for selective attack.
3. The virus is grown readily in tissue culture, and systems have been avail-

Antiviral Chemotherapy. Edited by D.J. Jeffries and E. De Clercq

able for several decades for assay of virus titre and hence for estimation of the activity of potential inhibitors.

4. Laboratory animal models have also been available in which to demonstrate antiviral effectiveness *in vivo* prior to use in man.
5. The lesions produced by HSV are common and often recurrent, resulting in a large commercial market for effective anti-herpetics.
6. The production of a safe and effective vaccine for HSV has proved difficult and, to date, no vaccine has been developed for general use.

THE HERPESVIRUS FAMILY

HSV is the archetypal member of the Herpesviridae, a family which includes many viruses of medical and veterinary importance (1). Herpes simplex virus types 1 and 2 (HSV-1 and HSV-2) are among at least six human herpesviruses characterized to date. In man, diseases associated with HSV are found to be caused by one of the two distinct virus types: HSV-1 and HSV-2. These two viruses, both of which belong to the subfamily Alphaherpesvirinae, were originally distinguished serologically, but they also have different biochemical and biological properties (and different susceptibilities to particular inhibitors). Today HSV isolates may readily be identified using type-specific monoclonal antibody in an enzyme-linked immunosorbent assay (ELISA) or neutralization test, or by their DNA restriction fragment polymorphism, the latter reflecting significant differences in the genomic organization of the virus types. Preliminary typing can also be done by testing the ability of virus isolates to grow in the presence or absence of a fixed concentration of the nucleoside analogue bromovinyldeoxyuridine (BVDU), to which strains of HSV-2 are relatively resistant.

THE MORPHOGENESIS OF VIRUS REPLICATION

When thin sections of virus-infected cells are studied under the electron microscope, characteristic changes are observed. Within a few hours the chromatin of the infected cell becomes disrupted and marginated. Capsids are assembled in the nucleus, empty at first, then filled with an electron-dense nucleoprotein core. The maturing nucleocapsids approach the inner lamella of the nuclear membrane through which they bud, thus acquiring the lipid envelope which is characteristic of the mature, infectious particles. Mature particles with DNA-containing cores are thus released into the extracellular space. The infection is cytolytic, and productive virus replication is inevitably accompanied by cell death. Cells adjacent to infected cells are often induced to fuse and form multinucleate cells or syncytia. Virus may thus pass from cell to cell without necessarily entering the extracellular fluid. Primary and reactivated infections *in vivo* produce inflammatory lesions which contain multinucleate, inclusion-bearing and pyknotic cells, with necrosis often accompanied by a profuse mononuclear cell infiltration.

THE BIOCHEMICAL NATURE OF HSV

The virion comprises an icosahedral capsid with a diameter of approximately 100 nm formed from 150 hexon and 12 penton capsomers. These surround the DNA genome which, in association with protein, forms the toroidal core of the virion. An amorphous tegument lies between the capsid and a lipid envelope (Figure 5.1). The envelope is derived from the nuclear membrane of the host cell, although this is modified in the infected cell by the insertion of virus-coded glycoproteins. These glycoproteins include the receptors which bring about the initial attachment of the infecting virion to the next host cell. The HSV genome is a linear, double-stranded molecule of approximately 150 kb and comprises a long (L) and a short (S) component each consisting of a unique region (U_l and U_s) bounded by inverted repeats (Figure 5.2). The genome of HSV-1 has been completely sequenced and contains at least 72 open reading frames (2), four of which correspond to two diploid genes mapping to the inverted repeats. Thus at least 70 different proteins are encoded of which 33, including eight envelope glycoproteins, are present in the intact virion.

THE BIOCHEMICAL EVENTS DURING REPLICATION IN PERMISSIVE CELLS

The replication of HSV in permissive cells results in the production of infectious virions and the inevitable destruction of the host cell. The replication

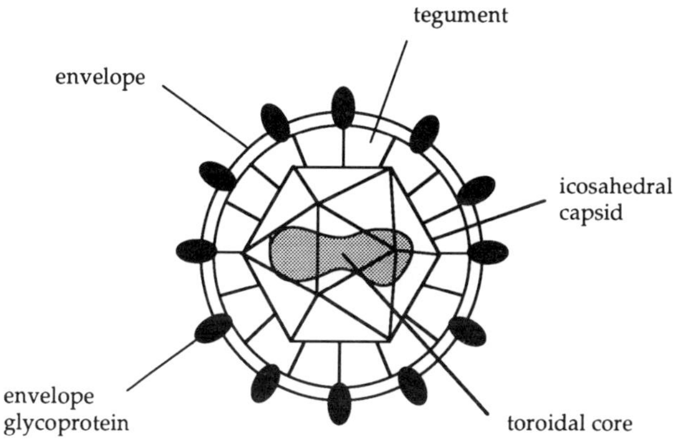

Figure 5.1. Structure of a herpes simplex virion

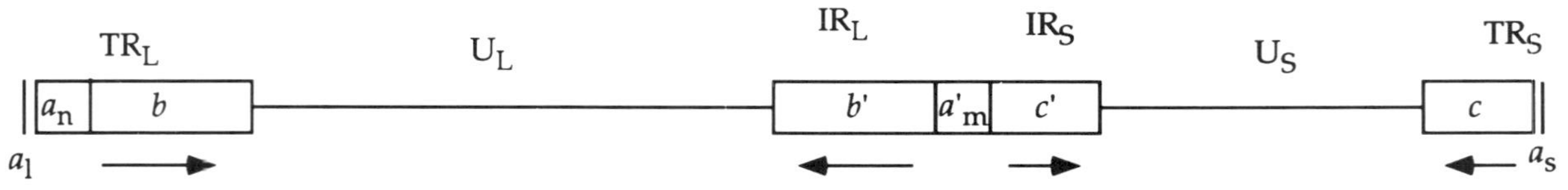

Figure 5.2. The structure of the HSV-1 genome, showing the unique sequences and inverted repeats (arrowed) of the long and short components. The repeats of the long component comprise *a* and *b* sequences, and the repeats of the short component comprise *a* and *c* sequences. When inverted, the *a*, *b* and *c* sequences become *a′*, *b′* and *c′*. U, unique sequences; TR, terminal repeats; IR, internal repeats; a_l and a_s, terminal *a* sequences; a_n and a_m, *a* sequence repeated *n* or *m* times

cycle of HSV-1, which has been extensively studied in cell culture, takes approximately 18 h and comprises stages of attachment, penetration, uncoating, genome replication and expression, assembly and release (Figure 5.3). The functions of individual gene products have been deter-

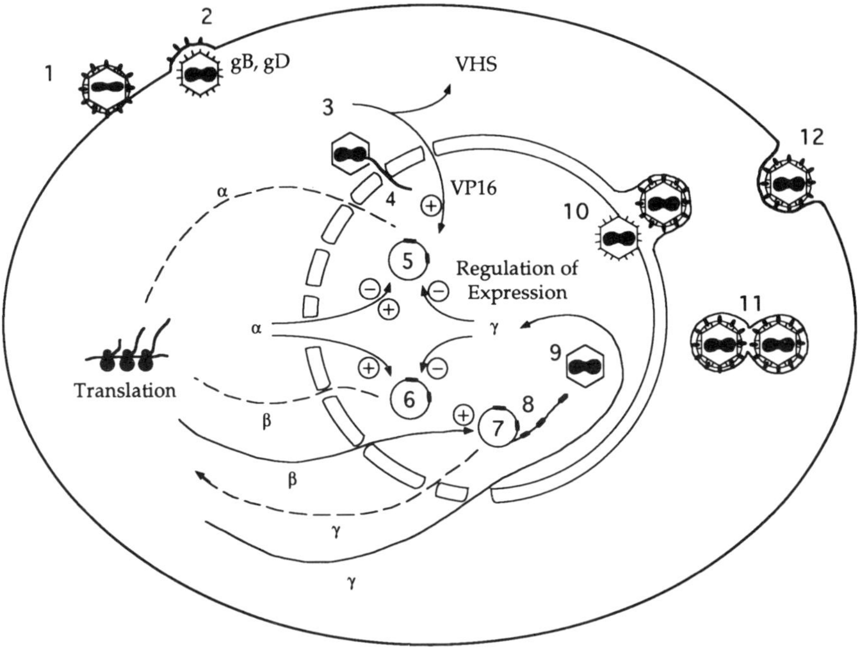

Figure 5.3. Schematic diagram summarizing HSV replication in a permissive cell (4). The dotted arrows refer to virus mRNAs, and the solid arrows refer to virus proteins. The circled + and – signs indicate the regulatory effects of virus gene products on virus gene expression. (1) *Attachment*: involves virus glycoproteins (possibly gB/gC), which are thought to interact initially with heparan sulphate proteoglycans on the cell surface. (2) *Penetration*: fusion of cell membrane and virus envelope, mediated by virus glycoproteins. (3) *Uncoating*: release of the virion host shut-off protein (VHS) and the virion transactivating protein (VP16). (4) *Release of viral DNA*: requires a viral function. (5) *α (immediate–early) gene expression*: see text. (6) *β (delayed–early) gene expression*: see text. (7) *γ (late) gene expression:* includes synthesis of the virus proteins required for genome replication (see text). Other virus proteins (including the envelope glycoproteins) are synthesized on membrane-bound polyribosomes, and are transported to the nuclear and/or plasma membrane (not indicated in diagram). (8) *Synthesis of virus DNA*: see text. (9) *Capsid assembly and packaging of virus genomes*: capsid assembly is poorly understood. Cleavage of virus DNA prior to packaging is directed by the *'a'* sequence (see text). (10) *Envelopment*: occurs at virally modified patches on the inner nuclear membrane. (11) *Transport through the cytoplasm*: accompanied by envelope glycoprotein maturation. (12) *Egress*

mined in various ways, for example by using conditional lethal (e.g. temperature-sensitive) mutants and in transient expression systems.

The first three stages of virus replication require functions mediated by virion proteins and glycoproteins. Another structural component of the virion, the tegument protein VP16 (Vmw 65), is a transactivator of virus genome expression (3). HSV genes are expressed in three groups: α, β and γ, forming a coordinately regulated cascade. Expression of the five α (or immediate–early (IE)) genes peaks between 2 and 4 h post infection. These genes have upstream, *cis*-acting regions containing the consensus nucleotide sequence TAATGARAT (where R = purine) to which the cellular transcription factor Oct-1 binds in conjunction with VP16, thereby activating gene transcription.

The products of IE genes regulate their own expression and that of other genes (4). In particular, ICP0 (Vmw 110) and ICP4 (Vmw 175) are major transactivators of the β (or delayed–early (DE)) genes. Expression of the DE genes peaks between 5 and 7 h after infection, and their products are responsible for nucleoside and nucleotide metabolism and DNA replication. Examples of such products are the virus-coded enzymes DNA polymerase, thymidine kinase (TK) and ribonucleotide reductase. These enzymes are of paramount importance in herpesvirus chemotherapy as targets for selective interaction with antiviral agents; in particular nucleoside analogues. Expression of the γ (late) genes is positively regulated by IE gene products (e.g. ICP27) and by DNA replication.

Replication of the HSV genome is thought to proceed by a rolling circle mechanism which follows circularization of the genome shortly after infection of the host cell. Consistent with this model are the observations that the free termini of the linear virion DNA disappear after infection and that nascent genomes take the form of 'head to tail' concatemers (5). Inversion of the L and S components and cleavage of concatemers into unit length genomes are directed by the 'a' sequence, one copy of which is present at the S terminus and several at the L terminus and the L–S junction (Figure 5.2).

Cleavage of the nascent DNA is linked to packaging of the viral capsids accumulating in the host cell nucleus late in infection. Full capsids then acquire envelopes from virus-modified patches of the inner lamella of the nuclear membrane and egress continues by a poorly understood mechanism in which virions are transported in membrane-bound structures (probably derived from the Golgi apparatus or endoplasmic reticulum) to the extracellular space.

During lytic HSV infection in cell culture, shut-off of host DNA and protein synthesis takes place—a process which ultimately leads to host cell death. Destabilization and degradation of host mRNA are under the influence of a virion component: the product of the *vhs* (viron host shut-off) gene. Various nuclear changes occur, such as disaggregation of the nucleolus, margination of chromatin and modification of the nuclear membrane. Other virus-induced changes in the host cell include the insertion of virus-specific glycoproteins into cell membranes. The branched *N*-linked oligosaccharides which accumulate in the herpesvirus-infected cell are considered to be potential targets of inhibition (6). Selective inhibition of terminal glycosylation by certain nucleoside analogues (see below) has been described and may contribute to their overall antiviral effect (7).

The events described above take place when a permissive cell is infected with a normal virus particle. If the cell is for some reason non-permissive, or the virus contains a disabling mutation, then the outcome of infection may be abortive with the destruction of the host cell (or in some cases cell survival) but without the release of infectious progeny. Similarly, when cells are infected with HSV in the presence of an effective inhibitor, the events leading to virus replication may be interrupted, such that no infectious progeny are released. Unless virus replication is prevented from the earliest stage, however, the host cell is unlikely to survive the abortive virus replication.

HSV AND DISEASE

The replication of HSV in man may proceed 'silently' and perhaps half or more of primary infections may be subclinical or pass unnoticed. However, HSV is associated with several different well-defined clinical syndromes (8). Typically the virus causes erythematous vesicles at or near mucocutaneous junctions. The vesicles may ulcerate and are often painful before healing over a period of a few days. The usual sites of these lesions are the mouth and lips for HSV-1 and the genitalia for HSV-2. HSV-1 also causes recurrent infection of the eye such as herpes keratitis—a major human eye disease. Another much feared manifestation of HSV-1 is herpes encephalitis, which has an incidence of between one in 250 000 and one in 500 000 per annum in the United States, and is the most important cause of acute encephalitis among adults in the Western world (9). The disease has a high mortality if untreated. Two other manifestations of HSV which deserve special mention are the generalized disease which may result from systemic infection of the newborn, and the severe chronic lesions which may occur in patients whose immune systems are compromised. The latter patients include those suffering from AIDS and those being treated for cancer or undergoing immunosuppressive therapy after organ transplantation.

LATENCY AND THE EPIDEMIOLOGY OF HSV INFECTION

Underlying these various manifestations of HSV in the human host are particular interactions between virus and differentiated cells which are less readily modelled in tissue culture systems. HSV appears to have a predilection for cells of ectodermal origin. The virus typically gains entry at a mucosal site (often the mucocutaneous junction), where it destroys cells in the vicinity and provokes inflammatory responses. It is the combination of virus destruction and host immune and inflammatory responses to the presence of virus antigens and virus-infected and damaged cells which result in the familiar and sometimes painful blisters of cold sores and genital herpes. Virus translocates to the associated nerve ganglion and remains there in a state of latency. A variety of stimuli including trauma, menstruation and exposure to strong sunlight may give rise to reactivation, recurrent virus shedding and sometimes to recrudescent lesions (8).

It seems that virions gain access to the neurone cell bodies in the peripheral nerve ganglia by travelling from the original infection site within the axons. There is evidence that in the neurone cell body molecular pathways of productive and latent infection diverge early (10,11). In other words, the normal productive virus replication cycle may be modified at an early stage, and virus DNA then persists in the nucleus in a potentially infectious but quiescent form while the neurone appears to remain undamaged. Certain stimuli then produce reactivation of the quiescent virus resulting in the full replication cycle. Infectious virus then flows, by means of axonal transport, to the peripheral site. It is assumed that the reactivating neurone is destroyed during this phase. While latent virus in the neurones of the trigeminal and sacral ganglia appears to give rise to the typical patterns of labial and genital recurrent disease respectively in man, non-neural sites of latency, such as the cornea, have also been identified (12), and the possibility remains that latency may also be established within the human central nervous system (CNS). Experiments in laboratory animals have demonstrated latency in cells of the CNS (13–15) suggesting that the brain is also a possible site of latency in man. The ability of HSV to establish latency means that the infection does not depend on regular transmission to maintain the infection among a population. Indeed isolated groups containing less than 1000 individuals may continue to harbour the infection, whilst acute infections like the common cold are unsustainable in such populations. Furthermore, latent HSV is not susceptible to nucleoside analogue inhibitors, because such inhibitors depend for their activity on the expression of DE gene products (for example DNA polymerase) in the infected cells (16,17). These facts, together with the difficulties which have been encountered in developing safe and effective vaccines, make HSV a very difficult virus to eradicate.

THE NATURE OF LATENT HSV IN NEURONES

Stevens and Cook (18) were the first to demonstrate that, when latently infected mouse ganglia were explanted and maintained in culture for a few days, virus reactivation occurred spontaneously with the release of infectious virus into the culture medium. Virus reactivation by culture of explanted neural tissue was later demonstrated in human trigeminal (19,20) and sacral ganglia (21) and this provided useful direct evidence of the presence of latent HSV in those tissues. However, further analysis of latency relies on the detection of the latent virus itself. Molecular hybridization techniques have therefore been employed to detect virus nucleic acids in infected tissue. These studies have shown that latent HSV exists during latency in an 'endless' non-integrated form, most likely as closed circles or head-to-tail concatemers (22).

There appears to be limited transcription of the HSV genome in latently infected neurones. Latency-associated transcripts (LATs) map exclusively to the long terminal repeat of the genome, and are transcribed in the opposite direction to the ICP0 gene with which they overlap (23). The major LAT species is a stable intron of a larger primary transcript (24) which is generated by splicing in the neuronal nucleus. High-resolution *in situ* nucleic acid hybridization, using non-radioactive probes, has enabled accumulated spliced products to be localized to discrete intranuclear foci (25). Recent evidence suggests that neurones are better able to splice LATs than other cell types. There is no evidence that LATs are translated to give a latency-associated protein, but it seems that the LATs themselves may have a role in the maintenance and reactivation of latency (26). Mutant HSV with deletions in the LAT region and which lack the ability to produce LATs have been shown to establish latency, albeit with reduced frequency. Furthermore, it appears that many LAT^- mutants are impaired in reactivation. It has been suggested that LATs accumulate in latently infected neurones (27) and thereby have some role in triggering reactivation.

It seems, then, that the latently infected neurone contains no virus-induced enzymes with which antiviral agents such as nucleoside analogues (see section below) might interact. While such drugs may be effective against replicating virus in the treatment of acute infections, current knowledge of latency at the molecular level suggests that latent HSV is 'immune' from elimination by conventional antiviral drugs.

IN VITRO SYSTEMS FOR THE STUDY OF HSV LATENCY

Organ-derived systems

It is clearly a research goal to obtain simple and well-defined systems for the study of HSV latency *in vitro*. This is important in order to study the factors which govern the establishment, maintenance and reactivation of latent infections. It is also desirable to use such systems in the study of virus inhibitors which may affect HSV latency. One approach is to infect mice using an inoculation procedure which results in latent infections being established, then to explant the appropriate dorsal route ganglia and maintain these in culture. The influence of inhibitors on virus latency and reactivation may then be investigated. These methods suffer from the disadvantage that the explantation procedure itself, involving the severing of all axonal connections to the neurone cell bodies harbouring latent HSV, may provide a powerful reactivation stimulus. However, successful studies have been carried out using such procedures to investigate antiviral agents (28).

In vitro latency systems

Molecular and biochemical analysis of HSV latency *in vivo* is hampered by the small proportion of latently infected neurones available in nervous tissue as well as the complexity of experimental studies in the whole animal.

In vitro latency systems have been described in cell lines of neuronal and non-neuronal origin. In cells normally permissive for HSV replication, suppression of virus growth can be achieved by interferon or chemical inhibition (with or without a subsequent upward temperature shift) or by a temperature shift alone (29,30). Reactivation has been induced by downward temperature shift and/or superinfection with human cytomegalovirus.

The validity of such systems for modelling the reproducible establishment, maintenance and reactivation of HSV latency *in vivo* has been investigated. For example, as mentioned above, viral genomes in acutely infected cells are in linear configuration, whereas latent virus genomes in neurones *in vivo* are in an 'endless' configuration. The conformation of viral DNA has been analysed in two well-established latency systems: that of Wigdahl (31) and that of Preston and Russell (32). Wigdahl concluded that the predominant form of HSV-1 genomes in their system is as linear, unintegrated unit lengths, whereas Preston and Russell detect non-linear HSV-2 genomes in their system. On the basis of genome configuration, Preston and Russell's system seems to be the more accurate model of latency *in vivo*. However, there are several fundamental differences between the two systems, and it is possible that neither reproduce latency as seen *in vivo*.

Among the *in vitro* latency systems, those involving cells of neuronal origin are likely to be the most relevant to the understanding of the establishment and reactivation of latency *in vivo* and the possible influence of antiviral agents on these processes. Latency has been established in primary rat neurones following infection at low multiplicity, and the latent infection could be reactivated by removing nerve growth factor from the culture medium (33). Infection of non-permissive, proliferating neuroblastoma lines results in the establishment of latent infection in a high proportion of cells, but latent virus is not stably maintained (34). The technical difficulties associated with the study of latency in cultured neuronal cells mean that, at present, studies of gene function in *in vitro* latency are predominantly confined to the non-neuronal systems.

It is likely that in the future models similar to those described above will form an important part in the search for new strategies for HSV inhibitors, and for the elucidation of the mechanisms of action of those already available. However, to date, most of the work concerning the effects of inhibitors on virus pathogenesis (particularly their effects on the establishment and maintenance of latency and on reactivation from the latent state) has all come from the study of a variety of laboratory animal models for HSV, and these will be considered below.

INHIBITORS OF HSV: THE DESIGN OF ANTIVIRAL AGENTS

CELL CULTURE SYSTEMS FOR TESTING ANTIVIRAL ACTIVITY

Because of the difficulties described above with *in vitro* latency systems, most of the work carried out on HSV inhibitors employs conventional tissue culture methods. Under conditions of high multiplicity of infection, cells in culture are seen to release the first infectious progeny from a few hours after infection and the virus replication cycle is complete within 24 h. Up to a few hundred mature infectious virions may be released from each cell; the virus yield from culture fluid or from disrupted cells can then be measured readily. In addition, destruction of the infected cells is manifest as 'cytopathic effect' visible under the light microscope. For example, under conditions of low multiplicity infection, individual foci of cytopathic effect called plaques arise from each originally infected cell. This observation has given rise to the plaque assay—the most important method for quantifying infectivity. In recent years, however, other methods for detecting virus replication (for example, ELISA for virus antigen) have also been employed. All these methods for assessing virus growth have been adapted for measuring the activity of virus inhibitors. Thus antiviral assays have been based on plaque reduction (usually 50% or 90%), virus yield reduction and on the inhibition of cytopathic effect. In an attempt to make the latter method more objective, tests have been developed which depend on the uptake of dye by non-viable cells. Cultures are infected at high multiplicity and after two to three days the dye uptake by the culture is measured colorimetrically. This technique is well suited to automation and has been employed for large-scale screens of compounds and virus isolates (35).

LABORATORY ANIMAL MODELS OF HSV INFECTION

Current understanding of the highly complex virus–host relationship which follows initial infection with HSV in man owes much to the study of a variety of animal models. Indeed, a great deal of the basic knowledge of the tissue distribution of HSV in the host was acquired in the 1920s using infected rabbits, long before the infectious agent had been characterized (36). Today a variety of well-characterized animal models are available in which mice, rats, rabbits or guinea-pigs are infected so as to mimic the various human clinical syndromes (28). These include labial, genital and ocular lesions, encephalitis and latterly disease in the immunocompromised patient.

The most extraordinary aspect of such models is that, despite the fact that herpesviruses are generally regarded as host specific, the crucial features of latency and reactivation can be demonstrated reproducibly. Indeed, biochemical evidence to date suggests that the molecular state of virus in latently infected neurones of laboratory mice is identical or at least very similar to that which occurs in man (37). Such models have been widely employed in the study of chemotherapy for HSV infections (38–40). For example, the effects of antiviral chemotherapy can be studied by observing reduction in clinical signs, quantitative virus yield in target organs, histopathological changes and, in some cases, effects on immune responses. Molecular studies of virus distribution and latency are also becoming increasingly important. The findings obtained in this way in several laboratory animal systems have proved to be accurate predictors of antiviral activity in man (28,41). When misleading data have been reported, this is often through inadequate interpretation of the findings. In some cases, perhaps, had more factors been taken into account the results could have been better interpreted to more accurately reflect the human case.

A particularly important aspect of some animal systems is the ability to study not only the events which take place during the acute phase of virus growth (that is, during the first few days or weeks following inoculation), but also the establishment and reactivation of latent infections. There are a number of models in which latent infections can be observed to undergo reactivation with virus shedding, and these provide systems for studying the effects of inhibitors on recurrence. For example, guinea-pigs inoculated with HSV-2 undergo spontaneous reactivation of genital infection (42). Following inoculation of the ear pinnae of mice with HSV-1, reactivation can be induced by mild trauma to the ear such as Sellotape stripping (43). Ocular recurrence may be successfully precipitated in corneally infected rabbits given adrenaline (epinephrine) iontophoresis (44). These are all powerful models which have been used to study the effects of virus inhibitors such as acyclovir (ACV) and BVDU (see below) on complex aspects of HSV pathogenesis.

THE SEARCH FOR INHIBITORS OF HSV

The first inhibitors of herpesvirus were discovered without the detailed knowledge of virus replication at the molecular level described above. The first compounds to be usefully employed against HSV were nucleoside analogues whose antiviral activity had come to light as a by-product of the search for DNA inhibitors for use as antitumour agents. It was the study of such inhibitors which led to the first recognition of virus-coded enzymes such as thymidine kinase and DNA polymerase. It became possible to develop *in vitro* enzyme assays in order to study interactions between inhibitors and their targets directly. These cell-free systems have been developed during the course of several decades and are increasingly used in the search for novel compounds with specific targets.

NUCLEOSIDE ANALOGUES

A list of nucleoside analogues which have been licensed to date for use in man in the UK is shown in Table 5.1. Initially these were uncomplicated molecules which resembled, more or less, the natural pyrimidine and purine nucleosides. The earliest compounds to be described were IDU, which has a halogen atom at the 5- position in the pyrimidine ring, and ara-A in which the configuration of the sugar moiety is changed by virtue of having the —OH in the 3′- position of the sugar ring in the unnatural 'ara' configuration.

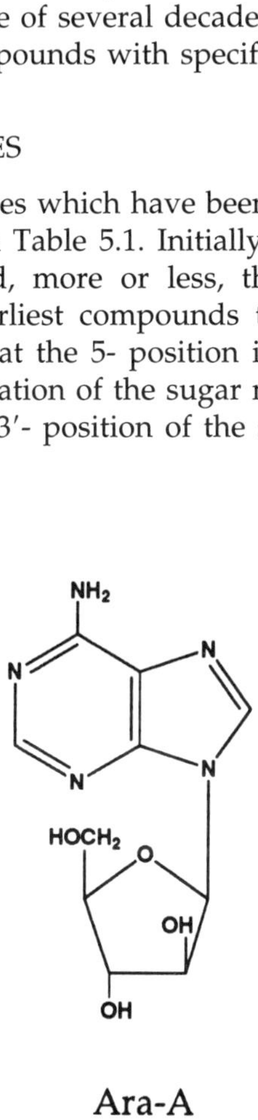

Ara-A

THE MODE OF ACTION OF NUCLEOSIDE ANALOGUES

The activity of all the useful nucleoside analogue inhibitors of HSV depends on their phosphorylation to their respective mono-, di- and triphosphates (45). The nucleotide then interferes with DNA metabolism in the infected cells. Several synthetic pathways are theoretical targets, but apparently the

Table 5.1. Nucleoside analogues licensed in the UK for use in man

Compound	Type of infection	Administration
Adenine arabinoside (ara-A)	Herpes simplex virus (HSV) encephalitis	Systemic
	Ophthalmic HSV infections	Topical
Iododeoxyuridine (IDU)	Labial, genital and ophthalmic HSV infections	Topical
	Shingles (varicella zoster virus (VZV))	Topical
Trifluorothymidine (TFT)	Ophthalmic HSV infections	Topical
Acyclovir (ACV)	Herpes simplex encephalitis	Systemic
	Labial, genital and ophthalmic HSV infection	Systemic/topical
	Shingles (VZV)	Systemic/topical
Ganciclovir (GCV)	Cytomegalovirus retinitis in the immunocompromised	Systemic
Famciclovir	Shingles (VZV)	Systemic

dominant effect is interference with DNA replication. This has been found to be of different types, for example the nucleoside triphosphate may inhibit the polymerase enzyme and thus prevent the incorporation of normal nucleotides into DNA. This is the case with acyclovir (ACV), which lacks the OH group in the 3′-position of the sugar. This OH group is necessary to form the diester bond with the next nucleotide to be incorporated into the growing DNA molecule, and its absence thus causes premature chain termination (46). Alternatively, the nucleoside triphosphate may be incorporated into virus DNA itself, rendering the substituted DNA non-functional, as is the case with iododeoxyuridine (see below) (47). As stated above, the nucleoside analogue triphosphates could have a variety of alternative effects on synthetic pathways in the cell, and some have been reported, such as inhibition of glycoprotein synthesis (7). Although such mechanisms may be demonstrated *in vitro*, the evidence from the characterization of resistant mutants, whose genetic lesions habitually map to the virus thymidine kinase and DNA polymerase genes (see below), suggests that glycoprotein synthesis is a relatively unimportant site of inhibition. It remains to be seen if these more minor targets of nucleoside analogue action make a contribution to the overall inhibition of virus replication, and whether such mechanisms could take on even more significance *in vivo* where, of course, such effects are very difficult to assess.

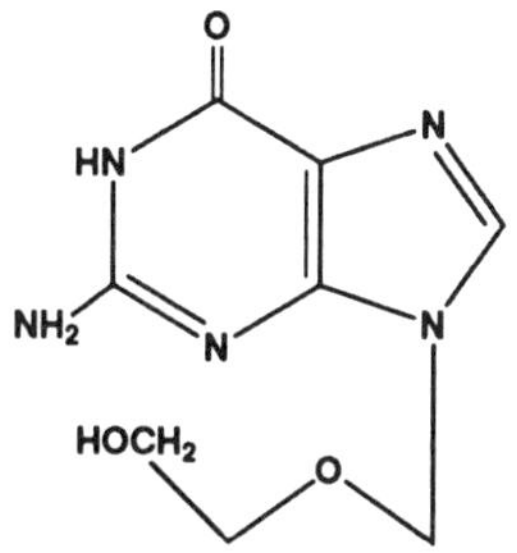

ACV

THE DEVELOPMENT OF NUCLEOSIDE ANALOGUES WITH IMPROVED SELECTIVE TOXICITY

Two early inhibitors of HSV to be used in man were iododeoxyuridine (IDU) and trifluorothymidine (TFT). These compounds lack specificity for virus-coded activation and are readily activated by cellular kinases—enzymes which phosphorylate the compounds in uninfected cells (although the rate of nucleoside analogue activation may be higher in infected cells). As a result, these two compounds are too toxic for systemic administration and have been useful for topical application only. Such compounds are now referred to as first-generation nucleoside analogues.

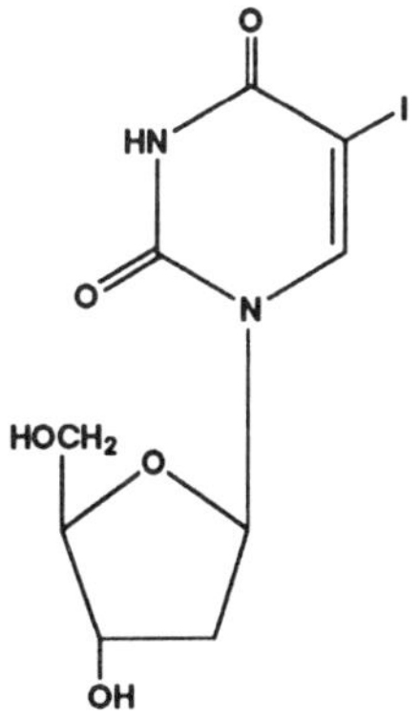

IDU

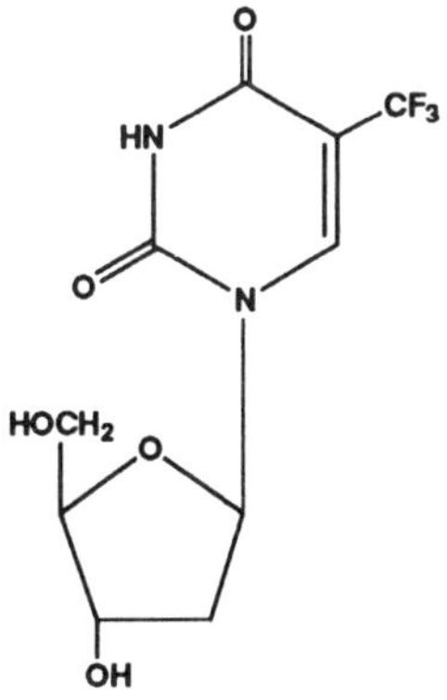

TFT

In contrast to TFT and IDU, some more recently discovered compounds, for example acyclovir (ACV) and penciclovir (PCV), are selectively phosphorylated by means of the viral enzyme thymidine kinase (TK) (48,49).

Actively dividing mammalian cells express TK activity themselves in both the cytoplasmic and mitochondrial cell compartments. However, the properties of the cellular enzymes have been shown to differ significantly from those which are virus-coded (50). Predictions on the relative selectivity of potential nucleosides can thus be obtained by kinetic analysis of their interactions with the relevant virus- and cell-coded enzymes in cell-free systems. The herpesvirus TK can generally accept a wider range of nucleoside substrates than the cellular enzymes, and will also phosphorylate ACV and PCV, whereas the cellular enzymes less readily accept these molecules as substrates. Highly selective compounds such as ACV and PCV have been termed second-generation nucleoside analogues.

HSV TK therefore provides the essential key to selective antiviral activity of ACV, since only cells containing actively replicating virus are able to convert ACV to ACV monophosphate. Cellular enzymes then convert the monophosphate to the diphosphate, and ACV diphosphate to ACV triphosphate (ACV-TP). Although ACV is a thymidine analogue, ACV-TP competes with dGTP to interfere with the herpesvirus DNA polymerase. It may be worth mentioning here that ACV is not a particularly good substrate for HSV TK, and the rate of phosphorylation is reckoned to be slow. However, the triphosphate, once formed, is a potent inhibitor of HSV DNA polymerase and the inhibition constant (K_i value) for ACV-TP versus the natural substrate, dGTP, has been reported to be as low as 0.1 μM (51). Moreover, cellular DNA polymerase α is found to be significantly less sensitive to ACV-TP than is HSV DNA polymerase (52), thus providing a second level of selectivity in the mechanism of action.

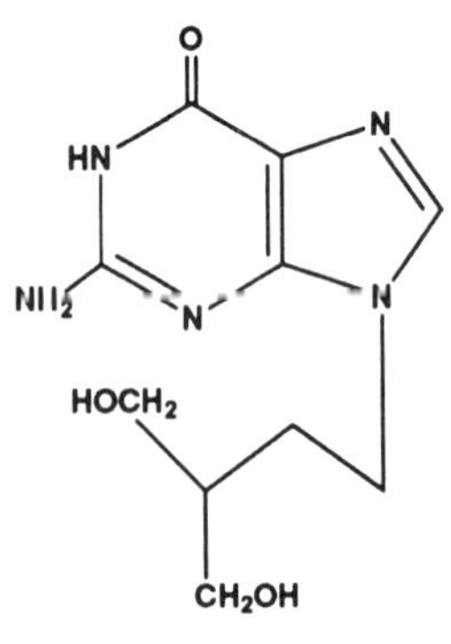

PCV

THE THYMIDYLATE KINASE ACTIVITY OF HSV-1 TK

HSV-1 TK differs from cellular TKs in that it is also capable of converting dTMP to dTDP, that is, it has thymidylate kinase activity. As a consequence, certain nucleoside analogues, for example BVDU, are converted by HSV TK directly to their respective nucleoside diphosphates in infected cells (53). In the case of BVDU this is thought to be a major factor in the relative insensitivity of HSV-2 strains compared to HSV-1. In other words, HSV-2-infected cells can convert BVDU to BVDU-MP but the diphosphate of the nucleoside analogue is not produced because the substrate specificity of the HSV-2 thymidylate kinase activity appears to be more restricted (54).

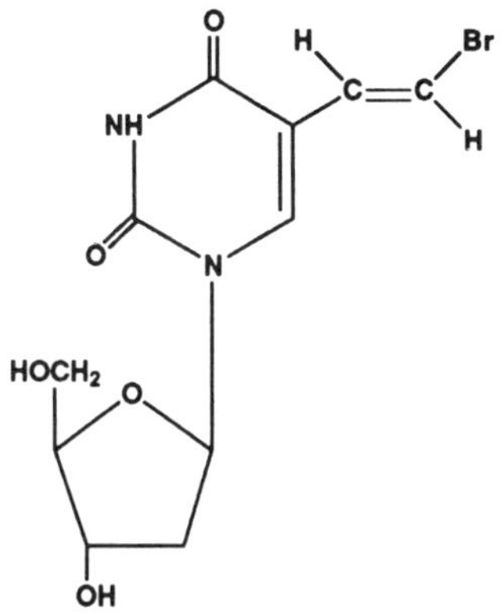

BVDU

ACTIVE NUCLEOSIDE ANALOGUES WITH NO OBVIOUS CLINICAL POTENTIAL

Chemical synthetic programmes have generated literally hundreds of alternative nucleoside analogues many of which have been shown, either in enzyme screens or tissue culture systems, to be potential inhibitors of HSV. Many compounds with putative antiviral activity have structures far removed from the original nucleosides from which they were derived, yet they may be phosphorylated by the HSV TK and/or inhibit virus DNA polymerase. Despite their antiviral activity, however, some compounds have been rejected because they are dangerous: for example 5-bromo-2′-deoxyuridine (BDU), which has mutagenic properties (55). Others, like ara-C, are toxic for cells and have more use as cytostatic drugs for anticancer therapy. Several compounds have looked very promising during their early development, for example FIAC. However, FIAC has not progressed to clinical trials for the treatment of HSV infections in man. This is because the metabolism of the compound in the host results in the formation of several secondary products, some of which are toxic (56).

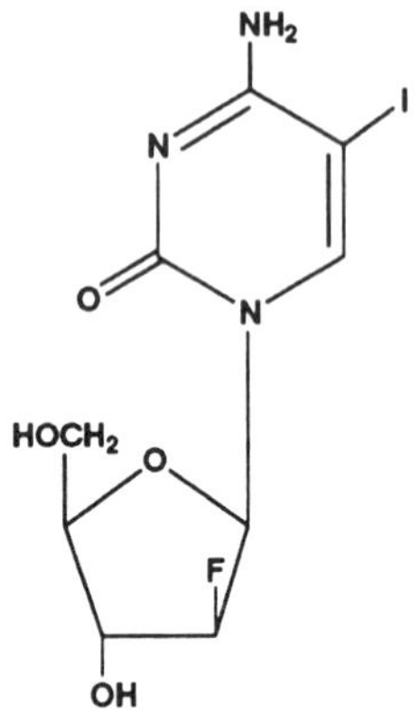

FIAC

STRUCTURE–ACTIVITY RELATIONSHIPS AND THE SELECTION OF COMPOUNDS FOR FURTHER INVESTIGATION

Attempts to develop a rational approach to the chemical design of new nucleoside analogues have involved the correlation of changes in a specific part of the molecule with changes in biological activity (that is, antiviral spectrum and toxicity). These are referred to as studies of structure–activity relationships and there are many published examples (57). It is likely that many compounds with less antiviral activity than the lead structure from which they are derived have yet to be widely tested *in vivo*, and further useful compounds may emerge from such lists in the future. This is in addition to a number of new potent second-generation nucleosides which are currently under intense development prior to possible use in man within the next few years.

Included among the newer compounds are several prodrugs of the second-generation nucleoside analogues. These compounds have no intrinsic antiviral activity, but are metabolized in the host to yield the active compound. The prodrug may have much better bioavailability than the active compound, for example as a result of improved gastrointestinal absorption. Two such prodrugs are 6-deoxy-6-aminoacylacyclovir valaciclovir (58), and famciclovir (49,59), the oral form of PCV.

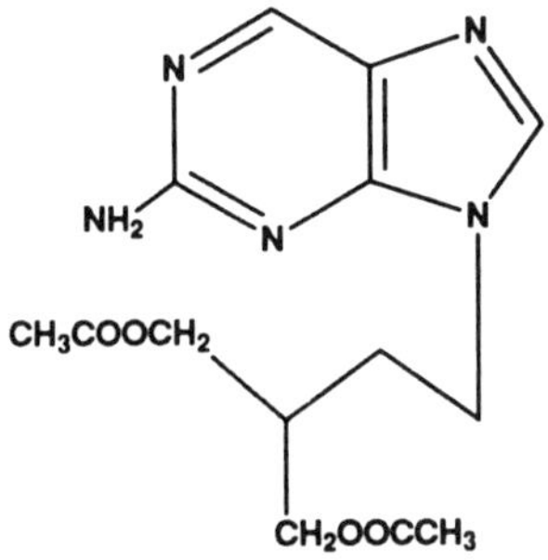

FCV

PYROPHOSPHATE ANALOGUE INHIBITORS OF HSV

These compounds are not nucleoside analogues, but they share with the nucleoside analogues the ability to inhibit the replication of HSV by interfering with its DNA metabolism. The two pyrophosphate analogues phosphonoacetic acid (PAA) and phosphonoformic acid (PFA) inhibit the herpesvirus DNA polymerase, as demonstrated in a cell-free assay, apparently by interacting with the pyrophosphate binding site on the DNA polymerase enzyme (60,61). The compounds may not have much potential as first-line antiviral agents, but the spectrum of virus resistance to them is unusual (see below), and they may have a role as alternative compounds for treatment of drug-resistant HSV infections.

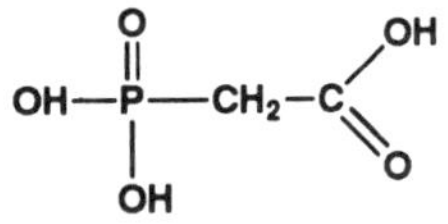

PAA

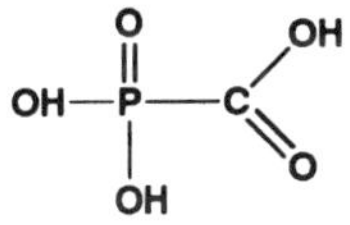

PFA

PROBLEMS IN HSV CHEMOTHERAPY: RESISTANCE AND LATENCY

THE STUDY OF HSV RESISTANCE TO ANTIVIRAL COMPOUNDS

One of the most important areas of fundamental research into the inhibitors of HSV has been, and remains, the study of resistance development. The reasons for this are as follows.

1. The demonstration of resistance development to a given drug gives direct evidence for a virus-specific mode of action which must be independent of anticellular effects or of host effects such as immunomodulation.
2. The characterization of resistant mutants reveals the genetic change leading to resistance and thus gives direct evidence for virus gene products involved in the mechanism of action.
3. The study of mutant viruses selected for drug resistance gives clues to the role of virus products in pathogenesis.
4. The study of laboratory mutants enables screening assays to be developed for the detection of resistant strains in clinical practice.
5. The investigation of resistance development in laboratory models enables strategies to be designed for the prevention or treatment of resistance.

Since the introduction of iododeoxyuridine (IDU) in the early 1960s, the laboratory study of resistant strains has fulfilled all the objectives listed above. This is best exemplified by the research which has accompanied the development of ACV. Isolation of resistant virus by passage of HSV-1 or HSV-2 in the presence of inhibitory concentrations of ACV have revealed two classes of mutants. In one class resistance maps to the *tk* gene, and in the other class DNA polymerase contains the genetic lesion (62,63). Mutants also exist in which resistance maps to both genes. The enzymes isolated from the resistant viruses have been found to be significantly reduced in their ability to interact with the nucleoside or, in the case of DNA polymerase mutants, the nucleoside triphosphate. HSV TK is not essential for virus replication in tissue culture and many TK mutants have lost completely the ability to induce this enzyme. Other mutants induce a modified form of the enzyme with altered substrate specificity (64–66). Mutants of both types (DNA polymerase and TK with altered substrate specificity) have been analysed by means of DNA sequencing and the respective genes found to contain single base substitutions, implying that single amino acid substitutions had been generated in the respective polymerase and TK polypeptides (67–70).

Thus, laboratory study enables the complete elucidation of the resistant phenotype in terms of the changed biochemical property of the enzyme and the underlying genetic change in the virus DNA. This provides a powerful approach to the design of new or alternative substrate analogues.

One intriguing aspect of laboratory studies of resistance is the finding that in animal model infections mutants are often reported to be attenuated (71). This applies in particular to the TK-defective mutant and, to a lesser extent, to the other types of mutant. Furthermore, it has proved very difficult to isolate resistant virus from animals undergoing treatment with the drug in question. To date, antiviral resistance has not emerged as a major problem in man, except in immunocompromised patients, and the explanation would seem to be that most resistant mutants show reduced pathogenicity.

In the immunocompromised patient, resistant viruses have been isolated with regularity and can give rise to infections which are intransigent to therapy (72). Virus isolates from such infections have been characterized and shown to conform exactly to the patterns of resistance predicted from the earlier laboratory studies. Moreover, viruses have been isolated from such clinical cases with identical nucleotide substitutions to those previously identified in laboratory mutants (67,73). One feature of drug resistance which was quickly established in laboratory models was the fact that resistant isolates may not be homogeneous but often comprise a mixture of sensitive and resistant strains, and this also appears to be the case in human infections, especially in the immunocompromised patient (74). The understanding of the significance of this phenomenon, and the development of alternative therapeutic regimens such as combination therapy, will rely heavily on the judicious use of cell culture systems and animal models.

LABORATORY ANIMAL MODELS OF THE CHEMOTHERAPY OF HSV INFECTION

As mentioned above, many models for HSV have been described at length in the literature. These include infections of the skin, genitalia, eye and CNS in both normal and immunologically compromised laboratory animals. Many of these models have also been employed extensively in the study of antiviral agents active against HSV, using topical or systemic administration. The resulting data, if subjected to an educated evaluation, may then yield conclusions which can be tentatively extrapolated to the clinical situation. It is particularly important to consider the following.

1. The uptake, metabolism and anatomical distribution of compounds can differ markedly in different species. The route of administration, dose, intervals between doses and duration of therapy must all be taken into account.
2. The activity of the drug in cell cultures derived from the animal species in question must be compared with activity in cells of human origin. Cells of different species may differ markedly in their response to particular compounds and apparent virus sensitivity thus may vary widely. Cells of different lineage, differentiation state and multiplication state may also have a bearing on virus sensitivity to a given drug.
3. Some methods of virus inoculation result in pathogenesis which varies widely from that which occurs naturally; for example, intracerebral or intraperitoneal inoculation gives rise to a rapidly fatal encephalitis in mice, whereas intranasal inoculation gives a pathogenesis which appears to resemble more closely the progression of the human disease.

The factors mentioned above may underlie significant differences between HSV infection and chemotherapy in animal models and that of man. However, if these differences can be taken into account quantitatively, then extrapolation to man is theoretically possible. In an attempt to bridge the gap between animal experiments and observations in tissue culture, parallel work is carried out using cells derived from the animal species in comparison with human cells. In some cases differences between resting and multiplying cells have been taken into account, and systems for maintaining skin *in vitro* have been described and employed with effect to study the uptake and penetration of topically applied agents (75). On the whole, the animal data obtained in the study of trifluorothymidine (TFT), IDU, ara-A and ACV have essentially been confirmed by observations made during the subsequent use of these drugs in clinical practice (76,77). With increased knowledge of species differences in the uptake and metabolism of drugs, the ability to predict efficacy will be further improved. Such models are now of the utmost importance when dealing with the more subtle effects which a drug may have upon herpesvirus pathogenesis, including the establishment and maintenance of latency, the suppression of recurrent infections or the modification of immune responses to infection (28).

Recently, interest in herpesvirus infections has focused on the particular problems which they can cause in the immunocompromised patient. Of particular importance is the finding that drug-resistant variants occur in such patients and cause lesions which are intransigent to therapy. Immunocompromised mice, for example athymic (nude) mice, or mice treated with immunosuppressive drugs such as cyclosporin A, have already been shown to yield drug-resistant virus isolates following therapy. Furthermore, these are powerful models in which to investigate treatment modalities which are less likely to yield resistance, as well as alternative drugs or drug combinations to treat the resistant infection once established (78).

CONCLUSION

In this chapter we have reviewed the current state of knowledge of HSV in relation to the development of antiviral chemotherapy. HSV infection has proved gratifyingly susceptible to chemotherapy. Some of the most spectacular successes have occurred in the therapy of particularly severe manifestations of HSV infection, such as encephalitis, generalized infections in the newborn, and severe infections in the immunocompromised. The fact that so much is known about the nature of HSV gives us confidence in the understanding of the modes of action of the drugs currently in use, and suggests strategies for the development of new compounds and drug combinations. However, research has also revealed the extraordinary complexity of virus–host relationships, both at the level of the single cell and in the milieu of the multicellular host. As we are able to interfere increasingly effectively with the normal processes of virus replication and disease, there will undoubtedly be unexpected observations in the clinic as the drugs are used ever more widely in man. Herpesvirus research over the greater part of this century provides a model for the close interplay between laboratory scientist and clinician.

REFERENCES

1. Roizman, B. (1990). Herpesviridae: a brief introduction. In *Virology*, B. N. Fields, D. M. Knipe *et al.* (eds), Raven Press, New York, pp. 1787–1794.
2. McGeoch, D. J. (1989). The genomes of the human herpesviruses: contents, relationship and evolution. *Annu. Rev. Microbiol.*, **43**, 235–265.
3. Campbell, M. E. M., Palfreyman, J. W. and Preston, C. M. (1984). Identification of herpes simplex virus DNA sequences which encode a trans-acting polypeptide responsible for stimulation of immediate early transcription. *J. Mol. Biol.*, **180**, 1–19.
4. Roizman, B. and Sears, A. E. (1990). Herpes simplex viruses and their replication. In *Virology*, B. N. Fields, D. M. Knipe *et al.* (eds), Raven Press, New York, pp. 1795–1842.
5. Jacob, R. J., Morse, L. S. and Roizman, B. (1979). Anatomy of herpes simplex virus DNA. XII. Accumulation of head to tail concatemers in the nuclei of infected cells and their role in the generation of four isomeric arrangements of viral DNA. *J. Virol.*, **29**, 448–457.
6. Datema, R., Olofsson, S. and Romero, P. (1987). Inhibitors of protein glycosylation and glycoprotein processing in viral systems. *Pharmacol. Ther.*, **33**, 221–286.
7. Olofsson, S. and Datema, R. (1990). New virus-selective inhibitor of terminal glycosylation increasing immunological reactivity of a viral glycoprotein. *Antiviral Chem. Chemother.*, **1**, 17–24.
8. Whitley, R. J. (1990). Herpes simplex viruses. In *Virology*, B. N. Fields, D. M. Knipe *et al.* (eds), Raven Press, New York, pp. 1843–1888.
9. Whitley, R. J. (1990). Viral encephalitis. *N. Engl. J. Med.*, **26**, 242–250.
10. Speck, P. G. and Simmons, A. (1991). Divergent molecular pathways of productive and latent infection with a virulent strain of herpes simplex virus type 1. *J. Virol.*, **65**, 4001–4005.
11. Speck, P. G. and Simmons, A. (1992). Synchronous appearance of antigen-positive and latently infected neurons in spinal ganglia of mice infected with a virulent strain of herpes simplex virus. *J. Gen. Virol.*, **73**, 1281–1285.
12. Tullo, A. B., Easty, D. L., Shimeld, C. *et al.* (1985). Isolation of herpes simplex virus from corneal discs of patients with chronic stromal keratitis. *Trans. Ophthalmol. Soc.*, **104**, 159–165.
13. Knotts, F. B., Cook, M. L. and Stevens, J. G. (1973). Latent herpes simplex virus in the central nervous system of rabbits and mice. *J. Exp. Med.*, **138**, 740–744.
14. Stroop, W. G. and Schaefer, D. C. (1986). Production of encephalitis restricted to the temporal lobes by experimental reactivation of herpes simplex virus. *J. Infect. Dis.*, **153**, 721–731.
15. Stroop, W. G., Rock, D. L. and Fraser, N. W. (1984). Localisation of herpes simplex virus in the trigeminal ganglia and olfactory systems of the mouse central nervous system during acute and latent infections by in situ hybridization. *Lab. Invest.*, **51**, 27–38.

16. Field, H. J., Bell, S. E., Elion, G. B. *et al.* (1979). Effect of acycloguanosine treatment on acute and latent herpes simplex infections in mice. *Antimicrob. Agents Chemother.*, **15**, 554–561.
17. Field, H. J. and De Clercq, E. (1981). Effects of oral treatment with acyclovir and bromovinyldeoxyuridine on the establishment and maintenance of latent herpes simplex virus. *J. Gen. Virol.*, **56**, 259–265.
18. Stevens, J. G. and Cook, M. L. (1971). Latent herpes simplex virus in spinal ganglia of mice. *Science*, **173**, 843–845.
19. Bastian, F. O., Rabson, A. S., Yee, C. L. and Tralka, T. S. (1972). Herpesvirus hominis: isolation from human trigeminal ganglion. *Science*, **178**, 306–307.
20. Baringer, J. R. and Swoveland, M. (1973). Recovery of herpes simplex virus from human trigeminal ganglions. *N. Engl. J. Med.*, **288**, 648–650.
21. Baringer, J. R. (1974). Recovery of herpes simplex virus from human sacral ganglia. *N. Engl. J. Med.*, **291**, 828–830.
22. Rock, D. L. and Fraser, N. W. (1983). Detection of herpes simplex virus genomes in the central nervous system of latently infected mice. *Nature*, **302**, 523–525.
23. Stevens, J. G. (1989). Human herpesviruses: a consideration of the latent state. *Microbiol. Rev.*, **53**, 318–332.
24. Farrell, M. J., Dobson, A. T. and Feldman, L. T. (1991). Herpes simplex virus latency-associated transcript is a stable intron. *Proc. Natl Acad. Sci. USA*, **88**, 790–794.
25. Arthur, J., Efstathiou, S. and Simmons, A. (1993). Intranuclear foci containing low abundance herpes simplex virus latency associated transcripts by non-isotopic *in situ* hybridization. *J. Gen. Virol.*, in press.
26. Nsiah, Y. A. and Rapp, F. (1991). Role of latency associated transcript in herpes simplex virus infection. *Intervirology*, **32**, 101–115.
27. Speck, P. G. (1992). Analysis of establishment of latent infection with a virulent strain of herpes simplex virus type 1. PhD thesis, University of Adelaide, Australia.
28. Field, H. J. and Brown, G. A. (1989). Animal models for antiviral chemotherapy. *Antiviral Res.*, **12**, 165–180.
29. Wigdahl, B. L., Scheck, A. C., De Clercq, E. and Rapp, R. (1982). High efficiency latency and activation of herpes simplex virus in human cells. *Science*, **217**, 1145–1146.
30. Russell, J. and Preston, C. M. (1986). An in vitro system for herpes simplex virus type 2. *J. Gen. Virol.*, **67**, 397–403.
31. Wigdahl, B. L., Scheck, A. C., Ziegler, R. J. *et al.* (1984). Analysis of the herpes simplex virus genome during in vitro latency in human diploid fibroblasts and rat sensory neurons. *J. Virol.*, **49**, 205–213.
32. Preston, C. M. and Russell, J. (1990). Retention of non-linear viral DNA during herpes simplex virus latency in vitro. *Intervirology*, **32**, 69–75.
33. Wilcox, C. L. and Johnson, E. M. (1988). Characterization of nerve growth factor-dependent herpes simplex virus latency in neurons. *J. Virol.*, **62**, 393–399.
34. Latchman, D. S. (1990). Current status review: molecular biology of herpes simplex virus latency. *J. Exp. Pathol.*, **71**, 133–141.
35. McLaren, C., Ellis, M. N. and Hunter, G. A. (1983). A colorimetric assay for the measurement of the sensitivity of herpes simplex virus to antiviral agents. *Antiviral Res.*, **3**, 223–234.
36. Goodpasture, E. W. and Teague, M. D. (1923). Experimental production of herpetic lesions in organs and tissues of the rabbit. *J. Med. Res.*, **44**, 121–199.
37. Efstathiou, S., Minson, A. C., Field, H. J. *et al.* (1986). Detection of herpes simplex

virus specific DNA sequences in latently infected mice and in man. *J. Virol.*, **57**, 446–455.

38. Field, H. J., Anderson, J. R. and Efstathiou, S. (1984). A quantitative study of the effects of several different nucleoside analogues on established herpes encephalitis in mice. *J. Gen. Virol.*, **65**, 707–719.
39. Datema, R., Ericson, A.-C., Field, H. J. *et al.* (1987). Critical determinants of antiherpes efficacy of buciclovir and related acyclic guanosine analogs. *Antiviral Res.*, **7**, 303–316.
40. Boyd, M. R., Bacon, T. H. and Sutton, D. (1988). Antiherpesvirus activity of 9-(4-hydroxy-3-hydroxymethyl-1-yl) guanine (BRL39123) in animals. *Antimicrob. Agents Chemother.*, **32**, 358–363.
41. Field, H. J. (1989). Persistent herpes simplex virus infection and mechanisms of virus drug resistance. *Eur. J. Clin. Microbiol.*, **8**, 671–680.
42. Stanberry, L. R., Harrison, C. J., Bravo, F. J. *et al.* (1990). Recurrent genital herpes in the guinea pig augmented by U.V. irradiation: effects of treatment with acyclovir. *Antiviral Res.*, **13**, 227–236.
43. Hill, T. J., Blyth, W. A. and Harbour, D. A. (1978). Trauma of the skin causes recurrence of herpes simplex in the mouse. *J. Gen. Virol.*, **39**, 21–28.
44. Hill, J. M. and Kwon, B. S. (1987). Effects of acyclovir therapy during simultaneous reactivation of latent HSV-1 in rabbits. *Antiviral Res.*, **7**, 237–243.
45. Elion, G. B. (1986). History, mechanism of action, spectrum and selectivity of nucleoside analogues. In *Antiviral Chemotherapy: New Directions for Clinical Application and Research*, J. Mills and L. Corey (eds), Elsevier, Amsterdam, pp. 118–137.
46. Furman, P. A., St Clair, M. H. and Spector, T. (1984). Acyclovir triphosphate is a suicide inactivator of the herpes simplex virus DNA polymerase. *J. Biol. Chem.*, **259**, 9575–9579.
47. Prusoff, W. H., Bakhle, Y. S. and Sekely, L. (1965). Cellular and antiviral effects of halogenated deoxyribonucleotides. *Ann. NY Acad. Sci.*, **130**, 135.
48. Fyfe, J. A., Keller, P. M., Furman, P. A. *et al.* (1978). Thymidine kinase from herpes simplex virus phosphorylates the new antiviral compound 9-(2-hydroxyethoxymethyl)guanine. *J. Biol. Chem.*, **253**, 8721–8727.
49. Vere Hodge, R. A., Sutton, D., Boyd, M. R. *et al.* (1989). Selection of an oral prodrug (BRL 42810; famciclovir) for the antiherpes agent BRL 39123 [9-(4-hydroxy-3-hydroxymethylbut-1-yl)guanine; penciclovir]. *Antimicrob. Agents Chemother.*, **33**, 1765–1773.
50. Cheng, Y.-C., Dutschman, G., De Clercq, E. *et al.* (1981). Differential affinities of 5-(2-halogenovinyl)-2′-deoxyuridines for deoxythymidine kinases of various origins. *Mol. Pharmacol.*, **20**, 230–233.
51. Elion, G. B. (1983). The biochemistry and mechanism of action of acyclovir. *J. Antimicrob. Chemother.*, **12** (Suppl. B), 9–17.
52. Derse, D., Cheng, Y.-C., Furman, P. A. *et al.* (1981). Inhibition of purified human and herpes simplex virus-induced DNA polymerase by 9-(2-hydroxyethoxymethyl)guanine triphosphate: effects on primer template function. *J. Biol. Chem.*, **256**, 11447–11451.
53. Prusoff, W. H. and Lin, T.-S. (1988). Experimental aspects of antiviral chemotherapy. In *Antiviral Drug Development*, E. De Clercq and R. T. Walker (eds), Plenum Press, New York, p. 175.
54. Fyfe, J. A. (1982). Differential phosphorylation of (*E*)-5-(2-bromovinyl-2′-deoxyuridine monophosphate by thymidylate kinases from herpes simplex viruses types 1 and 2 and varicella zoster virus. *Mol. Pharmacol.*, **21**, 432–437.

55. Perry, P. E. (1980). Chemical mutagenesis and sister chromatid exchange. In *Chemical Mutagens, Principles and Methods for their Detection*, F. J. de Seves and A. Hollaender (eds), Plenum Press, New York, p. 1.
56. Chou, T.-C., Feinberg, A., Grant, A. J. *et al.* (1981). Pharmacological disposition and metabolic fate of 2′-fluoro-5-iodo-1-β-D-arabinofuranosylcytosine in mice and rats. *Cancer Res.*, **41**, 3336.
57. De Clercq, E. (1983). Pyrimidine nucleoside analogues as antiviral agents. In *Targets for the Design of Antiviral Agents*, E. De Clercq and R. T. Walker (eds), Plenum Press, New York, pp. 203–230.
58. De Miranda, P. and Burnette, T. C. (1992). Metabolism and pharmacokinetics of the acyclovir prodrug BW 256U87 in cynomolgus monkeys. *Antiviral Res.*, **17** (Suppl. 1), 53.
59. Harnden, M. R., Jarvest, R. L., Boyd, M. R. *et al.* (1989). Prodrugs of the selective antiherpesvirus agent 9-[4-hydroxy-3-(hydroxymethyl)but-1-yl]guanine (BRL39123) with improved gastrointestinal absorption properties. *J. Med. Chem.*, **32**, 1738–1743.
60. Leinbach, S. S., Reno, G. M., Lee, L.F. *et al.* (1976). Mechanisms of phosphonoacetate inhibition of herpes virus-induced DNA polymerase. *Biochemistry*, **15**, 426–430.
61. Oberg, B. (1983). Antiviral effects of phosphonoformate (PFA, foscarnet sodium). *Pharmacol. Ther.*, **19**, 387–415.
62. Coen, D. M. and Schaffer, P. A. (1980). Two distinct loci confer resistance to acycloguanosine in herpes simplex virus type 1. *Proc. Natl Acad. Sci. USA*, **77**, 2265–2269.
63. Schnipper, L. E. and Crumpacker, C. S. (1980). Resistance of herpes simplex virus to acycloguanosine: role of viral thymidine kinase and DNA polymerase loci. *Proc. Natl Acad. Sci. USA*, **77**, 2270–2273.
64. Darby, G., Field, H. J. and Salisbury, S. A. (1981). Altered substrate specificity of herpes simplex virus thymidine kinase confers acyclovir resistance. *Nature*, **289**, 81–83.
65. Larder, B. A., Cheng, Y.-C. and Darby, G. (1983). Characterization of abnormal thymidine kinases induced by drug-resistant strains of herpes simplex virus type 1. *J. Gen. Virol.*, **64**, 523–532.
66. Veerisetty, V. and Gentry, G. A. (1983). Alterations in substrate specificity and physicochemical properties of deoxythymidine kinase of a drug-resistant herpes simplex virus type 1 mutant. *J. Virol.*, **46**, 901–908.
67. Darby, G., Larder, B. A. and Inglis, M. M. (1986). Evidence that the 'active centre' of the herpes simplex virus thymidine kinase involves an interaction between three distinct regions of the polypeptide. *J. Gen. Virol.*, **67**, 753–758.
68. Kit, S., Sheppard, M., Ichimura, H. *et al.* (1987). Nucleotide sequence changes in the thymidine kinase gene of herpes simplex virus type 2 clones from a patient treated with acyclovir. *Antimicrob. Agents Chemother.*, **31**, 1483–1490.
69. Honess, R. W., Purifoy, D. J. M., Young, D. *et al.* (1984). Single mutations at many sites within the DNA polymerase locus of herpes simplex viruses can confer hypersensitivity to aphidicolin and resistance to phosphonoacetic acid. *J. Gen. Virol.*, **65**, 1–17.
70. Larder, B. A., Kemp, S. D. and Darby, G. (1987). Related functional domains in virus DNA polymerase. *EMBO J.*, **6**, 169–175.
71. Coen, D. M. (1991). Antiviral drug resistance. *Ann. NY Acad. Sci.*, **616**, 224–237.
72. Field, H. J. and Goldthorpe, S. E. (1989). Virus drug resistance. *Trends Pharmacol. Sci.*, **10**, 333–337.
73. Nugier, F., Collins, P., Larder, B. A. *et al.* (1991). Herpes simplex virus isolates

from an immunocompromised patient who failed to respond to acyclovir treatment express thymidine kinase with altered substrate specificity. *Antiviral Chem. Chemother.*, **2**, 295–302.
74. Field, H. J. and Goldthorpe, S. E. (1992). The pathogenesis of drug resistant variants of herpes simplex virus. Forum on the clinical significance of drug resistant virus mutants. *Res. Virol.*, **143**, 115–148.
75. Spruance, S. L. and Freeman, D. J. (1990). Topical treatment of cutaneous herpes simplex virus infections. *Antiviral Res.*, **14**, 305–321.
76. de Miranda, P. and Good, S. S. (1992). Species differences in the metabolism and disposition of antiviral nucleoside analogues. 1. Acyclovir. *Antiviral Chem. Chemother.*, **3**, 1–8.
77. de Miranda, P. and Good, S. S. (1992). Species differences in the metabolism and disposition of antiviral nucleoside analogues. 2. Zidovudine. *Antiviral Chem. Chemother.*, **3**, 65–77.
78. Ellis, M. N., Martin, J. L., Lobe, D. C. *et al.* (1986). Induction of acyclovir-resistant mutants of herpes simplex virus type 1 in athymic nude mice. *J. Antimicrob. Chemother.*, **18** (Suppl. B), 95–101.

6 Epstein–Barr Virus: Therapy of Active and Latent Infection

JOSEPH S. PAGANO
UNC Lineberger Comprehensive Cancer Center, University of North Carolina at Chapel Hill, North Carolina, USA

INTRODUCTION

Despite the availability of effective antiviral drugs, treatment for Epstein–Barr virus (EBV) infections remains undeveloped. Why is it that although replication of the virus can be checked by many compounds there is not yet an accepted therapy in human beings? The problem comes about because the pathogenesis of EBV-associated diseases is complex. EBV infection has diverse effects leading to quite different diseases, partly because viral replication may stimulate aberrant host responses. EBV provides a paradigm of infection that causes pathology directly through cytolysis of infected cells, but also triggers immunopathological responses through an over-reaction to viral antigens. In addition when B lymphocytes are infected with EBV they proliferate; the cells mobilize through the bloodstream and distribute in many organs. In lymphocytes latent, as against productive, infection dominates, and so these cells are not destroyed by viral replication, but are immortalized. In immunodeficient hosts some proliferating cells may become neoplastic.

Since conventional antiviral drugs have no effect on latent infection or immunopathological responses, such drugs alone are unlikely to have much of an impact on EBV diseases, and treatment of infectious mononucleosis with acyclovir is only marginally beneficial. If viral replication could be checked early, triggering of the disease process might be diminished, but EBV diseases are insidious or occur after a long period of latency and reactivation, so that early treatment is generally not practicable. It might be best, therefore, to think of multi-modal treatments for EBV diseases, directed at both viral and reactive host processes. The components would be selected based on steps in molecular pathogenesis.

Treatment of EBV infections is challenging because it requires approaches that are still hypothetical. This chapter will deal with viral targets and antiviral agents that are available as well as with interventions being designed, but not yet developed.

Antiviral Chemotherapy. Edited by D.J. Jeffries and E. De Clercq

VIROLOGY

EBV, a human herpesvirus, produces productive and latent infections that are based on alternative ways the viral genome can replicate. Because of this duality of mechanisms different means of inhibition are needed. Encapsidated in the virion is a 178–190 kb linear double-stranded DNA genome with features typical of herpesvirus genomes such as internal and terminal repeats; deletions in different strains of EBV account for the variation in size (Figure 6.1) (1,2). The linear genome can circularize because the terminal repeats are complementary in sequence and form the EBV episome (Figure 6.2) (3–5). The episome is the basis for latent EBV infection, and its replication is accomplished by cellular DNA polymerase, whereas replication of linear genomes in the virus-productive state is accomplished by a virally encoded DNA polymerase (6). EBV episomes are unit-length genomic forms only found intracellularly, where they are arranged as nucleosomes within the chromatin (7). EBV episomes are present in cells in limited copy number that remains faithful in a given cell line from one generation to the next (8,9). Although EBV episomes exist in cells without producing virus they do express at least 10 of the virus's hundred or so genes (10); these are called latency genes, and at least one, Epstein–Barr antigen 1 (EBNA-1), is essential to maintain latent infection. Since latently infected B lymphocytes are also 'immortalized' by EBV, some of the latency genes propel cellular proliferation. When virus reactivates there is a transition from exclusive replication of episomes to replication of linear genomes.

REPLICATION OF EBV EPISOMES

The discovery and characterization of EBV episomes and hypotheses about their function raised the question of how they replicated (8). First attempts to identify an origin of replication for the EBV episome uncovered three autonomous replicating segments (*ars*) that could supply replication of plasmids containing fragments of the EBV genome in yeast (11). This experiment established the concept that EBV episomes might replicate via unique origins, but the discovery of the actual origins of EBV replication came later (12).

The origin of replication of the EBV episome, called *ori*-P, is used exclusively to replicate viral genomes that persist during latent infection. For production of virus itself another origin of replication is used, called *ori*-Lyt (13), discussed later. *Ori*-P consists of two *cis*-acting components located near the left end of the genome (Figure 6.2). Its components are a motif of repeated nucleotide sequences, 20×30 bp, and four additional repeat units arranged as a dyad separated by about 1 kb (14). The two *cis*-acting elements are essential, but the spacer DNA is largely dispensable. DNA replication initiated in the dyad proceeds bidirectionally and asymmetri-

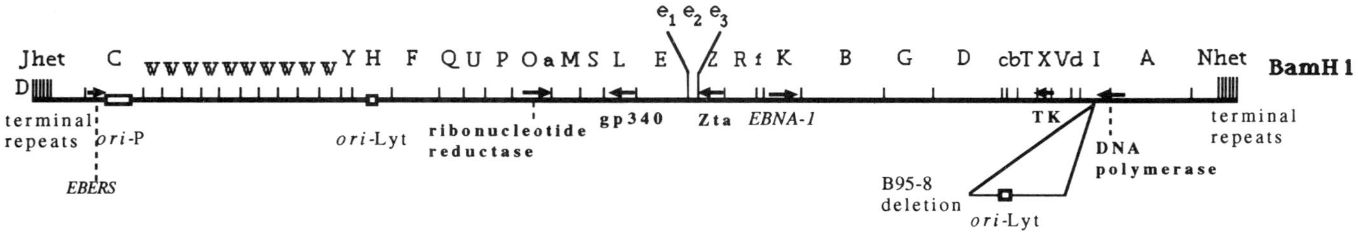

Figure 6.1. The EBV genome: a physical map of replication-related features. Positions of origins of replication for episomes (*ori*-P) and productive infection (*ori*-Lyt) are shown. The terminal repeated sequences are complementary and may be involved in a replication step. EBERS are small RNA polymerase III transcripts, probably having a regulatory function and expressed only in latent infection. EBNA-1 is a latency gene that activates *ori*-P *in trans*. BZLF-1 (Zta) is an immediate–early AP-1-like gene that triggers reactivation of latent infection. gp340 is a viral envelope glycoprotein that mediates attachment to the cellular receptor for EBV. In addition to DNA polymerase EBV encodes ribonucleotide reductase and thymidine kinase enzymes

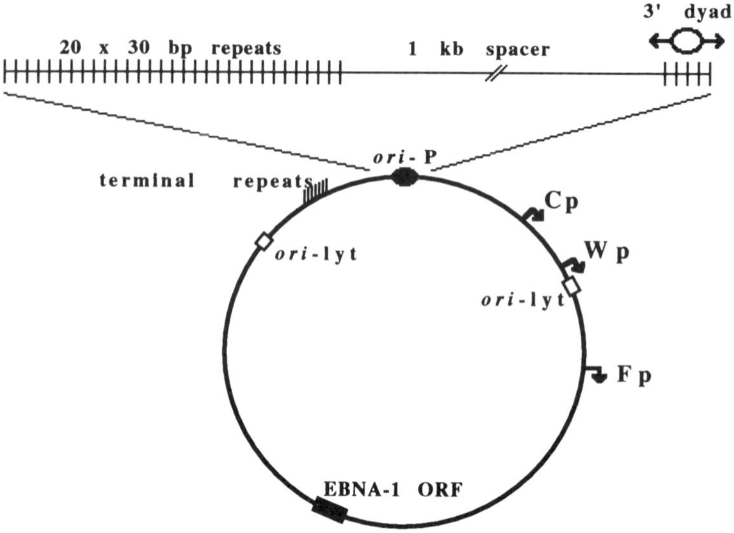

Figure 6.2. The EBV episome: a physical map. The episome is a unit-length circularized form of the linear EBV genome found in latently infected cells. Circularization occurs via fusion of the terminal repeat sequences, which are preserved in characteristic numbers in different viral strains. The origin of replication (*ori*-P) consists of two *cis*-acting elements, a motif of 20 × 30 bp repeats spaced 1000 bp from an area of dyad symmetry containing four similar repeat units. The motif of repeats functions *in vitro* as a transcriptional enhancer whose function is unknown. DNA replication initiates in the dyad and proceeds bidirectionally and asymmetrically, stalling in the motif of repeats. For *ori*-P function binding of the *trans*-acting latency protein, EBNA-1, to the *cis* elements is essential. At least three promoters (Cp, Wp, Fp) for the EBNA-1 open reading frame and other EBNAs are used in different cell types and states

cally, and stalls in the repeated units—one of the functions of the motif (15). The motif also serves as a transcriptional enhancer, although the promoter it affects has not been positively identified (16–18). The closest known latency gene promoter, Cp, is the principal promoter used for transcription of EBNA-1 (19,20). Fp is used for transcription of EBNA-1 in Type 1 latency (21) and in epithelial cells (22). Fp contains the only other EBNA-1 binding sites in the EBV genome, at the 'Q locus'. Here EBNA-1 functions as a repressor, the effect of which can be overcome by E2F, a cell-cycle regulated protein (22).

The simian EBV-like agent, *Herpesvirus papio*, contains an *ori*-P of similar but simpler general structure (23,24). A consensus sequence is conserved in the *ori*-Ps of both viruses. Other simian herpesviruses (*H. saimiri*, *H. ateles*) contain episomes, but other human herpesviruses do not seem to produce episomes despite the potential for their formation. Understanding the importance of episomes in EBV infection has been made easy because of the existence of latently infected cell lines.

Essential for *ori*-P function is the *trans*-acting viral latency protein, EBNA-1. This protein, whose open reading frame is in the BamH1 K fragment of the genome (Figure 6.1), is present in small amounts in cells, translated from an mRNA of low abundance (25). EBNA-1 is essential both for initiation and maintenance of replication of EBV episomes (17). The protein works by binding directly to the repeat units of *ori*-P apparently causing bending of the genome at the replication initiation site when it binds (26–28). *In vitro*, there is reduced assembly of nucleosomes at the initiation site (29). Binding of EBNA-1 to the two *cis*-acting elements *in vitro* causes looping of the DNA in *ori*-P so that the motif and the dyad element are brought into contact through contact with EBNA-1 homodimers (30–32). Recently cellular proteins that are induced during viral reactivation and displace EBNA-1 from binding to *ori*-P have been detected (32–35).

Details of molecular function of *ori*-P should provide a rationale for ways to design treatment of latent infection. EBV episomes not only serve as a template for episomal replication once each cell cycle early in S phase, but may also serve as templates for circular replicative intermediate forms and generation of linear genomes (9,36,37), in which case *ori*-Lyt is used. Thus, latent infection may reactivate and produce virus. Virus-producing cell lines are mostly latently infected; only 5–10% of the population of such lines produce virus, but there is continual spontaneous transition to the productive state. The transition is induced by many agents that trigger the action of immediate–early viral transactivators.

Integrated copies of the linear genome, usually intact but sometimes with *ori*-P deleted, have been detected in some cell lines (38). The significance of EBV integration is unknown since such forms have not been detected in primary infected tissues (39).

CELLULAR EFFECTS OF EBV INFECTION

The cellular receptor used by the virus for infection is C_2R (CD-21), the receptor used for the C_3D component of complement (40, 41). Primary infection takes place in mucosal epithelial cells where the outcome is cytolysis and replication of virus (42–44). B lymphocytes are also infected early in pathogenesis. In B lymphocytes infected *in vitro*, at first there is replication of virus and cytolysis, but later proliferating cells emerge that contain a small number of episomes and are not producing virus. These cells become immortalized latently infected lines; they are at first polyclonal, but later, through selective growth advantage, a monoclonal cell line may emerge (45–47). Thus there are two different outcomes of virus infection: cytolysis, usually in epithelial cells, the seat of productive infection; and cell proliferation, usually in B lymphocytes that harbour latent infection. Recently, infection of T cells that is apparently abortive has been reported (48–50).

IMMORTALIZATION OF CELLS BY EBV

The process of cell immortalization (51–55), which is unique among the human herpesviruses, mirrors pathogenesis *in vivo* where a similar latently infected B lymphocyte population is created. However, *in vivo* proliferation of this population is ordinarily limited by cytolytic T cell and natural killer (NK) cell responses recognized clinically as atypical lymphocytosis (46). The host cellular immune responses are evoked by viral neoantigens released from the nucleus or expressed in the plasma membrane of the infected B lymphocyte. Virally encoded membrane proteins (LMP1, LMP2 and LMP2A) and nuclear proteins (EBNA-1, EBNA-2a and EBNA-2b) have been identified, and processed derivatives of some of these antigens may be targets for cytolytic T cells (53,56). After the acute infection infected cells subside to $< 0.5\%$ of circulating B lymphocytes as a persistent subpopulation. Since such cells have the C_2R receptor, viral proteins at their surface and viral episomes, selected methods for targeting and destruction of these infected cells could be designed.

VIRUS REPLICATION

Replication of linear viral genomes and production of virus require virally encoded DNA polymerase, replication cofactors and viral proteins used for encapsidation of the genome. In latently infected persons or cell lines, viral reactivation is triggered by a *trans*-acting immediate–early viral protein, the BZLF-1 gene product (57–59). This key transactivator, a transcription factor that is a member of the B-Zip family, acts with other immediate–early gene products to activate promoters for early genes, such as those for the early-antigen-diffuse form (EA-D) and the EBV DNA polymerase. During latent infection the early genes are silent.

The BZLF-1 protein functions by binding to AP-1-like sites on these and other replication-associated promoters (60). BZLF-1 acts directly by augmenting constitutive promoter activity and also by recruitment of the transcription factor, TFIID, so that transcription can be initiated (61). Modulation of the BZLF-1 transactivation effects by cellular transcription factors that belong to the retinoic acid receptor family as well as by the p53 cell regulatory protein have been described recently (62,63). The effect of the BZLF-1 protein is intricately regulated by the virus itself, being first augmented by another EBV immediate–early transactivator, BRLF-1, and then negatively regulated by a novel chimeric gene product, RAZ, which acts as a transdominant repressor (64). RAZ is a decoy for the BZLF-1 protein which it inactivates by heterodimerization. In biological assays of induction by BZLF-1 of viral reactivation in latently infected cells, cotransfection with RAZ diminishes and can abort the reactivation. The mode of action of RAZ is novel and specific and may provide a model for an antiviral approach directed at inhibiting the first EBV-programmed step in viral reactivation, which is triggered by BZLF-1 protein.

The gene for the EBV DNA polymerase, which is encoded by BALF5, the fifth leftward open reading frame of the BAMH1 series of restriction fragments of the EBV genome, is homologous to the herpes simplex and cytomegalovirus DNA polymerase genes (Figure 6.3) (65–70). The EBV polymerase is a 110 kDa polypeptide that displays core enzymatic activity when translated *in vitro* and expressed in *Escherichia coli* (6,66). The polymerase purified from P_3HR1 cells (71) and superinfected Raji cells (66) also has a molecular weight of 110 kDa. Recently an EBV cofactor for the polymerase, EA-D (BMRF-1 gene product), has been shown to increase the processivity of the holoenzyme (72). In the HSV system, there is a direct interaction between the HSV polymerase and the HSV cofactor, UL42, and domains of interaction have been mapped (73,74). Specific peptides corresponding to the domain in UL42 that interacts with the polymerase can block the interaction of UL42 with the protein, thereby inhibiting efficient polymerase activity (75). To block the action of EBV DNA polymerase it may be possible to design analogous mimetic peptides to model specific antiviral drugs that block interaction with BMRF-1 protein. BMRF-1 protein copurified with EBV polymerase from infected cells appeared to stabilize enzymatic activity (76). The two proteins co-localize to the nucleus (77). Tsurumi *et al.* have expressed the EBV DNA polymerase and the EA-D (BMRF-1) cofactor in the baculovirus expression system (72,78). Most of the expressed polymerase localized to the nucleus and is insoluble. However, a small amount remains in the cytoplasm as a soluble fraction and can be purified. Similar results have been obtained by Lin *et al.* (79). This soluble fraction is not stimulated by high concentrations of salt. However, the addition of the cofactor to the polymerase renders the enzyme preparation stimulated by salt, which is characteristic of EBV and other herpesvirus polymerases (71,78); the cofactor also increases the processivity of the enzyme (72). The EBV DNA polymerase has an intrinsic 3′ to 5′ exonuclease activity and is sensitive to aphidicolin and phosphonoacetic acid like the holoenzyme purified from the infected cells (78). One of the conspicuous enzymatic properties of herpesvirus DNA polymerases, including the EBV polymerase, is a template-primer reference for poly(dC)/oligo (dG). The single subunit does not show any template preference, suggesting that the preference is conferred by the cofactor. Interaction between the polymerase and antiviral drugs is discussed later.

For replication of EBV six viral genes that serve as replication cofactors are thought to be essential: BALF5, the DNA polymerase; BALF2, the single-stranded DNA-binding protein homologue; BMRF1, the DNA polymerase processivity factor; BSLF1 and BBLF4, the primase and helicase homologues; and BBLF2/3, a potential homologue of the third component of the helicase/primase complex. In addition, a uracil DNA glycosylase homologue may augment replication (118). All these genes have HSV homologues (80). Finally, an alkaline deoxyribonuclease encoded by BGLF5 may participate in the replication complex (81). In the case of HSV replication cellular proteins such as topoisomerase II are also required. They are likely to be needed for EBV replication as well. Topoisomerase II has been exploited as a target for inhibition of human cytomegalovirus (HCMV) replication (82), but the available inhibitors have not been tested against EBV because they are toxic for P3HR1 cells (M. Smith and J. Pagano, unpublished data). Recently, the effect of the topoisomerase I and II inhibitors, camptothectin and ellipticine, on EBV replication has been reported (84).

For optimal utilization of *ori*-Lyt the two EBV immediate–early transactivators, BZLF-1 and BRLF-1, as well as the EBV early gene, BMLF-1, are needed (13,84). Finally an unconventional feature of the processing of the mRNA for the EBV DNA polymerase may provide a new target for antiviral therapy. The EBV pol message appears to be polyadenylated without the use of a canonical polyadenylation signal (85). Cleavage and polyadenylation of the 3′ end of the pol mRNA is accomplished through the intervention of a protein induced during the pre-replicative activation cascade. This induced protein, either cellular or viral, probably the latter, is thought to act *in trans* to guide cleavage/polyadenylation in the absence of a conventional signal (86). An EBV pre-early protein BMLF-1 gene product that acts post-transcriptionally is a candidate for this function (86,87). Thus a process thought to be entirely cellular may be modified by the virus. Features of the 5′ and 3′ control regions for the EBV DNA polymerase gene are schematized in Figure 6.3 (85,86,88,89).

The origin of DNA replication used by the EBV DNA polymerase is *ori*-Lyt, which has been localized to two sites in the EBV genome in most strains (only one in the deleted B95-8 strain) (Figure 6.1); these are the origins used in the cytolytic cycle for productive EBV infection (13). *Ori*-Lyt has a complex structure and requires viral and auxiliary factors including cellular DNA transcription factors and a transcriptional enhancer. The BZLF-1 gene product also binds directly to *ori*-Lyt and may serve as the origin-binding protein. The product of this origin is a concatameric DNA molecule. The combination of *ori*-P, *ori*-Lyt and the terminal repeats of the genome may comprise an EBV amplicon (13).

EBV-ASSOCIATED DISEASES

There are three phases of EBV infection: acute, latent, and reactivated. Latently EBV-infected lymphocytes ordinarily remain dormant in the peri-

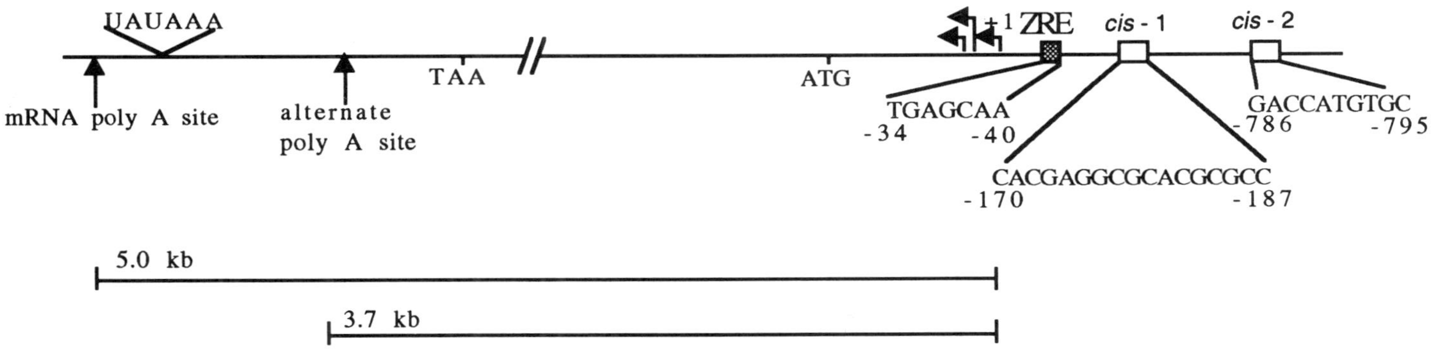

Figure 6.3. The EBV DNA polymerase gene and its control regions. The BALF-5 ORF encodes a 5.1 kb polymerase mRNA that is apparently polyadenylated via a non-canonical polyadenylation signal (UAUAAA); this is the authentic mRNA in most EBV-producing cell lines and in wild-type virus-infected cells. An alternative polyadenylation site upstream is used in B95-8 cells to produce a 3.7 kb mRNA because the downstream terminus is deleted in the B95-8 genome; there is no recognizable polyadenylation signal for this site. Message formation in both cases may involve a virally encoded pre-replicative protein. The upstream regulatory region of the promoter for the polymerase gene is TATA-less and contains a response element (ZRE) for the BZLF-1 gene product near the transcription initiation region. There are at least two *cis*-acting regions (*cis*-1 and *cis*-2) required for promoter activity, to which the cellular stimulatory proteins, USF-1 and bZip-268 bind; the viral immediate-early proteins also activate these elements. Thus this gene, which is only expressed when cells are replicating virus, is regulated both transcriptionally at its 5′ end and post-transcriptionally at its 3′ end (85, 88 and C. Liu and J. S. Pagano, unpublished data).

pheral blood and in lymphoid organs. However, if the host becomes immunosuppressed there is a reactivation process, and cellular proliferation and viral replication resume. Symptoms of reactivated EBV infection differ from those of the primary infection, being associated mainly with malignancies (90).

The virus infects the oropharynx, where it replicates initially in epithelial cells lining the pharynx and parotid ducts. Virus is chronically shed in saliva from these sites (91,92). The epithelial cytolysis and lymphoproliferation caused by EBV infections are self-limiting except in rare persons with specific genetic defects (93–95). The virus also replicates in epithelial cells in the cervix (96,97).

EBV is best known as the causative agent for infectious mononucleosis (98–100). Classically the virus is associated with African Burkitt's lymphoma, where the virus was discovered (101), and with carcinoma of the posterior nasopharynx in China (102,103). Other lymphoproliferative disorders arise in immunodeficient states and appear to be EBV induced (45). The most recent associations, T cell lymphomas and oral hairy leukoplakia, were quite unexpected (48–50,104,105). This seemingly disparate collection has common molecular pathobiological features (90,106).

Burkitt's lymphoma (BL) (Table 6.1) is a rapidly growing B cell lymphoma that presents in children as a tumour of the jaw. It is endemic in East and West Africa at lower elevations (107). However, in Western countries BL is sporadic in incidence and rare. Although over 98% of African BL contain hybridizable EBV DNA present as the EBV episome, only about one-seventh of the North American cases of BL contains EBV genomes (103,108–110). In Africa EBV infection precedes the development of the lymphoma

Table 6.1. EBV-associated diseases

Tissues affected and diseases	Role of EBV
Lymphoid	
Burkitt's lymphoma	Cofactor, non-essential
B cell immunoblastic lymphomas	Causal
T cell lymphomas	Clonal association
Hodgkin's disease	Clonal association, Reed–Sternberg cells infected
Epithelial	
Nasopharyngeal carcinoma	Essential factor
Parotid carcinoma	Clonal association
Hairy leukoplakia	Causal
Lymphoid and epithelial	
Infectious mononucleosis	Causal

(111), and monoclonal EBV episomes are found in the tumour (112,113). In BL characteristic translocations (t8;14, t22;8 and t2;8) that cause disregulation of *c-myc* expression are distinctive and confer an independent growth advantage for B lymphocytes resulting in a monoclonal malignancy either with or without EBV infection (114). Chromosomes 14, 22 and 2 contain immunoglobulin genes and their regulatory elements, and chromosome 8 contains the *c-myc* locus (55). EBV may contribute by stimulating B cell growth, increasing the likelihood of the critical translocations. A search for EBV gene products that may interact directly with the *c-myc* locus has recently uncovered several leads (115,116). Holoendemic malaria is thought also to contribute by stimulating B cell growth and depressing cytolytic T cell responses (117).

Immunoblastic sarcomas form a distinct class of B cell tumours that arise in immunodeficient patients who receive intensive immunosuppressive treatment for organ transplantation, and patients with AIDS (45,115,117–124). These tumours do not have translocations or lesions in oncogenes or growth suppressor genes, but are probably propelled by latent EBV infection alone; however, sometimes there is viral reactivation in the proliferating cells. The lymphomas are usually localized as solitary lymphomas in the brain or in the gut, but sometimes proliferation is diffuse and fulminant, especially if it is a primary infection. These neoplasms are at first polyclonal, but there may be monoclonal evolution. It has been suggested that reactivation of latent EBV infection may trigger some of these proliferations and that antiviral treatment may suppress such episodes (47,125). Recently *T cell lymphomas* containing monoclonal EBV episomes have been described (48–50), and EBV gene products have been detected in *Hodgkin's disease* in the Reed–Sternberg cells in up to 50% of cases (126–128). These associations are unexpected because the pathological cell type is not the B lymphocyte in these conditions, and the significance is unknown (106).

Nasopharyngeal carcinoma (NPC): carcinoma of the posterior nasopharynx is an epithelial malignancy with extraordinarily high incidence in southern China and in Chinese who migrate elsewhere from this area. The incidence is intermediate in North Africa, where the disease occurs in Caucasians, in black Africans in the endemic regions for BL, and in Alaskan Inuits (111,113). The incidence is low and sporadic in the United States and Europe. Monoclonal EBV episomes are detected in 100% of NPC specimens regardless of histological type or geographical area (102,103,113,129–131) and in dysplasias, the earliest preneoplastic lesion of NPC (113,132). Early stages of NPC are distinguished by appearance of circulating IgA antibodies to EBV replicative antigens (EA/VCA); these antibodies herald the appearance of the tumour and suggest that reactivation of latent virus infection triggers the malignancy (90,133,134). The IgA antibodies may facilitate entry of the virus into epithelial cells in the nasopharynx (135). Cofactors in the endemic regions might be dietary or environmental carcinogens and genetic predisposition (111,112).

Other epithelial tumours are linked to EBV infection including *parotid carcinomas*, some *supraglottal* and *laryngeal carcinomas* and *thymomas* of epithelial origin. These tissues, as well as NPC, have a common origin in the primitive oropharynx. The parotid gland is a site of EBV replication (136). The latest EBV-associated disease is *hairy leukoplakia*, which produces distinctive lesions on the side of the tongue. First recognized in patients with AIDS, the disease is characterized by epithelial proliferation and epithelial cells that contain enormous numbers of Epstein–Barr virions (104,105). The lesions present EBV infection in a virtually completely replicative state without hallmarks of latent infection such as EBER gene expression or episomes (137). Hairy leukoplakia responds to treatment with acyclovir, but the disease recurs.

Infectious mononucleosis (IM) is a syndrome with EBV the sole cause in over 90% of cases. The onset is insidious, and symptoms are caused not only by direct viral invasion and cytolysis resulting in pharyngitis, but also by secondary immunopathology of the lymph nodes, the spleen, and sometimes the brain, spinal cord, liver and bone marrow in complicated IM (90). The disease is marked by an atypical lymphocyte response in the peripheral blood which represents a cytolytic T cell response to EBV-infected cells. Trials of treatment of infectious mononucleosis with acyclovir are discussed under 'Conclusions', below.

ANTIVIRAL DRUGS

Currently drugs active against EBV replication are agents that inhibit replication of other human herpesviruses, the single exception being azidothymidine (AZT); of the seven human herpesviruses this drug inhibits only the replication of EBV. Most of these drugs are nucleoside analogues, with the primary target being the EBV DNA polymerase. Other classes of drugs that inhibit EBV replication are pyrophosphate analogues, thymidine kinase analogues and ribonucleoside reductase inhibitors (Table 6.2). Compounds of all these classes affect only productive infection, not latent infection or cell immortalization.

ASSAY SYSTEMS

Most EBV assay systems depend upon the use of cell lines that are already infected with EBV; such lines are either exclusively latently infected or continuously virus producing (138). The most precise assay measures reduction of EBV genome copy numbers as detected by cRNA–DNA or DNA–DNA hybridization in solution (139). More recently Southern blot hybridization

Table 6.2. Virally encoded EBV targets for antiviral agents

Productive infection
Receptor, C_2R (CD-21); and viral glycoprotein, gp340
DNA polymerase
Pyrophosphate binding site
Thymidine kinase
Ribonucleotide reductase
Latent infection
Epstein–Barr virus nuclear antigen 1 (EBNA-1)

with an EBV probe of unique genomic sequence has been used to measure copy numbers. Since the amount of virus and the number of EBV genomes produced by the P3HR1 cell line, which has been most used for antiviral assays, fluctuates greatly, high-producer clones have been developed (168). The total number of genomes measured includes both linear forms and the minor contribution coming from episomes since at any given moment the line consists of two cell populations: one that is virus producing and the other that is still latently infected (140). For quantitation of EBV genomes dot or slot-blot hybridization methods are not recommended; they tend to be unreliable because of high non-specific background hybridization and give less quantitative results (141).

A second assay system is based on superinfection with exogenous P3HR1 virus of the latently infected Raji cell line (142,143). Superinfection induces a relatively acute infection that can be quantitated by separation of viral DNA from cellular DNA by density-gradient centrifugation and hybridization methods. Superinfection also induces EBV productive antigens (EA/VCA) detected by immunofluorescence assays or immunoblotting. These methods are cumbersome and imprecise.

Third, many EBV strains will immortalize B lymphocytes obtained from umbilical cord blood; this was the viral property first exploited to assay EBV (55). However, the cord blood lymphocyte immortalization assay is not used for studies of inhibition of viral replication since cell immortalization will take place despite the presence of drugs that inhibit viral replication (144). The cord blood assay can, however, be used for studies of agents that inhibit the immortalization process itself.

Fourth, simian and rodent animal models have been developed. EBV infection of marmosets leads to disease, including occasionally lymphoma in a variable number of animals (145). Cottontop tamarins have been used more recently in EBV vaccine studies; in these animals EBV infection produces B cell lymphomas with high frequency after a latency period of a few weeks (146). Finally, transplantation of EBV-infected B lymphocytes into SCID mice produces lymphoproliferative disease in the animals that is a tractable model for prevention and treatment of this aspect of EBV infection (147). Interleukin 2 prevents this disease in SCID mice (148).

NUCLEOSIDE ANALOGUES

The first compound shown to inhibit herpes simplex virus replication, 5-iodo-2′-deoxyuridine (149), induces rather than inhibits replication of EBV as do other such analogues (150).

9-β-D-Arabinofuranosyladenine (ara-A) was the first nucleoside analogue found to inhibit EBV replication *in vitro* (151,152). Arabinofuranosylthymine, which also inhibited EBV replication, was thought to act by substrate competition for EBV thymidine kinase (TK) (153).

The first nucleoside analogue with selective activity against herpes simplex viruses, 9-(2-hydroxyethyoxymethyl)guanine (acyclovir or ACV), is a potent inhibitor of EBV replication. This is the only drug that has been tested in clinical trials for treatment of infectious mononucleosis. Other nucleoside analogues that are potent inhibitors in EBV-infected cell cultures include a series of halogenated compounds represented by 1-(2-fluoro-2-deoxy-β-D-arabinofuranosyl)-5-iodocytosine (FIAC) and bromovinyl derivatives such as *E*-5-(2-bromovinyl)-2′-deoxyuridine (BVDU). Recently, members of a new class of adenine analogues typified by (*S*)-9-(3-hydroxy-2-phosphonylmethoxypropyl)adenine (HPMPA), which are active against a broad spectrum of DNA viruses, have been shown to be potent inhibitors of EBV replication. This series of compounds has uncovered structure–activity relations involved in the inhibition of EBV replication.

ACYCLOVIR

Estimations of the inhibitory effect of ACV (154) on EBV replication were made in the virus-producing P3HR1 cell line (155). Based on reduction of EBV genome copy numbers the ED_{50} of ACV for EBV was estimated to be 6 μM—an underestimation due to failure to take into account already synthesized linear genomes and lack of drug effect on episomal forms. Later measurements of the ED_{50} of ACV for EBV were in the range of 0.3 μM (Table 6.3) (140). The ED_{90} was estimated to be 9 μM (Figure 6.4A). Although these values cannot be compared directly with the results of plaque assays of herpes simplex virus, sensitivity of EBV to ACV appears to be in the same general range as HSV.

Unlike ACV in HSV-infected cells there is little evidence that the drug is phosphorylated more efficiently in EBV-infected cells than in non-infected lymphocytes, which suggests that monophosphorylation of ACV in EBV infection does not require EBV TK (156,157). Moreover, monophosphorylation of ACV *in vitro* by EBV TK (158–161) has not been demonstrated (E. Littler and J. Fyfe, personal communications). It appears that very low

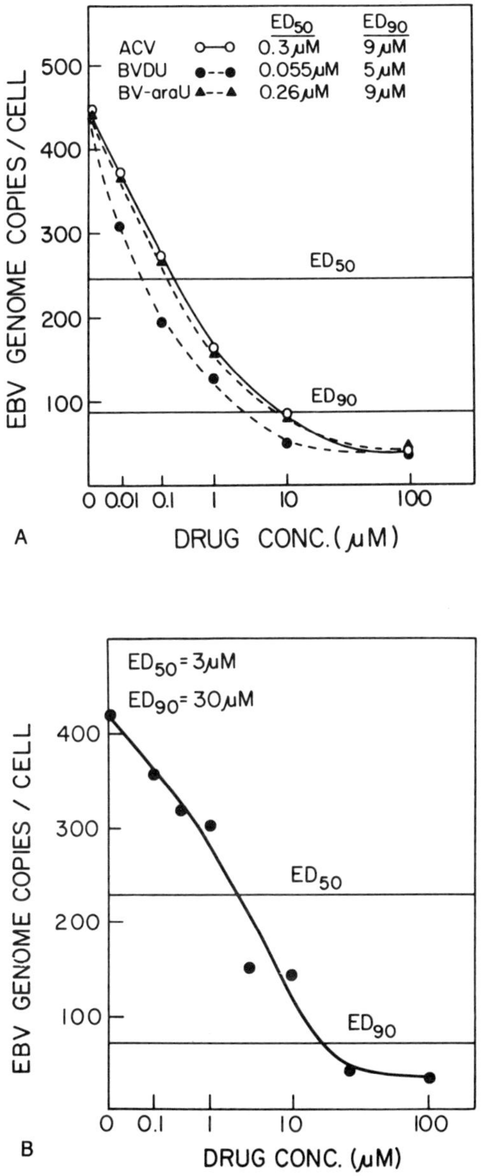

Figure 6.4. Inhibitors of replication of EBV DNA in a virus-producing cell line. Typical dose–response curves with four inhibitors are constructed by measurement of total average EBV genome copy numbers, linear and episomal, per cell by cRNA–DNA hybridization. The curves are biphasic with a plateau caused by residual viral genomes in the form of episomes whose replication is not inhibited. (A) Acyclovir, BVDU and BV-araU; (B) AZT

levels of ACV monophosphate (ACV-MP), perhaps produced by cellular kinases, are sufficient for inhibition of EBV replication (162).

The antiviral effect of ACV is due to interaction of ACV triphosphate (ACV-TP) with EBV-encoded DNA polymerase. With partially purified enzyme from EBV-infected cells, an apparent K_i for ACV-TP of 0.015 μM compared with 1.5 μM for lymphoblastoid cell DNA polymerase α was obtained (78,163). ACV-TP acted as a classical competitive inhibitor for dGTP for binding to polymerase with a K_m of 0.025 for the viral compared with the cellular enzyme. Thus the affinity of ACV-TP for EBV polymerase was approximately 100 times greater than for polymerase α; presumably, pure viral enzyme would have greater affinity and a lower K_i.

ACV-TP is preferentially incorporated into viral DNA by viral polymerase. In the case of HSV, ACV-MP is not excised from the primer template by HSV-1 3′,5′-exonuclease (which is associated with the HSV DNA polymerase), because of the acyclic nature of ACV-MP. The lack of a 3′-hydroxyl moiety prevents DNA chain elongation; however, ACV-TP is not a suicide substrate, nor is template primer containing ACV-MP a potent inhibitor in the absence of the next required nucleotide (dCTP). Rather incorporation of the analogue forms a tight dead-end complex (164).

Structure–activity relations with acyclic pyrimidine nucleosides with either base modifications or substitutions have demonstrated that base structure modifications reduce antiviral activity whereas substitutions on or in the pyrimidine ring exhibit selective activity against EBV (165).

Antiviral drug resistance of EBV must arise in persons chronically treated with ACV, since there is chronic, superficial replication of multiple viral strains (137), especially in patients with AIDS. However, there are no ready means to detect resistant virus since a plaque assay system for screening and detection of such mutants is not available for EBV. Since the EBV TK does not seem to serve an essential function in activation of ACV, any mutations that confer drug resistance should arise in the EBV DNA polymerase gene. Regions II and III of the HSV DNA polymerase where mutations producing ACV resistance have been mapped are conserved in the EBV DNA polymerase (166) with the use of the PCR-based technique called single-strand conformation polymorphism (SSCP) (167). This technique can detect single point mutations, but so far no significant mutations in these regions have been detected in several cell lines established from patients treated with ACV (Chunnan Liu and J. S. Pagano, unpublished data). Introduced mutations that are preserved in recombinant virus (169,171) will provide a way to study this largely unexplored issue.

9-(1,3-DIHYDROXY-2-PROPOXYMETHYL)GUANINE (GANCICLOVIR)

Ganciclovir (GCV) or DHPG is a more potent inhibitor of EBV replication in the same systems used to measure the effect of ACV (Table 6.3). The

Table 6.3. Relative efficacy of drugs active against EBV replication in infected cell culture

Drug	Antiviral effect ED_{50} (μM)	Anticellular effect ID_{50} (μM)	Therapeutic index ID_{50}/ED_{50}
ACV	0.3	250	850
DHPG	0.05	200	
BVdU	0.06	360	6500
BVara-U	0.26	390	1500
V-ara-U	0.005	20	4000
FMAU	0.0065	1	150
FIAC	0.005	5	1000
FIAU	0.005	1	200
(*S*)-DHPA	> 100		–
(*S*)-HPMPA	0.08	80	1000
PMEA	1.1		
PMEDAP	0.16	160	1000
(*S*)-HPMPC	0.03	150	5000
(*S*)-HPMPDAP	2.0	150	75
AZT	3	> 50	–

ED_{50} was determined by measurement of reduction of EBV genome copy number in the virus-producing lymphoblastoid P3HR1 cell line; ID_{50} was also determined in these cells.

ED_{50} of DHPG is 0.05 μM and the ED_{90}, 3 μM (168). In tissue culture the therapeutic index for this drug is very favourable; however, the drug does have significant toxicity in human beings, which precludes its use for the treatment of EBV infection in otherwise normal persons.

The inhibitory effect of ACV is rapidly lifted after removal of the drug from virus-producing cell cultures (Figure 6.5A). However, DHPG has a more persistent effect (140). These observations led to a study of the metabolism of DHPG in EBV-superinfected Raji cells which revealed that DHPG is 100-fold more efficiently phosphorylated in the superinfected cells than is ACV; at least part of the increase in drug-phosphorylating activity seemed to be caused by EBV infection (168). DHPG-TP tended to accumulate in the superinfected cells. The enzymes that accomplished phosphorylation of DHPG were not identified. Whether there is a homologue to the HCMV viral gene product thought to be responsible for phosphorylation of DHPG is unknown (170). Based on measurements of rate of decrease of DHPG-TP between days 1 and 5 after drug removal it would have taken more than two weeks for drug levels to diminish below the concentration sufficient for inhibition of EBV DNA polymerase. Thus persistence of DHPG-TP may account in part for the prolonged inhibitory effect. Also, the greater abundance of DHPG-TP compared with ACV-TP in infected cells might account for the greater sensitivity of the virus to DHPG by facilitating incorporation of the analogue into viral DNA both internally and terminally. Another guanine nucleoside analogue with activity against EBV is penciclovir (PCV), a 9-hydroxyalkyl-guanine which is both potent and selective (171). PCV-triphosphate has a long half-life in herpesvirus-infected cells, which may be advantageous for long-term treatment and prophylaxis provided that toxicity proves to be low. Famciclovir is the well-absorbed oral form of the drug (172).

E-5-(2-BROMOVINYL)-2′-DEOXYURIDINE (BVDU)

BVDU is a potent selective inhibitor of replication of EBV *in vitro*; concentrations of 10–20 μM effectively inhibit replication of EBV DNA both in the virus-producing P3HR1 cells and superinfected Raji cells (174,175). The ED_{50} of the drug is 0.06 μM, and the calculated therapeutic index is 6500, the drug being relatively non-toxic in the EBV cell line tested (Table 6.3). Inhibition of EBV replication is not reversed until about 10 days after removal of the drug from the culture medium.

Additional bromovinyl nucleoside analogues have been tested (176). One of these drugs, 1-β-D-arabinofuranosyl-*E*-5(2-bromovinyl)uracil (BV-ara-U), is less active active against EBV replication than BVDU (ED_{50} of 0.26 versus 0.06 μM) (Figure 6.4A), and hence its *in vitro* therapeutic index is decreased (1500), as compared to that of BVDU (Table 6.3). The ED_{50} of V-ara-U is 0.005 μM, and the *in vitro* therapeutic index 4000 (Table 6.3). The inhibitory effect of V-ara-U after drug removal was less prolonged than it was for BV-ara-U. Thus substitution of the H with the Br atom in the 5-vinyl group reduced anti-EBV activity while prolonging drug effect and diminishing cytotoxicity.

EBV DNA polymerase has an associated nuclease activity (78,177–181). Excision of the terminally incorporated drug triphosphate by exonuclease may affect drug potency so that the effect of nucleoside analogues that cause chain termination due to lack of the 3′ OH group might be more reversible than with drugs such as BVDU, BV-ara-U and V-ara-U analogues that incorporate into DNA, but do not terminate chain elongation. In the

Figure 6.5. (opposite) Reversibility of inhibition of viral DNA replication in EBV-producing cell cultures. Treatment with antiviral drugs for 7–14 days reduces total genome copy numbers to a residual number (~30) accounted for by episomal forms. The kinetics of recovery of viral replication differs depending on the inhibitor. (A) Acyclovir; (B) FMAU. Viral replication is suppressed due to inhibition of synthesis of linear genomes, but infection is not cured because the episomes can serve as a template for replication of linear genomes once the viral DNA polymerase inhibitors are dissipated

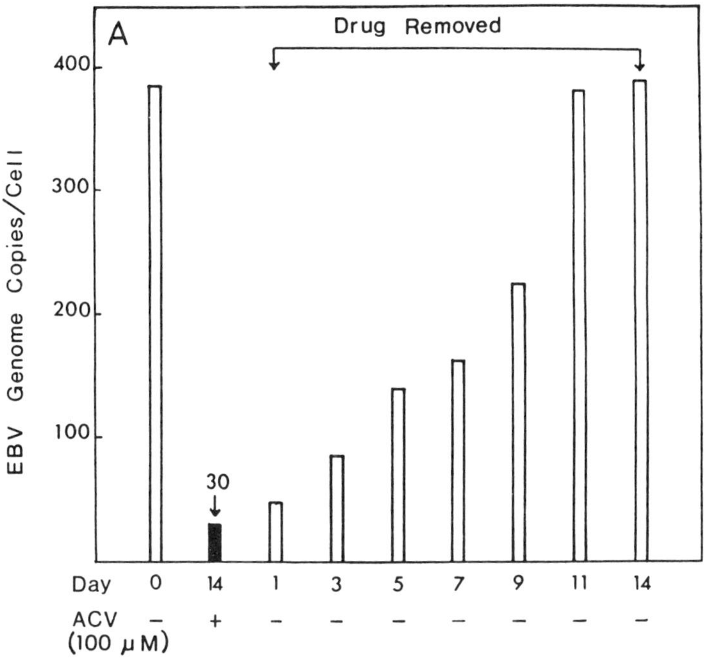
A
Drug Removed
EBV Genome Copies/Cell
400
300
200
100
30
Day 0 14 1 3 5 7 9 11 14
ACV – + – – – – – – –
(100 μM)

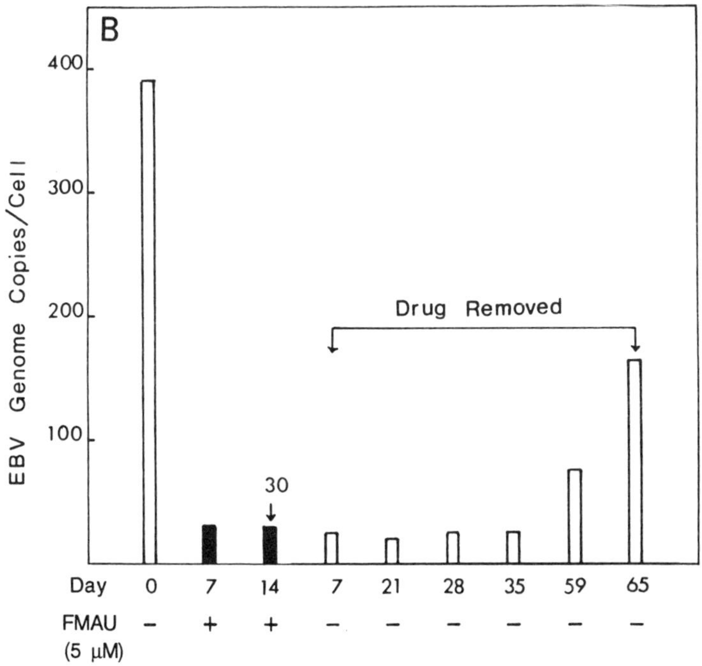
B
Drug Removed
EBV Genome Copies/Cell
400
300
200
100
30
Day 0 7 14 7 21 28 35 59 65
FMAU – + + – – – – – –
(5 μM)

case of BV-ara-U and BVDU, the bromine atom may render the incorporated analogue less accessible to excision by exonuclease due to steric hindrance of the enzyme (176). A new class of deoxyuridine analogues with antiherpes activity includes 5-(1-azido-2-haloethyl)-2′-deoxyuridine 3a–c, reported to be active against EBV (182).

OTHER HALOGENATED NUCLEOSIDE ANALOGUES

Three additional drugs, (2-deoxy-2-fluoro-β-D-arabinofuranosyl)-5-iodocytosine (FIAC), 1-(2-deoxy-2-fluoro-β-D-arabinofuranosyl)-5-methyluridine (FMAU) and 1-(2-deoxy-2-fluoro-β-D-arabinofuranosyl)-5-iodouridine (FIAU), have also been tested for activity against EBV (150,183). All three drugs have very high potency. However, they are also quite cytotoxic. The ED_{50}s for these drugs are in the range of 0.005 μM, and their ID_{50}s are 1–5 μM (Table 6.3). The therapeutic indices are thus not as favourable as drug potency would indicate. Of the three, FIAC may be the most promising, with a therapeutic index of 1000. All three of these drugs have remarkably persistent inhibitory effects in EBV-producing cell cultures (Figure 6.5B).

The relative potencies of these drugs based on anti-EBV activity were FIAC=FIAU>FMAU>DHPG>BVDU>ACV. On the basis of a more favourable therapeutic index the ranking was as follows: BVDU>DHPG>FIAC>ACV>FIAU>FMAU. These results suggest that FIAC might be worth additional investigation in view of its high potency and persistent effects, perhaps in reduced dosage (160).

ACYCLIC ADENOSINE ANALOGUES

This series of drugs includes (*S*)-9-(3-hydroxy-2-phosphonyl-methoxypropyl)adenine (HPMPA), 9-(2-phosphonylmethoxyethyl)adenine (PMEA) and (*S*)-9-(2,3-dihydroxypropyl)adenine (DHPA) (184). In this series DHPA is the parental compound. Only HPMPA and PMEA were effective inhibitors of EBV DNA replication, with ED_{50}s of 0.08 μM for HPMPA and 1.1 μM for PMEA (Table 6.3) (185). Both of these drugs are cytostatic but not clearly cytotoxic at concentrations as high as 100 μM.

New acyclic nucleoside phosphonate analogues in this series synthesized recently made possible evaluation of structure–activity relations in the inhibition of EBV replication. These drugs include (*S*)-9-(3-hydroxy-2-phos- phonylmethoxypropyl)-2, 6-diaminopurine (HPMPDAP), cyclic (*S*)-HPMPA (cHPMPA), 9-(2-phosphonylmethoxyethoxyethyl)-2,6-diaminopurine (PMEDAP), and (*S*)-1-(3-hydroxy-2-phosphonylmethoxypropyl)-cytosine (HPMPC) (186). Compared with the prototype drug (HPMPA), which had an ED_{50} of 0.08 μM, the ED_{50} for PMEDAP was 0.16; for HPMPC, 0.03; for HPMPDAP, 2.0; and for cHPMPA, 1.5 μM (Table 6.3). The therapeutic indices *in vitro* ranged from 5000 to 78, with HPMPC, PMEDAP and HPMPA having the most favourable indices.

Interestingly, certain ratios of combinations of HPMPC with AZT produced a synergistic inhibitory effect on EBV genome replication, but other combinations were antagonistic (186). In cell culture the most potent and selective of this series of acyclic nucleoside phosphonate analogues was HPMPC. These compounds are promising drug candidates because of their broad antiviral spectrum as well as their potency against EBV replication.

3′-AZIDO-3′-DEOXYTHYMIDINE (AZT)

AZT is inhibitory to EBV replication (187). This is surprising in that there is no significant inhibition of the other human herpesviruses. The ED_{50} and ED_{90} of AZT for EBV replication are 3 and 30 μM, respectively (Figure 6.4B). In patients with AIDS the plasma concentration of AZT reaches levels of 6–10 μM 1 h after an intravenous dose of 5 mg/kg. In the EBV-infected cell cultures concentrations of AZT as high as 100 μM were cytostatic but not cytotoxic. Combinations of AZT and ACV appear to be additive, but not synergistic, in inhibiting EBV replication. The basis for the action of AZT on EBV replication is unknown, but it is unlikely that the EBV-encoded TK accounts for the selective inhibition of EBV replication by AZT since the initial monophosphorylation of AZT is carried out by cellular TK rather than viral enzyme, and the levels of AZT-TP in HIV-infected and uninfected cells are similar (188).

Since AZT-TP is a potent inhibitor of HIV reverse transcriptase, the question arises whether EBV DNA polymerase shares with the reverse transcriptase common binding sites for the phosphorylated drug. If so, these sites are not available in polymerase α, since AZT-TP has low affinity for this cellular enzyme (189). Treatment of EBV-infected cells with AZT may cause a reduction in the intracellular level of dTTP, which is a competing substrate for EBV DNA polymerase. This effect would facilitate the binding of AZT-TP to viral polymerase. AZT with its 3′-azido group would also cause termination of DNA chain elongation upon incorporation of AZT-MP into viral DNA (188).

OTHER DRUGS

Phosphonoformic acid (PFA) and phosphonoacetic acid (PAA), pyrophosphate (PPi) analogues that were among the earliest drugs shown to inhibit HSV replication by inhibiting the viral DNA polymerase, also inhibit EBV replication (190–195). PFA inhibits EBV DNA polymerase in a linear non-competitive fashion with the four dNTPs as variable substrate and a saturating concentration of activated DNA, and produces kinetics of uncompetitive inhibition with variable concentrations of activated DNA as substrate and saturating deoxytriphosphate concentrations (195). The

Table 6.4. Inhibition of EBV DNA replication by a ribonucleotide reductase inhibitor (A111OU)

Dose (μM)	EBV genome equivalents/cell
0	331
0.01	268
0.1	273
1.0	95
5.0	67

J. C. Lin and J. S. Pagano, unpublished data. A111OU was the gift of Dr Tom Spector, Burroughs Wellcome Company.

apparent inhibitory constant for partially purified EBV polymerase is in the range of 2–3 μM.

The ribonucleotide reductase inhibitor, 2-acetylpyridine 5-[(dimethylamino)thiocarbonyl]thiocarbonohydrazone (A111OU) inhibits replication of a number of herpesviruses (196). The EBV genome contains a gene that encodes an 85 kDa polypeptide associated with EBV-induced ribonucleotide reductase activity (197). This polypeptide is a component of the early antigen-restricted (EA-R) complex. A111OU also inhibits replication of EBV genomes in the virus-producing P3HR1 cell line (Table 6.4). Synergy between ACV and A111OU in inhibiting EBV replication has not been demonstrated (J.-C. Lin and J. Pagano, unpublished data). The inhibitory levels (1–5 μM) are close to cytotoxic levels of the drug for P3HR1 cells.

REVERSIBILITY OF DRUG ACTION

Since herpesviral infections lead to persistent replication or latent infection, what happens after removal of drug from infected cells is relevant to treatment outcome. When ACV is applied to a cell line that chronically produces EBV, replication of linear viral genomes is abolished, and production of virus ceases after exhaustion of already synthesized viral constituents. However, in such treated cell cultures a fraction of viral DNA persists as EBV episomes; when the drug is removed, replication of linear viral genomes and virus production resume rapidly and reach pre-treatment levels. In P3HR1 cells treated up to two years, virus replication was suppressed as long as the drug was present, but the replication of episomes was unaffected (198). This reversibility of inhibition may suggest that the drug triphosphate is reversibly bound to the viral DNA polymerase. Probably a better explanation is that DNA chain termination does not affect the EBV episomes which persist as templates not only for episomal replication, but also as potential templates for replication of linear genomes (see section on 'Virology', above) presumably in cells that have been activated by the

BZLF-1 transactivator. The second pathway can only be utilized for virus production when the viral polymerase inhibitor is removed. These observations in persistently infected cell cultures were used to predict that administration of ACV to patients excreting EBV would suppress viral replication only transiently while drug was administered.

Different inhibitors behave differently with respect to the duration of the drug effect after removal with each drug having a characteristic profile. DHPG is a more potent inhibitor of EBV replication than is ACV, and FMAU is significantly more potent than either drug; the ranking of persistent drug effect is the same. However, correlation between potency of drug and persistence of drug effect is inconsistent. After removal of DHPG the kinetics of recovery of virus production are slower than with ACV, taking about 21 days for restoration to 25% of pre-drug exposure levels. The persistence of drug effect is most remarkable for FMAU—more than 58 days (Figure 6.5B). These different kinetics of recovery of viral replication point to different modes of action of the drugs that are probably related both to analogue incorporation into viral DNA and to differences in drug metabolism. The different effects may also suggest subtle effects on the cells that support viral replication. One possibility is that the triphosphates of the less selective drugs may be incorporated to a significant degree into cellular DNA and produce cellular effects that favour more prolonged viral inhibition. Theoretically a drug with long-lasting effect might be a useful agent, particularly for prophylactic treatment regimens as in persons with IgA responses at high risk for NPC in endemic regions (see 'Conclusions', below).

LATENT INFECTION

None of the antiviral drugs has any effect on replication of the episomal form of the EBV genome in Raji cells regardless of the differences in potency and mode of action. The lack of effect is independent of drug phosphorylation; neither ACV, which is poorly phosphorylated in lymphoblastoid cells, nor DHPG, which is 100-fold better phosphorylated, has any effect on latent infection.

Phosphonoformate, which does not require phosphorylation, is without effect on the replication of EBV episomes. Ribonucleotide reductase inhibitors also do not affect episomal replication. Since episomes are replicated by host DNA polymerase and ACV spares host polymerase while inhibiting synthesis of linear genomes by the viral enzyme, and all other drugs tested have a similar if not identical dichotomy of effect, it appears that only cytotoxic drugs are liable to have any effect on the maintenance of EBV episomal forms—at the cost of non-selective effects on cellular replication and viability.

Therefore a new conceptual approach for treatment of latent EBV infection has been devised. The strategy focuses on blocking the synthesis of a single viral protein, the EBNA-1 protein, which is essential to initiate and maintain replication of EBV episomes (6). EBNA-1 functions by binding to the origin of DNA replication of the episomes, *ori*-P. For this purpose oligodeoxynucleotides antisense to EBNA-1 mRNA were designed and tested in non-virus-producing latently EBV cell lines. The most effective oligomers were two sequential 18-mers beginning immediately after the AUG of the EBNA-1 open reading frame (ORF). In a single experiment treatment of Raji cells every three days with 40 μM of the unmodified oligomers over a 23-day period led to a significant reduction in both expression of EBNA-1 and number of EBV episomes in the continuously cultured cells (199). However, this experiment could not be reproduced despite efforts to control likely variables such as oligonucleotide uptake and stability, serum DNAse activity and Raji cell strain variability (200). More promising results have been obtained using a different shorter-term assay, discussed in the next section. Recently, antisense oligonucleotides directed against the BZLF-1 gene product have also been used to inhibit reactivation of productive infection (201).

INHIBITION OF GROWTH OF EBV-IMMORTALIZED CELLS

The cord lymphocyte immortalization assay provides a means of gauging the effects of agents that might inhibit EBV-induced lymphoproliferation in immunodeficiency states. A more sensitive and quantitative variation of the assay is based on counting microscopic transformed foci in each well in microtitre plates. Such assays have revealed that interferon α (IFN-α) can prevent EBV-induced B cell outgrowth and that combinations of interferons are synergistic (202). The IC_{50} for preventing focus formation was 10 U/ml for IFN-α and 1 U/ml for IFN-γ. Larger doses produced more than 90% inhibition of focus formation. Dosage levels that were not directly cytotoxic were 30 U/ml for IFN-α and 3 U/ml for IFN-γ. Thus the effective concentrations were lower than but close to cytotoxic doses. However, combinations of very low doses of the two interferons produced striking synergistic effects. As little as 1 U/ml of IFN-α and 0.1 U/ml of IFN-γ reduced focus formation by 80%. The combination indices are summarized in Table 6.5. These low doses of interferons may be non-toxic in human beings and useful for treatment of B cell lymphoproliferative conditions. There are anecdotal reports of the utility of IFN-α combined with intravenous γ-globulin for treatment of such conditions (203,204).

There are no means for specific inhibition of growth of cells that have already been immortalized by EBV. Freshly immortalized cord cell lines provide a good model for investigation because they are often polyclonal and rarely exhibit chromosomal translocations or significant oncogene activation. Whether cell growth might cease if the episomes could be removed

Table 6.5. Synergistic inhibition of human cord lymphocyte immortalization by EBV by IFN-α and -γ

Combination (U/ml)	Combination index (CI) at different effect (f_a) levels[a]	
	f_a	CI
IFN-α + IFN-γ		
1 + 0.05	0.73	0.021 (0.021)
1 + 0.1	0.83	0.010 (0.011)
3 + 0.05	0.77	0.031 (0.031)
3 + 0.1	0.85	0.014 (0.014)

[a] CI values were calculated from experimental data with the use of computer simulation of the classic isobologram equation. CI values in parentheses were calculated on the basis of the conservative isobologram equation, assuming independent modes of action. CI values of < 1, = 1 and > 1 indicate synergism, additivity and antagonism, respectively.

in such immortalized cell lines is a long-standing question (205). The kinetics of growth of such cells permit growth curve assays over a 5–10-day period in microtitre plates. Such cell lines are good targets for treatment with antisense oligomers to the EBV EBNA-1 ORF, the gene needed for episomal maintenance. Phosphorothioated oligomers of the same sequence described in the preceding section produced results such as those shown in Figure 6.6. By day 7 the scrambled-sense oligomers reduced cell numbers by 55%, the sense oligomers produced 86% reduction, whereas the antisense oligomers produced complete cytostasis with essentially complete inhibition of cell growth at 20 μM concentrations (Figure 6.6A) (200). In typical dose–response curves (Figure 6.6B), 20 μM of the antisense oligomers produced 100% inhibition, 10 μM produced 87%, and 5 μM produced 63% inhibition of cell growth. Although both sense and scrambled-sense oligonucleotides when phosphorothioated also have significant non-specific effects, the antisense compounds consistently produce a greater inhibitory effect on cell growth. It is difficult to measure whether episomal copy numbers are reduced in the treated cultures because of the cytostasis in the treated cultures. Treatment of the Raji BL cell line with the same compounds did not affect cell growth, which is expected since Raji cells have an 8;14 translocation, and their growth is driven by disregulation of *c-myc* expression.

Phosphorothioated oligomers have non-specific effects, shown by the partial inhibition of cell growth produced by the scrambled-sense oligomers (Figure 6.6A). Nonspecific effects are underscored by the report of inhibition of EBV DNA polymerase by phosphorothioated oligomers without sequence specificity (206). Further development in this emerging field of therapeutics will focus on design of new, more selective compounds and

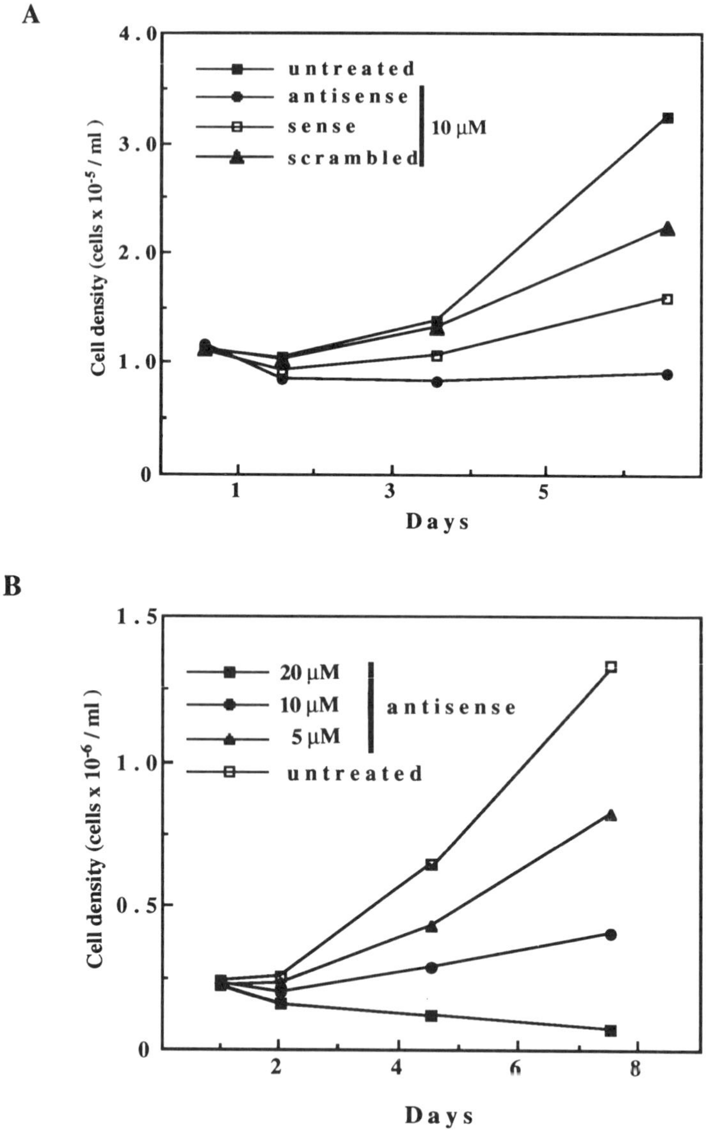

Figure 6.6. Specific inhibition of the growth of EBV-immortalized lymphocytes by antisense oligodeoxynucleotides to EBNA-1 mRNA. (A) The growth of a recently established EBV cord-lymphocyte line is significantly inhibited by scrambled-sense phosphorothioated oligomers, but cell growth is inhibited completely by the antisense oligomers. (B) Dose–response to the same antisense oligomers. The cell line, which carries EBV episomes, is a culture model for EBV-induced lymphoproliferative conditions

on improvements in cell uptake and stability of modified oligomers. Finally selection of key molecular targets is crucial. For example, EBNA-1 is not only the single critical product needed for episomal replication, it is also a *trans*-acting latency gene product entirely specific to the virus, and it is transcribed from an mRNA of low abundance in the cell (25). Thus EBNA-1 mRNA is in all respects an ideal target for this antiviral approach. As to the gene itself, oligomers that are antisense to other regions such as a splice acceptor site or the AUG might provide complementary inhibitory effects.

CONCLUSIONS

Specific treatment of persons with EBV infections has remained elusive. Although numerous compounds inhibit EBV replication, none has an effect on latent infection which is key in most EBV-associated diseases. The actual role of the virus in most of the diseases—causal, essential cofactor or contributory agent—remains uncertain (106). *Hairy leukoplakia* (HL) should be the simplest of the conditions to treat because latent infection seems not to be involved (Table 6.6). However, this disease, while it responds promptly to ACV (207), recurs after therapy, perhaps because HL is caused by multiple strains of EBV that co-infect the lesions and sometimes produce viral recombinants (137). Perhaps treatment of the lesions leaves a residuum of latent infection, not detectable during the active viral replication characteristic of the disease. This disease, once treated, should not recur if the underlying immunodeficiency were to be corrected.

Two trials of treatment of *infectious mononucleosis* (IM) with ACV given intravenously or orally have suggested marginal benefit that was, however, not statistically significant (208,209), although virus excretion in the oropharynx was transiently suppressed, an effect also produced by the drug

Table 6.6. Possible multi-modal therapies for diseases caused by or associated with EBV infection

Disease	Strategy, agents
Hairy leukoplakia	Viral DNA pol inhibitor
Infectious mononucleosis	Viral DNA pol inhibitor Immune modulator
Polyclonal B cell lymphomas	Episomal disruption, cytokines
Nasopharyngeal carcinoma	Viral DNA pol inhibitor, cytokines, differentiation promoters
Burkitt's lymphoma	*c-myc* gene product inhibitor; episomal disruption?

in patients with AIDS (210). In another trial significant benefit was reported (211). There are reasons for these ambiguous results: (i) unlike herpes genitalis or labialis, IM is an insidious disease, and in the trials ACV was given relatively late in the infection; (ii) the dosages of ACV were probably inadequate; (iii) most of the symptoms of IM are probably not due to direct effects of viral replication, but to secondary immunopathological responses of the host. Dealing with these problems is a challenge calling for methods to diagnose IM earlier, use of the new oral ACV prodrug (212,213) or other agents convenient to give for four to six weeks during the subacute phase, and agents such as corticosteroids that moderate cell-mediated immune responses, especially when organs or tissues such as central nervous system, liver and bone marrow that do not support viral replication are affected. IM is a disease of otherwise normal young persons, and any therapy would need to be non-toxic and without long-term side-effects.

Chronic fatigue syndrome (CFS) has been associated with EBV infection, but there is little solid evidence for such an association; CFS appears to be a collection of syndromes (141,214). A trial of treatment with ACV was without effect in a rather heterogeneous set of such patients (215,218).

Polyclonal B cell lymphomas appear to be driven by latent EBV infection, and therefore the principal antiviral target is the EBV episome. However, there is both virological and therapeutic evidence that viral replication may contribute to the disease process since these lymphomas occur in immunocompromised patients who have reactivated EBV infection, sometimes in the lymphoma cells themselves (216,217). Therefore the first line of therapy would be episomal disruption and use of cytokines such as interferons—perhaps IFN-α and IFN-γ in a synergistic combination—plus ACV or its equivalent in order to prevent immortalization of new cell populations. Trials guided by such strategies are timely since the incidence of lymphomas is rising in patients with AIDS, even after HIV infection is suppressed, and because of the serious, sometimes fulminant lymphoproliferation that occurs in allograft recipients, particularly cardiac.

Nasopharyngeal carcinoma (NPC) presents an intriguing and novel circumstance in which antiviral therapy might be used prophylactically. Although NPC occurs after decades of EBV infection there is compelling circumstantial evidence of a role for reactivation of EBV infection in triggering the onset of the disease. This evidence rests on the appearance of IgA antibodies to EBV replicative antigens preceding or accompanying disease onset in endemic areas (111,133). Moreover, although infection is latent in the NPC tumour cells and even in the early dysplastic lesions, islands of tumour cells sometimes display replicative antigens in contrast to the bulk of the tumour cell population in which a profile of latent EBV genome products is expressed (113). It may therefore make sense to give a viral DNA polymerase inhibitor orally to persons who have such IgA responses. Since, however, dysplasia or carcinoma *in situ* may already be present, agents such as cytokines and promoters of cell differentiation such as retinoids may be invoked, guided by the results of biopsy. More sensitive molecularly based EBV diagnostics are crucial for detection of NPC at its earliest, curable stages. A promising approach is based on detection of EBER RNA in immortalized B cells (219,220).

Treatment of *Burkitt's lymphoma* (BL) in the endemic regions with cancer chemotherapeutic agents is remarkably successful. North American patients with the sporadic form of BL may not respond so well, and the disease tends to relapse. Theoretically specific treatment for BL should be directed at the *c-myc* gene product, which is overexpressed in this disease and seems to be the single common molecular lesion. Transient suppression of cell growth has been produced in BL cell lines transfected with a construct expressing transcripts antisense to *c-myc* mRNA (115). Indeed transplants of BL in SCID mice regress upon induction of expression of anti-*c-myc* mRNA. Presumably in EBV-infected BL, disruption of episomal replication would also be necessary inasmuch as EBV episomes alone are sufficient to drive B cells. In antiviral therapy, as in therapy of most diseases, empiricism still reigns and inhibition of only one or two components that contribute to the pathogenesis of the disease may be enough to tip the balance in favour of the host's own corrective mechanisms. Now may be the time to become more venturesome in combating EBV infection not only with available viral inhibitors, but guided also by insights into the molecular pathogenesis of this remarkable array of diseases.

ACKNOWLEDGEMENTS

I am indebted to my colleague and former associate, Dr Jung-Chung Lin, for his expertise and good work that laid the basis for much of this chapter, and for the technical assistance of Miss Carolyn Smith, now deceased, to whom this chapter is dedicated. This work was supported by grants from the National Institutes of Health (RO1-AI-17205-13), the National Cancer Institute (P01-CA-19014-16 and R01-CA-56695-01), and the Burroughs Wellcome Company.

REFERENCES

1. Kieff, E. and Liebowitz, D. (1990). Epstein–Barr virus and its replication. In *Virology*, 2nd edn, B. N. Fields, D. M. Knipe *et al.* (eds), Raven Press, New York, pp. 1889-1920.
2. Baer, R., Bankier, A. T., Beggin, M. D. *et al.* (1984). DNA sequence and expression of the B95-8 Epstein–Barr virus genome. *Nature*, **310**, 207–211.
3. Pagano, J. S., Nonoyama, M. and Huang, C.-H. (1973). Epstein–Barr virus in human cells. In *Possible Episomes in Eukaryotes: Proceedings of the Fourth Lepetit Colloquium*, North-Holland, Amsterdam, pp. 218–228.

4. Adams, A. and Lindahl, T. (1975). Epstein–Barr virus genomes with properties of circular DNA molecules in carrier cells, *Proc. Natl Acad. Sci. USA*, **72**, 1477–1481.
5. Pagano, J. S. (1979). The Epstein–Barr virus plasmid. In *Extrachromosomal DNA*, D. J. Cummings, P. Borst, I. B. Dawid, S. M. Weissman and C. F. Fox (eds), Academic Press, New York, vol XV, pp. 235–248.
6. Pagano, J. S. (1991). Gertrude and Werner Henle lecture on viral oncology. From latency to replication: recent studies of the Epstein–Barr virus. In *Epstein–Barr Virus and Human Disease 1990*, D. V. Ablashi *et al.* (eds), Humana Press, Totowa, NJ, pp. 19–32.
7. Shaw, J., Levinger, L. and Carter, C., Jr (1979). Nucleosomal structure of Epstein–Barr virus DNA in transformed cell lines. *J. Virol.*, **29**, 657–665.
8. Nonoyama, M. and Pagano, J. S. (1972). Separation of Epstein–Barr virus DNA from large chromosomal DNA in nonvirus-producing cells. *Nature New Biol.*, **238**, 169–171.
9. Adams, A. (1987). Replication of latent Epstein–Barr virus genomes in Raji cells. *J. Virol.*, **61**, 1743–1746.
10. Sample, J. and Kieff, E. (1990). Transcription of the Epstein–Barr virus genome during latency in growth-transformed lymphocytes. *J. Virol.*, **64**, 1667–1674.
11. Henry, B. E., Raab-Traub, N.J. and Pagano, J. S. (1983). Detection of autonomous replicating sequences (ars) in the genome of Epstein–Barr virus (EBV). *Proc. Natl Acad. Sci. USA*, **80**, 1096–1100.
12. Yates, J., Warren, N., Reisman, D. and Sugden, B. (1984). A *cis*-acting element from the Epstein–Barr viral genome that permits stable replication of recombinant plasmids in latently infected cells. *Proc. Natl Acad. Sci. USA*, **81**, 3806–3810.
13. Hammerschmidt, W. and Sugden, B. (1988). Identification and characterization of oriLyt, a lytic origin of DNA replication of Epstein–Barr virus. *Cell*, **55**, 427–433.
14. Reisman, D., Yates, J. and Sugden, B. (1985). A putative origin of replication of plasmids derived from Epstein–Barr virus is composed of two *cis*-acting components. *Mol. Cell. Biol.*, **5**, 1822–1832.
15. Gahn, T. A. and Schildkraut, C. L. (1989). The Epstein–Barr virus origin of plasmid replication, *ori*-P, contains both the initiation and termination sites of DNA replication. *Cell*, **58**, 527–535.
16. Lupton, S. and Levine, A. (1985). Mapping genetic elements of Epstein–Barr virus that facilitate extrachromosomal persistence of Epstein–Barr virus-derived plasmids in human cells. *Mol. Cell. Biol.*, **5**, 2533–2542.
17. Reisman, D. and Sugden, B. (1986). *Trans* activation of an Epstein–Barr viral transcriptional enhancer by the Epstein–Barr viral nuclear antigen 1. *Mol. Cell. Biol.*, **6**, 3838–3846.
18. Sugden, B. and Warren, N. (1989). A promoter of Epstein–Barr virus that can function during latent infection can be transactivated by EBNA-1, a viral protein required for viral DNA replication during latent infection. *J. Virol.*, **63**, 2644–2649.
19. Woisetschlaeger, M., Yandava, C. N., Furmanski, L. A. *et al.* (1990). Promoter switching in Epstein–Barr virus during the initial stages of infection of B lymphocytes. *Proc. Natl Acad. Sci. USA*, **87**, 1725–1729.
20. Sung, N. S., Kenney, S., Gutsch, D. and Pagano, J. S. (1991). EBNA-2 transactivates a lymphoid-specific enhancer in the BamHI C promoter of Epstein–Barr virus. *J. Virol.*, **65**, 2164–2169.
21. Kerr, B. M., Lear, A. L., Rowe, M. *et al.* (1992). Three transcriptionally distinct

forms of Epstein–Barr virus latency somatic cell hybrids: cell phenotype dependence of promoter usage *Virol.*, **187**, 189–201.
22. Sung, N. S., Wilson, J., Davenport, M. *et al.* (1994). Reciprocal regulation of the Epstein–Barr Virus Bam H1-F promoter by EBNA-1 and an E2F transcription factor. *MCB*, **14**, in press.
23. Pesano, R. L. and Pagano, J. S. (1986). Herpesvirus papio contains a plasmid origin of replication that acts in cis interspecies with an Epstein–Barr virus transacting function. *J. Virol.*, **60**, 1159–1162.
24. Loeb, D., Sung, N. S., Pesano, R. L. *et al.* (1990). Plasmid origin of replication of herpesvirus papio: DNA sequence and enhancer function. *J. Virol.*, **64**, 2876–2883.
25. Sternas, L., Middleton, T. and Sugden, B. (1990). The average number of molecules of Epstein–Barr nuclear antigen 1 per cell does not correlate with the average number of Epstein–Barr virus (EBV) DNA molecules per cell among different clones of EBV-immortalized cells. *J. Virol.*, **64**, 2407–2410.
26. Rawlins, D., Milman, G., Hayward, S. D. and Hayward, G. S. (1985). Sequence-specific DNA-binding of the Epstein–Barr virus nuclear antigen (EBNA-1) to clustered sites in the plasmid maintenance region. *Cell*, **42**, 859–868.
27. Hearing, J., Mulhaupt, Y. and Harper, S. (1992). Interaction of Epstein–Barr virus nuclear antigen 1 with the viral latent origin of replication. *J. Virol.*, **66**, 694–705.
28. Frappier, L. and O'Donnell, M. (1992). EBNA1 distorts *oriP*, the Epstein–Barr virus latent replication origin. *J. Virol.*, **66**, 1786–1790.
29. Sexton, C. J. and Pagano, J. S. (1989). Analysis of the Epstein–Barr virus origin of plasmid replication (*ori*P) reveals an area of nucleosome sparing spanning the 3′ dyad. *J. Virol.*, **63**, 5505–5508.
30. Sexton, C. J. (1989). Structural analysis of the Epstein–Barr virus origin of plasmid replication and its interaction with the EBV nuclear antigen, EBNA-1. PhD dissertation, University of North Carolina.
31. Middleton, T. and Sugden, B. (1992). EBNA1 can link the enhancer element to the initiator's element of the Epstein–Barr virus plasmid origin of DNA replication. *J. Virol.*, **66**, 489–495.
32. Frappier, L. and O'Donnell, M. (1991). Epstein–Barr nuclear antigen 1 mediates a DNA loop within the latent replication origin of Epstein–Barr virus. *Proc. Natl Acad. Sci. USA*, **88**, 10875–10879.
33. Wen, L. T., Tanaka, A. and Nonoyama, M. (1989). Induction of anti-EBNA-1 protein by 12-*O*-tetradecanoylphorbol-13-acetate treatment of human lymphoblastoid cells. *J. Virol.*, **63**, 3315–3322.
34. Oh, S. J., Chittenden, T. and Levine, A. J. (1991). Identification of cellular factors that bind specifically to the Epstein–Barr virus origin of DNA replication. *J. Virol.*, **65**, 514–519.
35. Zhang, S. and Nonoyama, M. (1994). The cellular proteins that bind specifically to the Epstein–Barr virus origin of plasmid DNA replication belong to a gene family. *Proc. Natl Acad. Sci. USA*, **91**, 2843–2847.
36. Sato, H., Pagano, J. S. and Raab-Traub, R. (1988). Amplification of Epstein–Barr virus (EBV) DNA by superinfection with a strain of EBV derived from nasopharyngeal carcinoma. *J. Virol.*, **62**, 3288–3294.
37. Sato, H., Takimoto, T., Tanaka, S. *et al.* (1990). Concatameric replication of Epstein–Barr virus: structure of the termini in virus-producer and newly transformed cell lines. *J. Virol.*, **64**, 5295–5300.
38. Hurley, E. A., Agger, S., McNeil, J. A. *et al.* (1991). When Epstein–Barr virus persistently infects B-cell lines, it frequently integrates. *J. Virol.*, **65**, 1245–1254.

39. Gulley, M. L., Raphael, M., Lutz, C. T. *et al.* (1992). Epstein–Barr virus integration in human lymphomas and lymphoid cell lines. *Cancer*, **70**, 185–191.
40. Sixbey, J. W., Davis, D. S., Young, L. S. *et al.* (1987). Human epithelial cell expression of an Epstein–Barr virus receptor. *J. Gen. Virol.*, **68**, 805–811.
41. Frade, R., Barel, M., Ehlin-Henrikson, B. and Klein, G. (1985). gp140, the C3d receptor of human B lymphocytes, is the Epstein–Barr virus receptor. *Proc. Natl Acad. Sci. USA*, **82**, 1490–1493.
42. Sixbey, J. W., Nedrud, J. G., Raab-Traub, N. *et al.* (1984). Epstein–Barr virus replication in oropharyngeal epithelial cells. *N. Engl. J. Med.*, **310**, 1225–1230.
43. Pagano, J. S. (1984). Epithelial cell interactions of the Epstein–Barr virus. In *Concepts in Viral Pathogenesis*, A. Notkins and M. Oldstone (eds), Springer-Verlag, Berlin, pp. 307–314.
44. Li, Q. X., Young, L. S., Niedobitek, G. *et al.* (1992). Epstein–Barr virus infection and replication in a human epithelial cell system. *Nature*, **356**, 347–350.
45. Sixbey, J. W. and Pagano, J. S. (1984). New perspectives on the Epstein–Barr virus in the pathogenesis of lymphoproliferative disorders. In *Current Clinical Topics in Infectious Diseases*, J. Remington and M. Swartz (eds), McGraw-Hill, New York, pp. 146–176.
46. Raab-Traub, N. and Pagano, J. S. (1989). The Epstein–Barr virus and its antigens. *Hum. Immunogenet.*, **43**, 477–498.
47. Hanto, D. W., Frizzera, G., Gajl-Peczalska, K. J. *et al.* (1982). Epstein–Barr virus-induced B-cell lymphoma after renal transplantation: acyclovir therapy and transition from polyclonal to monoclonal B-cell proliferation. *N. Engl. J. Med.*, **306**, 913–918.
48. Kikuta, H., Taguchi, Y., Tomizawa, K. *et al.* (1988). Epstein–Barr virus genome-positive T lymphocytes in a boy with chronic active EBV infection associated with Kawasaki-like disease. *Nature*, **333**, 455–457.
49. Jones, J. F., Shurin, S., Abramowsky, C. *et al.* (1988). T-cell lymphomas containing Epstein–Barr viral DNA in patients with chronic Epstein–Barr virus infections. *N. Engl. J. Med.*, **318**, 733–740.
50. Su, I. J., Hsieh, H. C., Lin, K. H. *et al.* (1991). Aggressive peripheral T-cell lymphomas containing Epstein–Barr viral DNA: a clinicopathologic and molecular analysis. *Blood*, **77**, 799–808.
51. Pulvertaft, R. J. V. (1965). A study of malignant tumors in Nigeria by short term tissue culture. *J. Clin. Pathol.*, **18**, 261–273.
52. Pope, J. H., Achong, B. and Epstein, M. (1968). Transformation of fetal human leucocytes *in vitro* by filtrates of a human leukemic cell line containing herpes-like virus. *Int. J. Cancer*, **3**, 857–866.
53. Klein, G. (1989). Viral latency and transformation: the strategy of Epstein–Barr virus. *Cell*, **58**, 5–8.
54. Sugden, B. (1989). An intricate route to immortality. *Cell*, **57**, 5–7.
55. Miller, G. (1990). Epstein–Barr virus. In *Virology*, 2nd edn, B. N. Fields, D. M. Knipe *et al.* (eds), Raven Press, New York, pp. 1921–1958.
56. Moss, D. J., Misko, I. S., Burrows, S. R. *et al.* (1988). Cytotoxic T-cell clones discriminate between A- and B-type Epstein-Barr virus transformants. *Nature*, **331**, 719–721.
57. Countryman, J. and Miller, G. (1985). Activation of expression of latent Epstein–Barr herpesvirus after gene transfer with a small cloned subfragment of heterogeneous DNA. *Proc. Natl Acad. Sci. USA*, **82**, 4085–4089.
58. Rooney, C. M., Rowe, D. T., Ragot, T. and Farrell, P. J. (1989). The spliced BZLF1 gene of Epstein–Barr virus (EBV) transactivates an early promoter and induces the virus lytic cycle. *J. Virol.*, **63**, 3109–3116.

59. Kenney, D., Kamine, J., Holley, G. E. *et al.* (1989). The Epstein–Barr virus (EBV) BZLF1 immediate–early gene product differentially affects latent versus productive EBV promoters. *J. Virol.*, **63**, 1729–1736.
60. Farrell, P. J., Rowe, D. T., Rooney, C. M. and Kouzarides, T. (1989). Epstein–Barr virus BZLF1 transactivator specifically binds to a consensus AP-1 site and is related to c-fos. *EMBO J.*, **8**, 127–132.
61. Lieberman, P. M. and Berk, A. J. (1990). In vitro transcriptional activation, dimerization, and DNA-binding specificity of the Epstein–Barr virus Zta protein. *J. Virol.*, **64**, 2560–2568.
62. Sista, N. D., Pagano, J. S., Liao, W. and Kenney, S. (1993). Retinoic acid is a negative regulator of the Epstein–Barr virus protein (BZLF1) that mediates disruption of latent infection. *Proc. Natl Acad. Sci. USA*, **90**, 3894–3898.
63. Zhang, Q., Gutsch, D. and Kenney, S. (1994). Functional and physical interaction between p53 and BZLF1: implications for Epstein–Barr virus latency. *MCB*, **14**, 1929–1938.
64. Furnari, F., Zacny, V., Quinlivan, E. B., *et al.* (1993). RAZ, an Epstein–Barr virus transdominant repressor that modulates the viral reactivation mechanism. *Cell, J. Virol.*, **68**, 1827–1836.
65. Wang, T. S. E., Wong, S. W. and Korn, D. (1989). Human DNA polymerase α: predicted functional domains and relationships with viral DNA polymerases. *FASEB J.*, **3**, 14–21.
66. Lin, J. C., Sista, N. D., Besencon, F. *et al.* (1991). Identification and functional characterization of Epstein–Barr virus DNA polymerase by in vitro transcription–translation of a cloned gene. *J. Virol.*, **65**, 2728–2731.
67. Miller, R. L., Glaser, R. and Rapp, F. (1977). Studies of an Epstein–Barr virus-induced DNA polymerase. *Virology*, **76**, 494–502.
68. Goodman, S. R., Prezyna, C. and Benz, W. C. (1978). Two Epstein–Barr virus associated DNA polymerase activities. *J. Biol. Chem.*, **253**, 8617–8628.
69. Ooka, T., Lenoir, G. and Daillie, J. (1979). Characterization of an Epstein–Barr virus-induced DNA polymerase. *J. Virol.*, **29**, 1–10.
70. Allaudeen, H. S. and Rani, G. (1982). Cellular and Epstein–Barr virus specific DNA polymerase in virus-producing Burkitt's lymphoma cell lines. *Nucleic Acids Res.*, **10**, 2453–2465.
71. Kallin, B., Sternas, L., Saemundssen, A. K. *et al.* (1985). Purification of Epstein–Barr virus DNA polymerase from P3HR-1 cells. *J. Virol.*, **54**, 561–568.
72. Tsurumi, T., Daikoku, T., Kurachi, R. and Nishiyama, Y. (1993). Functional interaction between Epstein–Barr Virus DNA polymerase catalytic subunit and its accessory subunit. *In Vitro. J. Virol.*, **67**, 7648–7653.
73. Digard, P., Bebrin, W. R., Weisshart, K. and Coen, D. M. (1993). The extreme C terminus of herpes simplex virus DNA polymerase is crucial for functional interaction with processivity factor UL42 and for viral replication. *J. Virol.*, **67**, 398–406.
74. Digard, P., Chow, C. S., Pirrit, L. and Coen, D. M. (1993). Functional analysis of the herpes simplex virus UL42 protein. *J. Virol.*, **67**, 1159–1168.
75. Gottlieb, J. and Challberg, M. D. (1994). Interaction of herpes simplex virus type 1 DNA polymerase and the UL42 accessory protein with a model primer template. *J. Virol.*, **68**, 4937–4945.
76. Li, J. S., Zhou, B. S., Dutchman, G. E. *et al.* (1987). Association of Epstein–Barr virus early antigen diffuse component and virus-specified DNA polymerase activity. *J. Virol.*, **61**, 2947–2949.
77. Kiehl, A. and Dorsky, D. I. (1991). Cooperation of DNA polymerase and EA-D (BMRF1) *in vitro* and colocalization in nuclei of infected cells. *Virology*, **184**, 330–340.

78. Tsurumi, T., Kobayashi, A., Tamai, K., *et al.* (1993). Functional expression and characterization of the Epstein–Barr Virus DNA polymerase catalytic subunit. *J. Virol.*, **67**, 4651–4658.
79. Lin, J. C., De, B. K. and Mar, E. C. (1994). Functional characterization of partially purified Epstein–Barr Virus DNA polymerase expressed in the baculovirus system. *Virus Genes*, **8**, 3, 231–241.
80. Crute, J. J., Tsurumi, T., Zhu, L. *et al.* (1989). Herpes simplex virus 1 helicase-primase: a complex of three herpes-encoded gene products. *Proc. Natl Acad. Sci. USA*, **86**, 2186–2189.
81. Daibata, M. and Sairenji, T. (1993). Epstein–Barr Virus (EBV) replication and expressions of EA-D (BMRF1 gene product), virus-specific deoxyribonuclease, and DNA polymerase in EBV-activated akata cells. *Virol.*, **196**, 900-904.
82. Benson, J. D. and Huang, E.-S. (1988). Two specific topoisomerase II inhibitors prevent replication of human cytomegalovirus DNA: an implied role in replication of the viral genome. *J. Virol.*, **62**, 4797–4800.
83. Kawanishi, M. (1993). Topoisomerase I and II activities are required for Epstein–Barr virus replication. *J. Gen. Virol.*, **74**, 2263–2268.
84. Gruffat, H., Moreno, N. and Sergeant, A. (1990). The Epstein–Barr virus (EBV) ORI_{lyt} enhancer is not B-cell specific and does not respond synergistically to the EBV transcription factors R and Z. *J. Virol.*, **64**, 2810–2818.
85. Furnari, F. B., Adams, M. D. and Pagano, J. S. (1993). Unconventional processing of the 3′ termini of the Epstein–Barr virus DNA polymerase mRNA. *Proc. Natl Acad. Sci. USA*, **90**, 378–382.
86. Furnari, F. B. (1993). Mechanisms regulating the expression of the Epstein–Barr virus DNA polymerase gene. PhD dissertation, University of North Carolina.
87. Kenney, S., Kamine, J., Holley-Guthrie, E. *et al.* (1989). The EBV immediate–early gene product, BMLF1, acts *in trans* by a post-transcriptional mechanism which is reporter gene dependent. *J. Virol.*, **63**, 3870–3877.
88. Furnari, F., Adams, M. D. and Pagano, J. S. (1992). Regulation of the Epstein–Barr virus (EBV) DNA polymerase gene. *J. Virol.*, **66**, 2837–2845.
89. Furnari, F. B., Adams, M. and Pagano, J. S. (1993). The 3′ ends of the EBV DNA polymerase mRNA are processed without canonical polyadenylation signals. In *The Epstein–Barr Virus and Associated Diseases*, T. Tursz, J. S. Pagano, D. V. Ablashi, *et al.* (eds), INSERM and John Libbey Eurotext, London, pp. 175–180.
90. Pagano, J. S. (1991). Epstein–Barr virus. In *Textbook of Internal Medicine*, 2nd edn, N. Kelley (ed.), Lippincott, Philadelphia, pp. 1499–1503.
91. Miller, G., Niederman, J. C. and Andrews, L. L. (1973). Prolonged oropharyngeal excretion of Epstein–Barr virus after infectious mononucleosis. *N. Engl. J. Med.*, **288**, 229–232.
92. Niederman, J. C., Miller, G., Pearson, G. A. and Pagano, J. S. (1976). Infectious mononucleosis: Epstein–Barr virus shedding in saliva and oropharynx. *N. Engl J. Med.*, **294**, 1355–1359.
93. Purtilo, D. T., Brichacek, B., Luka, J., *et al.* (1993). Non-Hodgkin's lymphomas in X-linked lymphoproliferative disease. In *The Epstein–Barr Virus and Associated Diseases*, T. Tursz, J. S. Pagano, D. V. Ablashi, *et al.* (eds), INSERM and John Libbey Eurotext, London, pp. 411–414.
94. Mori, M., Kurozumi, H., Akagi, K. *et al.* (1992). Monoclonal proliferation of T cells containing Epstein–Barr virus in fatal mononucleosis. *N. Engl. J. Med.*, **327**, 58.
95. Mroczek, E. C., Weisenburger, D. D., Grierson, H. L. *et al.* (1987). Fatal infectious mononucleosis and virus-associated hemophagocytic syndrome. *Arch. Pathol. Lab. Med.*, **111**, 530–535.

96. Sixbey, J. W., Vesterinen, E. H., Nedrud, J. G. *et al.* (1983). EBV replication in human epithelial cells infected in vitro. *Nature*, **306**, 480–483.
97. Sixbey, J. W., Lemon, S. M. and Pagano, J. S. (1986). A second site for Epstein–Barr virus shedding: the uterine cervix. *Lancet*, **2**, 1122–1124.
98. Henle, G., Henle, W. and Diehl, V. (1968). Relation of Burkitt's tumor-associated herpes-type virus to infectious mononucleosis. *Proc. Natl Acad. Sci. USA*, **59**, 94–101.
99. Evans, A. S., Niederman, J. C. and McCollum, R. W. (1968). Seroepidemiologic studies of infectious mononucleosis with EB virus. *N. Engl. J. Med.*, **279**, 1121–1127.
100. Henle, G., Henle, W. and Horwitz, C. A. (1974). Antibodies to Epstein–Barr virus-associated nuclear antigen in infectious mononucleosis. *J. Infect. Dis.*, **130**, 231–239.
101. Epstein, M. A., Achong, B. G. and Barr, Y. M. (1964). Virus particles in cultured lymphoblasts from Burkitt's lymphoma. *Lancet*, **i**, 702–703.
102. Wolf, H., zur Hausen, H. and Becker, Y. (1973). EBV viral genomes in epithelial nasopharyngeal carcinoma cells. *Nature Biol.*, **244**, 245–257.
103. Nonoyama, M., Huang, C.-H., Pagano, J. S. *et al.* (1973). DNA of Epstein–Barr virus detected in tissue of Burkitt's lymphoma and nasopharyngeal carcinoma. *Proc. Natl Acad. Sci. USA*, **70**, 3265–3268.
104. Greenspan, J. S., Greenspan, D., Lennette, E. T. *et al.* (1985). Replication of Epstein–Barr virus within the epithelial cells of oral 'hairy' leukoplakia, an AIDS-associated lesion. *N. Engl. J. Med.*, **313**, 1564–1571.
105. Sandvej, K., Krenacs, L., Hamilton-Dutoit, S. J. *et al.* (1992). Epstein–Barr virus latent and replicative gene expression in oral hairy leukoplakia. *Histopathology*, **20**, 387–395.
106. Pagano, J. S. (1992). Epstein–Barr virus: culprit or consort. *N. Engl. J. Med.*, **327**, 1750–1752.
107. Burkitt, D. (1962). A children's cancer dependent on climatic factors. *Nature*, **194**, 232.
108. Pagano, J. S., Huang, C.-H. and Levine, P. (1973). Absence of Epstein–Barr viral DNA in American Burkitt's lymphoma. *N. Engl. J. Med.*, **289**, 1395–1399.
109. Pagano, J. S. (1975). The Epstein–Barr virus and malignancy: molecular evidence. In *Cold Spring Harbor Symposium on Quantitative Biology: Tumor Viruses*, XXIX, Cold Spring Harbor Laboratory, Cold Spring Harbor, New York, pp. 797–805.
110. Gravell, M., Levine, P. H., McIntyre, R. F. *et al.* (1976). Epstein–Barr virus in an American patient with Burkitt's lymphoma: detection of viral genome in tumor tissue and establishment of a tumor-derived cell line. *J. Natl Cancer Inst.*, **56**, 7001–7004.
111. De The, G. (1982). Epidemiology of Epstein–Barr virus and associated diseases in man. In *The Herpesviruses*, B. Roizman (ed.), Plenum Press, New York, pp. 25–103.
112. Raab-Traub, N. and Flynn, K. (1986). The structure of the termini of the Epstein–Barr virus as a marker of clonal cellular proliferation. *Cell*, **47**, 883–889.
113. Raab-Traub, N. (1992). Epstein–Barr virus and nasopharyngeal carcinoma. *Semin. Cancer Biol.*, **3**, 297–307.
114. Dalla-Favera, R., Bregni, M., Erikson, J. *et al.* (1982). Human c-myc oncogene is located on the region of chromosome 8 that is translocated in Burkitt lymphoma cells. *Proc. Natl Acad. Sci. USA*, **79**, 7824–7827.
115. Magrath, I. T., Jain, V. and Bhatia, K. (1993). Molecular epidemiology of Burkitt's lymphoma. In *The Epstein–Barr Virus and Associated Diseases*, T. Tursz, J. S.

Pagano, D. V. Ablashi, *et al.* (eds), INSERM and John Libbey Eurotext, London, pp. 377–396.
116. Kenney, S. C. (1993). Interactions of the Z protein with cellular proteins. In *The Epstein–Barr Virus and Associated Diseases*, T. Tursz, J. S. Pagano, D. V. Ablashi, *et al.* (eds), INSERM and John Libbey Eurotext, London, pp. 127–136.
117. Lam, K. M. C., Syed, N., Whittle, H. and Crawford, D. H. (1991). Circulating Epstein–Barr virus-carrying B cells in acute malaria. *Lancet*, **337**, 876–878.
118. Fixman, E. D., Hayward, G. S. and Hayward, D. (1992). Transacting requirements for replication of Epstein–Barr virus *ori-Lyt*. *J. Virol.*, **54**, 561–568.
119. Young, L., Alfieri, C., Hennessy, K. *et al.* (1989). Expression of Epstein–Barr virus transformation-associated genes in tissues of patients with EBV lymphoproliferative disease. *N. Engl. J. Med.*, **321**, 1080–1085.
120. Thomas, J. A., Hotchin, N. A., Allday, M. J. *et al.* (1990). Immunohistology of Epstein–Barr virus-associated antigens in B cell disorders from immunocompromised individuals. *Transplantation*, **49**, 944–953.
121. Randhawa, P. S., Jaffe, R., Demetris, A. J. *et al.* (1991). The systemic distribution of Epstein–Barr virus genomes in fatal post-transplantation lymphoproliferative disorders: an in situ hybridization study. *Am. J. Pathol.*, **138**, 1027–1033.
122. Katz, B. Z., Raab-Traub, N. and Miller, G. (1989). Latent and replicating forms of Epstein–Barr virus DNA in lymphomas and lymphoproliferative disease, *J. Infect. Dis.*, **160**, 589–598.
123. Randhawa, P. S., Markin, R. S., Starzl, T. E. and Demetris, A. J. (1990). Epstein–Barr virus-associated syndromes in immunosuppressed liver transplant recipients: clinical profile and recognition on routine allograft biopsy. *Am. J. Surg. Pathol.*, **14**, 538–547.
124. Penn, I. (1990). Cancers complicating organ transplantation. *N. Engl. J. Med.*, **323**, 1767–1769.
125. Katz, B. Z., Raab-Traub, N. and Miller, G. (1989). Latent and replicating forms of Epstein–Barr virus DNA in lymphomas and lymphoproliferative diseases. *J. Infect. Dis.*, **160**, 589–598.
126. Weiss, L. M., Movahed, L. A., Warnke, R. A. and Sklar, J. (1989). Detection of Epstein–Barr viral genomes in Reed–Sternberg cells of Hodgkin's disease. *N. Engl. J. Med.*, **320**, 502–506.
127. Weiss, L. M., Chen, Y. Y., Liu, X. F. and Shibata, D. (1991). Epstein–Barr virus and Hodgkin's disease: a correlative in situ hybridization and polymerase chain reaction study. *Am. J. Pathol.*, **139**, 1259–1265.
128. Herbst, H., Dallenbach, F., Hummel, M. *et al.* (1991). Epstein–Barr virus latent membrane protein expression in Hodgkin and Reed–Sternberg cells. *Proc. Natl Acad. Sci. USA*, **88**, 4766–4770.
129. Nonoyama, M. and Pagano, J. S. (1973). Homology between Epstein–Barr virus DNA and viral DNA from Burkitt's lymphoma and nasopharyngeal carcinoma determined by DNA–DNA reassociation kinetics. *Nature*, **242**, 44–47
130. Pagano, J. S., Huang, C. H., Klein, G. *et al.* (1975). Homology of Epstein–Barr virus DNA in nasopharyngeal carcinomas from Kenya, Taiwan, Singapore, and Tunis. In *Proceedings of the Second International Symposium on Oncogenesis and Herpesviruses*, Nuremberg, Germany. IARC, Lyon, Publication No. 11, Part II, pp. 179–190.
131. Desgranges, C., Wolf, H., de The, G. *et al.* (1975). Nasopharyngeal carcinoma. X. Presence of Epstein–Barr virus genomes in epithelial cells of tumors from high and medium risk areas. *Int. J. Cancer*, **16**, 7–15.
132. Li, Z. Q., Chen, J. J. and Li, W. J. (1983). Early detection of nasopharyngeal carcinoma (NPC) and nasopharyngeal mucosal hyperplastic lesion (NPHC)

with its relationship to carcinomatous change. In *Nasopharyngeal Carcinoma: Current Concepts*, D. Ablashi, U. Prasad and P. H. Levine (eds), University of Malaya Press, Kuala Lumpur, pp. 17–23.
133. Henle, G. and Henle, W. (1976). Epstein–Barr virus-specific IgA serum antibodies as an outstanding feature of nasopharyngeal carcinoma. *Int. J. Cancer*, **17**, 1–7.
134. Pearson, G. R., Weiland, L. H. and Neel, H. B. (1983). Application of Epstein–Barr virus (EBV) serology to the diagnosis of North American nasopharyngeal carcinoma. *Cancer*, **51**, 260–268.
135. Sixbey, J. W. and Yao, Q. Y. (1992). Immunoglobulin A-induced shift of Epstein–Barr virus tissue tropism. *Science*, **255**, 1578–1580.
136. Raab-Traub, N., Rajadurai, P., Flynn, K. and Lanier, A. P. (1991). Epstein–Barr virus infection in carcinoma of the salivary gland. *J. Virol.*, **65**, 7032–7036.
137. Walling, D. M., Edmiston, S. N., Sixbey, J. W. *et al.* (1992). Coinfection with multiple strains of the Epstein–Barr virus in human immunodeficiency virus-associated hairy leukoplakia. *Proc. Natl Acad. Sci. USA*, **89**, 6560–6564.
138. Pagano, J. S. and Shaw, J. E. (1979). Molecular probes and genome homology. In *The Epstein–Barr Virus*, M. A. Epstein and B. G. Achong (eds), Springer-Verlag, New York, pp. 109–146.
139. Nonoyama, M. and Pagano, J. S. (1971). Complementary RNA specific to the DNA of the Epstein–Barr virus: detection of EB viral genome in nonproductive cells. *Nature New Biol.*, **233**, 103–106.
140. Lin, J. C., Smith, M. C. and Pagano, J. S. (1984). Prolonged inhibitory effect of 9-(1,3-dihydroxy-2-propoxymethyl)guanine against replication of Epstein–Barr virus. *J. Virol.*, **50**, 50–55.
141. Pagano, J. S. (1991). Detection of Epstein–Barr virus with molecular hybridization techniques. *Rev. Infect. Dis.*, **13** (Suppl. 1), S123–128.
142. Shaw, J. E., Seebeck, T., Li, J.-L. H. and Pagano, J. S. (1977). The Epstein–Barr virus DNA synthesized in superinfected Raji cells. *Virology*, **77**, 762–771.
143. Lin, J.-C. and Machida, H. (1988). Comparison of two bromovinyl nucleoside analogs, 1-β-D-arabinofuranosyl-*E*-5-(2-bromovinyl)uracil and *E*-5-(2-bromovinyl)-2′-deoxyuridine, with acyclovir in inhibition of Epstein–Barr virus replication. *Antimicrob. Agents Chemother.*, **32**, 1068–1072.
144. Sixbey, J. W. and Pagano, J. S. (1985). Epstein–Barr virus transformation of human B-lymphocytes despite inhibition of viral polymerase. *J. Virol.*, **53**, 299–301.
145. Miller, G., Shope, T., Coope, D. *et al.* (1977). Lymphoma in cotton-top marmosets after inoculation with Epstein–Barr virus: tumor incidence, histologic spectrum, antibody responses, demonstration of viral DNA, and characterization of viruses. *J. Exp. Med.*, **45**, 948–967.
146. Morgan, A. J. (1993). Recent progress in EBV vaccine development. In *The Epstein–Barr Virus and Associated Diseases*, T. Tursz, J. S. Pagano, D. V. Ablashi, *et al.* (eds), INSERM and John Libbey Eurotext, London, pp. 549–555.
147. Cannon, M. J., Pisa, P., Fox, R. I. and Cooper, N. R. (1990). Epstein–Barr virus induces aggressive lymphoproliferative disorders of human B cell origin in SCID/hu chimeric mice. *J. Clin. Invest.*, **85**, 1333–1337.
148. Baiocchi, R. A. and Caligiuri, M. A. (1994). Low-dose interleukin 2 prevents the development of Epstein–Barr virus (EBV)-associated lymphoproliferative disease in scid/scid mice reconstituted i.p. with EBV-seropositive human peripheral blood lymphocytes. *Natl. Acad. Sci. USA*, **91**, 5577–5581.
149. Prusoff, W. H. (1959). Synthesis and biological activities of iododeoxyuridine, an analog of thymidine. *Biochim. Biophys. Acta*, **32**, 295–296.

150. Lin, J. C., Smith, M. C., Cheng, Y. C. and Pagano, J. S. (1983). Epstein–Barr virus: inhibition of replication by three new drugs. *Science*, **221**, 578–579.
151. Coker-Vann, J. and Dolin, R. (1977). Effect of adenine arabinoside on Epstein–Barr virus *in vitro*. *J. Infect. Dis.*, **135**, 447–453.
152. Benz, W. C., Siegel, P. J. and Baer, J. (1978). Effects of adenine arabinoside on lymphocytes infected with Epstein–Barr virus. *J. Virol.*, **27**, 475–482.
153. Ooka, T., Calander, A., de Turenne, M. and Daillee, J. (1983). Effect of arabinofuranosylthymine on the replication of Epstein–Barr virus and relationship with a new induced thymidine kinase activity. *J. Virol.*, **46**, 187–195.
154. Elion, G. B., Furman, P. A., Fyfe, J. A. *et al.* (1977). Selectivity of action of an antiherpetic agent, 9-(2-hydroxyethoxymethyl)guanine. *Proc. Natl Acad. Sci. USA*, **74**, 5716–5720.
155. Colby, B. M., Shaw, J. E., Elion, G. B. and Pagano, J. S. (1980). The effect of acyclovir [9-(2-hydroxyethoxymethyl) guanine] on Epstein–Barr virus DNA replication. *J. Virol.*, **34**, 560–568.
156. Colby, B . M., Furman, P. A., Shaw, J. E. *et al.* (1981). Phosphorylation of acyclovir [9-(2-hydroxy-ethoxymethyl guanine] in Epstein–Barr virus-infected lymphoblastoid cell lines. *J. Virol.*, **38**, 606–611.
157. Datta, A. K. and Pagano, J. S. (1983). Phosphorylation of acyclovir (9-(2-hydroxyethoxymethyl guanine) in vitro in activated Burkitt somatic cell hybrids. *Antimicrob. Agents Chemother.*, **24**, 10–14.
158. De Turenne-Tessier, M., Ooka, T., De The, G. and Daillie, J. (1986). Characterization of an Epstein–Barr virus-induced thymidine kinase. *J. Virol.*, **57**, 1105–1112.
159. Littler, E. and Arrand, J. R. (1988). Characterization of the Epstein–Barr virus-encoded thymidine kinase expressed in heterologous eucaryotic and procaryotic systems. *J. Virol.*, **62**, 3892–3895.
160. Littler, E., Zeuthen, J., *et al.* (1986). Identification of an Epstein–Barr virus-coded thymidine kinase. *EMBO J.*, **5**, 1959–1966.
161. Povey, A. C., Cooper, D. P. and Littler, E. (1991). 32P-postlabelling of alkylated thymidines using Epstein–Barr virus encoded thymidine kinase. *Carcinogenesis*, **12**, 709–712.
162. Pagano, J. S. and Datta, A. K. (1982). Perspectives on interactions of acyclovir with Epstein–Barr virus and other herpesviruses. *Am. J. Med.* (Acyclovir Symposium), 18–26.
163. Datta, A. K., Colby, B. M., Shaw, J. E. and Pagano, J. S. (1980). Acyclovir inhibition of Epstein–Barr virus replication. *Proc. Natl Acad. Sci. USA*, **77**, 5163–5166.
164. Reardon, J. E. and Spector, T. (1989). Herpes simplex virus type 1 DNA polymerase. *J. Biol. Chem.*, **264**, 7405–7411.
165. Beauchamp, L. M., Serling, B. L., Kelsey, J. E. *et al.* (1988). Effect of acyclic pyrimidines related to 9-[(1,3-dihydroxy-2-propoxy)methyl]guanine on herpesviruses. *J. Med. Chem.*, **31**, 144–149.
166. Wang, T. S. F., Wong, S. W. and Korn, D. (1989). Human DNA polymerase α: predicted functional domains and relationships with viral DNA polymerases. *FASEB J.*, **3**, 14–21.
167. Orita, M., Suzuki, Y., Sekiya, T. and Hayashi, K. (1989). Rapid and sensitive detection of point mutations and DNA polymorphisms using the polymerase chain reaction. *Genomics*, **5**, 874–879.
168. Lin, J.-C., Nelson, D. J., Lambe, C. U. and Cho, E. I. (1986). Metabolic activation of 9([2-hydroxy-1-(hydroxymethyl)ethoxy]methyl)guanine in human lymphoblastoid cell lines infected with Epstein–Barr virus. *J. Virol.*, **60**, 569–573.

169. Wang, F., Marchini, A. and Kieff, E. (1991). Epstein–Barr virus recombinants: use of positive selection markers to rescue mutants in EBV-negative B-lymphoma cells. *J. Virol.*, **65**, 1701–1709.
170. Sullivan, V., Talarico, C. L., Stanat, S. C. *et al.* (1992). A protein kinase homologue controls phosphorylation of ganciclovir in human cytomegalovirus-infected cells. *Nature*, **358**, 162–164.
171. Bacon, T. H. and Boyd, M. R. (1994). Comparative activity of penciclovir and acyclovir against Epstein–Barr Virus. *Antiviral Res.*, **23**, 99.
172. Littler, E., Sangar, D., Miller, W. *et al.* (1994). Studies on the *in vivo* synthesis and *in vitro* biochemical properties of penciclovir triphosphate. *Antiviral Res.*, **23**, 102.
173. Lee, M. A., Kim, O. J. and Yates, J. L. (1992). Targeted gene disruption in Epstein–Barr virus. *Virology*, **189**, 253–265.
174. Lin, J. C., Smith, M. C. and Pagano, J. S. (1985). Comparative efficacy and selectivity of some nucleoside analogs against Epstein–Barr virus. *Antimicrob. Agents Chemother.*, **27**, 971–973.
175. Lin, J.-C., Smith, M. C., Choi, E. I. *et al.* (1985). Effect of (*E*)-5-(2-bromovinyl)-2′-deoxyuridine on replication of Epstein–Barr virus in human lymphoblastoid cell lines. *Antiviral Res.*, **Suppl. 1**, 121–126.
176. Lin, J. C., Reefschlager, J., Herrmann, G. and Pagano, J. S. (1991). Evaluation of structure–activity relations between (*E*)-5-(2-bromovinyl) and 5-vinyl-1-β-D-arabinofuranosyluracil (BV-araU, V-araU) in inhibition of Epstein–Barr virus replication. *Antiviral Res.*, **17**, 43–52.
177. Clough, W. (1980). An endonuclease isolated from Epstein–Barr virus-producing human lymphoblastoid cells. *Proc. Natl Acad. Sci. USA*, **77**, 6194–6198.
178. Stinchcombe, T. and Clough, W. (1985). Epstein–Barr virus induces a unique pyrimidine deoxynucleoside kinase activity in superinfected and virus-producer B cell lines. *Biochemistry*, **24**, 2027–2033.
179. Baylis, S. A., Purifoy, D. J. M. and Littler, E. (1991). High-level expression of the Epstein–Barr virus alkaline deoxyribonuclease using a recombinant baculovirus: application to the diagnosis of nasopharyngeal carcinoma. *Virology*, **181**, 390–394.
180. Chen, M. R., Hsu, T. Y., Chen, J. Y. and Yang, C. S. (1990). Molecular characterization of a cDNA clone encoding the Epstein–Barr virus (EBV) Dnase. *J. Virol.*, **29**, 127–141.
181. Feighny, R. J., Henry, B. E., II and Pagano, J. S. (1982). Epstein–Barr virus-induced deoxynuclease and the reutilization of host cell DNA degradation products in viral DNA replication. *Virology*, **115**, 395–400.
182. Kumar, R., Wiebe, L. I. and Knaus, E. E. (1993). Synthesis and antiviral activity of novel 5-(1-azido-2-haloethyl) and 5-(1-azido-, amino-, or methoxyethyl) analogs of 2′-deoxyuridine. *J. Med. Chem.*, **36**, 2470–2474.
183. Lopez, C., Watanabe, K. A. and Fox, J. J. (1980). 2′-Fluoro-5-iodo-aracytosine, a potent and selective anti-herpesvirus agent. *Antimicrob. Agents Chemother.*, **17**, 803–806.
184. De Clercq, E. (1991). Broad-spectrum anti-DNA virus and anti-retrovirus activity of phosphonylmethoxyalkylpurines and -pyrimidines. *Biochem. Pharmacol.*, **42**, 963–972.
185. Lin, J.-C., De Clercq, E. and Pagano, J. S. (1987). Novel acyclic adenosine analogs inhibit Epstein–Barr virus replication. *Antimicrob. Agents Chemother.*, **31**, 1431–1433.
186. Lin, J. C., De Clercq, E. and Pagano, J. S. (1991). Inhibitory effects of acyclic nucleoside phosphate analogs, including (*S*)-1-(3-hydroxy-2-phosphonyl-

methoxypropyl)-cytosine, on Epstein–Barr virus replication. *Antimicrob. Agents Chemother.*, **35**, 2440–2443.

187. Lin, J.-C., Zhang, Z.-X., Smith, M. C. *et al.* (1988). Anti-human immunodeficiency virus agent 3′-azido-3′-deoxythymidine inhibits replication of Epstein–Barr virus. *Antimicrob. Agents Chemother.*, **32**, 265–267.
188. Furman, P. A., Fyfe, J. A., St. Clair, M. H. *et al.* (1986). Phosphorylation of 3′-azido-3′-deoxythymidine and selective interaction of the 5′-triphosphate with human immunodeficiency virus reverse transcriptase. *Proc. Natl Acad. Sci. USA*, **83**, 8333–8337.
189. Nickel, W., Austermann, S., Bialek, G. and Grosse, F. (1992). Interactions of azidothymidine triphosphate with the cellular DNA polymerae α, δ, and ϵ and with DNA primase. *J. Biol. Chem.*, **267**, 848–854.
190. Leinbach, S. S., Reno, R. M., Lee, L. F. *et al.* (1976). Mechanism of phosphonoacetate inhibition of herpesvirus-induced DNA polymerase. *Biochemistry*, **15**, 426–430.
191. Mao, J. C.-H., Robishaw, E. E. and Overby, L. R. (1975). Inhibition of DNA polymerase from herpes simplex virus-infected WI-38 cells by phosphonoacetic acid. *J. Virol.*, **15**, 1281–1283.
192. Summers, W. C. and Klein, G. (1976). Inhibition of Epstein–Barr virus DNA synthesis and late gene expression by phosphonoacetic acid. *J. Virol.*, **18**, 151–155.
193. Yajima, Y., Tanaka, A. and Nonoyama, M. (1976). Inhibition of productive replication of Epstein–Barr virus DNA by phosphonoacetic acid. *Virology*, **71**, 352–354.
194. Rickinson, A. B. and Epstein, M. A. (1978). Sensitivity of the transforming and replicative functions of Epstein–Barr virus to inhibition by phosphonoacetate. *J. Gen. Virol.*, **40**, 409–420.
195. Datta, A. K. and Hoop, R. E. (1981). Mechanism of inhibition of Epstein–Barr virus replication by phosphonoformic acid. *Virology*, **114**, 52–59.
196. Spector, T., Harrington, J. A., Morrison, R. W., Jr *et al.* (1989). 2-Acetylpyridine 5-[(dimethylamino)thiocarbonyl]-thiocarbonohydrazone (A1110U), a potent inactivator of ribonucleotide reductases of herpes simplex and varicella-zoster viruses and a potentiator of acyclovir. *Proc. Natl Acad. Sci. USA*, **86**, 1051–1055.
197. Goldschmidts, W. L., Ginsburg, M. and Pearson, G. R. (1989). Neutralization of Epstein–Barr virus-induced ribonucleotide reductase with antibody to the major restricted early antigen polypeptide. *Virology*, **170**, 330–333.
198. Colby, B. M., Shaw, J. E., Datta, A. K. and Pagano, J. S. (1982). Replication of Epstein–Barr virus DNA in lymphoblastoid cells treated for extended periods with acyclovir. *Am. J. Med.*, **73** (1A) (Acyclovir Symposium), 77–81.
199. Lin, J. C., Raab-Traub, N. and Pagano, J. S. (1990). Disruption of Epstein–Barr virus episomal DNA maintenance by a specific oligodeoxyribonucleotide. *Antiviral Res.*, **70**, (Suppl. 1), 76.
200. Pagano, J. S., Jimenez, G., Sung, N. *et al.* (1992). Epstein–Barr latency and cell immortalization as targets for antisense oligomers. *Ann. NY Acad. Sci.*, **660**, 107–116.
201. Daibata, M., Monroe, J. E., Kilkuskie, R. *et al.* (1994). Antisense oligonucleotides against BZLF-1 inhibit induction of the productive replication of EBV. *Antiviral Res.*, **23**, 70.
202. Lin, J.-C., Zhang, Z.-X., Chou, T.-C. *et al.* (1989). Synergistic inhibition of Epstein–Barr virus: transformation of B lymphocytes by α and γ interferon and by 3′-azido-3′-deoxythymidine. *J. Infect. Dis.*, **159**, 248–254.
203. Shapiro, R. S., Chauvenet, A., McGuire, W. *et al.* (1988). Treatment of B-cell

lymphoproliferative disorders with interferon alpha and intravenous gamma globulin. *N Engl. J. Med.*, **318**, 1334.
204. Filipovich, A. H., Mathur, A., Kamat, D. and Shapiro, R. S. (1992). Primary immunodeficiencies: genetic risk factors for lymphoma. *Cancer Res.*, **52**, 5465s–5467s.
205. Nilsson, K., Klein, E., Klein, G. *et al.* (1971). The establishment of lymphoblastoid lines from adult and fetal human lymphoid tissue and its dependence on EBV. *Int. J. Cancer*, **8**, 443–450.
206. Yao, G. Q., Grill, S., Egan, W. and Cheng, Y. C. (1993). Potent inhibition of Epstein–Barr virus by phosphorothioate oligodeoxynucleotides without sequence specification. *Antimicrob. Agents Chemother.*, **37**, 1420–1425.
207. Herbst, J. S., Morgan, J., Raab-Traub, N. and Resnick, L. (1989). Comparison of the efficacy of surgery and acyclovir therapy in oral hairy leukoplakia. *J. Am. Acad. Dermatol.*, **21**, 753–756.
208. Pagano, J. S., Sixbey, J. W. and Lin, J. C. (1983). Acyclovir and Epstein–Barr virus infection. *J. Antimicrob. Chemother.*, **12** (Suppl. B), 113–121.
209. van der Horst, C., Joncas, J., Ahronheim, G. *et al.* (1991). Lack of effect of peroral acyclovir for the treatment of acute infectious mononucleosis. *J. Infect. Dis.*, **164**, 788–792.
210. Luxton, J. C., Williams, I., Weller, I. and Crawford, D. H. (1993). Epstein–Barr virus infection of HIV-seropositive individuals is transiently suppressed by high-dose acyclovir treatment. *AIDS*, **7**, 1337–1343.
211. Andersson, J., Britton, S., Ernberg, I. *et al.* (1986). Effect of acyclovir on infectious mononucleosis: a double-blind, placebo-controlled study. *J. Infect. Dis.*, **153**, 283–290.
212. Beauchamp, L. M., Orr, G. F., de Miranda, P. *et al.* (1992). Amino acid ester prodrugs of acyclovir. *Antiviral Chem. Chemother.*, **3**, 157–164.
213. Nusinoff-Lehrman, S., Smiley, L. and Szczech, G. (1993). Update on acyclovir prodrugs. In *Antiviral Chemotherapy: New Directions for Clinical Applications and Research*, Vol. 3, J. Mills (ed.), **3**, 97–104.
214. Swartz, M. N. (1989). Acyclovir treatment of the chronic fatigue syndrome. *N. Engl. J. Med.*, **321**, 187.
215. Strauss, S. E. (1989). Acyclovir treatment of the chronic fatigue syndrome. *N. Engl. J. Med.*, **321**, 188.
216. Sullivan, J. L., Medveczky, P., Forman, S. J. *et al.* (1984). Epstein–Barr virus induced lymphoproliferation: implications for antiviral chemotherapy. *N. Engl. J. Med.*, **311**, 1163–1167.
217. Sullivan, J. L., Byron, K. S., Brewster, F. E. *et al.* (1982). Treatment of life-threatening Epstein–Barr virus infections with acyclovir. *Am. J. Med.*, **73** (1A) (Acyclovir Symposium), 262–266.
218. Pagano, J. S. (1989). Acyclovir treatment of the chronic fatigue syndrome: letter to the editor. *N. Engl. J. Med.*, **321**, 188.
219. Lerner, M. R., Andrews, N. C., Miller, G. and Steitz, J. A. (1981). Two small RNAs encoded by Epstein–Barr virus and complexed with protein are precipitated by antibodies from patients with systemic lupus erythematosus. *Proc. Natl Acad. Sci. USA*, **78**, 805–809.
220. Randhawa, P. S., Jaffe, R., Demetris, A. J. *et al.* (1992). Expression of Epstein–Barr virus-encoded small RNA (by the EBER-1 gene) in liver specimens from transplant recipients with post-transplantation lymphoproliferative disease. *N. Engl. J. Med.*, **327**, 1710–1714.

7 The Treatment of Herpes Simplex Virus Infections

ADRIAN MINDEL and PETER BROCKLEHURST
Academic Department of Genitourinary Medicine, Middlesex Hospital, London, UK

INTRODUCTION

Infections caused by herpes simplex virus (HSV) are amongst the commonest human viral diseases. In a small minority of individuals exposed to HSV, particularly the very young or the immunosuppressed, infection may be life threatening but for many others the ability of the virus to establish latency and cause symptomatic recurrences may lead to great distress and anxiety. However, for perhaps the majority of infected individuals the manifestations of their infection are either so mild as to be unrecognized or truly asymptomatic.

With the advent of effective and well-tolerated antiviral agents, particularly acyclovir (ACV), there has been a resurgence of interest in HSV infections and treatment. Unlike the situation in the past where treatment was toxic and reserved for severe infections, it is now used for all manner of HSV infection, usually with great success.

This chapter assesses the many clinical trials which have been conducted for the treatment of HSV infections, and offers some guidelines for the most appropriate therapy for each condition. Where controlled trials have not been performed, for example in very uncommon conditions, then an attempt has been made to adapt the conclusions drawn from treating related herpes infections so that some form of therapy can be recommended. This situation will hopefully be rectified as controlled trials of antiviral therapy covering every aspect of HSV infection are published.

MUCOCUTANEOUS INFECTIONS IN THE IMMUNOCOMPETENT HOST

GENITAL HERPES

Symptomatic genital herpes infection may affect as many as 2–3% of the sexually active population. First-episode genital herpes can be a severe and

Antiviral Chemotherapy. Edited by D.J. Jeffries and E. De Clercq

prolonged illness, particularly in those who have not been previously exposed to HSV; however, the manifestations are varied. In general, first-episode infection lasts from 16 to 21 days (1).

First-episode infection may be followed by intermittent reactivation of latent virus to cause recurrent episodes of genital lesions. The frequency, severity and duration of recurrences are variable between different individuals and are also variable within one individual over time; however, recurrences are usually less severe and of shorter duration than the first episode (1).

Numerous and diverse therapies have been suggested for the treatment of genital herpes (2). However, the only drug that has consistently shown any efficacy in a series of clinical trials is ACV.

First-episode infection

There have been numerous randomized double-blind placebo-controlled trials using ACV in patients with first episodes of genital herpes infection with several different formulations of the drug, including intravenous, oral and topical preparations (3–15) (Table 7.1). These studies have shown that patients treated with ACV have a statistically significant reduction in the time to healing, the duration of viral shedding, pain and other associated symptoms, compared with placebo recipients. The reduction in viral shedding is the most dramatic and consistent finding, with ACV-treated individuals shedding virus for a mean of two to three days compared with 8–10 days in the placebo recipients. Patients with true primary genital herpes who usually have more severe and prolonged symptoms appear to respond better to oral ACV than those with non-primary first episode (11).

Systemic ACV therapy appears to be superior to topical (13) and there is no apparent advantage in combining systemic and topical therapy (15).

Kinghorn *et al.* in 1986 (12) suggested that the combination of ACV with cotrimoxazole may produce a significantly shorter time to healing than ACV alone. However, the numbers in this study were small.

The treatment, therefore, of first-episode genital herpes infection should be with oral ACV 200 mg × 5 per day for five days, particularly if administered early in the natural history of the illness. The earlier the drug is administered the more dramatic will be the response, whereas if ACV is administered when there is already extensive ulceration the reduction in viral shedding will only have a minimal effect on the total duration of symptoms and the time to healing (16).

One of the disappointing aspects of treatment with ACV has been the observation that ACV does not prevent or reduce the likelihood of the development of recurrences, nor does it decrease their frequency (17). Even prolonged treatment of the first episode fails to achieve this objective (18). It is suggested that this failure to influence recurrence rates is explained by the very early establishment of latency of the virus in the sacral ganglia, even before the commencement of symptoms (19). ACV given at this time would, therefore, have no effect on the latent virus and hence on subsequent recurrence rates.

Recurrent genital herpes

The treatment of each individual recurrence with either topical or oral ACV has proved disappointing. Although several studies have shown a statistically significant reduction in the duration of viral shedding and the time to healing there has usually been little effect on duration of symptoms such as pain (6,9,20–26). In almost all of these studies there is little clinically significant decrease in symptoms or severity of the recurrence, even though some of the parameters of investigation such as viral shedding may be reduced.

A Scandinavian study comparing patient-initiated therapy and physician-initiated therapy showed no advantage for either (22). A small uncontrolled trial has suggested that treatment started early in the prodrome may abort or shorten recurrences (23). However, not all patients have prodromal symptoms and not all prodromes lead to clinical recurrences.

Early studies of new topical therapy regimes are beginning to be published. A large multi-centre Canadian study (27) employing Edoxudine (5-ethyl 2′-deoxyuridine) 3.0% cream for the treatment of recurrent genital herpes infection in a placebo-controlled trial has demonstrated improvements in parameters such as viral shedding and lesion tenderness.

Shupack *et al.* in 1990 (28) investigated the use of topical human interferon α (IFN-α) in the management of recurrent genital herpes infection in a placebo-controlled trial. The authors noticed improvement in symptoms of pain, itching and burning with the high-dose preparation, although there was no difference between high-dose IFN, low-dose IFN and placebo in time to crusting and time to complete healing. Further studies combining topical IFNs and systemic antiviral therapy were suggested.

It is evident that treatment of individual recurrences with ACV is of limited benefit. An alternative approach is to use continuous suppressive ACV to prevent recurrences. Several double-blind placebo-controlled trials using suppressive ACV therapy have been conducted in patients with frequently recurring genital herpes (29–38). The initial studies showed that continuous oral ACV used for periods of three to six months and at doses of 600–1000 mg daily was highly effective. The majority of patients on ACV had either no recurrences or very few minor episodes, whereas those treated with placebo continued to have recurrences at the same frequency and with similar severity as before. There are several additional benefits of suppressive therapy, including a decrease in prodromal symptoms and neuralgia, a decreased risk of transmission to sexual partners, and an improvement

Table 7.1. Double-blind, placebo-controlled trials of ACV in the treatment of first-episode genital herpes infection

Ref.	Number of patients in study	Dose		Time to healing (days) A	Time to healing (days) P	Viral shedding (days) A	Viral shedding (days) P	Symptom duration (days) A	Symptom duration (days) P
Topical ACV									
3	69	Ointment 5% × 4–6/day (7 days)		11.2* (mean)	15.8	2.0* (mean)	4.6	3.6* (mean)	6.7
4	77	Ointment 5% × 4/day (7 days)	Primary	10.9	14.3	4.1*	7.0	6.2 (pain)	8.8
			First episode non-primary	10.9 (mean)	11.3	0.9 (mean)	3.5	3.6 (pain) (mean)	4.9
5	101	Cream 5% × 5/day (10 days)		8*** (median)	13	3*** (median)	9	5** (median)	8
6	53	Cream 5% × 5/day (10 days)		8*** (median)	14	4*** (median)	11	4* (pain) (median)	8
7	40	Ointment 5% × 5/day		9** (median)	13.5	2*** (median)	9	5** (median)	10
8	30	Ointment 5% × 5/day (10 days)		8** (median)	13	4* (median)	6	8 (median)	7

Oral ACV									
9	31	200 mg × 5/day (5 days)		6** (median)	11	1*** (median)	13	4* (median)	9
10	48	200 mg × 5/day (10 days)	Male	12	15	4	8	2** (pain)	3.8
			Female	9.5* (mean)	13.7	3.9*** (mean)	13.4	2.8 (pain) (mean)	3.4
11	150	200 mg × 5/day (10 days)	Primary	12**	16	2**	9	5* (pain)	7
			First episode non-primary	9 (median)	13	0** (median)	6	2 (pain) (median)	4
12	38	200 mg × 5/day (5 days)		9.0* (mean)	12.5	2.3*** (mean)	11.5	8.2 (mean)	13.4
Intravenous									
13	30	5 mg/kg × 3/day (7 days)		7*** (median)	14	2.0*** (median)	8.5	6.5* (median)	8.5
14	31	5 mg/kg × 3/day (5 days)		9** (median)	21	2*** (median)	13	3* (pain) (median)	7

* $p < 0.05$; ** $p < 0.01$; *** $p < 0.001$. A = acyclovir; P = placebo.

in both psychological and psychosexual well-being (39). Although symptomatic recurrences are greatly reduced with suppressive therapy, there remains the problem of asymptomatic viral shedding. Bowman *et al.* in 1990 (40) demonstrated that seven out of 48 patients on suppressive therapy shed virus asymptomatically during a 12-month period. Hence, the advice given to patients embarking on suppressive therapy in terms of their infectivity may need to be cautious.

Kaplowitz *et al.* in 1991 (36) demonstrated the efficacy of long-term suppressive therapy with ACV in a three-year open-label study involving 525 patients. ACV suppression maintained efficacy over the three-year period and was safe and was well tolerated (Figure 7.1). The efficacy and safety of continuous suppressive acyclovir therapy has now been confirmed for up to six years (41, 41a).

Two studies have been conducted to determine the most efficacious dose for commencing and maintaining suppressive ACV therapy (42,43). These two studies have shown that the most effective dose for commencing suppression is 200 mg q.d.s. Patients on 400 mg b.d., 200 mg t.d.s., 200 mg b.d., 800 mg o.d., 400 mg o.d. and 200 mg o.d. are all statistically significantly more likely to have recurrences than those on 200 mg × 4 per day. In these studies as the total daily dose and/or the frequency of tablet taking were lowered so the likelihood of having a recurrence was increased. For example, Mindel *et al.* in 1988 (42) (Figure 7.2) showed that at the end of the 60 days on suppressive therapy 7% of patients taking 200 mg × 4 per day

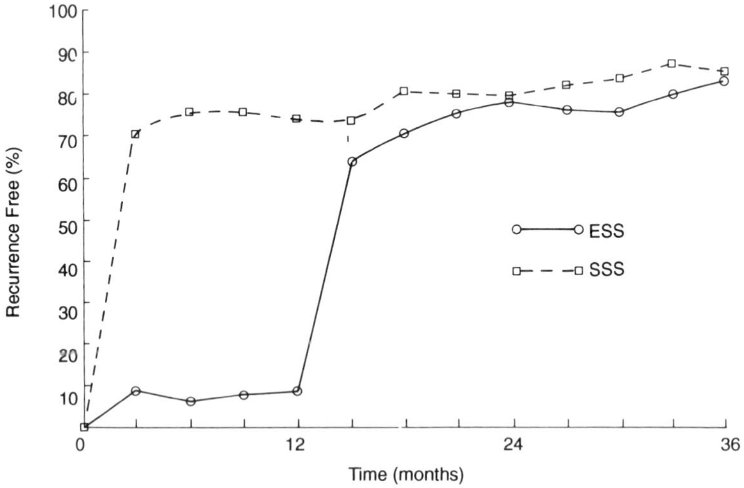

Figure 7.1. Percentage of patients recurrence free during the three years of the study. ESS indicates one year of acute therapy followed by two years of suppressive therapy. SSS, three years of suppressive therapy (from Kaplowitz *et al.* (36); reproduced by permission of the *Journal of the American Medical Association*, **265**, 747–751. Copyright 1991, American Medical Association)

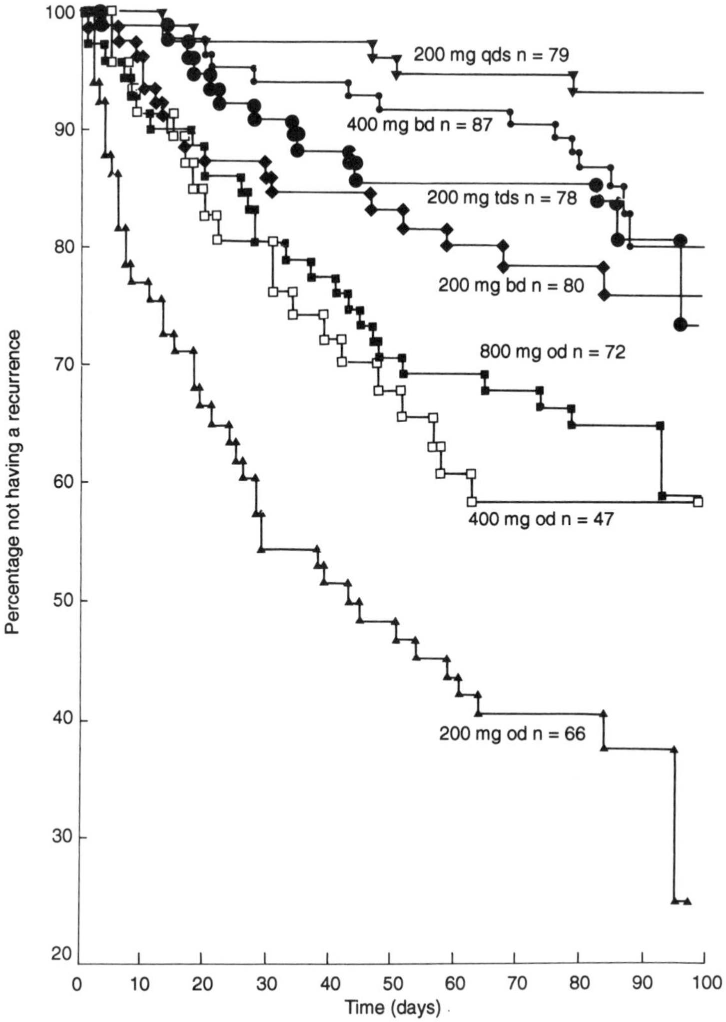

Figure 7.2. Time to first recurrence with different doses of acyclovir. od, once daily; bd, twice a day; tds, thrice a day; qds, four times a day (from Mindel *et al.* (42); reproduced by permission of *The Lancet*, 1988, **i**, 926–928)

had had a recurrence compared with 14% on 200 mg × 3 per day, 19% on 200 mg × 2 per day and 56% on 200 mg × 1 per day. Once-daily therapy is particularly likely to lead to breakthrough recurrences irrespective of dose. On 800 mg × 1 per day 30% of individuals will have recurred after 60 days compared with 41% on 400 mg × 1 per day and 56% on 200 mg × 1 per day. Whilst breakthrough recurrences can occur on all doses, virus-positive episodes are more common on once-daily therapy. On the basis of these studies we recommend that all patients should commence therapy on 200 mg × 4 per day and this should be reduced to 200 mg × 3 per day after two to three months if the patient is recurrence free. Further reductions may then be possible until breakthrough recurrences occur. Some patients may be successfully treated with 400 mg twice daily.

The length of time patients should receive suppressive therapy remains unresolved. It is not yet known whether long-term suppressive ACV therapy alters the natural history of the infection, although a study comparing the efficacy of placebo, intermittent ACV, and continuous ACV therapy over a one-year period failed to demonstrate any difference in the frequency of recurrences on withdrawal of treatment (44) (Figure 7.3). However, other studies have noted that the frequency of recurrences tends to decline after one or two years of suppressive treatment (41,45). On this assumption it may be appropriate to treat patients with suppressive ACV for one year and then to stop therapy to assess the recurrence rate. If the frequency of recurrences remains as it was before treatment then further therapy should be offered.

Because of the protracted course of treatment with suppressive therapy and also the expense of treatment the question of who to treat remains controversial. When assessing an individual for consideration of suppressive ACV therapy the following factors need to be taken into consideration: the frequency of recurrences; the duration of the recurrences; the severity of the symptoms; any associated psychological or psychosexual morbidity; the total duration of the infection; and the likelihood of transmission to sexual partners (16). Different centres have used different criteria for selecting patients for suppression. One view is that all patients with eight or more recurrences per year should be offered suppression irrespective of the severity. However, patients with fewer than six recurrences a year may have severe or prolonged symptoms and would likewise benefit from suppressive therapy.

PRIMARY HERPES GINGIVOSTOMATITIS AND HERPES LABIALIS

Herpes labialis is a common infection and frequently affects young children and adults. In the majority of patients the initial episode is mild and short lived (2) and recurrent episodes are infrequent, minor and self-limiting (46). Many preparations to treat herpes labialis have been tried; however, most of these have not been evaluated in double-blind placebo-controlled trials and the results of those that have are generally disappointing (2). However, of all the preparations tested so far, ACV appears to be the most useful.

Initial infection

There has been very little published on the treatment of primary gingivostomatitis. Ducoulombier *et al.* in 1988 (47) conducted a randomized double-blind placebo-controlled trial in 20 children with acute herpetic gingivostomatitis using oral ACV 200 mg × 5 per day. There was a significant improvement in pain and hypersalivation in the ACV-treated group. However, there was no difference in the duration of lesions between the two groups.

Recurrent herpes labialis

Topical ACV has been employed in several double-blind placebo-controlled trials to assess the use of physician- or patient-initiated treatment of recurrences. Two different preparations have been tested: a polyethylene glycol base as an ointment, or a modified aqueous cream (48–53). In most of the studies, the cream appears to perform better than the ointment. However, in all the clinical studies topical ACV has only a marginal clinical advantage over placebo (Table 7.2).

More recently, Spruance *et al.* in 1990 (54) published the results of a large multi-centre study to assess the use of 15% idoxuridine in a dimethyl sulphoxide (DMSO) base applied topically six times a day for four days in a double-blind placebo-controlled patient-initiated trial. They found that 15% idoxuridine in DMSO decreased pain by 35% ($p = 0.01$) and decreased mean healing time to loss of crust by 21% ($p = 0.004$). In those who began treatment in the prodrome or erythema stage, pain was reduced by 42% and mean healing time to loss of crust by 38%. The authors explained this difference between idoxuridine and previous trials with ACV by postulating that topical idoxuridine in DMSO is able to overcome the difficulties in drug penetration found with the ACV preparations and therefore is able to inhibit HSV replication at an earlier stage.

Oral therapy using ACV 200 mg × 5 per day for five days, whether initiated by the physician or the patient, has likewise proved of only marginal clinical benefit. Raborn *et al.* in 1987 (55) conducted a placebo-controlled trial using oral ACV and showed that the treated group healed more quickly and had a shorter duration of viral shedding. Although statistically significant the clinical significance is marginal as the time to healing was not vastly different. Similarly, Spruance *et al.* in 1990 (56) performed a double-blind placebo-controlled patient-initiated study in 174 patients with culture-proven herpes labialis. They were able to demonstrate that, if started early, oral ACV could hasten lesion resolution and decrease pain by up to 36% and the mean healing time to crusting by 27%. However, this was only in those who initiated treatment in the prodrome or erythema stage.

These studies suggest that only in those patients who regularly suffer second crops of vesicles or who have prolonged recurrences may the use of intermittent oral ACV be justified.

A

	Mean recurrences		
	Placebo	Intermittent	Suppressive
Number of patients[a]	28	29	47
Treatment interval			
0–3 months	2.57	2.55	0.42
4–6 months	1.54	2.14	0.23
7–9 months	1.75	2.07	0.13
10–12 months	1.71	2.62	0.21
Overall	7.57	9.38	1.00

[a]Includes only those patients completing study and excludes recurrences in first study week.

B

	Combined placebo and intermittent group	*vs*	Suppressive group	p value[a]
Number of patients[b]	56		29	
Median duration (days)	6.0		5.0	0.001[a]
	Intermittent group	*vs*	Suppressive group	
Number of patients[b]	29		29	
Median duration (days)	6.0		5.0	0.03[a]
	Placebo group	*vs*	Intermittent group	
Number of patients[b]	27		29	
Median duration (days)	7.0		6.0	0.05

[a]p value based on Wilcoxon rank-sum test.
[b]Includes only those patients completing the study and excludes recurrences in first study week.

C

	Intermittent treatment group		
	Completed study	Withdrew from study	p values[a]
Number of patients[b]	29	20	
Median duration of recurrences (days)	6.0	7.0	0.05

[a]Wilcoxon rank-sum test.
[b]Excludes recurrences in the first study week.

Suppressive therapy

A small cross-over trial using continuous therapy with 5% ACV cream for 16 weeks showed a significant decrease in the number of days with symptoms or cold sores from 12.4 in placebo recipients to 9.5 days in ACV recipients (57). The number of doctor-confirmed recurrences was 0.5 in the treated group and 1.1 in the placebo group. However, a similar placebo-controlled trial (58) using twice-daily topical ACV failed to show any significant differences.

In a cross-over trial using oral ACV 200 mg × 4 per day for non-genital herpes simplex infections (of which nine were labial), only two out of 11 patients taking ACV compared with nine out of 11 taking placebo experienced a recurrence over a period of 12 weeks (59).

The benefit of short-term ACV suppression has been demonstrated in skiers with a history of recurrences on exposure to sunlight. Spruance in 1988 (60) found that only 7% of those taking 400 mg ACV × 2 per day experienced a recurrence compared with 26% of those on placebo ($p < 0.001$).

Spruance and co-workers (61) have developed a model for studying herpes labialis using ultraviolet (UV) light. Using this model they irradiated, with UV light, the lips of 196 patients with a history of sun-induced herpes labialis, and used ACV either orally or as a cream and compared the results with placebo. They found that after exposure to UV light there was a subgroup of individuals who experienced lesions within 48 h (immediate subgroup) and a further group who develop lesions two to seven days after exposure (delayed subgroup). No therapy effectively prevented the appearance of lesions in the immediate subgroup. Also, topical ACV begun at the time of exposure did not alter the subsequent frequency or severity of recurrences. However, oral ACV 200 mg × 5 per day for five days, started either at the time of UV exposure or seven days beforehand, significantly reduced the frequency of recurrences.

Schadelin *et al.* in 1988 (62), in a randomized blinded study, showed that following trigeminal nerve surgery only three out of 14 patients taking 400 mg ACV twice a day for five days experienced a recurrence of herpes labialis, compared with 12 out of 16 taking placebo.

Figure 7.3. (opposite) (A) Mean number of recurrences during treatment period. (B) Duration of recurrences during treatment among the three treatment groups. (C) Duration of recurrences comparing intermittent treatment group patients completing or not completing the study (from Mattison *et al.* (44); reproduced by permission of the *American Journal of Medicine*, 1988, **85** (Suppl. 2A), 20–25)

Table 7.2. Double-blind, placebo-controlled trials of topical ACV in the treatment of recurrent herpes labialis

Ref.	Number of patients in study	Preparation and dose	Time to healing (days)		Viral shedding (days)		Pain (days)	
			A	P	A	P	A	P
48	208	ACV ointment 5% × 5/day (5 days)	7.8 (mean)	7.3	1.7 (mean)	1.9	2.5 (mean)	2.6
49	13	ACV ointment 5% × 5/day (5 days)	6** (median)	8	Not reported		Not reported	
50	49	ACV cream 5% × 5/day (5 days)	4** (median)	6	Not reported		1 (median)	3
51	30	ACV cream 5% × 5/day (5 days)	5.4* (mean)	6.6	Not reported		1.7 (mean)	1.7
52	69	ACV ointment 10% × 8/day (5 days)	6.0 (median)	5.2	1.1 (median)	1.9	2.0 (median)	2.3
53	45	ACV cream 5% × 5/day (5 days)	9 (median)	10	Not reported		5 (all symptoms) (median)	6

* $p < 0.05$; ** $p < 0.01$. A = acyclovir; P = placebo.

Prophylaxis

First-episode infection

The possible benefit of primary prophylaxis for herpes labialis using oral ACV has been suggested in a study by Kuzushima *et al.* (63). During three outbreaks of HSV-1 infection in a day nursery the authors gave ACV 30–60 mg/kg in three to five divided doses to unaffected children as soon as the first cases of primary infection were diagnosed and no new cases occurred. This compared with 82% new symptomatic infections occurring in two historical control groups studied during two earlier outbreaks within the same nursery.

Conclusions

Topical ACV appears to have limited efficacy in the management of recurrent herpes labialis. Suppressive oral ACV should be reserved for those patients with severe and/or frequent recurrences. There is no evidence as yet that the cessation of long-term therapy allows a subgroup of individuals to be identified in whom no further therapy is necessary, as has been demonstrated with suppressive therapy for genital herpes infection (45). However, this policy would seem sensible and, as is the case with genital herpes infection, therapy should be ceased after one to two years to assess the recurrence rate. Should recurrences continue to be frequent, further suppression may be necessary. However, in some patients recurrences may be less frequent or less severe, making further suppression unnecessary. Primary prophylaxis may be considered in institutions such as nurseries to prevent episodes in susceptible children.

CUTANEOUS HERPES INFECTION

Eczema herpeticum

Eczema herpeticum or Kaposi's varicelliform eruption is a widespread cutaneous HSV infection which usually affects individuals with atopic dermatitis (64), although it may occur with a variety of other dermatological conditions, including mycosis fungoides and Sézary syndrome (65,66), keratosis follicularis (67), burns (68), pemphigus foliaceus (69) and ichthyosis vulgaris (70).

Eczema herpeticum appears to be increasing in incidence, which is presumed to mirror the increase in incidence of HSV infections in general (64).

There are a number of anecdotal reports of the efficacy of ACV in the management of this condition (71–74) but no good controlled studies, presumably due to the infrequency of the condition in any one centre. A retrospective review of 75 episodes of eczema herpeticum in 63 patients stated that by using intravenous ACV 15 mg/kg per day for five days a rapid improvement was achieved, with drying and involution of the vesicles (64). This was an observational study and there was no control group. The authors suggested that other types of therapy that had been tried in the past in their unit were without merit. These included immunoglobulin infusions, systemic antibiotics and 'immunostimulating' agents.

There is a suggestion that recurrent eczema herpeticum occurs more commonly than was initially thought. Bork *et al.* in their retrospective series (64) found that five out of 75 cases had one recurrence, two had two recurrences and one patient had three recurrences. In total just over 10% had more than the initial outbreak. The majority of recurrences were managed in the same way as the first episode.

In summary, there are no controlled data concerning the efficacy of ACV in the treatment of recurrent eczema herpeticum, although oral and intravenous ACV have been found to be effective in individual case reports.

Other cutaneous infections

Herpetic whitlow describes a condition whereby the lateral or proximal nail-fold of the finger becomes infected with HSV (75). It is considered particularly hazardous when it occurs in health care workers because of the possibility of transmission to susceptible patients (76–78).

Intravenous and oral ACV (79,80) have both been used for the treatment of first-episode herpetic whitlow, and oral ACV has been used for the treatment of recurrent infections (81,82); however, no controlled trials have been published. Suppressive ACV has been used in one patient with frequently recurring herpetic whitlow and appeared to be effective in a dose of 200 mg × 3 per day (81).

Herpes gladiatorum occurs amongst wrestlers, rugby players and other sportsmen where close bodily contact is common, and presents as cutaneous or occasionally ocular infection with what is usually HSV type 1 (83–86). Straus *et al.* treated patients with ACV 200 mg five times daily for five days during an outbreak in a wrestling camp and suggested that this limited the severity of the disease (87). However, there are no published controlled trials for this condition.

ERYTHEMA MULTIFORME

Erythema multiforme has been described in association with cutaneous HSV infection regardless of the site of initial infection, and it is thought that HSV is the commonest precipitating factor for erythema multiforme (88). The condition tends to recur with each recurrence of infection, and treatment has been aimed at preventing recurrences. Of interest is the observation that ACV can prevent erythema multiforme in patients with or without an overt preceding episode of HSV infection, suggesting that asymptomatic recurrences may be enough to trigger erythema multiforme (89).

Several uncontrolled studies have reported success with doses of oral ACV between 400 mg and 1 g per day for periods up to 12 months (90–94). The use of topical ACV has been less successful (95,96). Recently, Williams *et al.* (97) reported the successful suppression of post-herpetic erythema multiforme with ACV 200 mg once daily, after gradually decreasing from 200 mg four times daily. Defining the lowest dose possible to prevent recurrent disease is obviously an advantage in terms of patient compliance and cost. However, work with genital herpes would suggest that only a few individuals with recurrent herpes infection can be adequately suppressed on such low doses (42).

HERPES SIMPLEX ENCEPHALITIS

Herpes simplex encephalitis is a severe illness which has an untreated mortality approaching 80% (98). HSV accounts for 10–20% of all cases of viral infections of the central nervous system in the United States, making it the single most common cause of encephalitis (99). Over 95% of infections are due to HSV type 1 (100).

The diagnosis of herpes simplex encephalitis remains difficult. Until recently there was little argument that prompt stereotactic brain biopsy was essential to establish correctly the diagnosis before commencing therapy (101). This was because symptoms and non-invasive investigations were unreliable (102), and as therapy was not without considerable toxicity (103) a definitive diagnosis was almost always obtained before therapy was instituted. Since the advent of well-tolerated antiviral therapy and improvements in less invasive methods of diagnosis of herpes simplex encephalitis (104), brain biopsy is less commonly performed and therapy can be instituted immediately a diagnosis of encephalitis is suspected, with a definitive diagnosis being made at a later stage.

TREATMENT

Idoxuridine was reported as being clinically useful in the treatment of herpes simplex encephalitis in 1966 when a single patient showed clinical improvement (105). Subsequently there were several case reports or small series to suggest that idoxuridine, although toxic, was clinically efficacious (106). In 1975, comparative trials of idoxuridine, vidarabine and placebo were undertaken which showed that idoxuridine was no different from placebo in outcome and was extremely toxic (103). Consequently idoxuridine is no longer used.

A double-blind placebo-controlled trial of vidarabine for biopsy-proven HSV encephalitis showed a decreased mortality from 70% with placebo to 28% with vidarabine ($p = 0.03$). In the treated group 50% of the survivors had either no, or only moderately, debilitating neurological sequelae compared with 20% of those taking placebo (100).

Skoldenberg *et al.* in 1984 (107), in an open-label randomized controlled trial, looked at 51 patients with herpes simplex encephalitis who received either ACV 10 mg/kg eight hourly for 10 days or vidarabine 15 mg/kg per day for 10 days. She demonstrated a marked reduction in mortality with ACV; from 50% in the patients treated with vidarabine to 19% in those treated with ACV ($p = 0.04$). In addition, the majority of patients who received ACV had either no or mild sequelae compared with only a small number in the vidarabine group. In patients who entered the trial with more severe disease (i.e. those patients who were comatose), ACV was even more striking in its benefit over vidarabine, with 40% of the ACV group and none of the vidarabine group surviving with minimal sequelae.

Similarly in 1986 Whitley *et al.* (108) looked at 69 patients with biopsy-proven herpes simplex encephalitis and again compared ACV with vidarabine (Figure 7.4). As was expected, the outcome in the ACV group was improved when compared with the vidarabine group, with 38% of the ACV group recovering to near normality when compared with only 15% of the vidarabine group. In this study it was noted that in the elderly or in those with severe disease at entry to the trial the outcome was poor, regardless of treatment used.

In all the trials to date ACV has been given intravenously for 10 days. However, recently there have been reports of clinical deterioration in patients with herpes simplex encephalitis after cessation of treatment and this has been shown in one case to be associated with ACV-sensitive HSV (109,110). It may therefore be appropriate to continue treatment for 14–21 days.

Apart from specific antiviral therapy for herpes simplex encephalitis many of these patients will require general supportive measures, which may include ventilation, careful control of fluid balance and correction of electrolyte disturbances (98).

The use of dexamethasone to prevent development of cerebral oedema, or at least control it once it has become established, has not been shown to be of any benefit (111). However, in the Swedish collaborative trial of ACV and vidarabine, three-quarters of the patients were treated with dexamethasone at an initial dose of 16 mg daily (107).

OCULAR HERPES INFECTION

HSV can cause a wide spectrum of disease in the eye, including blepharitis, conjunctivitis, superficial keratitis, stromal herpetic disease, keratouveitis

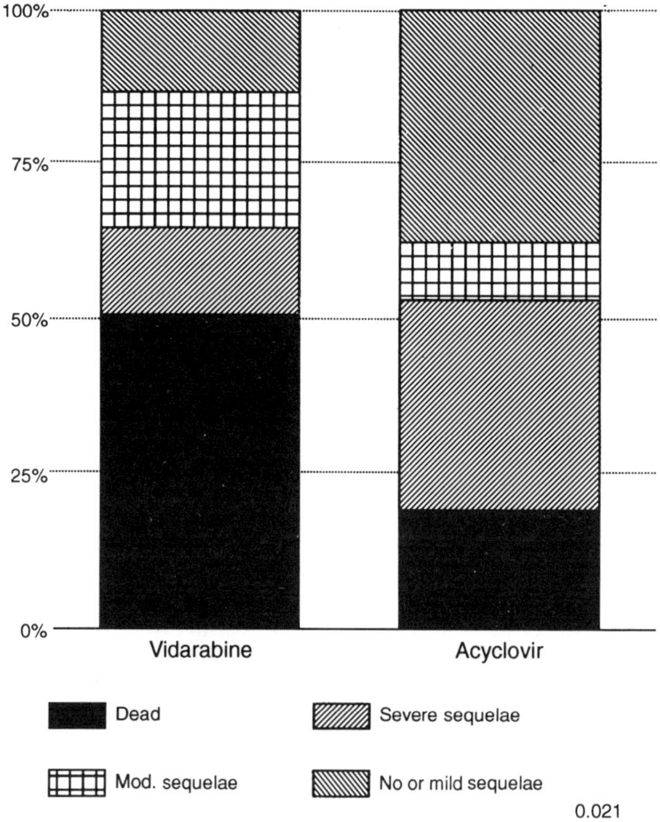

Figure 7.4. Mortality and morbidity of biopsy proven herpes simplex encephalitis comparing vidarabine with acyclovir (adapted from Whitley *et al.* (108); reprinted by permission of the *New England Journal of Medicine*, 1986, **324**, 444–449)

and, in its most severe form, acute retinal necrosis (112–114). Herpes simplex keratitis is the most frequent cause of blindness due to corneal disease in the developed world (115).

SUPERFICIAL HERPETIC KERATITIS

Superficial dendritic corneal ulcers are relatively simple to treat and mechanical debridement remains an important therapeutic procedure (114). Topical antivirals are used to eliminate the virus from the cornea and so improve healing. ACV, trifluorothymidine (116), vidarabine (117) and idoxuridine (118) have all been tried and have all been shown to be effective, with no single agent assuming obvious superiority (119,120). However, as ACV and trifluorothymidine are less toxic than vidarabine and idoxuridine, their use is probably favoured. ACV is applied as a 3% ophthalmic ointment five times a day for up to 14 days. In this setting 95–100% of dendritic ulcers will heal in approximately five days. Similar efficacy has been found with idoxuridine 0.5% and 1% ointments, trifluorothymidine 2% and vidarabine 3% ointment (121).

Two controlled trials have suggested that the combination of topical ACV and IFN-α is superior to ACV alone (122,123).

With the more difficult geographical corneal ulceration, Collum *et al.* (124) in 1985 compared ACV 3% ophthalmic ointment and vidarabine 3% ophthalmic ointment in a double-blind study. The ointments were applied five times a day until three days after the completion of healing. There was no statistically significant difference between mean time to healing in the two groups.

Oral and topical ACV appear to be equally effective (125,126). In patients on oral ACV 400 mg × 5 per day the mean tear fluid concentration of ACV was 0.64 mmol/l, which is well inside the 50% inhibitory concentration for HSV type 1 (125).

STROMAL DISEASE

Superficial herpetic keratitis may progress to produce stromal damage. This is thought to be as a result of an inflammatory process in response to viral antigens within the stroma rather than direct viral proliferation (127), and certainly most of the studies looking at the treatment of stromal disease have shown the importance of using topical corticosteroid therapy in combination with topical antiviral therapy. Sanitato *et al.* (128) in 1984 showed that neither topical ACV 3% ophthalmic ointment nor oral ACV 400 mg × 5 per day healed patients with disciform keratitis or necrotizing stromal keratitis, and less than 50% of patients showed any improvement. However, studies comparing ACV ointment alone with ACV and local corticosteroids have demonstrated more rapid resolution of disease with the latter (129,130).

Other topical antivirals including idoxuridine, trifluorothymidine and vidarabine appear to be of similar efficacy to ACV (120,130). However, topical vidarabine has been associated with the development of superficial punctate keratopathy (131).

At present the treatment of choice for stromal disease is ACV 3% ophthalmic ointment five times a day and betamethasone ophthalmic drops 0.1% five times a day until after healing has occurred.

KERATOUVEITIS

The mainstay of treatment for herpetic keratouveitis is ACV 3% ophthalmic ointment applied five times a day. In a non-randomized study ACV was said to be superior to trifluorothymidine although the use of corticosteroids by the two groups was variable (132).

In a small uncontrolled study by Schwab in 1988 (115) the use of systemic oral ACV 200 mg × 5 per day for two to three weeks was said to produce a consistent improvement in the disease. However, 16 of these 20 patients were also receiving topical corticosteroid therapy. The authors concluded that oral ACV was a useful adjunct to standard therapy for the treatment of recalcitrant herpetic eye disease.

There are no published studies on the use of suppressive ACV in patients with recurrent herpetic keratouveitis or stromal disease despite the fact that each recurrence is likely to cause further ocular damage.

ACUTE RETINAL NECROSIS

Acute retinal necrosis is the most severe ocular manifestation of herpes infection and frequently leads to retinal detachment and blindness (133). There are a few case reports demonstrating the successful use of intravenous ACV with or without vitrectomy or intravitreal infusion of ACV (134,135).

CONCLUSION

Herpetic ocular disease remains a frequent problem which may lead to loss of vision. The use of topical and systemic ACV appears to have advantages over the use of other antiviral therapies and may need to be employed with topical corticosteroid or IFN-α therapy for maximal effect, particularly in the treatment of stromal disease.

HERPES IN PREGNANCY AND NEONATAL HERPES

HERPES INFECTION IN PREGNANCY

HSV infection may present as either first-episode infection or as recurrent disease during pregnancy, when the most troublesome site of infection is genital.

There appears to be an increased risk of local and generalized dissemination of infection if a pregnant woman acquires a new herpes infection (136), and there have been a variety of case reports of herpes hepatitis (137,138) and encephalitis (139) occurring during pregnancy or in the puerperium.

There is, however, little firm evidence that the natural history of pre-existing HSV infections is altered during pregnancy, although one study

(140) has indicated a slight increase in the frequency of genital herpes recurrences in the last trimester.

Treatment

First-episode infection

In the UK ACV is not yet licensed for use in pregnancy (141) and for obvious reasons no clinical trials using antivirals in pregnancy have been published. To date there is no evidence that ACV is teratogenic, or in any other way harmful to the fetus, when used during pregnancy (138,142–144). The Acyclovir in Pregnancy Registry (145) collects all prospective and retrospective reports of ACV used during pregnancy (mostly inadvertent use during the first trimester), and analyses neonatal outcome. From this registry ACV appears to be well tolerated in both mother and fetus. However, more safety information will need to be collected before ACV can be recommended for routine use during pregnancy.

The risk to both mother and fetus from disseminated herpetic infections is considerable and anecdotal reports suggest that intravenous ACV may be extremely effective. The doses used and duration of therapy are identical to those used in non-pregnant patients (138,142,143), and are based on the patient's weight, as the fetus and amniotic fluid are included in the drug's volume of distribution and so total doses will need to be increased in line with the increase in weight with advancing pregnancy (146).

First-episode genital herpes infection acquired during pregnancy is associated with an increased risk of intrauterine growth retardation and premature labour (147), which seems to be unrelated to the development of neonatal herpes infection. The mechanism for this is not understood and there is as yet no information as to whether antiviral therapy influences pregnancy outcome.

Recurrent genital herpes infection in pregnancy

Recurrent genital herpes infection in pregnancy is probably only a problem if there are active genital lesions present at the time of vaginal delivery which is associated with 3–8% risk of neonatal infection (148–150). Recurrent disease does not predispose to intrauterine infection and has no effect on the length of pregnancy or on neonatal weight (151). In order to avoid neonatal infection, the presence of lesions around the genitalia at the time of labour may be an indication for Caesarean section (152,153).

The possibility of using ACV during the last few weeks of pregnancy to prevent recurrent episodes of genital herpes and therefore the need for

Caesarean section is an attractive one (154). A study by Stray-Pederson (155) reported on 100 women with recurrent genital herpes infection who had been given ACV 200 mg × 4 per day for an average 12 days before the onset of labour. None of these women required a Caesarean section for recurrent genital herpes infection. However, this study was not randomized or placebo controlled. Subsequent follow-up of these women and their neonates showed no detrimental effect from the administration of ACV. A properly controlled and randomized placebo-controlled trial is necessary before any firm conclusions about the efficacy and safety of suppressive ACV in late pregnancy can be made (156). An alternative suggestion is to use ACV in all neonates following known vaginal exposure at the time of delivery (157).

NEONATAL HERPES

Neonatal herpes infection occurs most commonly from the infected birth canal of the mother; however, infection can also occur post-natally from relatives or birth attendants with active herpetic lesions (158).

When it does occur, neonatal herpes infection has a wide variety of manifestations with infection localized to skin, eye or mouth, central nervous system (CNS) infection or disseminated to involve multiple organ systems (159).

Overall the mortality, if untreated, is 40–60% with approximately 50% of the survivors having residual, predominantly neurological sequelae (158,159). Patients with CNS or disseminated disease have a worse prognosis.

The true incidence of neonatal herpes infection is not known, although in the United States the incidence rose from 2.6 per 100 000 live births between 1966 and 1969 to 11.9 cases per 100 000 live births in 1981 (160). In Sweden six cases of neonatal herpes infection per 100 000 live births were reported from a ten-year period, 1979–1989 (161). In the UK from July 1986 to December 1991 there were 72 confirmed cases reported to the British Paediatric Surveillance Unit (P. Tookey, personal communication), which gives an incidence of two per 100 000 live births. However, it is recognized that this may represent a considerable under-diagnosis of the condition.

Treatment

Early placebo-controlled trials for neonatal herpes infection using vidarabine 15 or 30 mg/kg daily for 10 days showed a reduction in mortality from 74% with placebo to 40% with vidarabine (162).

In 1991 Whitley *et al.* (163) reported on a large multi-centre study comparing vidarabine with ACV. The doses used were vidarabine 30 mg/kg per day or ACV 30 mg/kg per day, both for 10 days. A total of 210 babies with virologically proven neonatal herpes infection were entered into the study. There were no statistically significant differences between vidarabine or ACV with respect to mortality or morbidity (Figure 7.5), and little difference in toxicity between the two drugs. The authors concluded that because of its ease of administration ACV in a dosage of 30 mg/kg per day for 10 days was the treatment of choice.

Although both ACV and vidarabine reduce mortality, a considerable number of babies are left with serious long-term sequelae which are mainly CNS damage. The reasons for this probably include late initiation of treatment in some cases and difficulty with diagnosis. Consequently prevention of this potentially devastating infection remains a major therapeutic objective.

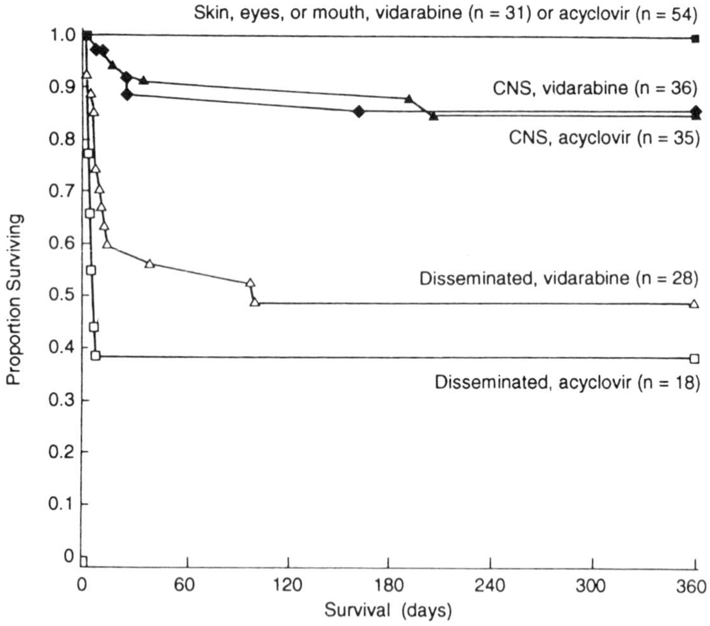

Figure 7.5. Survival of babies with neonatal HSV infection, according to treatment and the extent of disease. The infection was classified as confined to the skin, eyes or mouth; affecting the central nervous system (CNS); or producing disseminated disease. After adjustment for the extent of disease with use of a stratified analysis, the overall comparison of vidarabine with acyclovir was not statistically significant ($p = 0.27$) by a log-rank test. No comparison of treatments within disease categories was statistically significant

HSV INFECTION AND IMMUNOSUPPRESSION

HERPES INFECTION AND MALIGNANCY

Treatment

The majority of infections caused by HSV in patients immunocompromised by malignancy, and more specifically by antitumour therapy, are in general recurrences of pre-existing latent infection (164). Primary infections in this group of patients are more commonly seen in children with lymphoreticular malignancies, who by virtue of their age are less liable to have been exposed to HSV in the past.

Infections are often severe and prolonged; viral shedding is prolonged and dissemination to other cutaneous and visceral sites may occur. Mortality is high (164).

The use of antiviral therapy in these individuals differs from those with other acquired immunodeficiency states in that prevention of disease may be possible. This is because the cause of the immunosuppression, i.e. bone marrow transplantation (BMT) or induction chemotherapy (IC), is controlled and reversible and so reactivation of herpes infection can be anticipated.

In the case of patients undergoing BMT approximately 80% of those with antibodies to HSV will develop symptomatic HSV disease at some point during their course of therapy (165). By using suppressive antiviral therapy before the initiation of treatment and throughout the period of treatment (and immunosuppression), this may be completely prevented. Once normal immune function is restored antiviral therapy can be stopped. ACV is the drug of choice. Vidarabine has been used but appears to be less effective than ACV (166).

Established infection

Several double-blind, placebo-controlled studies have demonstrated that intravenous and oral ACV are effective in patients with mild to moderate HSV disease (121,167–169). Topical ACV (170) has been used in patients with mild cutaneous disease and, although significant differences were found in healing times and duration of pain when compared with placebo, topical therapy did not appear to be as effective as oral or intravenous therapy, particularly in the management of intra-oral, vaginal and visceral herpes infection.

Prophylaxis

Intravenous ACV has been compared with placebo in groups of patients undergoing BMT (171,172). The majority of the patients recruited to these studies were seropositive for HSV antibodies. The dosage regimens employed have been from 250 mg/m^2 to 5 mg/kg twice daily starting a week to a day before BMT and continuing for the period of immunosuppression, which ranged from a few weeks to 24 months. In these studies, which involved relatively small numbers of patients, ACV was found to produce a statistically significant decrease in the number of symptomatic infections during the period of prophylaxis when compared with placebo. This effect was also seen with oral ACV (Table 7.3). Similarly, intravenous and oral ACV have both been used successfully to decrease episodes of herpes in patients undergoing induction chemotherapy (172,176,177)*.

In all the above studies the overall length of treatment has varied, but the aim is to cover the time of immunosuppression, which may be as long as 24 months. Continuous intravenous therapy three times daily for this time period has considerable disadvantages, and Ljungren *et al.* administered 250 mg/m^2 ACV intravenously for six weeks, starting five days before BMT, and followed this with 400 mg ACV orally twice daily for six months (178). This has the advantage of providing high serum levels of ACV at the time of the most profound immunosuppression, but changing to an oral regime after six weeks decreases the inconvenience to the patient while maintaining treatment for an appropriate time. This study, involving 42

Table 7.3. Randomized, placebo-controlled trials of ACV prophylaxis in immunocompromised patients undergoing bone marrow transplantation

Ref.	Number of patients in study	Dose	Percentage of patients having symptomatic recurrence during treatment period (%)		p value
			A	P	
Intravenous					
171	20	25 mg/m^2 t.d.s. for 18 days	0	70	< 0.01
172	20	5 mg/kg b.d. during neutropenia	0	50	< 0.05
Oral					
173	39	200 mg × 4/day (43 days)	0	68	< 0.0001
174	51	400 mg × 5/day (35 days)	21	68	< 0.01
175	51	800 mg × 2/day (31–75 days)	0	13	< 0.001

A = acyclovir; P = placebo.

*Table 7.4 added in proof, page 237

patients, decreased HSV infection from 32% in the placebo group to 5% in the treatment group.

Conclusion

In view of the efficacy and safety of ACV in profoundly immunocompromised states and the high frequency with which symptomatic disease may develop in this group, some recommendations for the management of patients undergoing BMT and IC can be made. All prospective BMT or IC patients should be screened for the presence of HSV antibodies. In those who are seropositive, prophylactic ACV should be offered during the period of immunosuppression either orally or intravenously, preferably commencing before BMT or chemotherapy. Treatment should be continued until immune function is thought to be normal—probably for at least six months.

HERPES INFECTION AND ORGAN TRANSPLANTATION

Up to 60% of patients undergoing renal transplantation who have HSV antibodies will have a clinical recurrence of HSV infection during the period of profound immunosuppression (179) and both intravenous (for severe recurrences) and oral ACV (for mild to moderate recurrences) may be useful to treat outbreaks (121).

In a controlled trial, intravenous ACV was shown to be of benefit for the treatment of mucocutaneous HSV infections in patients undergoing heart transplants (180). As with bone marrow transplantation or induction chemotherapy, prophylaxis with oral ACV may be useful. Studies using 200 mg ACV × 3 per day or × 4 per day for four to six weeks post transplant in patients with HSV antibodies have shown a highly significant decrease in the number of herpes episodes during the treatment period when compared with placebo (181–183).

There are as yet no published clinical trials using ACV prophylaxis in patients undergoing other forms of organ transplantation although, from the evidence available, it may be appropriate to suggest that patients undergoing liver, heart or heart and lung transplantation who have antibodies to HSV should have prophylactic treatment with ACV to cover them during the period of immunosuppression.

HERPES INFECTION IN HUMAN IMMUNODEFICIENCY VIRUS (HIV) DISEASE

Introduction

Infection with HSV in patients with HIV infection may have a variety of clinical manifestations. The majority of patients, particularly those in the asymptomatic stage of HIV infection, will present with mucocutaneous herpes similar in manifestation and severity to that seen in the immunocompetent (184), although there have been suggestions that recurrences may be longer and more severe (185,186).

Other manifestations of HSV infection include retinitis (187,188); atypical or slowly progressive encephalitis (189); persistent or progressive oral (190) and oesophageal ulceration; and perianal ulceration (191), which is a particular problem, occurring in up to 13% of homosexual men with AIDS (192).

Treatment

HIV-positive patients who are asymptomatic and have normal immune function who present with first-episode HSV infection should be managed in the same way as immunocompetent patients.

In patients with frequently recurrent herpes simplex infection, long-term suppressive therapy with ACV (initially at 200 mg × 4 per day) is usually effective (184,192). The indications for therapy are similar to those for immunocompetent patients and include frequent or prolonged recurrences (16).

In patients with persistent mucocutaneous ulceration, which occurs predominantly in those with advanced HIV disease, there have been several reports of treatment failures usually due to ACV-resistant HSV (193–197). Three different ACV-resistant mutants have been described: first, those mutants with an absent thymidine kinase (TK); second, those with altered TK substrate specificity; and finally those with altered DNA polymerase (198–200). The majority of clinically significant ACV-resistant isolates are TK negative.

Foscarnet acts directly on the viral DNA polymerase without the need for viral TK and has been used in doses up to 180 mg/kg per day (in divided doses) to successfully treat ACV-resistant herpes ulceration (194,196,201–204). However, foscarnet is not without significant toxicity, e.g. nephrotoxicity, anaemia, hypo- and hyperphosphataemia, hypo- and hypercalcaemia, nausea, vomiting and seizures (205), and should not be administered unless ACV resistance is confirmed. A suggested treatment algorithm is presented in Figure 7.6. Unfortunately, foscarnet-resistant isolates are now being described (205a).

Vidarabine has been tried but was inferior to foscarnet (206), and topical trifluorothymidine 1% ophthalmic ointment has been assessed in nine patients with ACV-resistant herpes and appears to be of benefit (207).

Following successful healing of ulcers in patients with resistant HSV the most appropriate form of maintenance therapy has yet to be established. Isolates from subsequent symptomatic recurrences may be sensitive to ACV; however, the majority of patients will go on to develop further recurrences resistant to ACV and will require further treatment with foscarnet

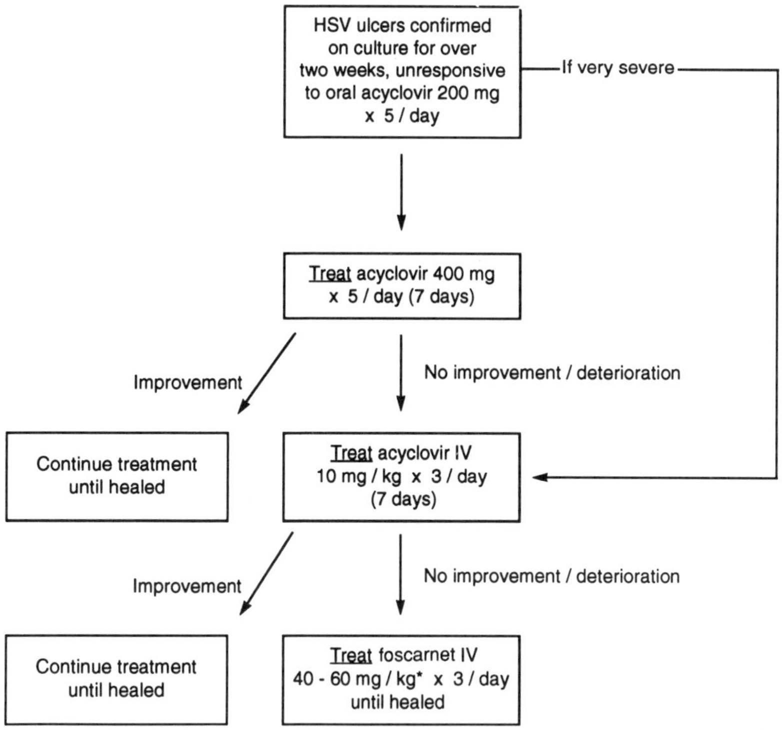

* dose dependent upon renal function

Figure 7.6. Treatment algorithm for persistent herpes simplex virus ulceration in HIV infected individuals

(203,206). A trial comparing daily intravenous foscarnet with oral ACV as maintenance therapy in patients with a previously resistant infection is at present under way (204).

FAILURE TO RESPOND TO ACV THERAPY

There are many reasons why patients may fail to respond to therapy with ACV (16).

1. The diagnosis may be incorrect and the patient may not have HSV disease.
2. Compliance with therapy may be poor.
3. An insufficient dose is being used.
4. There is malabsorption of the drug.
5. There is drug resistance.

Selective malabsorption of ACV was demonstrated by Mindel and Carney in 1988 (208), who reported a patient who had undergone previous surgery with removal of a section of terminal ileum and, despite large doses of oral ACV, was failing to absorb it. This is an uncommon cause of failure to respond.

SUMMARY OF TREATMENT REGIMENS

Herpes labialis

First episode	Oral ACV 200 mg × 5 per day for five days.
Recurrent	Suppressive therapy with ACV 200 mg × 4 per day if necessary (see text).
Prophylaxis	400 mg × 2 per day starting before exposure to sunlight and continuing for duration of exposure.

Genital herpes

First episode	Oral ACV 200 mg × 5 per day for five days. Intravenous ACV 5 mg/kg t.i.d. for 5–10 days, if severe.
Recurrent	Suppressive therapy with ACV 200 mg × 4 per day if necessary (see text).
Prophylaxis	No evaluated method known.

Cutaneous herpes infection

First episode	Intravenous ACV 5 mg/kg t.i.d. for 5–10 days if severe *or* oral ACV 200 mg × 5 per day for five days.
Recurrent	Not enough information on which to base recommendation. ACV 200 mg × 4 per day as suppressive therapy may be useful.

Erythema multiforme

For frequently recurrent erythema multiforme in association with recurrent herpes infection, suppressive therapy starting at ACV 200 mg × 4 per day and decreasing to the minimum dose to prevent recurrences. This may also be useful in those who do not have identifiable recurrences.

Herpes encephalitis

Intravenous ACV 10 mg/kg t.i.d. for 10–14 days, started promptly.

Ocular herpes

Blepharitis/ conjunctivitis	ACV 3% ophthalmic ointment five times daily to affected eye until lesions have healed.
Superficial keratitis	ACV 3% ophthalmic ointment five times daily to affected eye until three days after lesions have healed.
Stromal disease	ACV 3% ophthalmic ointment plus betamethasone 0.1% eye-drops five times daily to affected eye until healed. Consider oral ACV 200 mg × 5 per day if progress slow.
Keratouveitis	ACV 3% ophthalmic ointment five times daily to affected eye *or* oral ACV 200 × 5 per day until healed. ?Consider suppressive ACV 200 mg × 4 per day in patients with frequently recurrent infection.
Acute retinal necrosis	?Oral ACV 200 mg × 5 per day until disease is quiescent.

Herpes and pregnancy

In pregnancy	Only use antiviral therapy if infection in mother is severe or life threatening. In disseminated disease intravenous ACV 10 mg/kg t.i.d. for 10 days.
Neonatal herpes	Intravenous ACV 30 mg/kg per day for 10 days *or* intravenous vidarabine 30 mg/kg per day for 10 days.

Herpes and immunosuppression

Malignancy

Established infection	Intravenous ACV 5–10 mg/kg t.i.d. for 10 days for severe disease, oral ACV 400 mg × 5 per day for five days for mild to moderate disease.

Prophylaxis before bone marrow transplant or induction chemotherapy for patients with HSV antibodies

Intravenous ACV 5–10 mg/kg t.i.d. starting before the procedure and continuing for six weeks, followed by oral ACV 200 mg × 4 per day or 400 mg b.i.d. for the remaining period of immunosuppression.

Organ transplantation

Established infection	Intravenous ACV 5–10 mg/kg t.i.d. for 5–10 days if severe, oral ACV 200 mg × 5 per day for 5–10 days if mild to moderate.
Prophylaxis	Oral ACV 200 mg × 3 to × 4 per day for four to six weeks (efficacy only demonstrated in renal transplant recipients).

HIV disease

First episode	Intravenous ACV 5 mg/kg t.i.d. for 10 days if severe, oral ACV 200 mg × 5 per day for five days if mild to moderate.
Recurrent	Suppressive therapy with oral ACV 200 mg × 4 per day indefinitely if necessary.
ACV-resistant herpes	Intravenous foscarnet 40 mg/kg t.d.s. increasing to 60 mg/kg t.d.s. if there is no response after one week's therapy. Dose depends on renal function.

REFERENCES

1. Corey, L., Adams, H. G., Brown, Z. A. and Holmes, K. K. (1983). Genital herpes simplex virus infections: clinical manifestations, course and complications. *Ann. Intern. Med.*, **98**, 958–972.
2. Overall, J. C. (1984). Dermatologic viral diseases. In *Antiviral Agents and Viral Diseases of Man*, 2nd edn, G. J. Galasso, T. C. Merigan and R. A. Buchanan (eds), Raven Press, New York, pp. 247–312.
3. Corey, L., Benedetti, J., Critchlow, C. W. *et al.* (1982). Double-blind controlled trial of topical acyclovir in genital herpes simplex virus infections: Acyclovir Symposium, *Am. J. Med.*, **73**, 326–334.
4. Corey, L., Nahmias, A. J., Guinan, M. E. *et al.* (1982). Trial of topical acyclovir in genital herpes simplex virus infections. *N. Engl. J. Med.*, **306**, 1313–1319.
5. Fiddian, A. P., Kinghorn, G. R., Goldmeier, D. *et al.* (1983). Topical acyclovir in the treatment of genital herpes: a comparison with systemic therapy. *J. Antimicrob. Chemother.*, **12** (B), 67–77.
6. Kinghorn, G. R., Turner, E. B., Barton, I. G. *et al.* (1983). Efficacy of topical acyclovir cream in first and recurrent episodes of genital herpes. *Antiviral Res.*, **3**, 291–301.
7. Thin, R. N., Nabarro, J. M., Parker, J. D. and Fiddian, A. P. (1983). Topical acyclovir in the treatment of initial genital herpes. *Br. J. Vener. Dis.*, **59**, 116–119.
8. Lacey, C. J. N., Meaden, J. D., Darville, J. M. *et al.* (1985). Topical acyclovir ointment in the treatment of genital herpes simplex virus infections. *Eur. J. Sex Trans. Dis.*, **2**, 167–170.
9. Nilsen, A. E., Assen, T., Halsos, A. M. *et al.* (1982). Efficacy of oral acyclovir in the treatment of initial and recurrent genital herpes. *Lancet*, **ii**, 571–573.

10. Bryson, Y. J., Dillon, M., Lovett, M. *et al.* (1983). Treatment of first episodes of genital herpes simplex virus infections with oral acyclovir. *N. Engl. J. Med.*, **308**, 916–921.
11. Mertz, G. J., Critchlow, C. J., Benedetti, J. *et al.* (1984). Double-blind placebo-controlled trial of oral acyclovir in first-episode genital herpes simplex virus infection. *JAMA*, **252**, 1147–1151.
12. Kinghorn, G. R., Abeywickreme, I., Jeavons, M. *et al.* (1986). Efficacy of oral treatment with acyclovir and co-trimoxazole in first episode genital herpes. *Genitourin. Med.*, **62**, 33–37.
13. Mindel, A., Adler, M., Sutherland, S. and Fiddian, P. (1982). Intravenous acyclovir for primary genital herpes. *Lancet*, **i**, 697–700.
14. Corey, L., Benedetti, J., Critchlow, C. *et al.* (1983). Treatment of primary first-episode genital herpes simplex virus infections with acyclovir: results of topical, intravenous and oral therapy. *J. Antimicrob. Chemother.*, **12** (B), 79–88.
15. Kinghorn, G. R., Abeywickreme, I., Jeavons, M. *et al.* (1986). Efficacy of combined treatment with oral and topical acyclovir in first episode genital herpes. *Genitourin. Med.*, **62**, 186–188.
16. Mindel, A. (1991). Antiviral chemotherapy for genital herpes. *Rev. Med. Virol.*, **1**, 111–118.
17. Corey, L., Mindel, A., Fife, K. H. *et al.* (1985). Risk of recurrence after treatment of first episode genital herpes with intravenous acyclovir. *Sex. Transm. Dis.*, **12**, 215–218.
18. Mindel, A., Weller, I. V. D., Faherty, A. *et al.* (1986). Acyclovir in first attack of genital herpes and prevention of recurrences. *Genitourin. Med.*, **62**, 28–32.
19. Wildy, P. (1985). Herpes viruses: a background. *Br. Med. Bull.*, **41**, 339–344.
20. Goldberg, L. H., Kaufman, R., Contant, M. A. *et al.* (1986). Oral acyclovir for episodic treatment of recurrent genital herpes. *J. Am. Acad. Dermatol.*, **15**, 256–264.
21. Reichman, R. C., Badger, G. J., Mertz, G. J. *et al.* (1984). Treatment of recurrent genital herpes simplex infections with oral acyclovir. *JAMA*, **251**, 2103–2107.
22. Ruhnek-Forsbeck, M., Sandstrom, E., Andersson, B. *et al.* (1985). Treatment of recurrent genital herpes simplex infections with oral acyclovir. *J. Antimicrob. Chemother.*, **16**, 621–628.
23. Whatley, J. D. and Thin, R. N. (1991). Episodic acyclovir therapy to abort recurrent attacks of genital herpes simplex infection. *J. Antimicrob. Chemother.*, **27**, 677–681.
24. Salo, O. P., Lassus, A. and Hovi, T. (1983). Double-blind placebo-controlled trial of oral acyclovir in recurrent genital herpes. *Eur. J. Sex. Transm. Dis.*, **1**, 95–98.
25. Kinghorn, G. R. (1984). Topical acyclovir in the treatment of recurrent herpes simplex virus infections. *Scand. J. Infect. Dis.*, **47** (Suppl.), 58–62.
26. Luby, J. P., Gnann, J. W., Alexander, W. J. *et al.* (1984). A collaborative study of patient-initiated treatment of recurrent genital herpes with topical acyclovir or placebo. *J. Infect. Dis.*, **150**, 1–6.
27. Sacks, S. L., Tyrrell, L. D., Lawee, D. *et al.* (1991). Randomised, double-blind, placebo-controlled, clinic-initiated, Canadian multicenter trial of topical Edoxudine 3.0% cream in the treatment of recurrent genital herpes. *J. Infect. Dis.*, **164**, 665–672.
28. Shupack, J., Stiller, M., Knobler, E. *et al.* (1990). Topical alpha-interferon in recurrent genital herpes simplex infection. *Dermatology*, **181**, 134–138.
29. Blom, I., Back, O., Egelrud, T. *et al.* (1986). Long-term oral acyclovir treatment prevents recurrent genital herpes. *Dermatology*, **173**, 220–223.

30. Douglas, J. M., Critchlow, C., Benedetti, J. *et al.* (1984). A double-blind study of oral acyclovir for suppression of recurrences of genital herpes simplex virus infection. *N. Engl. J. Med.*, **310**, 1551–1556.
31. Halsos, A. M., Salo, A. P., Lassus, A. *et al.* (1985). Oral acyclovir suppression of recurrent genital herpes: a double-blind, placebo controlled, crossover study. *Acta Derm. Venereol.*, **65**, 59–63.
32. Mertz, G. J., Jones, C. C., Mills, J. *et al.* (1988). Long-term acyclovir suppression of frequently recurring genital herpes simplex virus infection: a multicentre double-blind trial. *JAMA*, **260**, 201–206.
33. Mindel, A., Weller, I. V. D., Faherty, A. *et al.* (1984). Prophylactic oral acyclovir in recurrent genital herpes. *Lancet*, **ii**, 56–59.
34. Straus, S. E., Takiff, H. E., Seidlin, M. *et al.* (1984). Suppression of frequently recurring genital herpes: a placebo-controlled double-blind trial of oral acyclovir. *N. Engl. J. Med.*, **310**, 1545–1550.
35. Thin, R. N., Jeffries, D. J., Taylor, P. K. *et al.* (1985). Recurrent genital herpes suppression by oral acyclovir: a multicentre double blind trial. *J. Antimicrob. Chemother.*, **59**, 116–119.
36. Kaplowitz, L. G., Baker, D., Gelb, L. *et al.* (1991). Prolonged continuous acyclovir treatment of normal adults with frequently recurring genital herpes simplex virus infection. *JAMA*, **265**, 747–751.
37. Mertz, G. J., Eron, L., Kaufman, R. *et al.* (1988). Prolonged continuous versus intermittent oral acyclovir treatment in normal adults with frequently recurring genital herpes simplex infection. *Am. J. Med.*, **85** (2A), 14–19.
38. Clive, D., Corey, L., Reichman, R. C. *et al.* (1991). A double-blind, placebo-controlled cytogenetic study of oral acyclovir in patients with recurrent genital herpes. *J. Infect. Dis.*, **164**, 753–757.
39. Carney, O., Ross, E., Ikos, G. and Mindel, A. (1993). The effect of acyclovir on the psychological morbidity associated with recurrent genital herpes. *Genitourin. Med.*, **69**, 457–459.
40. Bowman, C. A., Wooley, P. D., Herman, S. *et al.* (1990). Asymptomatic herpes simplex virus shedding from the genital tract whilst on suppressive doses of acyclovir. *Int. J. STD AIDS*, **1**, 174–177.
41. Fife, K. H., Crumpacker, C. S., Mertz, G. J. *et al.* (1994). Recurrences and resistance patterns of herpes simplex virus following cessation of equal to or greater than 6 years of chronic suppression with acyclovir. *J. Infect. Dis.*, **169**, 1388–1441.
41a. Goldberg, L. H., Kaufman, R., Kurtz, T. O. *et al.* (1993). Long term suppression of recurrent genital herpes with acyclovir. A five year bench mark. *Arch. Dermatol.*, **129**, 582–587.
42. Mindel, A., Faherty, A., Carney, O. *et al.* (1988). Dosage and safety of long-term suppressive acyclovir therapy for recurrent genital herpes. *Lancet*, **i**, 926–928.
43. Kroon, S., Peterson, C. S., Andersen, L. P. *et al.* (1990). Long-term suppression of severe recurrent genital herpes simplex infections with oral acyclovir: a dose titration study. *Genitourin. Med.*, **66**, 101–104.
44. Mattison, H. R., Reichman, R. C., Bolgiano, D. *et al.* (1988). Double-blind, placebo-controlled trial comparing long term suppressive therapy with short term oral acyclovir therapy for the management of recurrent genital herpes. *Am. J. Med.*, **85**, 20s–25s.
45. Straus, S. E., Croen, K. D., Sawyer, M. H. *et al.* (1988). Acyclovir suppression of frequently recurring genital herpes: efficacy and diminishing need during successive years of treatment. *JAMA*, **260**, 2227–2230.
46. Spruance, S. L., Overall, J. C., Kern, E. R. *et al.* (1977). The natural history of recurrent herpes simplex labialis. *N. Engl. J. Med.*, **297**, 69–75.

47. Ducoulombier, H., Cousin, J., DeWilde, A. *et al.* (1988). La stomato-gingivite herpetique de l'enfant: essai a controlle aciclovir versus placebo. *Ann. Pediatr.*, **35**, 212–216.
48. Spruance, S. L. and Crumpacker, C. S. (1982). Topical 5 percent acyclovir in polyethylene glycol for herpes simplex labialis: antiviral effect without clinical benefit. Acyclovir symposium. *Am. J. Med.*, **73**, 315–318.
49. Fiddian, A. P. and Ivanyi, L. (1983). Topical acyclovir in the management of recurrent herpes labialis. *Br. J. Dermatol.*, **109**, 321–326.
50. Fiddian, A. P., Yeo, J. M., Stubbings, R. and Dean, D. (1983). Successful treatment of herpes labialis with topical acyclovir. *Br. Med. J.*, **286**, 1699–1701.
51. Van Vloten, W. A., Swart, R. N. J. and Pot, F. (1983). Topical acyclovir therapy in patients with recurrent orofacial herpes simplex infections. *J. Antimicrob. Chemother.*, **12** (B), 89–93.
52. Spruance, S. L., Crumpacker, C. S., Schnipper, L. E. *et al.* (1984). Early, patient initiated treatment of herpes labialis with topical 10% acyclovir. *Antimicrob. Agents Chemother.*, **25**, 553–555.
53. Shaw, M., King, M., Best, J. M. *et al.* (1985). Failure of acyclovir cream in treatment of recurrent herpes labialis. *Br. Med. J.*, **291**, 7–9.
54. Spruance, S. L., Stewart, J. C. B., Freeman, D. J. *et al.* (1990). Early application of topical 15% idoxuridine in dimethyl sulfoxide shortens the course of herpes simplex labialis: a multicenter placebo-controlled trial. *J. Infect. Dis.*, **161**, 191–197.
55. Raborn, G. W., McGaw, W. T., Grace, M. *et al.* (1987). Oral acyclovir and herpes labialis: a randomised double blind placebo controlled study. *J. Am. Dent. Assoc.*, **115**, 38–42.
56. Spruance, S. L., Stewart, J. C. B., Rowe, N. H. *et al.* (1990). Treatment of recurrent herpes simplex labialis with oral acyclovir. *J. Infect. Dis.*, **161**, 185–190.
57. Gibson, J. R., Klaber, M. R., Harvey, S. G. *et al.* (1986). Prophylaxis against herpes labialis with acyclovir cream: a placebo controlled study. *Dermatology*, **172**, 104–107.
58. Fawcett, H. A., Wansbrough-Jones, M. H., Clark, A. E. and Leigh, I. M. (1983). Prophylactic topical acyclovir for frequent herpes simplex infection with and without erythema multiforme. *Br. Med. J.*, **287**, 798–799.
59. Thomas, R. H. M., Dodd, H. J., Yeo, J. M. and Kirby, J. D. T. (1985). Oral acyclovir in the suppression of recurrent non-genital herpes simplex virus infection. *Br. J. Dermatol.*, **113**, 731–735.
60. Spruance, S. L. (1988). Cutaneous herpes simplex virus lesions induced by ultraviolet radiation: a review of model systems and prophylactic therapy with oral acyclovir. *Am. J. Med.*, **85** (2A), 43–45.
61. Spruance, S. L., Freeman, D. J., Stewart, J. C. B. *et al.* (1991). The natural history of ultraviolet radiation-induced herpes simplex labialis and response to therapy with peroral and topical formulations of acyclovir. *J. Infect. Dis.*, **163**, 728–734.
62. Schadelin, J., Schilt, U. and Rohner, M. (1988). Prevention of herpes labialis following trigeminal surgery. *Am. J. Med.*, **85** (2A), 46–48.
63. Kuzushima, K., Kudo, T., Kimura, H. *et al.* (1992). Prophylactic oral acyclovir in outbreaks of primary herpes simplex virus type 1 infection in a closed community. *Pediatrics*, **89**, 379–383.
64. Bork, K. and Brauninger, W. (1988). Increasing incidence of eczema herpeticum: analysis of seventy-five cases. *J. Am. Acad. Dermatol.*, **19**, 1024–1029.
65. Axelrod, P. I., Lorber, B. and Vonderheid, E. C. (1992). Infections complicating mycosis fungoides and Sezary syndrome. *JAMA*, **267**, 1354–1358.
66. Taulbee, K. S. and Johnson, S. C. (1981). Disseminated cutaneous herpes simplex infection in cutaneous T-cell lymphoma. *Arch. Dermatol.*, **117**, 114–115.

67. Higgins, P. G. and Crow, K. D. (1973). Recurrent kaposis varicelliform eruption in Dariers disease. *Br. J. Dermatol.*, **88**, 391–394.
68. Nishimura, M., Maekawa, M., Hino, Y. *et al.* (1984). Kaposis varicelliform eruption: development in a patient with a healing second-degree burn. *Arch. Dermatol.*, **120**, 799–800.
69. Silverstein, E. H. and Burnett, J. W. (1967). Kaposis varicelliform eruption complicating pemphigus foliaceus. *Arch. Dermatol.*, **95**, 214–216.
70. Verbor, J., Munro, D. D. and Miller, A. (1972). Recurrent eczema herpeticum associated with icthyosis vulgaris. *Br. J. Dermatol.*, **86**, 638–640.
71. Mullerman, P. J., Doyle, J. A. and House, R. F. (1986). Eczema herpeticum treated with oral acyclovir. *J. Am. Acad. Dermatol.*, **15**, 716–717.
72. Swart, R. N. J., Vermeer, B. J., Van Der Meer, J. W. M. *et al.* (1983). Treatment of eczema herpeticum with acyclovir. *Arch. Dermatol.*, **119**, 13–16.
73. Jawitz, J. C., Hines, H. C. and Marshall, A. N. (1985). Treatment of eczema herpeticum with systemic acyclovir. *Arch. Dermatol.*, **121**, 274–275.
74. Atherton, D. J. and Harper, J. I. (1981). Management of eczema herpeticum. *J. Am. Acad. Dermatol.*, **4**, 757–758.
75. Louis, D. S. and Silva, J. (1979). Herpetic whitlow infections of the digits. *Am. J. Hand Surg.*, **4**, 90–93.
76. Manzella, J. P., McConville, J. H., Valenti, W. *et al.* (1984). An outbreak of HSV type 1 gingivostomatitis in a dental hygiene practice. *JAMA*, **252**, 2019–2022.
77. Rowe, H. N., Heine, C. S. and Kowalski, C. J. (1982). Herpetic whitlow: an occupational disease of practising dentists. *J. Am. Dent. Assoc.*, **105**, 471–473.
78. Rosato, F. E., Rosato, E. F. and Plotkin, S. A. (1970). Herpetic paronychia: an occupational hazard of medical personnel. *N. Engl. J. Med.*, **283**, 804–805.
79. Schwandt, N. W., Mjos, D. P. and Lubow, R. W. (1987). Acyclovir and the treatment of herpetic whitlow. *Oral Pathol.*, **64**, 255–258.
80. Tschen, E. H. and Baack, B. (1987). Treatment of herpetic whitlow in pregnancy with acyclovir. *J. Am. Acad. Dermatol.*, **17**, 1059–1060.
81. Laskin, O. L. (1985). Acyclovir and suppression of frequently recurring herpetic whitlow. *Ann. Int. Med.*, **102**, 494–495.
82. Gill, M. J., Arlette, J., Buckan, K. and Tyrrell, L. (1986). Therapy for recurrent herpetic whitlow. *Ann. Int. Med.*, **105**, 631.
83. Selling, B. and Kilbrick, S. (1964). An outbreak of herpes simplex among wrestlers (herpes gladiatorum). *N. Engl. J. Med.*, **270**, 979–982.
84. Porter, P. S. and Baughman, R. D. (1965). Epidemiology of herpes simplex among wrestlers. *JAMA*, **194**, 998–1000.
85. White, W. B. and Grant-Kels, J. M. (1984). Transmission of herpes simplex virus type 1 infection in rugby players. *JAMA*, **252**, 533–535.
86. Belongia, E. A., Goodman, J. L., Holland, E. J. *et al.* (1991). An outbreak of herpes gladiatorum at a high school wrestling camp. *N. Engl. J. Med.*, **325**, 906–910.
87. Strauss, R. H., Leizman, D. J., Lanese, R. R. and Para, M. F. (1989). Abrasive shirts may contribute to herpes gladiatorum among wrestlers. *N. Engl. J. Med.*, **320**, 598–599.
88. Huff, J. C., Weston, W. L. and Tonnesen, M. G. (1983). Erythema multiforme: a critical review of characteristics, diagnostic criteria and causes. *J. Am. Acad. Dermatol.*, **8**, 763–775.
89. Leigh, I. M. (1988). The management of nongenital herpes simplex virus infection in immunocompetent patients. *Am. J. Med.*, **85**, 34s–38s.
90. Goldberg, L. H. and Sperber, J. (1986). Erythema multiforme due to herpes simplex: treatment with oral acyclovir. *South. Med. J.*, **79**, 757–759.

91. Green, J. A., Spruance, S. L., Wenerstrom, G. and Piepkorn, M. W. (1985). Post-herpetic erythema multiforme prevented with prophylactic acyclovir. *Ann. Int. Med.*, **102**, 632–633.
92. Lemak, M. A., Duvik, M. and Bean, S. F. (1986). Oral acyclovir for the prevention of herpes associated erythema multiforme. *J. Am. Acad. Dermatol.*, **15**, 50–54.
93. Molin, L. (1987). Oral acyclovir prevents herpes simplex virus-associated erythema multiforme. *Br. J. Dermatol.*, **116**, 109–111.
94. Huff, J. C. (1988). Acyclovir for recurrent erythema multiforme caused by herpes simplex. *J. Am. Acad. Dermatol.*, **18**, 197–199.
95. Fawcett, H. A., Wansbrough-Jones, M. H., Clark, A. E. and Leigh, I. M. (1983). Prophylactic topical acyclovir for frequently recurrent herpes simplex with and without erythema multiforme. *Br. Med. J.*, **287**, 798–799.
96. Kennedy, C. T. C., Leigh, I. M., Ridgway, H. A. *et al.* (1981). Treatment of erythema multiforme secondary to herpes simplex by prophylactic topical acyclovir. *Br. Med. J.*, **283**, 1360–1361.
97. Williams, R. E. A. and Lever, R. (1990). Very low dose acyclovir can be effective as prophylaxis for post-herpetic erythema multiforme. *Br. J. Dermatol.*, **124**, 111.
98. Longson, M. (1984). Herpes simplex encephalitis. In *Recent Advances in Clinical Neurology*, W. B. Matthews and G. H. Glaser (eds), Churchill Livingstone, Edinburgh, pp. 123–140.
99. Corey, L. and Spear, P. G. (1986). Infections with herpes simplex viruses. *N. Engl. J. Med.*, **314**, 749–757.
100. Whitley, R. J., Soong, S.-J., Dolin, R. *et al.* (1977). Adenosine arabinoside therapy of biopsy-proved herpes simplex encephalitis. *N. Engl. J. Med.*, **297**, 289–294.
101. Whitley, R. J., Soong, S.-J., Hirsch, M. *et al.* (1981). Herpes simplex encephalitis: vidarabine therapy and diagnostic problems. *N. Engl. J. Med.*, **304**, 313–318.
102. Johnson, R. T., Olson, L. C. and Buescher, E. L. (1968). Herpes simplex virus infections of the nervous system: problems in laboratory diagnosis. *Arch. Neurol.*, **18**, 823–932.
103. Boston Interhospital Virus Study Group (1975). Failure of high dose 5-iodo-2-deoxyuridine in the therapy of herpes simplex virus encephalitis. *N. Engl. J. Med.*, **292**, 600–603.
104. Skoldenberg, B. (1991). Herpes simplex encephalitis. *Scand. J. Infect. Dis.*, **78**, 15–20.
105. Breedon, C. J., Hall, T. C. and Tyler, H. R. (1966). Herpes simplex encephalitis treated with systemic 5-iodo-2-deoxyuridine. *Ann. Int. Med.*, **65**, 1050–1056.
106. Johnson, R. T. (1972). Treatment of herpes simplex encephalitis. *Arch. Neurol.*, **27**, 97–98.
107. Skoldenberg, B., Forsgren, M., Alestig, K. *et al.* (1984). Acyclovir versus vidarabine in herpes simplex encephalitis: randomised multicentre study in consecutive Swedish patients. *Lancet*, **ii**, 707–711.
108. Whitley, R. J., Alford, C. A., Hirsch, M. S. *et al.* (1986). Collaborative antiviral study group: vidarabine versus acyclovir therapy in herpes simplex encephalitis. *N. Engl. J. Med.*, **314**, 144–149.
109. VanLandingham, K. E., Marstellar, H. B., Ross, G. W. and Hayden, F. G. (1988). Relapse of herpes simplex encephalitis after conventional acyclovir therapy. *JAMA*, **259**, 1051–1053.
110. Rothman, A. L., Cheesman, S. H., Lehrman, S. N. *et al.* (1988). Herpes simplex encephalitis in a patient with lymphoma: relapse following acyclovir therapy. *JAMA*, **259**, 1056–1057.

111. Longson, M. (1983). Antiviral and corticosteroid therapy in herpes simplex encephalitis. In *Dilemmas in the Management of the Neurological Patient*, C. Warlow and J. Garfield (eds), Churchill Livingstone, Edinburgh, pp. 196–201.
112. Pavan-Langston, D. (1984). Ocular viral diseases. In *Antiviral Agents and Viral Diseases of Man*, 2nd edn, G. J. Galasso, T. C. Merigan and R. A. Buchanan (eds), Raven Press, New York, pp. 207–245.
113. Dawson, C. R. (1984). Ocular herpes simplex virus infections. *Clin. Dermatol.*, **2**, 56–66.
114. Liesegang, T. J. (1988). Ocular herpes simplex infection: pathogenesis and current therapy. *Mayo Clin. Proc.*, **63**, 1092–1105.
115. Schwab, I. R. (1988). Oral acyclovir in the management of herpes simplex ocular infections. *Ophthalmology*, **95**, 423–429.
116. Sugar, J. and Kaufman, H. E. (1973). Halogenated pyrimidines in antiviral therapy. In *Selective Inhibitors of Viral Functions*, W. A. Carter (ed.), CRC Press, Cleveland, pp. 295–311.
117. Whitley, R., Alford, C., Hess, F. and Buchanan, R. (1980). Vidarabine: a preliminary review of its pharmacological properties and therapeutic use. *Drugs*, **20**, 267–282.
118. Kaufman, H. E. and Maloney, E. D. (1963). IDU and cytosine arabinoside in experimental herpetic keratitis. *Arch. Ophthalmol.*, **69**, 626–629.
119. Jackson, W. B., Breslin, C. W., Lorenzetti, D. W. C. and Michaud, R. (1984). Treatment of herpes simplex keratitis: comparison of acyclovir and vidarabine. *Can. J. Ophthalmol.*, **19**, 107–111.
120. Klauber, A. and Ottovay, E. (1982). Acyclovir and idoxuridine treatment of herpes simplex keratitis: a double-blind clinical study. *Acta Ophthalmol.*, **60**, 838–844.
121. Richards, D. M., Carmine, A. A., Brogden, R. N. *et al.* (1983). Acyclovir: a review of its pharmacodynamic properties and therapeutic efficacy. *Drugs*, **26**, 378–438.
122. Colin, J., Chastel, C., Renard, G. and Cantell, K. (1983). Combination therapy for dendritic keratitis with human leucocyte interferon and acyclovir. *Am. J. Ophthalmol.*, **95**, 346–348.
123. de Koning, E. W. J., van Bijsteveld, P. and Cantell, K. (1983). Combination therapy for dendritic keratitis with acyclovir and alpha-interferon. *Arch. Ophthalmol.*, **101**, 1866–1869.
124. Collum, L. M. T., Logan, P., McAuliffe-Curtin, D. *et al.* (1985). Randomised double-blind trial of acyclovir and adenine arabinoside in herpes simplex amoeboid corneal ulceration. *Br. J. Ophthalmol.*, **69**, 847–850.
125. Collum, L. M. T., Akhtar, J. and McGettrick, P. (1985). Oral acyclovir in herpetic keratitis. *Trans. Ophthalmolog. Soc. UK*, **104** (6), 629–631.
126. Porter, S. M., Patterson, A. and Kho, P. (1990). A comparison of local and systemic acyclovir in the management of herpetic disciform keratitis. *Br. J. Ophthalmol.*, **74**, 283–285.
127. Swyers, J. S., Lausch, R. N. and Kaufman, H. E. (1976). Corneal hypersensitivity to herpes simplex. *Br. J. Ophthalmol.*, **51**, 843–846.
128. Sanitato, J. J., Asbell, P., Varnell, E. D. *et al.* (1984). Acyclovir in the treatment of herpetic stromal disease. *Am. J. Ophthalmol.*, **98**, 537–547.
129. Collum, L. M. T., Logan, P. and Ravenscroft, T. (1983). Acyclovir in herpetic disciform keratitis. *Br. J. Ophthalmol.*, **67**, 115–118.
130. Collum, L. M. T. and Logan, P. (1982). Acyclovir in complicated herpetic disciform keratitis. Abstract. *Irish J. Med. Sci.*, **151**, 291–292.

131. Collum, L. M. T. and Grant, D. M. (1987). A double-blind comparative trial of acyclovir and adenine arabinoside in combination with dilute betamethasone in the management of herpetic disciform keratitis. *Curr. Eye Res.*, **6**, 221–224.
132. Hoang-Xuan, T., Frot, P. and Pouliquen, Y. (1984). Aciclovir et trifluorothymidine dans la kerato-uveite herpetique: une étude comparative en clinique humaine. Indications de la corticothérapie. *J. Fr. Ophtalmol.*, **7**, 445–448.
133. Urayama, A., Yamada, N., Sasaki, T. *et al.* (1971). Unilateral acute uveitis with periarteritis and detachment. *Jpn. J. Clin. Ophthalmol.*, **25**, 607–619.
134. Hirst, L. W., Beyer, T. L., Waters, D. and Fleischman, J. (1987). Successful management of acute retinal necrosis with intravenous acyclovir. *Ann. Ophthalmol.*, **19**, 445–448.
135. Peyman, G. A., Goldberg, M. F., Uninsky, E. *et al.* (1984). Vitrectomy and intravitreal drug therapy in acute retinal necrosis syndrome. *Arch. Ophthalmol.*, **102**, 1618–1621.
136. Peacock, J. E. and Sarubbi, F. A. (1983). Disseminated herpes simplex virus infection during pregnancy. *Obstet. Gynecol.*, **61**, 13s–17s.
137. Wertheim, R. A., Brooks, B. J., Rodriguez, F. H. *et al.* (1983). Fatal herpetic hepatitis in pregnancy. *Obstet. Gynecol.*, **62**, 38s–42s.
138. Klein, N. A., Mabie, W. C., Shaver, D. C. *et al.* (1991). Herpes simplex virus hepatitis in pregnancy: two patients successfully treated with acyclovir. *Gastroenterology*, **100**, 239–244.
139. Anderson, J. M. and Nicholls, N. W. N. (1972). Herpes encephalitis in pregnancy. *Br. Med. J.*, **i**, 632.
140. Harger, J. H., Amortegui, A. J., Meyer, M. P. and Pazin, W. (1989). Characteristics of recurrent genital herpes infections in pregnant women. *Obstet. Gynecol.*, **73**, 367–372.
141. Acyclovir Data Sheet (1991–92). *ABPI Data Sheet Compendium.*
142. Grover, L., Kane, J., Kravitz, J. and Cruz, A. (1985). Systemic acyclovir in pregnancy: a case report. *Obstet. Gynecol.*, **65**, 284–287.
143. Cox, S. M., Phillips, L. E., DePaolo, H. D. and Faro, S. (1986). Treatment of disseminated herpes simplex virus in pregnancy with parenteral acyclovir. *J. Reprod. Med.*, **31**, 1005–1007.
144. Brown, Z. A., Corey, L., Unadkat, J. *et al.* (1987). Pharmacokinetics of acyclovir in the term human pregnancy and neonate. *28th Interscience Conference on Antimicrobial Agents and Chemotherapy*, New York, Abstr. 1154.
145. Andrews, E. B., Tilson, H. H., Hurn, B. A. L. and Cordero, J. F. (1988). Acyclovir in pregnancy registry. *Am. J. Med.* **85** (2A), 123–128.
146. Brown, Z. A. and Baker, D. A. (1989). Acyclovir therapy during pregnancy. *Obstet. Gynecol.*, **73**, 526–531.
147. Brown, Z. A., Vontver, L. A., Benedetti, J. *et al.* (1987). Effects of first episode genital herpes during pregnancy. *N. Engl. J. Med.*, **317**, 1246–1251.
148. Prober, C. G., Sullender, W. M., Yasukawa, L. C. *et al.* (1987). Low risk of herpes simplex virus in neonates exposed to the virus at the time of vaginal delivery to mothers with recurrent genital herpes simplex virus infections. *N. Engl. J. Med.*, **316**, 240–244.
149. Arvin, A. M., Hensleigh, P. A., Prober, C. G. *et al.* (1986). Failure of antepartum maternal cultures to predict the infant's risk of exposure to herpes simplex virus at delivery. *N. Engl. J. Med.*, **315**, 796–800.
150. Nahmias, A. J., Josey, W. E., Naib, Z. M. *et al.* (1971). Perinatal risk associated with maternal genital herpes simplex virus infection. *Am. J. Obstet. Gynecol.*, **110**, 825–837.

151. Harger, J. H., Amortegui, A. J., Meyer, M. P. and Pazin, G. J. (1989). Characteristics of recurrent genital herpes simplex infections in pregnant women. *Obstet. Gynecol.*, **73**, 367–372.
152. Vontver, L. A., Hickok, D. E., Brown, Z. A. *et al.* (1982). Recurrent genital herpes simplex virus infection in pregnancy: infant outcome and frequency of asymptomatic recurrences. *Am. J. Obstet. Gynecol.*, **143**, 75–84.
153. Binkin, N. J., Koplan, J. P. and Cates, W. (1983). Preventing neonatal herpes: the value of weekly viral cultures in pregnant women with recurrent genital herpes. *JAMA*, **251**, 2816–2821.
154. Gibbs, R. S. and Mead, P. B. (1992). Preventing neonatal herpes: current strategies. *N. Engl. J. Med.*, **326**, 946–947.
155. Stray-Pedersen, B. (1992). Genital herpes in pregnant women in Oslo. *7th Meeting of the Scandinavian Society for Genitourinary Medicine*, Trondheim, Abstr. 17.
156. Brocklehurst, P., Carney, O., Helson, K. *et al.* (1990). Acyclovir, herpes and pregnancy. *Lancet*, **336**, 1595–1596.
157. Lissaur, T. and Jeffries, D. (1989). Preventing neonatal herpes infection. *Br. J. Obstet. Gynaecol.*, **98**, 1015–1023.
158. Whitley, R. J., Nahmias, A. J., Visintine, A. M. *et al.* (1980). The natural history of herpes simplex virus infection of mother and newborn. *Pediatrics*, **66**, 489–494.
159. Nahmias, A. J., Keyserling, H. H. and Kerrick, G. (1983). Herpes simplex. In *Infectious Diseases of the Fetus and Newborn Infant*, J. S. Remington and J. O. Klein (eds), Saunders, Philadelphia, pp. 156–190.
160. Sullivan-Bolyai, H., Hull, H. F., Wilson, C. and Corey, L. (1983). Neonatal herpes simplex infection in King County, Washington. *JAMA*, **250**, 3059–3062.
161. Forsgren, M. (1990). Genital herpes simplex virus infection and incidence of neonatal diseases in Sweden. *Scand. J. Infect. Dis.*, **69**, 37s–41s.
162. Whitley, R. J., Nahmias, A. J., Soong, S. J. *et al.* (1980). Vidarabine therapy of neonatal herpes simplex virus infection. *Pediatrics*, **66**, 495–501.
163. Whitley, R. J., Arvin, A., Prober, C. *et al.* (1991). A controlled trial comparing vidarabine with acyclovir in neonatal herpes simplex virus infection. *N. Engl. J. Med.*, **324**, 444–449.
164. Meyers, J. D. (1985). Treatment of herpesvirus infections in the immunocompromised host. *Scand. J. Infect. Dis.*, **47** (Suppl.), 128–136.
165. Meyers, J. D., Flourney, N. and Thomas, E. D. (1980). Infections with herpes simplex virus and cell-mediated immunity after marrow transplants. *J. Infect. Dis.*, **142**, 338–346.
166. Whitley, R. J., Spruance, S., Hayden, F. G. *et al.* (1984). Vidarabine therapy for mucocutaneous herpes simplex infections in the immunocompromised host. *J. Infect. Dis.*, **149**, 1–8.
167. Mitchell, C. D., Gentry, S. R., Boen, J. R. *et al.* (1981). Acyclovir therapy for mucocutaneous herpes simplex infections in immunocompromised patients. *Lancet*, **i**, 1389–1392.
168. Wade, J. C., Newton, B., McLaren, C. *et al.* (1982). Intravenous acyclovir to treat mucocutaneous herpes simplex virus infection after marrow transplantation: a double-blind trial. *Ann. Intern. Med.*, **96**, 265–269.
169. Meyers, J. D., Wade, J. C., Mitchell, C. D. *et al.* (1982). Multicenter collaborative trial of intravenous acyclovir for the treatment of mucocutaneous herpes simplex virus infection in the immunocompromised host. *Am. J. Med.*, **73**, 229–235.
170. Whitley, R. J., Levin, M., Barton, H. *et al.* (1984). Infections caused by herpes simplex virus in the immunocompromised host: natural history and topical acyclovir therapy. *J. Infect. Dis.*, **150**, 323–329.

171. Saral, R., Burns, W. H., Laskin, O. L. *et al.* (1981). Acyclovir prophylaxis of herpes-simplex virus infections: a randomised double-blind controlled trial in bone-marrow-transplant recipients. *N. Engl. J. Med.*, **305**, 63–67.
172. Hann, I. M., Prentice, H. G., Blacklock, H. A. *et al.* (1983). Acyclovir prophylaxis against herpes virus infections in severely immunocompromised patients: randomised double-blind trial. *Br. Med. J.*, **287**, 384–388.
173. Gluckman, E., Lotsberg, J., Devergie, A. *et al.* (1983). Prophylaxis of herpes infections after bone marrow transplantation by oral acyclovir. *Lancet*, **ii**, 706–708.
174. Wade, J. C., Newton, B., Flournoy, N. and Meyers, J. D. (1984). Oral acyclovir for prevention of herpes simplex virus reactivation after marrow transplantation. *Ann. Intern. Med.*, **100**, 823–828.
175. Shepp, D. H., Dandliker, P. S., Flournoy, N. and Meyers, J. D. (1987). Sequential intravenous and twice-daily oral acyclovir for extended prophylaxis of herpes simplex virus infection in marrow transplant patients. *Transplantation*, **43**, 654–657.
176. Saral, R., Ambinder, R. F., Burns, W. H. *et al.* (1983). Acyclovir prophylaxis against herpes simplex virus infection in patients with leukaemia. *Ann. Intern. Med.*, **99**, 773–776.
177. Anderson, H., Scarffe, J. H., Sutton, R. N. *et al.* (1984). Oral acyclovir prophylaxis against herpes simplex virus in non-Hodgkin lymphoma and acute lymphoblastic leukaemia patients receiving remission induction chemotherapy: a randomised double-blind, placebo controlled trial. *Br. J. Cancer*, **50**, 45–49.
178. Ljungren, P., Wilczek, H., Gahrton, G. *et al.* (1986). Long-term acyclovir prophylaxis in bone marrow transplant recipients and lymphocyte proliferation responses to herpes virus antigens in vitro. *Bone Marrow Transplant.*, **1**, 185–192.
179. Ho, M. (1977). Virus infections after transplantation in man: brief review. *Arch. Virol.*, **55**, 1–24.
180. Chou, S., Gallagher, J. G. and Merigan, T. C. (1981). Controlled clinical trial of intravenous acyclovir in heart transplant patients with mucocutaneous herpes simplex infections. *Lancet*, **i**, 1392–1394.
181. Pettersson, E., Hovi, T., Ahonen, J. *et al.* (1985). Prophylactic oral acyclovir after renal transplantation. *Transplantation*, **39**, 279–281.
182. Seale, L., Jones, C. L., Kathpalia, S. *et al.* (1985). Prevention of herpes simplex virus infections in renal allograft recipients by low-dose oral acyclovir. *JAMA*, **254**, 3435–3438.
183. Stoffel, M., Squifflet, J. P., Pirson, Y. *et al.* (1987). Effectiveness of oral acyclovir prophylaxis in renal transplant recipients. *Transplant. Proc.*, **19**, 2190–2193.
184. Safrin, S., Ashley, R., Houlihan, C. *et al.* (1991). Clinical and serologic features of herpes simplex virus infection in patients with AIDS. *AIDS*, **5**, 1107–1110.
185. Erlich, K. S. and Mills, J. (1990). Herpes simplex virus. In *The AIDS Knowledge Base*, P. T. Cohen, M. A. Sande and P. A. Volberding (eds), Massachusetts Medical Society, Waltham, pp. 6.42.1.–6.42.16.
186. Corey, L. (1990). Genital herpes. In *Sexually Transmitted Diseases*, 2nd edn, K. K. Holmes, P.-A. Mardh, P. F. Sparling *et al.* (eds), McGraw-Hill, New York, pp. 391–413.
187. Mildvan, D., Mathur, U., Enslow, R. W. *et al.* (1982). Opportunistic infection and immune deficiency in homosexual men. *Ann. Intern. Med.*, **96**, 700–704.
188. Gold, J. W. M. (1985). Clinical spectrum of infection in patients with HTLV-III associated disease. *Cancer Res.*, **45**, 4652–4654.

189. Levy, R. M., Bredesen, D. E. and Rosenblum, M. L. (1985). Neurological manifestations of the acquired immunodeficiency syndrome (AIDS): experience of UCSF and review of the literature. *J. Neurosurg.*, **62**, 475–495.
190. Barr, C. E. and Torosian, J. P. (1985). Oral manifestation in patients with AIDS or AIDS-related complex. *Lancet*, **ii**, 288.
191. Siegal, F. P., Lopez, C., Hammer, G. S. *et al.* (1981). Severe acquired immunodeficiency in male homosexuals manifested by chronic perianal ulcerative herpes simplex lesions. *N. Engl. J. Med.*, **305**, 1439–1444.
192. Conant, M. A. (1988). Prophylactic and suppressive treatment with acyclovir and the management of herpes in patients with acquired immunodeficiency syndrome. *J. Am. Acad. Dermatol.*, **18**, 186–188.
193. Bevilacqua, F., Marcello, A., Toni, M. *et al.* (1991). Acyclovir resistance/susceptibility in herpes simplex virus type 2 sequential isolates from an AIDS patient. *J. AIDS*, **4**, 967–969.
194. Birch, C. J., Tachedjian, G., Docherty, R. R. *et al.* (1990). Altered sensitivity to antiviral drugs of herpes simplex virus isolates from a patient with the acquired immune deficiency syndrome. *J. Infect. Dis.*, **162**, 731–734.
195. Englund, J. A., Zimmerman, M. E., Swierkosz, E. M. *et al.* (1990). Herpes simplex virus resistant to acyclovir: a study in a tertiary care centre. *Ann. Intern. Med.*, **112**, 416–422.
196. Youle, M. M., Hawkins, D. A., Collins, P. *et al.* (1988). Acyclovir-resistant herpes in AIDS treated with foscarnet. *Lancet*, **ii**, 341–342.
197. Erlick, K. S., Mills, J., Chatis, P. *et al.* (1989). Acyclovir-resistant herpes simplex virus in patients with the acquired immune deficiency syndrome, *N. Engl. J. Med.*, **320**, 293–296.
198. Coen, C. M. and Schaffer, P. A. (1981). Two distinct loci confer resistance to acycloguanosine in herpes simplex virus type 1. *Proc. Natl Acad. Sci. USA*, **77**, 2265–2269.
199. Schaipper, L. E. and Crumpacker, C. S. (1980). Resistance of herpes simplex virus to acycloguanosine: role of viral thymidine kinase and DNA polymerase loci. *Proc. Natl Acad. Sci. USA*, **77**, 2270–2273.
200. Field, H. J., Darby, G. and Wildy, P. (1980). Isolation and characterisation of acyclovir-resistant mutants of herpes simplex virus. *J. Gen. Virol.*, **49**, 115–124.
201. Ehrlich, K. S., Jacobson, M. A., Kochler, J. E. *et al.* (1989). Foscarnet therapy of severe acyclovir-resistant herpes simplex virus type 2 infections in patients with the acquired immunodeficiency syndrome (AIDS). *Ann. Intern. Med.*, **110**, 710–713.
202. Chatis, P. A., Miller, C. H., Schrager, L. E. and Crumpacker, C. S. (1989). Successful treatment with foscarnet of an acyclovir resistant mucocutaneous infection with herpes simplex virus in a patient with acquired immunodeficiency syndrome. *N. Engl. J. Med.*, **320**, 297–300.
203. Safrin, S., Assaykeen, T., Follansbee, S. and Mills, J. (1990). Foscarnet therapy for acyclovir resistant mucocutaneous herpes simplex virus infection in 26 AIDS patients: preliminary data. *J. Infect. Dis.*, **161**, 1078–1084.
204. Hardy, W. D. (1992). Foscarnet treatment of acyclovir resistant herpes simplex virus infection in patients with acquired immunodeficiency syndrome: preliminary results of a controlled, randomised, regimen-comparative trial. *Am. J. Med.*, **92** (2A), 30s–35s.
205. Jacobson, M. A., O'Donnell, J. J. and Mills, J. (1989). Foscarnet treatment of cytomegalovirus retinitis in patients with the acquired immune deficiency syndrome. *Antimicrob. Agents Chemother.*, **33**, 736–741.

205a. Safrin, S., Kemmerly, S., Plotkin, B., *et al.* (1994). Foscarnet resistant herpes simplex virus infection in patients with AIDS. *J. Infect. Dis.*, **169**, 193–196.
206. Safrin, S. V., Crumpacker, C., Chatis, P. *et al.* (1991). A controlled trial comparing foscarnet with vidarabine for acyclovir resistant mucocutaneous herpes simplex in the acquired immunodeficiency syndrome. *N. Engl. J. Med.*, **325**, 551–555.
207. Kessler, H., Weaver, D., Benson, C. *et al.* (1992). ACTG 172: treatment of acyclovir resistant mucocutaneous herpes simplex virus infection in patients with AIDS. Open label pilot study of topical trifluridine. Abstract. *VIII International Conference on AIDS/III STD World Congress*, Amsterdam, The Netherlands.
208. Mindel, A. and Carney, O. (1988). Acyclovir malabsorption. *Br. Med. J.*, **296**, 1605.

Table 7.4. Randomized, placebo-controlled trials of acyclovir prophylaxis in immunocompromised patients undergoing induction chemotherapy for haematological malignancies

Ref.	Number of patients in study	Dose	Percentage of patients having symptomatic recurrences during treatment period (%) A	P	*p* value
Intravenous					
172	39	5 mg/kg × 2/day during neutropenia	11	50	<0.05
176	31	250 mg/m^2 × 3/day (32 days)	0	73	<0.0001
Oral					
177	40	200 mg × 4/day (42 days)	5	60	<0.001

A = acyclovir; P = placebo.

8 The Treatment of Varicella Zoster Virus Disease

HILLAR O. KANGRO and DONALD J. JEFFRIES
Department of Virology, The Medical College of St. Bartholomew's Hospital, London, UK

INTRODUCTION

Two common diseases are caused by varicella-zoster virus (VZV): chickenpox (varicella) and shingles (herpes zoster). The association between varicella and herpes zoster was first reported at the beginning of this century when it was noticed that a case of zoster in a household was often followed by a minor outbreak of varicella in the younger members of the family and their friends. It was further demonstrated that it was possible to induce chickenpox in young volunteers by inoculating vesicle fluid from zoster cases. Confirmation that the two diseases are due to the same virus was provided by Weller in 1953 when he isolated the virus. It has now been proved by restriction endonuclease analysis of viral DNA from clinical isolates that the same virus causes varicella, as the manifestation of primary infection, and zoster as the manifestation of reactivation (1).

VIRUS STRUCTURE AND REPLICATION

VZV is classified as an alphaherpesvirus, as is herpes simplex virus (HSV). In fact, much of the knowledge about VZV has been obtained by reference to HSV, although recent years have seen major advances in the understanding of VZV at the molecular level. The complete DNA sequence of VZV was published in 1986 by Davison and Scott (2) and a general review of the molecular biology of VZV is given by Davison (3).

The organization of the VZV genome shows distinct similarities with HSV DNA and the two viruses have sufficient sequence homology to permit hybridization under non-stringent conditions. However, there is substantial local variation in the extent of this homology. The similarities between the HSV and VZV genomes would be compatible with a common ancestry (4). Sixty-eight open reading frames (ORF) have been identified in the VZV genome, and nearly half of the genes have been, at least tenta-

Antiviral Chemotherapy. Edited by D.J. Jeffries and E. De Clercq

tively, identified (Table 8.1) mostly by analogy with HSV. However, five of the VZV genes, including a gene for a thymidylate synthetase, are not found in HSV, while three HSV genes have no VZV equivalent. In common with other herpesviruses, the synthesis of VZV proteins broadly involves three phases, designated immediate early (alpha), early (beta) and late (gamma), where only the synthesis of the late proteins requires prior DNA replication. Many VZV proteins are involved in virus replication, including the thymidine kinase and thymidylate synthetase enzymes, two virus-specified protein kinases, a range of DNA binding proteins including the viral DNA polymerase, and several immediate–early (IE) transcriptional regulators (see Table 8.1).

TARGETS FOR ANTIVIRAL CHEMOTHERAPY

The currently used drugs for the treatment of VZV infections, as well as new drugs undergoing phase II/III clinical trials, are listed in Table 8.2. All the currently used compounds are targeted against the virally encoded DNA polymerase and all, except foscarnet (a non-nucleoside pyrophosphate derivative), are nucleoside analogues. Acyclovir (ACV) and the other related compounds are only phosphorylated by the viral thymidine kinase (TK) and this gives these compounds very high selective indices. Famciclovir and valaciclovir have been modified to increase their bioavailability and penciclovir (PCV) has a longer intracellular half-life, compared with ACV, but their *in vitro* activity against VZV is not significantly higher than that of ACV. In fact, PCV-TP has approximately 100-fold lower affinity for viral DNA polymerase compared to ACV-TP. Conversely, the intracellular concentration of ACV-TP is approximately 100-fold less than PCV-TP. All these compounds are generally less active against VZV than they are against HSV. Conversely, BV-ara-U (bromovinyl arabinosyl uracil) and 882C (1-(β-D-arabinofuranosyl) 5-propynyl uracil) are especially active against VZV ($ID_{50} < 0.005$ μM and ≤ 1 μM respectively) with high selective indices. Both compounds are phosphorylated to mono- and diphosphates by the VZV TK, which has both thymidine- and thymidylate-phosphorylating activity. HSV TK is unable to generate the diphosphate of 882C and only HSV-1 TK is able to activate Bv-ara-U, which explains their difference in activity against VZV and HSV. Both compounds are currently undergoing clinical trials for the treatment of VZV disease, with particular emphasis on zoster in immunocompromised patients.

Drugs which are directly targeted against the herpesvirus TK have been developed but none has so far gone on to clinical trials (5). Since they would block TK activity they could not be used in combination with ACV and related drugs.

VZV, like HSV, encodes a ribonucleotide reductase which differs sufficiently from the cellular enzymes to provide a potential target for antiviral

Table 8.1. Identified products of VZV genes

Gene	HSV homologue	Protein identity (%)	Translation product (kDa)	Function
4	U_L54	29	51.5	Transcriptional activator (IE protein)
6	U_L52	37	122.5	DNA helicase/primase component
8	U_L50	25	44.8	Deoxyuridine triphosphatase
13	No homologue	—	34.5	Thymidylate synthetase
14	U_L44	23	61.4	Membrane glycoprotein gC
16	U_L42	21	46.1	Associated with DNA polymerase
17	U_L41	32	51.4	Host shut-off
18	U_L40	54	35.4	Ribonucleotide reductase small subunit
19	U_L39	30	86.8	Ribonucleotide reductase large subunit
28	U_L30	52	134.0	DNA polymerase
29	U_L29	50	132.1	Binds single-stranded DNA
31	U_L27	45	98.1	Membrane glycoprotein gB
33	U_L26	34	66.0	Assembly proteinase (immature nucleocapsids)
33.5[a]	$U_L26.5$[a]	24	32.8	Assembly protein (immature nucleocapsids)
36	U_L23	28	37.8	Pyrimidine deoxyribonucleotide kinase
37	U_L22	25	93.6	Membrane glycoprotein gH
40	U_L19	52	155.0	Major capsid protein
47	U_L13	33	54.3	Protein kinase
48	U_L12	29	61.3	Deoxyribonuclease
49	U_L11	26	8.9	Myristoylated protein
51	U_L9	44	94.4	ori_s binding protein
52	U_L8	28	86.3	DNA helicase/primase component
55	U_L5	56	98.8	DNA helicase/primase component
59	U_L2	39	34.4	Uracil-DNA glycosylase
60	U_L1	19	17.6	Membrane glycoprotein gL
61	IE110	Local only	50.9	Transcriptional repressor (IE protein)
62/71	IE175	Complex	140.0	Transcriptional activator (IE protein)
63/70	U_S1	Local only	30.5	Transcriptional activator (IE protein)
66	U_S3	33	43.7	Protein kinase
67	U_S7	23	39.4	Membrane glycoprotein gI
68	U_S8	22	70.0	Membrane glycoprotein gE

Data from references 2, 3 and 77. [a] Internal initiation within previously identified gene.

Table 8.2. Antiviral drugs currently used or under development for treatment of VZV disease

Drug	Target
Idoxuridine (IUDR)	DNA polymerase
Vidarabine (Ara-A)	DNA polymerase
Acyclovir (ACV)	DNA polymerase, via TK
Penciclovir/famciclovir[a] (PCV/FCV)	DNA polymerase, via TK
Valaciclovir[b]	DNA polymerase, via TK
Alkanyl pyrimidines (882C)[c]	DNA polymerase, via TK
Bromovinyl arabinosyl uracil (BV-ara-U)	DNA polymerase, via TK
Foscarnet (phosphonoformate sodium)	DNA polymerase

[a] Famciclovir is the orally active form (diacetyl ester) of penciclovir.
[b] Prodrug of ACV.
[c] Development of 882C has been suspended (Summer 1994).

drugs. Thiosemicarbazone derivatives are active against this enzyme at micromolar levels and have been shown to potentiate the activity of ACV against VZV (6). Cellular toxicity is a problem with these compounds but they may find a use as a topical agent in combination therapy. It has also been possible to synthesize small isosteric peptides (five to nine amino acids long) which inhibit the herpesvirus ribonucleotide reductases by dissociating the two subunits of the enzyme. Cellular uptake and stability are problems with these peptides but early clinical trials have started to evaluate their use as topical agents against VZV and HSV, in combination with ACV. VZV has also been shown to encode a proteinase and a myristoylated protein (lp7/orf 49) thought to be involved in nucleocapsid assembly and virus maturation, and these may provide novel targets for antiviral drugs. Thus, Harper *et al.* (7) have shown that myristoylation inhibitors can block VZV assembly and replication *in vitro*, without significant cellular toxicity, and proteinase inhibitors against HIV are currently undergoing phase II/III trials. All existing and new drugs are only active against replicating virus. Compounds active against latent virus, such as antisense oligonucleotides or ribozymes, are not yet available as serious contenders for the treatment of VZV infections.

PATHOGENESIS

Studies on the pathogenesis of human VZV diseases have long been hampered by the lack of a good animal model. A model for the pathogenesis of varicella, based on Fenner's mousepox model, has been proposed by Grose (8) and there is generally good support for this model, mainly derived from clinical observations. There is still, however, controversy about the source and route of transmission of the virus. It is presumed that the respiratory tract is the portal of entry and undoubtedly VZV is transmissible via the airborne route and does not require close personal contact. The skin lesions are teeming with infectious virus, even at the maculopapular stage, and are the most likely source of airborne virus. In contrast, it is virtually impossible to isolate virus at any stage from the upper respiratory tract of cases of varicella.

Leukoviraemia has been demonstrated during the incubation period in healthy, as well as in immunocompromised, patients (9) and apart from the target organ—the skin—it is likely that the virus spreads to and replicates in many other organs of the body. Normally the infection at these sites does not manifest clinically but in those cases when extensive infection involves organs such as the lung or brain serious disease can result.

Termination of the primary infection is brought about by both the humoral and the cellular arms of the immune response but the latter appears to be the most important. Large amounts of free and cell-associated virus can be detected in the skin lesions, which strongly suggests that the damage results from a lytic effect of the virus. In fact, the lesions in the immunocompromised are not modified in any way other than being more extensive and this makes it unlikely that immune mechanisms play an important part in their genesis. Only one serological type of VZV is known worldwide and, thus, recovery from the primary infection usually results in life-long immunity to exogenous infection.

Even less is known above VZV latency and reactivation than is known about the corresponding processes with HSV. VZV, unlike HSV, has not been rescued from ganglia during the latent interval. However, numerous recent reports have shown the presence and expression of VZV genetic material in normal human trigeminal and thoracic ganglia (10,11). During latency the viral DNA appears to exist in episomal form with only a small number of genes being transcribed. The mechanisms involved in reactivation are not understood but in approximately 20% of individuals the virus reactivates in the ganglion and then progresses peripherally down the sensory nerve to produce the typical skin lesions of herpes zoster. Most cases of zoster occur spontaneously but trauma, sunburn and stress are well-known triggers of reactivation. Inadequacy of cell-mediated immunity is likely to be of critical importance in the failure to contain the virus in the ganglia since patients with Hodgkin's and similar diseases are much more likely to experience severe forms of zoster and are also more likely to experience more than one attack of the disease. In recent years it has also been shown that the appearance of zoster correlates with increasing immunodeficiency in patients infected with human immunodeficiency virus (HIV), which primarily affects cellular immunity (12,13).

EPIDEMIOLOGY

Varicella is one of the classic diseases of childhood, with the highest prevalence occurring in the early school years in most industrialized countries in temperate climates (Figure 8.1). Varicella is highly communicable, with an attack rate of approximately 90% in close contacts (e.g. household or playfriend), and therefore most people become infected before adulthood. Even so, from Figure 8.1 it can be seen that about 10% of young adults are still susceptible to varicella. This is important in hospital practice since health care workers without immunity frequently become infected following contact with zoster patients and can further transmit the infection to patients and other staff.

In developing countries or countries with crowded living conditions, the peak attack rates can occur at an earlier age but even in these countries infections before the age of two years are relatively uncommon.

CLINICAL FEATURES

VARICELLA

The illness usually commences with the appearance of the characteristic vesicular rash but occasionally there are prodromal symptoms which

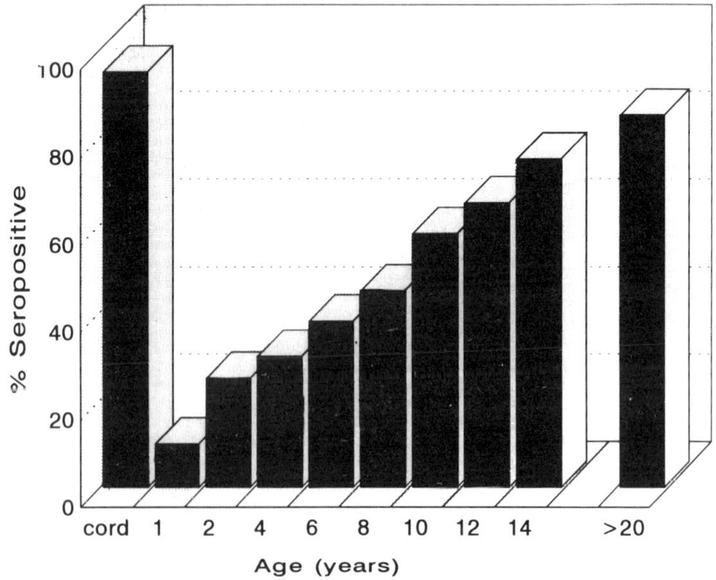

Figure 8.1. Age-related prevalence of antibodies to VZV in the UK (data from Kangro *et al.* (78))

resemble an influenza-like illness and appear a few days before the rash. The constitutional symptoms during varicella are typically mild in children. However, it is frequently observed that overall disease severity increases in secondary and tertiary cases as a result of serial transmission in outbreaks. Adults also tend to suffer more severe disease. Patients are generally considered to be infectious from a couple of days before the rash until new vesicle formation has ceased and existing vesicles have crusted, which usually occurs five to seven days after onset. Estimation of the period of infectivity forms an important basis for the management of nosocomial outbreaks.

COMPLICATIONS OF VARICELLA

The main complications of varicella are listed in Table 8.3.

Sepsis

Secondary bacterial infection of the skin lesions is by far the most common complication of varicella, and although rarely a serious problem it does increase scarring of the skin. Secondary bacterial pneumonia can occur but is very uncommon.

Haemorrhagic chickenpox

Haemorrhagic symptoms sometimes occur during the course of varicella, usually on the second or third day of the rash. Haemorrhage typically occurs into the skin but epistaxis, melaena or haematuria may be additional

Table 8.3. Complications of varicella

Bacterial skin infection
Pneumonitis
Cerebellar ataxia
Encephalitis
Meningitis
Transverse myelitis
Guillain–Barré syndrome
Reye's syndrome
Uveitis
Optic neuritis
Haemorrhage/bullae
Purpura
Hepatitis
Arthritis
Glomerulonephritis

presenting features. The haemorrhage may be so severe as to be life threatening. Thrombocytopenia and/or consumptive coagulopathy may be present.

Viral pneumonia

Overt viral pneumonitis is the most important complication of varicella and usually develops four to six days after onset of the rash. The patient presents with cough and chest pain and may then develop dyspnoea and cyanosis. The condition of the patient may be more serious than would be suspected from inspection of a chest X-ray. The distinction between this disease and bacterial pneumonia is difficult unless a biopsy is taken (14). The illness frequently runs a fulminating course and is the single most common cause of varicella-associated death (15). Pneumonitis can develop in up to 32% of children with leukaemia, with a mortality as high as 25% if untreated (16). Interestingly, cessation of immunosuppressive therapy during the incubation period of chickenpox in susceptible contacts does not appear to reduce the incidence of pneumonitis (16). It is also the commonest serious complication in previously healthy adults. Surviving patients may develop fibrosis of the lungs with permanent respiratory impairment.

Encephalitis

VZV is neurotropic and minor degrees of involvement of the central nervous system are probably common during the normal course of varicella. Mild ataxia suggesting cerebellar involvement is relatively common during varicella but has a good prognosis, and isolated cases of paralysis of oculomotor muscles have often been noted to follow varicella. Other neurological disorders, including meningitis, transverse myelitis and Guillain-Barré syndrome, have also been associated with the disease.

Varicella encephalitis is a rare but often fatal complication accounting for approximately 20% of varicella-associated deaths (15). It occurs most frequently in immunocompromised patients but it has not been firmly established whether varicella encephalitis is of the acute, or post-infectious, type (17).

VZV is also an important cause of Reye's syndrome and ranks second only to influenza in terms of frequency. This mainly affects children and is a form of encephalopathy secondary to liver damage, which carries a high mortality and can be confused with VZV encephalitis.

Other complications of varicella

VZV infection may involve virtually any organ of the body but, apart from the skin and occasionally the lung and brain, it is unusual for infection at other sites to manifest clinically. Nevertheless, myocarditis, arthritis and both renal and ureteric damage associated with varicella have been reported. An unusual chronic or recurrent form of varicella has been described in children infected with HIV (13).

VARICELLA IN PREGNANCY

From Figure 8.1 it can be seen that 10–20% of women entering childbearing age are susceptible to varicella. Several studies have shown that varicella occurs in 0.01–0.05% of pregnancies. Pregnant women are recognized as being at high risk of developing complications, especially pneumonitis, but it is not clear whether this is because of their age or the pregnancy. Varicella can also present two quite distinct problems to the fetus, depending on whether the infection is contracted in the early or late stages of the pregnancy. For a review of varicella in pregnancy, see Hanshaw *et al.* (18).

In the early stages of pregnancy the virus may cross the placenta and cause fetal defects, referred to as the 'congenital varicella syndrome' (14). Various studies have estimated the risk of fetal damage from maternal varicella early in pregnancy as between 0 and 9% (19–21). In a recent prospective study, Balducci *et al.* (22) found no cases of congenital varicella syndrome in 36 babies born to mothers who had varicella in the first trimester. Asymptomatic congenital VZV infection occurs more frequently than symptomatic infection and probably accounts for some cases of zoster during infancy (23). Varicella in the *late stages of pregnancy* can result in neonatal varicella. The risk of a baby acquiring varicella in this way is dependent on the time interval between the date of onset of the rash in the mother and the date of delivery. If the onset of the rash is less than seven days before delivery then no maternal antibody will have been transferred across the placenta and the severe disseminated form of neonatal varicella may develop. Case fatality rates of approximately 30% have been reported for neonatal varicella so this provides an important challenge for antiviral intervention.

The newborn baby may also be exposed to VZV shortly after birth, from the mother or other family members. Of particular importance are seronegative mothers whose babies contract varicella in the neonatal period and premature or very low birth-weight babies born to seropositive mothers. These babies do not have adequate levels of passive immunity from the mother, and therefore are also at risk of experiencing severe forms of the disease. Infected full-term children born to seropositive mothers are usually protected by humoral antibody and for this reason herpes zoster does not usually present a problem in pregnancy even when it occurs close to delivery. It is worth nothing that this protection is not complete since cases of mild varicella have been reported in babies born to seropositive mothers, and such babies could become a source of infection in neonatal or paediatric units. The protective efficacy of the maternal antibodies is maximal during the first two months of life (24).

HERPES ZOSTER

The average annual incidence of zoster is approximately 0.2% and it can occur at any age, although the vast majority of cases occur in individuals over 50 years old. Zoster is rare in children but may result either from underlying immunosuppressive illness or varicella acquired *in utero* or during infancy.

The siting of the skin lesion is dependent on the involved ganglia and two or more contiguous dermatomes may be affected. The trigeminal ganglion, lower cervical (particularly in children), thoracic and lumbar (T5–L2) posterior root ganglia are most frequently involved. Paraesthesia usually precedes the eruption and burning or shooting pains in the involved segment are often experienced. Over 90% of zoster patients experience a prodrome and this provides an opportunity for starting early treatment (25). The skin may be exquisitely tender to the touch (hyperaesthesia). In some cases the skin lesion is minimal or absent (zoster sine herpete) with pain localized to a particular dermatome.

The trigeminal ganglion is overall the most common site for reactivation of latent VZV infection and the ophthalmic branch is involved about 20 times more frequently than the maxillary and mandibular branches. Ramsay–Hunt syndrome is a form of aural zoster involving the geniculate ganglion of the seventh cranial nerve. It presents as facial palsy associated with vesicles in the external auditory meatus and is often accompanied by hearing loss and vertigo. The sacral ganglia may be involved and, in these cases, the skin lesions may be associated with retention of urine or symptoms suggestive of urinary tract infection and sometimes frank haemorrhagic cystitis.

The disease process is frequently prolonged in immunocompromised patients and they are most likely to experience the disseminated form of zoster. A minor degree of dissemination is probably common during VZV reactivation. Thus, in one study, asymptomatic VZV viraemia was detected in 19% of bone marrow transplant recipients, using the polymerase chain reaction (26). Extensive dissemination of the virus can occur in immunocompromised patients so that the appearance is similar to varicella but with the addition of the zoster lesion. Patients with such dissemination are usually extremely ill, often with visceral involvement, but there is rarely a fatal outcome.

COMPLICATIONS OF HERPES ZOSTER

Infection

As with varicella, secondary bacterial infection of the skin can occur and occasionally can lead to impetigo or cellulitis, but with appropriate antibiotic therapy this is rarely a serious problem.

Neuralgia

This is undoubtedly the most common and important complication of herpes zoster and affects some 10% of cases. Most patients experience pain at the site of the lesion but in approximately 90% of cases the acute pain remits within two to three weeks. In the remaining patients a severe disabling chronic neuralgia may ensue. Most of these patients recover within one year but in up to 20% of cases, depending on age, the pain may become intractable and can lead to exhaustion and even suicidal tendencies. Post-herpetic neuralgia is rarely seen in people under the age of 50 years. In a recent study in the UK the average age of patients with shingles was 58 years, while that of patients with prolonged post-herpetic neuralgia was 75 years (27). The same study showed that infection of the trigeminal ganglion was more likely to lead to post-herpetic neuralgia that at other sites.

Central nervous system

Encephalitis is a rare complication of zoster, even in immunocompromised patients. Typically in such cases the rash involves the cranial or upper cervical nerves.

Motor as well as sensory neurones may be involved in cases of herpes zoster as seen, for example, in ptosis associated with ophthalmic zoster or paralysis of the intrinsic muscles of the hand associated with skin lesions of the deltoid region. Most of the motor neuropathies are transient and serious sequelae are rarely seen. Guillain–Barré syndrome and myelitis with ascending paralysis have been reported in small numbers of cases. A rare but serious complication, particularly associated with ophthalmic zoster, is contralateral hemiparesis which is caused by a granulomatous inflammatory process in the brain with infarction of the cerebral arteries.

Ocular

Ophthalmic zoster is a particular problem because the risk of complications is high even in immunocompetent individuals. Between 50% and 70% of cases develop some form of ocular complication. Direct damage by zoster can involve any of the structures of the eye and its surrounds, such as the eyelid, conjunctiva, sclera, cornea and iris—iritis and keratitis being the most common complications. The risk of complications is particularly high if the nasociliary branch of the fifth cranial nerve is involved. Ophthalmic zoster can also lead to chronic eye disease due to inflammatory processes, such as anterior uveitis and stromal keratitis. Blindness following ophthalmic zoster is, however, rare even as a result of chronic eye disease.

TREATMENT

VARICELLA IN HEALTHY CHILDREN

The management of varicella in healthy children is normally uncomplicated because the illness is generally mild and complications are rare. For the typical case, no treatment is required apart, perhaps, for soothing lotions for itching, antipyretics (not salicylates because of the risk of Reye's disease) and antibiotics if there are signs of secondary bacterial infection. A small number of well-conducted trials have consistently demonstrated a clinical benefit from early ACV therapy in children with varicella (28,29). In the largest randomized, placebo-controlled study, involving 724 normal children with varicella, aged between two and 12 years, it was shown that oral ACV (20 mg/kg q6h for five days) started within 24 h after onset of the rash could significantly reduce the number of lesions and the duration of new vesicle formation and fever by two to four days (30). Overall, the ACV-treated group showed accelerated healing by one to two days compared with the placebo group. There was no significant difference in mean antibody levels or lymphocyte proliferation responses between the two groups up to one year after treatment, which indicates that the treatment is unlikely to compromise long-term immunity to VZV. In spite of the measurable effects of ACV treatment it did not, however, enable the children to return to school earlier. Thus the clinical benefits of ACV therapy in healthy children would appear to be minimal, reducing the duration of a generally mild disease by one to two days, and therefore difficult to justify on economic grounds. Surprisingly, in the above study there was no apparent reduction in the complication rate in the ACV-treated group compared to the placebo group.

The potential benefits of ACV may be age dependent since adolescents often have more severe disease and therefore could benefit more from treatment (30). Based on the available data, the American Academy of Pediatrics Committee on Infectious Diseases recently concluded (31) that:

1. Oral ACV is not indicated routinely for the treatment of varicella in otherwise healthy children because of the marginal therapeutic effect,

the cost and the low feasibility of administering the drug within 24 h after onset of illness.

2. ACV therapy should be considered in adolescents and in children over 12 months of age who have chronic cutaneous or pulmonary disorders, and in children on long-term salicylate therapy, although there is no evidence that this reduces the risk of Reye's syndrome in these children.

VARICELLA IN HEALTHY ADULTS

Whether the routine use of oral ACV is indicated in adults with chickenpox is currently an open question, although it is likely that the benefits would be greater than in children (32,33). In an open study involving 22 adolescents and adults, who were given oral ACV (4 g daily for five days), Feder (34) showed improvement in the overall severity (duration of fever and days to crusting) of varicella provided treatment was started within 24 h after onset. None of the cases in this study, however, had the severe form of varicella. A larger double-blind, placebo-controlled study at a US Naval Hospital in San Diego comprised 148 Marine and Navy Corps personnel with chickenpox who were given either oral ACV (800 mg five times a day for seven days) or placebo (35). Again the results showed that ACV therapy started within 24 h after onset of rash decreased healing time (Table 8.4) and duration of fever, but treatment started after the first day had no effect on uncomplicated cases. The complication rate was again low in this study group, possibly because of the low mean age (20 years), and did not permit any evaluation of the effects of ACV therapy on serious complications.

The results of the studies in healthy adults are thus very similar to those obtained in healthy children and adolescents. Therefore, on present evidence, the question of whether to treat healthy individuals with ACV is controversial and only clearly justified if there is a high risk or suspicion

Table 8.4. Comparison of rash progression in adults given ACV or placebo within 24 h after onset of varicella

Rash parameter	ACV ($n = 38$)	Placebo ($n = 38$)	p value
Total number of lesions	268	500	0.04
Time to 5% decrease in lesions (days)	2.6	3.3	< 0.001
Time to maximum number of lesions (days)	1.5	2.1	0.002
Time to full crusting (days)	5.6	7.4	0.001

From Wallace *et al.* (35).

of pneumonic involvement. In this context it is worth noting that ACV is not licensed for use in pregnant women, although there is no evidence that it is teratogenic, and it has now been used successfully without ill-effect in numerous women to treat serious VZV disease (36). Clearly the potential benefits of treatment have to be balanced against any possible hazards in pregnant women, and the decision to treat or not lies with the physician. The available clinical evidence clearly supports the use of intravenous (i.v.) ACV in women who show clinical or radiographic signs of lower respiratory tract involvement (37).

There are no clear data to show that ACV reduces the risk of complications of varicella in healthy individuals, even if this is likely to be the case. Unfortunately there are no reliable predictors of disease severity or complications in healthy individuals, other than age, early in the disease process. Thus, the effectiveness of any antiviral drugs against VZV will be limited by the time at which the treatment can be started. There is a danger that if the treatment is started too early during the incubation period it will prevent the development of an adequate immune response and long-term immunity. It is therefore reasonable to delay treatment in healthy individuals until symptoms appear. In this context it is encouraging that several studies have now shown that early ACV treatment does not significantly affect antibody titres or cell-mediated responses for up to three years after chickenpox (28,35,38–40).

The safety aspect is not a problem with ACV since all the above trials have shown that it can be used safely to treat varicella in healthy individuals. The high dosing level required and the cost are major disadvantages but the improved bioavailability of famciclovir and valaciclovir will probably permit a much lower dosing with the same or better efficacy.

VARICELLA IN PATIENTS AT HIGH RISK OF COMPLICATIONS

The management of varicella in immunocompromised individuals is very different from that in previously healthy individuals (Table 8.5). Both ACV and vidarabine have proved useful for the treatment of varicella and zoster in high-risk individuals.

Vidarabine (adenine arabinoside; ara-A) was the first drug proved to be useful for the treatment of varicella in immunocompromised patients but it often shows neurotoxicity (41). It is poorly soluble and therefore has to be administered by slow i.v. infusion at a dosage of 10 mg/kg per day for at least five days. ACV is now the treatment of choice for VZV disease as it is much less toxic than vidarabine and appears more effective in reducing both the incidence of pneumonia and mortality (16,42,43). Unfortunately, ACV is less active against VZV than HSV and a concentration approximately 10-fold higher is required for effective inhibition. The optimal dose for the treatment of VZV disease has still not been established but it is

Table 8.5. Summary of strategies for management of varicella in individuals at high risk of complications

Avoidance of contact:	School/playmates Relatives Hospital (staff, patients)
Prophylaxis:	VZIG (ACV?) (Vaccine)[a]
Treatment:	ACV (vidarabine) (i.v. to prevent visceral complications)

[a] Not licensed in most countries.

possible to obtain an adequate inhibitory concentration in the blood if a dose of 10 mg/kg is given i.v. over a 1 h period every 8 h (Table 8.6). This is the treatment of choice for immunocompromised patients and should be continued for at least five days. ACV is also well tolerated orally but only 15–25% is bioavailable. Consequently, 800 mg taken five times daily is required to maintain an inhibitory blood concentration. Anecdotal accounts, and several placebo-controlled trials, have demonstrated that both oral and i.v. ACV can bring about cessation of new vesicle formation and, more importantly, reduce the incidence of visceral involvement (39,44–46). In Feldman and Lott's retrospective study (16) on 228 children with cancer, none of the children treated with ACV ($n = 18$) developed pneumonitis,

Table 8.6. Dosage and administration of ACV

Indication	Patient's immune status	Dosage[a] Intravenous	Dosage[a] Oral
Primary and recurrent varicella zoster infections	Normal	10 mg/kg every 8 h for 5–7 days	800 mg 5 times daily for 7 days[b]
Primary and recurrent varicella zoster infection	Immuno-compromised	10 mg/kg every 8 h for 7 days	800 mg 5 times daily for 7–10 days
Encephalitis	Normal or immuno-compromised	10–15 mg/kg every 8 h for 10–14 days followed by oral ACV	–

[a]Should be reduced in patients with impaired renal function.
[b]Five days is sufficient in uncomplicated cases of varicella.

compared with 29% of the children treated with vidarabine ($n = 28$) and 28% of untreated children. There were no deaths among the ACV-treated children compared to an overall mortality of 7% in untreated children.

Unfortunately, there are also cases where ACV therapy had been commenced early but failed to prevent the development of a fatal pneumonic illness. There is a serious lack of data on penetration of the drug into tissues such as lung and particularly the levels and persistence of the active triphosphate.

Preliminary reports on the use of human leucocyte (alpha) interferon (IFN-α) for the treatment of varicella in children with cancer have shown a reduced number of days of new vesicle formation and a reduced risk of dissemination in treated children, but the toxicity of current preparations remains a major problem (47). The possibility of combining low-dose IFN with ACV, or other drugs, has been suggested (48) to reduce the adverse effects, but no trials are currently in progress with this regimen.

HERPES ZOSTER

This illness, occurring in a previously healthy individual, can be very unpleasant, but is not usually a serious cause for concern. It is the post-herpetic neuralgic pain, particularly when it is prolonged and intractable, which presents the main challenge for treatment in cases of zoster. In a large UK study on 376 zoster patients over 60 years old the proportion with pain after the rash was 61% after one month, 25% after three months and 13% at six months (25).

Analgesics are usually ineffective and the prolonged duration of the pain rules out the use of opiates. In a recent retrospective study, Bowsher (49) reviewed 87 patients with post-herpetic neuralgia of three or more months' duration and found that amitriptyline can offer significant pain relief if started early in zoster but has no effect on established neuralgia. There are reports of the successful use of steroids (prednisone or prednisolone), both locally on the rash and systemically in the convalescent period, to prevent the development of neuralgic pain (50). Such treatment must be given with great care because of the risk of dissemination and, perhaps, generalization of the infection due to the immunosuppressive effect of systemic steroids. Surgery involving removal of the dorsal roots may be required for those with the severe intractable forms of the pain.

The more severe forms of herpes zoster are seen in immunocompromised patients. Most recover satisfactorily from the infection, particularly if it is possible to suspend the immunosuppressive treatment for a short time. Nevertheless, antiviral chemotherapy is increasingly being prescribed for these cases to reduce dissemination and the duration of the illness. Idoxuridine was the first antiviral drug to be used for this purpose. It can be administered topically as a 40% suspension in dimethyl sulphoxide. This form of treatment is cumbersome and has now been replaced by systemic or oral treatment with the newer compounds, although it may still be of some use for combination therapy in patients with persisting zoster lesions.

The effectiveness of vidarabine for the treatment of herpes zoster has been assessed in a well-conducted multi-centre trial in the USA (51), where it was shown to reduce the time of virus shedding and to accelerate the cessation of new vesicle formation. Overall, the benefits of treatment were not impressive and, surprisingly, these benefits were not observed in those over the age of 38 years.

ACV (i.v.) has now replaced vidarabine as the treatment of choice for zoster in the immunocompromised. The treatment regimen should be continued for a period of at least seven days (Table 8.6). Placebo-controlled trials of the efficacy of ACV have shown that it is more effective than vidarabine and significantly reduces the duration of virus shedding and accelerates healing. However, Whitley *et al.* (52) found both drugs equally effective in a double-blind study of ACV versus vidarabine involving 73 patients with disseminated zoster. In this study, the patients were treated for seven or more days with either 30 mg ACV/kg per day i.v. or 10 mg vidarabine/kg per day by continuous infusion. Unfortunately, neither drug appears to have any effect on the incidence or severity of postherpetic neuralgia (25,43,53), although one American study has shown a reduction in pain up to three months after zoster (54).

Famciclovir (Famvir) has recently been licensed in several countries for the treatment of zoster and clinical trials have shown that a regimen of 250 mg three times a day is as effective as 800 mg ACV five times a day (60). The benefit of Famciclovir is derived from its better bioavailability (77%) and longer intra-cellular half-life (9 hrs), compared to ACV (20% and 0.8 hrs respectively), permitting an easier dosing schedule. Trials have also shown a significant effect of Famciclovir in reducing zoster-associated pain provided it is given within 48 hours after onset of rash (61,62). Preliminary results of clinical trials of i.v. penciclovir in patients with severe zoster have shown that it has a comparable clinical effect to i.v. ACV (63).

There are also encouraging preliminary reports of the use of leucocyte IFN and one report (55) of transfer factor for the treatment of zoster in immunocompromised patients, but varicella-zoster immunoglobulin (VZIG) has been shown to be ineffective for treatment. Following the promising results of the early trials with human leucocyte IFN (56) a randomized double-blind placebo-controlled trial in cancer patients with localized zoster showed that early interferon treatment significantly decreased dissemination and neuralgia (57,58). Fever and bone marrow depression were frequent problems in treated patients. Recombinant IFN has recently been used in zoster patients with a comparable effect to ACV (59) but the toxicity problems remain. Of the new drugs, BV-ara-U and 882C are particularly active against VZV. BV-ara-U (Brovavir) was released in Japan in 1993 for the treatment of severe zoster but was recently withdrawn again following a number of deaths in patients who were receiving concomitant treatment with 5-fluorouracil (5-FU). BV-ara-U is known to increase the toxicity of 5-FU and therefore the two drugs must not be given together. It does, however, also raise a question about the usefulness of BV-ara-U in patients who receive cytostatic drugs. Dihydroxypropoxymethyl-guanine (DHPG) is active against VZV but is associated with bone marrow depression and gonadal toxicity which make it unacceptable for the treatment of most VZV disease. Valaciclovir is currently undergoing phase III trials for the treatment of zoster in immunocompromised patients. Foscarnet is also active against VZV but since it has to be administered by infusion it will only be used to treat special cases of VZV infections (see below).

The outcome of current trials of established drugs and newer treatments is awaited with interest. Interestingly, there is no evidence as yet that these drugs will give a significantly greater clinical benefit in zoster patients compared to ACV. It is likely that any form of antiviral therapy is normally started too late in the disease process to have a dramatic effect on the initial lesions, but it would be of value if it regularly prevented dissemination from the affected dermatome(s) and this must be the aim of new drugs. A treatment which reduced the incidence or duration of post-herpetic neuralgia would of course also be of major benefit.

OPHTHALMIC ZOSTER

There is a clear indication for antiviral therapy in individuals with zoster involving the ophthalmic branch of the trigeminal nerve and, in view of the higher incidence of zoster-associated pain, a strong case can be made for treating zoster in any site in people over the age of 50 years. Disease involving the exterior of the eye, as well as dendritic keratitis, is normally self-limiting even without treatment but several trials have now shown that systemic or oral ACV reduces the severity of disease and the incidence of ocular complications (65,66). The treatment should, however, be started as soon as possible to be effective, preferably within 72 h of onset. A placebo-controlled trial of oral ACV (800 mg five times a day) in 46 patients with ophthalmic zoster showed significantly less active ocular disease six months after onset and significantly less pain at three to six months in the ACV-treated group (67). There is therefore clear evidence that early ACV treatment modifies the disease process in ophthalmic zoster and protects against long-term ocular complications. It is not known, however, how effective ACV is in treating chronic complications such as anterior uveitis and stromal keratitis, which often require systemic steroid therapy.

DRUG RESISTANCE

ACV-resistant strains of VZV have been isolated and clearly it will be important in the future to monitor anti-VZV therapy carefully with this in mind. Resistant VZV strains have so far only been isolated from immunocompromised patients on long-term ACV therapy and there is no evidence to suggest that these strains are transmissible (68). This may prove to be a particular problem in HIV-infected individuals who may develop a chronic type of zoster. Several isolates of ACV-resistant VZV from AIDS patients have been reported and characterized and the vesicular lesions may be associated with atypical hyperkeratotic papules (69–74). Most of these isolates contained either TK-deficient or TK-altered virus, although two of the isolates were found to have an altered DNA polymerase which conferred ACV resistance (71,72). Talarico *et al.* (74) characterized 12 ACV-resistant VZV isolates from AIDS patients on long-term oral ACV. All isolates showed reduced TK function which in five isolates was shown to be due to nucleotide deletions leading to a truncated protein. The other seven isolates showed single point mutations leading to amino acid substitutions, which were not restricted to the ATP or nucleotide binding sites. Some of the isolates showed cross-resistance to other TK-dependent drugs, viz. penciclovir and BV-ara-U, but all were sensitive to the DNA polymerase-dependent drugs foscarnet and vidarabine. Safrin *et al.* (72) used foscarnet, 40 mg/kg every 8 h in a 1 h infusion for at least 10 days, in an open study to treat five AIDS patients with ACV-resistant VZV infections. Four of the patients showed healing and became culture negative for VZV. In one patient, the virus also developed foscarnet resistance during treatment. Thus, foscarnet appears to be a tolerable drug for treating ACV-resistant VZV infections but the optimal dose and duration of treatment need to be defined.

PREVENTION

The prevention of varicella deserves a brief mention as it forms an important part of the overall management of VZV disease in high-risk individuals. It is currently aimed at those who are at risk of contracting the severe forms of the disease (Table 8.7) and for these individuals both passive and active prophylaxis are now available. In the first instance it is of considerable importance to counsel the patient, or the patient's parents, on the avoidance of any identifiable contact with the disease (Table 8.5). In children, this advice can have an appreciable disruptive effect on their education.

Many immunocompromised patients will cope normally with varicella, especially if the immunosuppressive therapy is withdrawn, but consider-

Table 8.7. Underlying or associated conditions which place patients at risk of severe forms of varicella and complications

Leukaemias, Hodgkin's disease and other neoplasms of the lymphoreticular system, whether or not treatment is being given
Other cancers but which are being treated with cytotoxic drugs or other regimens which are immunosuppressive
Primary immunodeficiency syndromes
Bone marrow transplant recipients irrespective of their own or the donor's VZV status
Diseases requiring systemic steroids at a dosage equivalent to at least 2 mg prednisone/kg per day
Susceptible pregnant women in close contact with VZV
Newborn infants of women who contracted varicella $\leq$ 7 days before or after delivery
Premature infants whose mothers have no history of varicella or any infant whose birth weight is less than 1000 g

ation should always be given to the possibility of administering human zoster immune globulin to these patients prophylactically if they come in contact with VZV. It is not possible, at the moment, to give guidelines on the prophylactic use of antivirals because there are no reports of placebo-controlled trials demonstrating the efficacy of such a strategy. Since the maximum beneficial effect of these drugs is likely to be achieved the earlier they are given, early recognition and diagnosis is important and it is not logical to restrict their use to those patients who are beginning to show the more severe manifestations of infection.

At present there is no means of inhibiting reactivation of VZV and thus preventing the onset of herpes zoster.

DRUGS

ACV is now used routinely for prophylaxis of HSV infection in immunocompromised patients. There is no evidence that high-dose oral ACV will prevent varicella or herpes zoster but clinical trials of this drug and the newer drugs which offer greater efficacy and/or bioavailability should provide further information.

PASSIVE IMMUNIZATION

Human immunoglobulin preparations with high titres of antibody to VZV are an established means of attempting to prevent varicella but have no role to play in the treatment of VZV disease, except possibly in conjunction with ACV in patients with poor antibody responses. Current preparations are obtained by processing pre-selected sera from blood donors with high titres of antibody to VZV. These preparations are referred to as varicella zoster immune globulin (VZIG) or human anti-varicella zoster immunoglobulin. Normal human immunoglobulin (NHIG) has been shown not to be effective in prevention of varicella (75) but antibody concentrations in the blood as high as those with VZIG have been obtained with i.v. NHIG and this may be used on an empirical basis as an alternative when VZIG is not available. However, nothing is known about the efficacy of NHIG. VZIG should be administered (Table 8.8) to any susceptible 'at risk' individual as soon as possible after contact, but studies have shown it to have some effect up to 10 days after contact with either varicella or herpes zoster. A convincing history of varicella or zoster from someone exposed to the virus, or the demonstration of antibody to VZV in serum, are reasonably reliable indicators of immunity and obviate the need to administer prophylactic immunoglobulin. Because of the severe degree of immunosuppression, recipients of bone marrow transplants should be assumed to be susceptible regardless of past history of varicella.

Unfortunately, the efficacy of VZIG is still not entirely clear and differences in the results of different studies may reflect different potencies of the preparations used. An early trial, involving only 12 children with family contact, indicated that VZIG gave complete protection whereas human normal immunoglobulin was totally ineffective. In a later study carried out in the UK it was shown that of 27 seronegative children who were in contact at home, 18 (67%) became infected—14 (52%) with symptoms—in spite of receiving VZIG. The rationale of administering VZIG to those at risk is therefore not so much to prevent infection but to prevent the serious forms of the disease with visceral involvement. Feldman and Lott (16) reviewed the impact of varicella in 280 children with cancer and the effectiveness of various forms of management. In their study group, passive immunization significantly reduced both the incidence and mortality of pneumonitis compared to untreated children. Even so, pneumonitis developed in 11% of

Table 8.8. Dose of VZIG recommended at different ages

Age (years)	Dose[a] of VZIG (mg)[b]
0–5	250
6–10	500
11–14	750
$\geqslant$ 15	1000

[a] Repeated after 3 weeks if necessary.
[b] Potency: approximately 1 IU VZV IgG/mg.

children who received VZIG, requiring intensive additional antiviral chemotherapy.

It is also recommended that VZIG be given to susceptible pregnant women in close contact with VZV infection in the hope that it will reduce the risk of transmission of infection to the fetus and also to ameliorate any potentially serious VZV disease which can occur in pregnant women. There are, however, no data on the efficacy of VZIG used in this way in immunocompetent individuals. Should a woman contract varicella perinatally, it is important to administer VZIG to the newborn baby, although a proportion of the infants can still be expected to develop chickenpox (76).

REFERENCES

1. Straus, S. E., Reinhold, W., Smith, H. A. *et al.* (1984). Endonuclease analysis of viral DNA from varicella and subsequent zoster infection in the same patient. *N. Engl. J. Med.*, **311**, 1362–1364.
2. Davison, A. J. and Scott, J. E. (1986). The complete DNA sequence of varicella-zoster virus. *J. Gen. Virol.*, **67**, 1759–1816.
3. Davison, A. J. (1991). Varicella-zoster virus. *J. Gen. Virol.*, **72**, 475–486.
4. Davison, A. J. and McGeoch, D. J. (1986). Evolutionary comparisons of the S segments in the genomes of herpes simplex virus type 1 and varicella-zoster virus. *J. Gen. Virol.*, **67**, 597–611.
5. Cameron, J. M. (1990). New developments in antiviral therapy. In *Control of Virus Diseases*, N. J. Dimmock, P. D. Griffiths and C. R. Madeley (eds), Cambridge University Press, Cambridge, pp. 341–373.
6. Spector, T., Harrington, J. A., Morrison, R. W., Jr *et al.* (1989). 2-Acetylpyridine 5-[(dimethylamino)thiocarbonyl]-thiocarbonohydrazone (A1110U), a potent inactivator of ribonucleotide reductases of herpes simplex and varicella zoster viruses and a potentiator of acyclovir. *Proc. Natl Acad. Sci. USA*, **86**, 1051–1055.
7. Harper, D. R., Gilbert, R. L., Blunt, C. and McIlhinney, R. A. J. (1993). Inhibition of varicella-zoster virus replication by an inhibitor of protein myristoylation. *J. Gen. Virol.*, **74**, 1181–1184.
8. Grose, C. (1987). Varicella-zoster virus: pathogenesis of the human disease, the virus and viral replication, and the major viral glycoproteins and proteins. In *Natural History of Varicella-Zoster Virus*, R. W. Hyman (ed.), CRC Press, Boca Raton, FL, Ch. 1.
9. Asano, Y., Itakura, N., Hiroishi, Y. *et al.* (1985). Viraemia is present in incubation period in immunocompromised children with varicella. *J. Pediatr.*, **106**, 69–71.
10. Gilden, D. H., Rozenman, Y., Murray, R. *et al.* (1987). Detection of varicella-zoster virus nucleic acid in neurons of normal human thoracic ganglia. *Ann. Neurol.*, **22**, 377–380.
11. Mahalingam, R., Wellish, M., Wolf, W. *et al.* (1990). Latent varicella-zoster viral DNA in human trigeminal and thoracic ganglia. *N. Engl. J. Med.*, **323**, 627–631.
12. Fletcher, C. V. (1992). Treatment of herpesvirus infections in HIV-infected individuals. *Ann. Pharmacother.*, **26**, 955–962.
13. Srugo, I., Israele, V., Wittek, A. E. *et al.* (1993). Clinical manifestations of varicella-zoster virus infections in human immunodeficiency virus-infected children. *Am. J. Dis. Child.*, **147**, 742–745.

14. Heath, R. B. and Kangro, H. O. (1990). Varicella zoster. In *Principles and Practice of Clinical Virology*, A. J. Zuckermann, J. E. Banatvala and J. R. Pattison (eds), John Wiley, Chichester, pp. 44–68.
15. Joseph, C. A. and Noah, D. N. (1988). Epidemiology of chickenpox in England and Wales, 1967–1985. *Br. Med. J.*, **296**, 673–676.
16. Feldman, S. and Lott, L. (1987). Varicella in children with cancer: impact of antiviral therapy and prophylaxis. *Pediatrics*, **80**, 465–472.
17. Kennedy, P. G. E., Barrass, J. D., Graham, D. I. and Clements, G. B. (1990). Studies on the pathogenesis of neuronal diseases associated with varicella-zoster virus. *Neuropathol. Appl. Neurobiol.*, **16**, 305–316.
18. Hanshaw, J. B., Dudgeon, J. A. and Marshall, W. C. (1985). Varicella-zoster infections. In *Viral Diseases of the Fetus and Newborn*, J. B. Hanshaw, J. A. Dudgeon and W. C. Marshall (eds) Saunders, Philadelphia, p. 161.
19. Siegel, M. (1973). Congenital malformations following chickenpox, measles, mumps and hepatitis: results of a cohort study. *JAMA*, **226**, 1521–1524.
20. Enders, G. (1984). Varicella-zoster virus infection in pregnancy. *Prog. Med. Virol.*, **29**, 166–196.
21. Paryani, S. G. and Arvin, A. M. (1986). Intrauterine infection with varicella-zoster virus after maternal varicella. *N. Engl. J. Med.*, **314**, 1542–1546.
22. Balducci, J., Rodis, J. F., Rosengren, S. *et al.* (1992). Pregnancy outcome following first-trimester varicella infection. *Obstet. Gynecol.*, **79**, 5–6.
23. Brunell, P. A. and Kotchmar, G. S. (1981). Zoster in infancy: failure to maintain virus latency following intrauterine infection. *J. Pediatr.*, **98**, 71–73.
24. Baba, K., Yabuuchi, H., Takahashi, M. and Ogra, P. L. (1982). Immunologic and epidemiologic aspects of varicella infection acquired during infancy and early childhood. *J. Pediatr.*, **100**, 881–885.
25. McKendrick, M. V., McGill, J. I. and Wood, M. J. (1989). Lack of effect of acyclovir on postherpetic neuralgia. *Br. Med. J.*, **298**, 431.
26. Wilson, A., Sharp, M., Koropchak, C. M. *et al.* (1992). Subclinical varicella-zoster virus viremia, herpes zoster, and T lymphocyte immunity to varicella-zoster viral antigens after bone marrow transplantation. *J. Infect. Dis.*, **165**, 119–126.
27. Glynn, C. (1992). Epidemiology of herpes zoster infection. In *The Management of Varicella Zoster*, D. Jeffries (ed.), Colwood House Medical Publications, Reading, UK, pp. 8–9.
28. Balfour, H. H., Jr, Kelley, J. M., Suarez, C. S. *et al.* (1990). Acyclovir treatment of varicella in otherwise healthy children. *J. Pediatr.*, **116**, 633–639.
29. Dunkle, L. M., Arvin, A. M., Whitley, R. J. *et al.* (1991). A controlled trial of acyclovir for chickenpox in normal children. *N. Engl. J. Med.*, **325**, 1539–1544.
30. Balfour, H. H., Jr, Rothbart, H. A., Feldman, S. *et al.* (1992). Acyclovir treatment of varicella in otherwise healthy adolescents. *J. Pediatr.*, **120**, 627–633.
31. Anonymous (1993). American Academy of Pediatrics Committee on Infectious Diseases: the use of oral acyclovir in otherwise healthy children with varicella. *Pediatrics*, **91**, 674–676.
32. Haake, D. A., Zakowski, P. C., Haake, D. L. and Bryson, Y. J. (1990). Early treatment with acyclovir for varicella pneumonia in otherwise healthy adults: retrospective controlled study and review. *Rev. Infect. Dis.*, **12**, 788–798.
33. Al-Nakib, W., Al-Kandari, S., El-Khalik, D. M. A. and El-Shirbiny, A. M. (1983). A randomized controlled study of intravenous acyclovir (Zovirax) against placebo in adults with chickenpox. *J. Infect.*, **6**, 549–556.
34. Feder, H. M. (1990). Treatment of adult chickenpox with oral acyclovir. *Arch. Int. Med.*, **150**, 2061–2065.

35. Wallace, M. R., Bowler, W. A., Murray, N. B. *et al.* (1992). Treatment of adult varicella with oral acyclovir: a randomized, placebo-controlled trial. *Ann. Intern. Med.*, **117**, 358–363.
36. Boyd, K. and Walker, E. (1988). Use of acyclovir to treat chickenpox in pregnancy. *Br. Med. J.*, **296**, 393–394.
37. Smego, R. A., Jr and Asperilla, M. O. (1991). Use of acyclovir for varicella pneumonia during pregnancy. *Obstet. Gynecol.*, **78**, 1112–1116.
38. England, J. A., Arvin, A. M. and Balfour, H. H. (1990). Acyclovir treatment for varicella does not lower gpI and IE-62 (p170) antibody response to varicella zoster virus in normal children. *J. Clin. Microbiol.*, **28**, 2327–2330.
39. Prober, C. G., Kirk, L. E. and Keeney, R. E. (1982). Acyclovir therapy of chickenpox in immunosuppressed children: a collaborative study. *J. Pediatr.*, **101**, 622–625.
40. Rotbart, H. A., Levin, M. J. and Hayward, A. R. (1993). Immune responses to varicella zoster virus infections in healthy children. *J. Infect. Dis.*, **167**, 195–199.
41. Feldman, S., Robertson, P. K., Lott, L. and Thornton, D. (1986). Neurotoxicity due to adenine arabinoside therapy during varicella-zoster virus infections in immunocompromised children. *J. Infect. Dis.*, **154**, 889–893.
42. Balfour, H. H., Jr (1991). Varicella-zoster virus infections in the immunocompromised host: natural history and treatment. *Scand. J. Infect. Dis.*, **80** (Suppl.), 69–74.
43. Shepp, D. H., Dandliker, P. S. and Meyers, J. D. (1986). Treatment of varicella-zoster virus infection in severely immunocompromised patients: a randomised comparison of acyclovir and vidarabine. *N. Engl. J. Med.*, **314**, 208–212.
44. Balfour, H. H., Jr (1984). Intravenous acyclovir therapy for varicella in immunocompromised children. *J. Pediatr.*, **104**, 134–136.
45. Meszner, Z., Nyerges, G. and Bell, A. R. (1993). Oral acyclovir to prevent dissemination of varicella in immunocompromised children. *J. Infect.*, **26**, 9–15.
46. Nyerges, G., Meszner, Z., Gyarmati, E. and Kerpel-Fronius, S. (1988). Acyclovir prevents dissemination of varicella in immunocompromised children. *J. Infect. Dis.*, **157**, 309–313.
47. Arvin, A. M., Kushner, J. H., Feldman, S. *et al.* (1982). Human leukocyte interferon for the treatment of varicella in children with cancer. *N. Engl. J. Med.*, **306**, 761–765.
48. Levin, M. J. and Leary, P. L. (1981). Inhibition of human herpesviruses by combinations of acyclovir and human leukocyte interferon. *Infect. Immun.*, **32**, 995–999.
49. Bowsher, D. (1992). Acute herpes zoster and postherpetic neuralgia: effects of acyclovir and outcome of treatment with amitriptyline. *Br. J. Gen. Pract.*, **42**, 244–246.
50. Benoldi, D., Mirizzi, S., Zucchi, A. and Allegra, F. (1991). Prevention of postherpetic neuralgia: evaluation of treatment with oral prednisone, oral acyclovir, and radiotherapy. *Int. J. Dermatol.*, **30**, 288–290.
51. Whitley, R. J., Chi'en, L. T., Dollin, R. *et al.* (1976). Adenine arabinoside therapy of herpes zoster in the immunosuppressed: NIAID collaborative antiviral study. *N. Engl. J. Med.*, **294**, 1193–1199.
52. Whitley, R. J., Gnann, J. W., Jr, Hinthorn, D. *et al.* (1992). Disseminated herpes zoster in the immunocompromised host: a comparative trial of acyclovir and vidarabine. The NIAID Collaborative Antiviral Study Group. *J. Infect. Dis.*, **165**, 450–455.
53. Bean, B., Aeppli, D. and Balfour, H. H. (1983). Acyclovir in shingles. *J. Antimicrob. Chemother.*, **12** (Suppl. B), 123–127.

54. Huff, J. C., Bean, B., Balfour, H. H., Jr *et al.* (1988). Therapy of herpes zoster with oral acyclovir. *Am. J. Med.*, **85** (Suppl. 1A), 84–89.
55. Wisnes, R., Froland, S. S. and Degré, M. I. (1978). Effect of transfer factor and zoster immunoglobulin in patients with varicella-zoster infection and malignancy. *Scand. J. Infect. Dis.*, **10**, 21–27.
56. Emödi, G., Rufli, T., Just, M. *et al.* (1975). Human interferon therapy for herpes zoster in adults. *Scand. J. Infect. Dis.*, **7**, 1–5.
57. Merigan, T. C., Rand, K. H., Pollard, R. B. *et al.* (1978). Human leukocyte interferon for the treatment of herpes zoster in patients with cancer. *N. Engl. J. Med.*, **298**, 981–987.
58. Merigan, T. C., Gallagher, J. G., Pollard, R. B. *et al.* (1981). Short-course human leukocyte interferon in treatment of herpes zoster in patients with cancer. *Antimicrob. Agents Chemother.*, **19**, 193–195.
59. Duschet, P., Schwarz, T., Soyer, P. *et al.* (1988). Treatment of herpes zoster: recombinant alpha interferon versus acyclovir. *Int. J. Dermatol.*, **27**, 193–197.
60. Delescluse, J. (1993). Famciclovir in the treatment of herpes zoster infections. In *Abstracts of Symposium on Herpesvirus Infections*, 3rd Congress of EADV, Adelphi Communications, Macclesfield, UK, pp. 8–9.
61. McKendrick, M., Wood, M., Degreef, H. *et al.* (1994). Reduction of zoster-associated pain (ZAP) by famciclovir. *Int. Conf. Antivir. Res.* 27 Feb–4 Mar, Poster 208.
62. Cunningham, A., Tyring, S., Nahlik, J. *et al.* (1994). Efficiency of famciclovir on herpes zoster rash resolution and post-herpetic neuralgia. *Int. Antivir. Symp.*, 7–10 June, Poster 28.
63. Duschet, P., Auer-Grumbach, P. and Gschnait, F. (1992). Efficacy and safety of penciclovir (PCV) in the treatment of patients with herpes zoster (HZ): a double-blind, randomised acyclovir (ACV)-controlled study. *Proc. 32nd Intersci. Conf. Antimicrob. Agents and Chemother.*, **395**, Abstract 1708.
64. Cobo, M. (1992). The treatment of zoster ophthalmicus. In *The Management of Varicella Zoster*, D. Jeffries (ed.), Colwood House Medical Publications, Reading, UK, pp. 10–11.
65. Harding, S. (1992). Oral acyclovir in herpes zoster ophthalmicus. In *The Management of Varicella Zoster*, D. Jeffries (ed.), Colwood House Medical Publications, Reading, UK, pp. 12–13.
66. Harding, S. P. and Porter, S. M. (1991). Oral acyclovir in herpes zoster ophthalmicus. *Curr. Eye Res.*, **10** (Suppl.), 177–182.
67. Cole, N. L. and Balfour, H. H., Jr (1986). Varicella-zoster virus does not become more resistant to acyclovir during therapy. *J. Infect. Dis.*, **153**, 605–608.
68. Jacobson, M. A., Berger, T. G., Fikrig, S. *et al.* (1990). Acyclovir-resistant varicella zoster virus infection after chronic oral acyclovir therapy in patients with the acquired immunodeficiency syndrome (AIDS). *Ann. Intern. Med.*, **112**, 187–191.
69. Leibovitz, E., Kaul, A., Rigaud, M. *et al.* (1992). Chronic varicella zoster in a child infected with human immunodeficiency virus: case report and review of the literature. *Cutis*, **49**, 27–31.
70. Linnemann, C. C., Jr, Biron, K. K., Hoppenjans, W. G. and Solinger, A. M. (1990). Emergence of acyclovir-resistant varicella zoster virus in an AIDS patient on prolonged acyclovir therapy. *AIDS*, **4**, 577–579.
71. Pahwa, S., Bioron, K., Lim, W. *et al.* (1988). Continuous varicella-zoster infection associated with acyclovir resistance in a child with AIDS. *JAMA*, **260**, 2879–2882.
72. Safrin, S., Berger, T. G., Gilson, I. *et al.* (1991). Foscarnet therapy in five patients with AIDS and acyclovir-resistant varicella-zoster virus infection. *Ann. Intern. Med.*, **115**, 19–21.

73. Sawyer, M. H., Inchauspe, G., Biron, K. K. *et al.* (1988). Molecular analysis of the pyrimidine deoxyribonucleoside kinase gene of wild-type and acyclovir resistant strains of varicella zoster virus. *J. Gen. Virol.*, **69**, 2585–2593.
74. Talarico, C. L., Phelps, W. C. and Biron, K. K. (1993). Analysis of the thymidine kinase genes from acyclovir-resistant mutants of varicella-zoster virus isolated from patients with AIDS. *J. Virol.*, **67**, 1024–1033.
75. Feldman, S., Hughes, W. T. and Daniel, C. B. (1975). Varicella in children with cancer: seventy-seven cases. *Pediatrics*, **56**, 388–397.
76. Miller, E., Cradock-Watson, J. E. and Ridhalgh, M. K. S. (1989). Outcome in newborn babies given anti-varicella-zoster immunoglobulin after perinatal maternal infections with varicella-zoster virus. *Lancet*, **ii**, 371–373.
77. McGeoch, D. J., Dalrymple, M. A., Davison, A. J. *et al.* (1988). The complete DNA sequence of the long unique region in the genome of herpes simplex virus type 1. *J. Gen. Virol.*, **69**, 1531–1574.
78. Kangro, H. O., Osman, H. K., Lau, Y. L. *et al.* (1994). Seroprevalence of antibodies to human herpesviruses in England and Hong Kong. *J. Med. Virol.*, **43**, 91–96.

9 Clinical Aspects of Treatment of Cytomegalovirus

D. PILLAY, V. C. EMERY and P. D. GRIFFITHS
Department of Virology, The Royal Free Hospital School of Medicine, London, UK

INTRODUCTION

Human cytomegalovirus (HCMV) is a member of the Herpesviridae. HCMV infection is ubiquitous with up to 100% of adults being infected, depending on their geographical location and other risk factors. In the majority of cases, infection is asymptomatic but if the host immune response is suboptimal through disease or following transplantation or AIDS, or through immaturity, HCMV can cause serious morbidity and mortality. The aim of this review is to highlight the clinical situations in which existing therapies offer significant control of HCMV disease.

MODE OF ACTION OF CURRENT ANTIVIRAL DRUGS

Like the DNA polymerases of both herpes simplex virus (HSV) and varicella zoster virus (VZV), the HCMV polymerase is optimally active under high salt conditions and is particularly sensitive to inhibition by phosphonoacetate and phosphonoformate (foscarnet) and to the nucleoside triphosphate analogues such as ganciclovir triphosphate (Figure 9.1). A mechanistic understanding of these data is not available. The HCMV polymerase complex consists of two proteins of M_r 140 000 and M_r 58 000 (1,2). The former protein is the DNA polymerase (3), whilst the latter is a DNA binding protein. Conservation of amino acid residues between the HCMV polymerase and the other herpesvirus polymerases is highest in the C-terminal portion of the protein. By analogy with other polymerases this region probably comprises the deoxynucleoside triphosphate and inorganic phosphate binding domains. Consistent with such data is the fact that mutations in the C-terminal region have been identified in viruses that are resistant to the effects of nucleoside analogues (4). The most widely used anti-CMV drug, ganciclovir (9-(1,3-dihydroxy-2-propoxymethyl)guanine) (GCV), is a potent inhibitor of the HCMV DNA polymerase (Figure 9.1).

All the nucleoside analogues have to be phosphorylated to their triphosphate form before they act as chain-terminating competitive inhibitors

Antiviral Chemotherapy. Edited by D.J. Jeffries and E. De Clercq

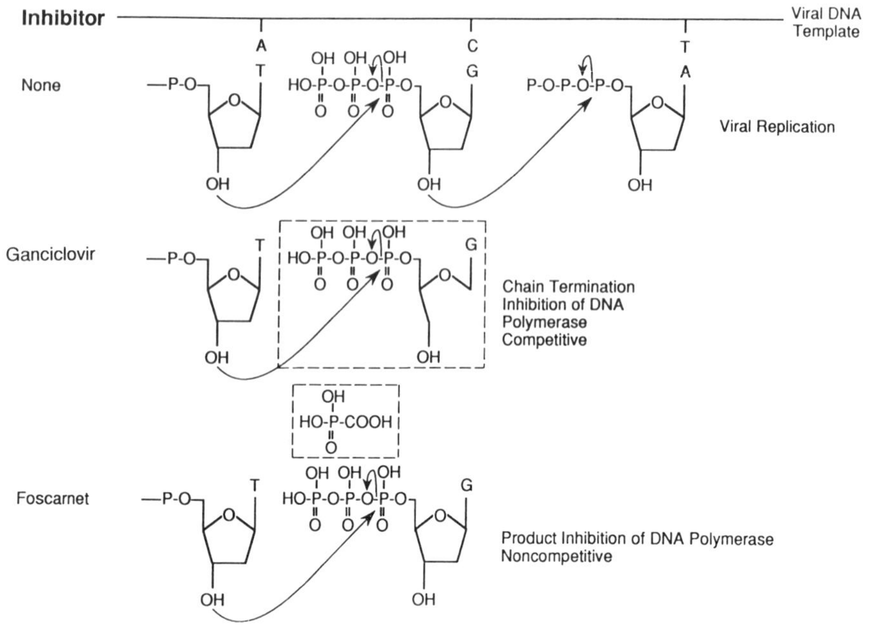

Figure 9.1. Sites of action of ganciclovir triphosphate (GCV-TP) and foscarnet. The active inhibitory species is boxed

of the HCMV DNA polymerase. In the case of acyclovir (ACV), HSV-1-infected cells catalyse the initial phosphorylation step by the viral-encoded thymidine kinase. To date, no such homologous gene or viral gene activity has been detected in HCMV-infected cells. However, more recent data have identified a putative protein kinase, *UL97*, that is encoded within the HCMV genome which functions to phosphorylate GCV directly (5). A 12 bp deletion encoding four amino acids has been shown to yield a virus that is resistant to GCV. The deletion is within a conserved region which in cyclic AMP-dependent protein kinases participates in substrate recognition (6). *UL97* has the ability to phosphorylate both ACV and GCV. Note that ACV triphosphate is a more potent inhibitor of CMV DNA polymerase than is GCV triphosphate (7). The relative efficacy of GCV over ACV in HCMV-infected cell cultures or *in vivo* may be due to the shorter half-life of intracellular ACV-triphosphate. These data will be important in future rational drug design for agents active against CMV.

PHARMACOLOGY OF LICENSED ANTI-CMV DRUGS

GANCICLOVIR

GCV is a synthetic acyclic purine (guanosine) analogue, similar in structure to ACV. It has *in vitro* activity against a range of herpesviruses. The drug is preferentially converted to the triphosphate within HCMV-infected cells, and competitively inhibits the binding of deoxyguanosine triphosphate to DNA polymerase, in the process causing chain termination and inhibition of DNA synthesis. At present, GCV is only licensed for intravenous (i.v.) use, although an orally available formulation is currently being assessed for efficacy. Intravitreal administration has also been reported but is not licensed in the UK (8). The recommended dosage for treatment of HCMV disease is 5 mg/kg i.v. twice daily for 14–21 days. If further maintenance therapy is required, as is the case for retinitis in AIDS, this dose can be given once daily. The drug undergoes renal excretion similar to ACV and therefore dosage requires adjustment for renal function. It has low penetration of the central nervous system (CNS), with around 40% of blood levels being achieved. The half-life of GCV is 2–3 h in plasma, but is estimated to reach 6 h for the intracellular triphosphate form. Neutropenia represents the major side-effect of GCV, which ranges in incidence from 13% to 67% (9), and may limit the ability to administer GCV in conjunction with other myelotoxic drugs such as zidovudine. Regular blood cell counts should be undertaken throughout the duration of treatment. Other adverse effects include abnormal liver function, thrombocytopenia, rashes, gastrointestinal disturbance and CNS abnormalities. An inhibitory effect on spermatogenesis in rodents has been observed so this potential effect must be considered before initiating therapy in humans.

FOSCARNET

Foscarnet is a pyrophosphate analogue which inhibits a number of viral polymerases, including those of the herpesviruses, retroviruses and influenza. It reversibly and non-competitively inhibits the HCMV DNA polymerase without requiring prior phosphorylation. Foscarnet is administered i.v. and is excreted unchanged through the kidneys. However, a small degree of 'non-renal clearance' reflects sequestration for long periods of time in bone. CNS availability reaches 40% of serum levels. Dosage is recommended at 60 mg/kg 8-hourly for 14 days, then reducing to once daily administration of 90 mg/kg for maintenance therapy. The major side-effect is renal failure, which is reduced if patients on treatment are kept well hydrated, due in part to an inhibition of phosphate excretion. Long periods of infusion are required for those receiving induction therapy, and this makes administration of the drug in an outpatient setting (as maintenance therapy) difficult. The precise dosage must be adjusted for pre-existing renal function. It is essential that regular assessments of electrolyte balance, especially for calcium and phosphate, are made during therapy. The incidence of renal dysfunction is estimated as up to 40%, and care must be taken when foscarnet is used in combination with other nephrotoxic drugs. Other adverse effects include gastrointestinal disturbance, anaemia and a fixed drug eruption on genital skin.

EPIDEMIOLOGY AND DISEASE SPECTRUM

HCMV infects between 50% and 100% of the adult population, depending on factors such as socio-economic status and degree of sexual activity. Thus, 60% of UK adults are seropositive, compared with 90–100% in many developing countries. On the other hand, around 80% of homosexual men in the UK have evidence of prior infection (10).

Infection can be acquired by intrauterine or perinatal transmission from the mother. Since young children who develop infection may excrete virus from urine and saliva for many months, or even years, they may be responsible for further spread among this age group and to adults in close contact with them (11). In immunocompromised individuals, transmission of virus with blood transfusions or donor organs is of particular concern in view of the risk for development of disease following HCMV infection. This has been well documented in premature babies, in whom HCMV is an important cause of morbidity and mortality (12).

Intrauterine HCMV infection may lead to severe fetal damage and represents the commonest cause of symptomatic congenital infection in the UK. In populations with a high prevalence of seropositivity, fetal infection is usually due to maternal reactivation. In low-prevalence populations, primary infection is more common and is more likely to lead to symptoms in the offspring (13). These include mental retardation, chorioretinitis and deafness.

Infection acquired perinatally or in infancy does not usually give rise to symptoms. However, HCMV is one of the commonest agents causing infantile atypical pneumonia. In later life, primary infection in the immunocompetent may lead to a self-limiting mononucleosis-type syndrome.

It is among those individuals with a compromised immune system, however, that HCMV infection causes major morbidity and mortality, and in whom antiviral therapy is usually indicated. A variety of HCMV-related diseases has been documented, including debilitating pyrexial illness, pneumonitis, gastrointestinal disease (colitis, oesophagitis, hepatitis, pancreatitis), retinitis, myelitis, encephalitis and polyradiculopathy, although HCMV has also been isolated from many other organs in the body (14). A discussion of the patterns of HCMV disease suffered and risk factors for development of disease is best approached by grouping immunocompromised individuals according to their underlying clinical condition.

RECIPIENTS OF SOLID ORGAN TRANSPLANTS

Kidney, liver, heart and heart/lung transplantation are now well-established procedures. However, HCMV disease remains a major cause of morbidity and mortality in such recipients. Of interest is the apparent predilection of HCMV for the transplanted organs, so that HCMV hepatitis and pneumonitis are particularly common in liver and lung recipients, respectively (15,16). Since this group of patients receive immunosuppressive therapy for a limited period, chronic complications of HCMV infection such as retinitis are rare. The use of high-dose steroids and specific anti-T cell drugs, such as anti-thymocyte globulin (ATG) and OKT3, is associated with an increased risk of HCMV reactivation (17), and reduction in dosage of immunosuppression is often a useful adjunct to specific antiviral therapy for the management of severe HCMV disease. In liver and heart transplant recipients, the perioperative blood demands are often high and transfusion volume has been associated with subsequent HCMV infection (18). In the UK, it is often difficult to guarantee a large supply of HCMV-seronegative blood from the Blood Transfusion Service, and filtration of blood may be required to minimize this risk (19). Perhaps the most important risk factor for post-transplant infection and disease is the receipt of an organ from a HCMV-seropositive donor. Although primary infection (donor seropositive, recipient seronegative) is most likely to give rise to symptoms, seropositive recipients of seropositive kidneys have been shown to develop disease due to reinfection from the donor, rather than reactivation of endogenous virus (20).

BONE MARROW TRANSPLANT RECIPIENTS

In contrast to solid organ transplant recipients, reactivation accounts for the bulk of HCMV infection and disease in those receiving bone marrow transplants. HCMV pneumonitis is a particular problem between the first and third post-transplant months in this group of individuals, especially in recipients of allografts, compared to autografts and syngeneic grafts. Pretransplant lung irradiation may increase the susceptibility of this organ to disease (21). Collection of T cell-depleted marrow from seropositive donors has been shown to lessen the severity of post-transplant pneumonitis (22), possibly due to an enhanced adoptive transfer of immunity against HCMV from HCMV-seropositive donors (23). If the marrow is not depleted of T cells, then it may transfer HCMV infection (24).

AIDS

Since HIV infection produces a relentless decline in immune function over a long period of time, the pattern of HCMV disease observed is different from that described for individuals in whom profound immunosuppression occurs for a limited time period. HCMV retinitis and colitis are common in those with low CD4 cell counts, and HCMV is often identified in post-mortem central nervous system (CNS) tissue, suggesting that at least a proportion of undiagnosed CNS-related symptoms may be attributable to this virus (13). On the other hand, pneumonitis is rare in AIDS patients, despite a high rate of HCMV recovery from bronchial washing samples (25,58) (see later). With the increased use of anti-retroviral drugs and prophylactic regimes against, for instance, *Pneumocystis carinii* pneumonia, it is likely that survival of these individuals will increase and new manifestations of HCMV infection may then become apparent. It is likely that infection in AIDS patients represents reactivation of endogenous virus, especially among homosexual men in whom the HCMV seroprevalence is high (10), although the possibility of exogenous reinfection has not been studied in detail.

CMV AS A COFACTOR FOR DISEASE PROGRESSION IN PATIENTS WITH HIV INFECTION

Following HIV infection, the range of incubation periods to the development of AIDS is remarkably variable (2–20 years or more). One possible explanation is that some patients harbour other virus(es), e.g. HCMV, human herpesvirus type 6 (HHV-6), which interact with HIV to drive the rate at which HIV causes AIDS.

It has been shown in a haemophilic cohort that those individuals with HCMV progressed to AIDS significantly faster than those without HCMV (26). In such studies, it is important that an AIDS diagnosis was not made as the basis of opportunistic disease due to HCMV. There are many possible interactions between HCMV and HIV at the molecular or cellular level, any one of which could explain the clinical findings described above (reviewed in reference 27). It will be important to study these in detail and identify potential inhibitors which could be subjected to controlled clinical trials. Recently, two placebo-controlled trials have reported significant reductions in mortality from high dose (800 mg q.d.s.) acyclovir prophylaxis (28,29).

OTHER CAUSES OF IMMUNOSUPPRESSION

HCMV infection and disease have been documented in cancer patients, and those receiving immunosuppressive therapy for both malignancy and autoimmune disease. Blood transfusion is common in leukaemics, and is a risk for primary infection in such individuals (30).

PATHOGENESIS OF HCMV DISEASE

It is evident that two different pathological processes are at play in the generation of HCMV-related disease. First, HCMV replication may produce a lytic infection, with subsequent tissue damage. In such instances, large amounts of virus can be detected at the site of disease. This is the case for gastrointestinal disease, CNS disease and chorioretinitis. It follows that treatment of such infections with GCV or foscarnet should limit the pathological process and produce clinical improvement. On the other hand, HCMV pneumonitis is thought to represent a host immune response to infection within the lung, rather than a lytic infection *per se*. (31). HCMV has the capacity to alter many aspects of host cell gene transcription, in addition to coding itself for homologues of HLA and G-binding proteins, and these factors may contribute to aberrant responses in infected cells. In addition, the presence of graft-versus-host disease increases the risk of post-transplant pneumonitis. In support of the hypothesis that host immune factors play a major role in the generation of this disease is the observation that HCMV isolated from lungs of AIDS patients with low CD4 cell counts ($< 100 \times 10^9/l$) is rarely associated with pathology (25,58).

DIAGNOSIS OF HCMV INFECTION

The availability of effective treatment of HCMV disease has heightened the requirement for rapid methods of HCMV diagnosis, which are both sensitive and specific. Serological methods of diagnosis in the immunocompromised host are unreliable since antibody responses to infection in this group of patients are often delayed or absent. Further, they are subject to interference by passively acquired immunoglobulin with transfusion of blood products.

Although conventional cell culture remains the 'gold standard' against which all other methods must be compared, a number of techniques based on monoclonal antibodies are now available for detecting virus in clinical samples within 24 h (32–34).

The polymerase chain reaction (PCR) promises to overshadow previous methodology, especially with regard to speed and sensitivity. The detection of viraemia by PCR has been shown to predict CMV disease in immunocompromised patients (35). It also has the potential for rapid quantification of virus in clinical samples which may be a more specific prognostic indicator for subsequent development of disease, or useful as an assessment of response to therapy (36).

Detection of viruses resistant to antiviral regimens will become important in the future. Culture-based methods are time consuming, whilst PCR potentially offers a more rapid approach once the molecular basis of drug resistance has been elucidated.

It is important to recognize that HCMV excretion in the immunocompromised is a common occurrence, especially from peripheral sites such as urine, and is not synonymous with disease. Diagnosis of disease requires, ideally, identification of virus from the tissue in question, in association with characteristic signs and symptoms. The only exception to this is HCMV retinitis, which is diagnosed purely on ophthalmological examination.

Surveillance cultures may be used at regular intervals in high-risk individuals. A typical protocol involves weekly sampling for virus excretion, from multiple sites, during the period in which HCMV disease is most likely to occur. Critical assessments of this approach, using rapid monoclonal antibody-based diagnostic methods, have concluded that, in renal, liver and bone marrow recipients, and in AIDS patients, HCMV viraemia is highly predictive of subsequent development of disease (relative risk 7.0), compared with virus detection in urine or saliva (37,38).

TREATMENT STRATEGIES

Given the natural history, pathogenesis and diagnosis of HCMV in immunocompromised patients described above, several potential strategies for the use of antiviral drugs can be envisaged. In the tables, we present details of all the placebo-controlled randomized trials using virological diagnosis which have been conducted to date. In the text, we will refer to some other trials which, although not placebo controlled, randomized some patients to receive no treatment.

PROPHYLAXIS

This strategy aims to reduce HCMV replication and/or dissemination to levels below which disease is common. It recognizes that HCMV represents a major threat to particular groups of patients, so that administration of a drug to cover the most vulnerable periods could be justified. Since many patients will be treated who would not be destined to develop HCMV disease, this approach should only be considered where the drug is known to have no or minimal side-effects.

In transplant recipients, the greatest incidence of HCMV disease is in the second and third months post-transplantation. In the first interferon (IFN) trial, prophylaxis was given from the time of transplantation until six weeks later (39). The results suggested that prophylaxis delayed the appearance of HCMV infection so that longer therapy may be required. In later trials, IFN, ACV and immunoglobulin were given for 11–14 weeks (see Table 9.1) (40–43), with better evidence of disease control. GCV reduced the incidence of CMV disease in heart transplant patients (44). However, in bone marrow

Table 9.1. Placebo-controlled trials of prophylaxis for CMV infection and disease

Patient group	Study drug	Dose	Planned duration of therapy (weeks)	Number of patients		Markers of efficacy				Ref.
				Placebo	Drug	Reduced viraemia	Delayed excretion	Reduced disease	Increased survival	
RT_x	IFN	3×10^6 U 2/w	6	20	21	+	+	–	–	39
RT_x	IFN	3×10^6 U 3/w 6 w 3×10^6 U 2/w 8 w	14	22	20	–	+	+	–	40
RT_x	IFN	3×10^6 U 3/w 6 w 3×10^6 U 2/w 8 w	14	36	32	–	+	–	–	41
RT_x	ACV	800–3200 mg/day	12	51	53	+	+	+	–	42
RT_x with rejection	Ig	100 mg/kg	15	16	11	–	–	–	+	43
HT_x	GCV	5 mg/kg b.d. 14 d 6 mg/kg o.d. 5/7 d	4	73	76	–	+	+	–	44
BMT_x with rejection	GCV	2.5 mg/kg t.d.s. days –7 to –1 then 6 mg/kg 5 d/week after engraftment	Median 13.5	45	40	–	+	–	–	45
BMT_x	GCV	After engraftment 5 mg/kg b.d. 5 d, then o.d.	Median 10.9	31	33	–	+	+	–	46
BMT_x	GCV	500 mg/m^2 t.d.s. 1 m then 800 mg q.d.s. 6 m or placebo Third arm: 200–400 mg 1 m then placebo	30	105	102	+	+	+	+	48

IFN = interferon α; ACV = acyclovir; Ig = immunoglobulin; GCV = ganciclovir; RT_x = renal transplant; HT_x = heart transplant; BMT_x = bone marrow transplant.

recipients, treatment was associated with significant toxicity and did not affect overall mortality, despite controlling CMV disease (45,46). The results to date therefore show that IFN, ACV and GCV provide some control of HCMV disease when given prophylactically (47). The effect of immunoglobulin is controversial, with only some studies reporting clinical benefit and others virological responses (49,50).

One study suggests that recombinant IFN-α2C may precipitate graft rejection in renal allograft patients (51). Such an effect has not been seen in the studies cited in Table 9.1, which used 'natural' IFN preparations.

Two ACV prophylaxis trials have been published in patients with HIV infection and no effect on CMV disease was seen (28,29).

SUPPRESSION

This strategy aims to give an antiviral drug only to those who have HCMV infection, as detected by surveillance cultures of urine or saliva, in the hope of reducing the development of HCMV disease. This approach should be considered carefully with a drug which is toxic and/or not orally bioavailable and/or expensive, so that it is not used in those without active infection.

The sensitivity of this approach obviously depends on the laboratory assays available for diagnosis. As described earlier, rapid methods using monoclonal antibodies do not detect all individuals at risk of future disease and those detected have a relative risk of disease of only 2. Nevertheless, one GCV trial has so far been conducted (see Table 9.2) (52), although it also encompassed the concept of pre-emptive therapy, as discussed below.

PRE-EMPTIVE THERAPY

This strategy aims to identify patients with HCMV infection disseminated in the bloodstream or which has already reached a target organ such as the lung.

Pre-emptive therapy of HCMV pneumonitis is predicated upon the immunopathological pathogenesis of this condition, as described earlier. The aim is to decrease HCMV replication in the lung so that cells are not rendered susceptible to immune attack. The time required to initiate the immunopathological response may be sufficient to allow effective therapeutic intervention. To date, one study suggests that performing bronchial lavage at day 35 post bone marrow transplantation can identify individuals with HCMV lung *infection* who have not yet developed HCMV *disease* and who have a decreased risk of pneumonitis if given GCV (53).

Table 9.2. Placebo-controlled trial of HCMV suppression

				Number of patients			Markers of efficacy			
Patient group	Study drug	Dose	Duration of therapy	Placebo	Drug	Indication for trial entry	Suppress excretion	Reduced disease	Increased survival	Ref.
BMT_x	GCV	5 mg/kg b.d. 7 d then 5 mg/kg o.d.	100 d	35	37	HCMV at any site	+	+	+	52

GCV = ganciclovir; BMT_x = bone marrow transplant.

TREATMENT OF ESTABLISHED DISEASE

This was the first strategy to be employed and dates from the era when available antiviral drugs were considered to be so highly toxic that their use would be justified only in people with established life-threatening disease.

In general, the treatment of disease rather than its prevention or curtailment has a major theoretical disadvantage in that tissue damage must have occurred following virus replication to allow disease to present and that further damage will occur while diagnostic investigations are performed. The best antiviral agent can only be expected to stop virus replication; it cannot directly cause tissue repair. In the specific case of HCMV pneumonitis, there is another disadvantage since, as discussed above, this condition has a significant immunopathological component so that removal of the viral 'trigger' for this response may not necessarily produce clinical benefit. Thus, a series of open clinical trials of various antiviral agents (including GCV) showed no evidence of improved survival in bone marrow transplant patients with HCMV pneumonitis, although serial lung biopsies often showed reduction in titres of HCMV within the lung (reviewed in reference 54).

There are no controlled trials of antiviral therapy in HCMV pneumonitis, but the results of two further open studies suggest that the combination of high-dose i.v. immunoglobulin with GCV reduces mortality in bone marrow transplant patients (54,55). Presumably, the immunoglobulin has immunomodulatory effects on the immunopathological response against HCMV-infected cells, whilst the GCV decreases the chances that neighbouring cells will become targets for the aberrant immune response.

Only two placebo-controlled trials of treatment of established HCMV disease have been published to date (see Table 9.3). One showed that GCV reduced HCMV excretion in bone marrow transplant patients but had no discernible clinical benefit (57). It is possible that this disappointing outcome resulted from the short duration of therapy. A 14-day induction course followed by maintenance GCV AIDS patients (59) did not reduce CMV disease by the primary endpoint assessment but did so on a subsidiary analysis.

CURRENTLY RECOMMENDED THERAPY

Depending upon the types of patients and the body site involved, it is possible to describe the therapy which is currently recommended for HCMV (see Table 9.4). Several points should be noted.

Although the open trials of the combination of immunoglobulin and GCV have so far involved bone marrow transplant patients only, this combination is recommended for all allograft patients. However, it is not appropriate for AIDS patients, who appear to be unable to mount the immuno-

Table 9.3. Controlled trials of therapy for CMV disease

Patient group	Organ affected	Drug 1	Drug 2	Planned duration of therapy (days)	Number of patients		Significant markers of efficacy reported					Ref.
					Drug 1	Drug 2	Reduced viraemia	Reduced excretion	Reduced disease	Reduced dissemination	Increased survival	
BMT_x	Upper GIT	GCV 2.5 mg/kg t.d.s.	Placebo	14	18	19	–	+	–	–	–	56
AIDS	Lower GIT	GCV 5 mg/kg b.d. 14 d then o.d.	Placebo	14	32	30	–	+	–	+	–	57
AIDS	Retina	GCV 5 mg/kg b.d. 14 d then o.d.	Fos. 60 mg/kg t.d.s. 14 d then maintenance 90 mg/kg o.d.	14	127	107	ND	ND	–	–	+	58

GCV = ganciclovir; Fos. = foscarnet; BMT_x = bone marrow transplant; GIT = gastrointestinal tract; ND = not determined.

Table 9.4. Suggested treatment of HCMV (1994)

	Patient group	
Site infected	Transplant	AIDS
Urine or saliva	None	None
Blood	GCV	GCV?
Lung	Ig + GCV	None
Retina	GCV	Fos. + maint.
GIT	GCV	GCV

GCV = ganciclovir; Ig = normal immunoglobulin; Fos. = foscarnet; maint. = maintenance therapy; GIT = gastrointestinal tract.

pathological response required to develop HCMV pneumonitis. One exception to this may be in patients who develop HIV seroconversion disease in whom HCMV pneumonitis may occur (58).

Allograft patients with HCMV retinitis who respond to treatment usually do not have recurrences. In contrast, AIDS patients with HCMV retinitis are at high risk of recurrence and so require maintenance therapy. A recent controlled trial has shown that GCV and foscarnet are equally effective at suppressing HCMV retinitis but that the latter is associated with significantly improved survival (59). This result is unexplained but may be related to the ability of foscarnet to inhibit the reverse transcriptase enzyme of HIV, or may be related to inhibition of a cofactor effect of HCMV in HIV-positive patients. Thus, for HCMV retinitis, foscarnet is recommended for first-line therapy in AIDS patients, whereas GCV is recommended in transplant patients.

POTENTIAL PROBLEMS WITH HCMV CHEMOTHERAPY STRATEGIES

Use of an antiviral agent active against viruses other than HCMV has the potential disadvantage of allowing the selection of cross-resistant virus populations. For example, ACV prophylaxis for HCMV could potentially allow an increase in HSV resistance to this drug. Although this is only a theoretical possibility, all trials should monitor for cross-resistance.

It should also be anticipated that prophylaxis will decrease the quantity of HCMV detectable in clinical samples, either because of reduced replication *in vivo* or because the drug (such as ACV) is excreted into clinical samples and so is present in the inoculum used for cell cultures. It follows that the sensitivity of diagnostic assays must be monitored prospectively as different policies of chemotherapy/prophylaxis are introduced.

Finally, individual trials report the efficacy of their approach in the patients selected for the study, without necessarily relating the study to the whole population at risk. For example, the trial of pre-emptive therapy following bronchial lavage at day 35 post bone marrow transplantation (53) reported that GCV was 93% effective at reducing disease attributable to HCMV because 15 cases occurred in placebo recipients, compared with one cases among drug recipients, by day 100. Yet, the 72 patients in this study came from a total population of 281, with 65 expected cases of HCMV disease by day 180, nine of which were prevented by GCV. Thus, the overall efficacy can be calculated to be 9/65 = 14%. Whilst acknowledging the contribution made by this important paper, the overall impact of any therapeutic strategy should be calculated.

It can be concluded that each treatment strategy will have something to offer, and that the best overall control of HCMV disease will probably come from the combined use of more than one approach. As described above, interactions between each approach and with diagnostic assays are to be expected, so future trials must provide full details and keep all other aspects constant, except the drug under study.

DRUG RESISTANCE

The increasing use of GCV and foscarnet in recent years has been accompanied by reports of drug-resistant HCMV isolates (60–62), mirroring the experience with other antiviral agents. Many of these isolates have been associated with both clinical and *in vitro* resistance. The possible molecular sites of resistance have been discussed previously.

We currently recommend that a switch to foscarnet therapy be considered where clinical resistance of HCMV disease to GCV is suspected and vice versa. Synergism exists between GCV and foscarnet *in vitro*, as would be expected from their different sites of antiviral action. However, any potential benefit to be obtained with concurrent therapy (63) must be balanced against the possibility of generating strains resistant to both agents, as has been demonstrated in a bone marrow transplant recipient (64).

FUTURE PROSPECTS

Given the importance of controlling HCMV disease in immunocompromised patients, the requirement for safe, effective antiviral agents is paramount. As yet, the antiviral agents available do not meet these criteria. The recognition of HCMV as a serious pathogen in these patients should stimulate further research into new nucleoside analogues with better bioavailability and therapeutic ratios, and the synthesis of phosphate ester derivatives which overcome the necessity for primary phosphorylation, as is discussed elsewhere. In all these cases, new agents *must* be evaluated in controlled, double-blind clinical trials, and the appearance of viruses resistant to the antiviral agent closely monitored. Presuming some of the lead compounds currently available will prove worthy of continued investigation, it can be hoped that we may possess an anti-HCMV drug that is as clinically useful and as safe as is ACV for HSV within the foreseeable future.

REFERENCES

1. Huang, E.-S. (1975). Human cytomegalovirus. III. Virus-induced DNA polymerase. *J. Virol.*, **16**, 298–310.
2. Nishiyama, Y., Maeno, K. and Yoshida, S. (1983). Characterization of human cytomegalovirus-induced DNA polymerase and the associated 3′-to-5′, exonuclease. *Virology*, **124**, 221–231.
3. Heilbronn, R., Jahn, G., Burkle, A. *et al.* (1987). Genomic localization, sequence analysis, and transcription of the putative human cytomegalovirus DNA polymerase gene. *J. Virol.*, **61**, 119–124.
4. Biron, K. K. (1991). GCV-resistant human CMV clinical isolates: resistance mechanisms and in vitro susceptibility to antiviral agents. *Transplant. Proc.*, **23** (3, Suppl. 3), 162–167.
5. Littler, E., Stuart, A. D. and Chee, M. S. (1992). Human cytomegalovirus *UL97* open reading frame encodes a protein that phosphorylates the antiviral nucleoside analogue ganciclovir. *Nature*, **358**, 160–162.
6. Sullivan, V., Talarico, C. L., Stanat, S. C. *et al.* (1992). A protein kinase homologue controls phosphorylation of ganciclovir in human cytomegalovirus-infected cells. *Nature*, **358**, 162–164.
7. Mar, E. C., Chiou, J. F., Cheng, Y. C. and Huang, E. S. (1985). Inhibition of cellular DNA polymerase alpha and human cytomegalovirus-induced DNA polymerase by the triphosphates of 9-(2-hydroxyethoxymethyl)guanine and 9-(1,3-dihydroxy-2-propoxymethyl)guanine. *J. Virol.*, **53**, 776–780.
8. Cantrill, H. L., Henry, K., Melroe, N. H. *et al.* (1989). Treatment of cytomegalovirus retinitis with intravitreal ganciclovir: long-term results. *Ophthalmology*, **96**, 367–374.
9. Balfour, H. H. J. (1990). Management of cytomegalovirus disease with antiviral drugs. *Rev. Infect. Dis.*, 12 (Suppl. 7), S849–S860.
10. Berry, N. J., Burns, D. M., Wannamethee, G. *et al.* (1988). Seroepidemiologic studies on the acquisition of antibodies to cytomegalovirus, herpes simplex virus, and human immunodeficiency virus among general hospital patients and those attending a clinic for sexually transmitted diseases. *J. Med. Virol.*, **24**, 385–393.
11. Pass, R. F., Little, E. A., Stagno, S. *et al.* (1987). Young children as a probable source of maternal and congenital cytomegalovirus infection. *N. Engl. J. Med.*, **316**, 1366–1370.
12. Yeager, A. S., Grumet, F. C., Hafleigh, E. B. *et al.* (1981). Prevention of transfusion-acquired cytomegalovirus infections in newborn infants. *J. Pediatr.*, **98**, 281–287.
13. Fowler, K. B., Stagno, S., Pass, R. F. *et al.* (1992). The outcome of congenital cytomegalovirus infection in relation to maternal antibody status. *N. Engl. J. Med.*, **326**, 663–667.
14. Pillay, D., Lipman, M. C., Lee, C. A. *et al.* (1993). A clinico-pathological audit of opportunistic viral infections in HIV-infected patients. *AIDS*, **7**, 969–974.
15. Bronsther, O., Makowka, L., Jaffe, R. *et al.* (1988). Occurrence of cytomegalovirus hepatitis in liver transplant patients. *J. Med. Virol.*, **24**, 423–434.

16. Bailey, T. C., Trulock, E. P., Ettinger, N. A. *et al.* (1992). Failure of prophylactic ganciclovir to prevent cytomegalovirus disease in recipients of lung transplants. *J. Infect. Dis.*, **165**, 548–552.
17. Singh, N., Dummer, J. S., Kusne, S. *et al.* (1988). Infections with cytomegalovirus and other herpesviruses in 121 liver transplant recipients: transmission by donated organ and the effect of OKT3 antibodies. *J. Infect. Dis.*, **158**, 124–131.
18. Pillay, D., Charman, H., Burroughs, A. K. *et al.* (1992). Surveillance for CMV infection in orthotopic liver transplant recipients. *Transplantation*, **53**, 1261–1265.
19. Gilbert, G. L., Hayes, K., Hudson, I. L. and James, J. (1989). Prevention of transfusion-acquired cytomegalovirus infection in infants by blood filtration to remove leucocytes. Neonatal Cytomegalovirus Infection Study Group. *Lancet*, **i**, 1228–1231.
20. Grundy, J. E., Lui, S. F., Super, M. *et al.* (1988). Symptomatic cytomegalovirus infection in seropositive kidney recipients: reinfection with donor virus rather than reactivation of recipient virus. *Lancet*, **ii**, 132–135.
21. Zaia, J. A. (1990). Viral infections associated with bone marrow transplantation. *Hematol. Oncol. Clin. North Am.*, **4**, 603–623.
22. Grob, J. P., Grundy, J. E., Prentice, H. G. *et al.* (1987). Immune donors can protect marrow-transplant recipients from severe cytomegalovirus infections. *Lancet*, **i**, 774–776.
23. Wimperis, J. Z., Brenner, M. K., Prentice, H. G. *et al.* (1986). Transfer of a functioning humoral immune system in transplantation of T-lymphocyte-depleted bone marrow. *Lancet*, **i**, 339–343.
24. Meyers, J. D. (1989). Prevention of cytomegalovirus infection after marrow transplantation. *Rev. Infect. Dis.*, **11** (Suppl. 7), S1691–S1705.
25. Bozzette, S. A., Arcia, J., Bartok, A. E. *et al.* (1992). Impact of Pneumocystis carinii and cytomegalovirus on the course and outcome of atypical pneumonia in advanced human immunodeficiency virus disease. *J. Infect. Dis.*, **165**, 93–98.
26. Webster, A., Cook, D. G., Emery, V. C. *et al.* (1989). Cytomegalovirus infection and progression towards AIDS in haemophiliacs with human immunodeficiency virus infection. *Lancet*, **ii**, 63–66.
27. Webster, A. (1992). Viral cofactors in acquired immune deficiency syndrome. *Rev. Med. Virol.*, **2**, 29–34.
28. Cooper, D. A., Pehrson, P. O., Pederson, C. *et al.* (1993). The efficacy and safety of zidovudine alone or as aotherapy with acyclovir for the treatment of patients with AIDS and AIDS-related complex. *AIDS*, **7**, 197–207.
29. Youli, M. S., Gozzard, B. G., Johnson, M. A. *et al.* (1994). Effects of high dose oral acyclovir on herpesvirus disease and survival in patients with advanced HIV disease: a double-blind, placebo-controlled study. *AIDS*, **8**, 641–649.
30. Murphy, M. F., Grint, P. C., Hardiman, A. E. *et al.* (1988). Use of leucocyte-poor blood components to prevent primary cytomegalovirus (CMV) infection in patients with acute leukaemia. *Br. J. Haematol.*, **70**, 253–254.
31. Grundy, J. E., Shanley, J. D. and Griffiths, P. D. (1987). Is cytomegalovirus interstitial pneumonitis in transplant recipients an immunopathological condition? *Lancet*, **ii**, 996–999.
32. Griffiths, P. D., Panjwani, D. D., Stirk, P. R. *et al.* (1984). Rapid diagnosis of cytomegalovirus infection in immunocompromised patients by detection of early antigen fluorescent foci. *Lancet*, **ii**, 1242–1245.
33. Gleaves, C. A., Smith, T. F., Shuster, E. A. and Pearson, G. R. (1984). Rapid detection of cytomegalovirus in MRC-5 cells inoculated with urine specimens by using low-speed centrifugation and monoclonal antibody to an early antigen. *J. Clin. Microbiol.*, **19**, 917–919.

34. van-der-Bij, W., Torensma, R., van-Son, W. J. *et al.* (1988). Rapid immunodiagnosis of active cytomegalovirus infection by monoclonal antibody staining of blood leucocytes. *J. Med. Virol.*, **25**, 179–188.
35. Kidd, I. M., Fox, J. C., Pillay, D. *et al.* (1993). Routine application of the polymerase chain reaction for cytomegalovirus provides prognostic information in immunocompromised patients. *Transplantation*, in press.
36. Fox, J. C., Griffiths, P. D. and Emery, V. C. (1992). Quantification of human cytomegalovirus DNA using the polymerase chain reaction. *J. Gen. Virol.*, **73**, 2405–2408.
37. Meyers, J. D., Ljungman, P. and Fisher, L. D. (1990). Cytomegalovirus excretion as a predictor of cytomegalovirus disease after marrow transplantation: importance of cytomegalovirus viremia. *J. Infect. Dis.*, **162**, 373–380.
38. Webster, A., Blizzard, B., Pillay, D. *et al.* (1993). The value of routine surveillance cultures for detection of CMV pneumonitis following bone marrow transplantation. *Bone Marrow Transplant.*, in press.
39. Cheeseman, S. H., Rubin, R. H., Stewart, J. A. *et al.* (1979). Controlled clinical trial of prophylactic human-leukocyte interferon in renal transplantation: effects on cytomegalovirus and herpes simplex virus infections. *N. Engl. J. Med.*, **300**, 1345–1349.
40. Hirsch, M. S., Schooley, R. T., Cosimi, A. B. *et al.* (1983). Effects of interferon-alpha on cytomegalovirus reactivation syndromes in renal-transplant recipients. *N. Engl. J. Med.*, **308**, 1489–1493.
41. Lui, S. F., Ali, A. A., Fernando, O. N. *et al.* (1992). Double-blind placebo-controlled trial of human lymphoblastoid interferon prophylaxis of cytomegalovirus infection in renal transplant recipients. *Nephrol. Dial. Transplant.*, in press.
42. Balfour, H. H. J., Chace, B. A., Stapleton, J. T. *et al.* (1989). A randomized, placebo-controlled trial of oral acyclovir for the prevention of cytomegalovirus disease in recipients of renal allografts. *N. Engl. J. Med.*, **320**, 1381–1387.
43. Metselaar, H. J., Rothbarth, P. H., Brouwer, R. M. *et al.* (1989). Prevention of cytomegalovirus-related death by passive immunization: a double-blind placebo-controlled study in kidney transplant recipients treated for rejection. *Transplantation*, **48**, 264–266.
44. Merigan, T. C., Renlund, D. G., Keay, S. *et al.* (1992). A controlled trial of ganciclovir to prevent cytomegalovirus disease after heart transplantation. *N. Engl. J. Med.*, **326**, 1182–1186.
45. Winston, D. J., Ho, W. G., Bartoni, K. *et al.* (1993). Ganciclovir prophylaxis of cytomegalovirus infection and disease in allogeneic bone marrow transplant recipients: results of a placebo-controlled, double-blind trial. *Ann. Intern. Med.*, **118**, 179–184.
46. Goodrich, J. M., Bowden, R. A., Fisher, L. *et al.* (1993). Ganciclovir prophylaxis to prevent cytomegalovirus disease after allogeneic marrow transplant. *Ann. Intern. Med.*, **118**, 173–178.
47. Meyers, J. D., Reed, E. C., Shepp, D. H. *et al.* (1988). Acyclovir for prevention of cytomegalovirus infection and disease after allogeneic marrow transplantation. *N. Engl. J. Med.*, **318**, 70–75.
48. Prentice, H. G., Gluckman, E., Powles, R. L. *et al.* (1994). Impact of long-term acyclovir on cytomegalovirus infection and survival after allogeneic bone marrow transplantation. *Lancet*, **343**, 749–753.
49. Snydman, D. R., Werner, B. G., Heinze-Lacey, B. *et al.* (1987). Use of cytomegalovirus immune globulin to prevent cytomegalovirus disease in renal-transplant recipients. *N. Engl. J. Med.*, **317**, 1049–1054.
50. Bowden, R. A., Fisher, L. D., Rogers, K. *et al.* (1991). Cytomegalovirus (CMV)-

specific intravenous immunoglobulin for the prevention of primary CMV infection and disease after marrow transplant. *J. Infect. Dis.*, **164**, 483–487.
51. Kovarik, J., Mayer, G., Pohanka, E. *et al.* (1988). Adverse effect of low-dose prophylactic human recombinant leukocyte interferon-alpha treatment in renal transplant recipients: cytomegalovirus infection prophylaxis leading to an increased incidence of irreversible rejections. *Transplantation*, **45**, 402–405.
52. Goodrich, J. M., Mori, M., Gleaves, C. A. *et al.* (1991). Early treatment with ganciclovir to prevent cytomegalovirus disease after allogeneic bone marrow transplantation. *N. Engl. J. Med.*, **325**, 1601–1607.
53. Schmidt, G. M., Horak, D. A., Niland, J. C. *et al.* (1991). A randomized, controlled trial of prophylactic ganciclovir for cytomegalovirus pulmonary infection in recipients of allogeneic bone marrow transplants. *N. Engl. J. Med.*, **324**, 1005–1011.
54. Reed, E. C., Bowden, R. A., Dandliker, P. S. *et al.* (1988). Treatment of cytomegalovirus pneumonia with ganciclovir and intravenous cytomegalovirus immunoglobulin in patients with bone marrow transplants. *Ann. Intern. Med.*, **109**, 783–788.
55. Emanuel, D., Cunningham, I., Jules-Elysee, K. *et al.* (1988). Cytomegalovirus pneumonia after bone marrow transplantation successfully treated with the combination of ganciclovir and high-dose intravenous immune globulin. *Ann. Intern. Med.*, **109**, 777–782.
56. Reed, E. C., Wolford, J. L., Kopecky, K. J. *et al.* (1990). Ganciclovir for the treatment of cytomegalovirus gastroenteritis in bone marrow transplant patients. A randomized, placebo-controlled trial. *Ann. Intern. Med.*, **112**, 505–510.
57. Dieterich, D. T., Kotler, D. P., Busch, D. F. *et al.* (1993). Ganciclovir treatment of cytomegalovirus colitis in AIDS: a randomised double-blind, placebo-controlled multicenter study. *J. Infect. Dis.*, **167**, 278–282.
58. Squire, S. B., Lipman, M. C. I., Bagdades, E. K. *et al.* (1992). Severe cytomegalovirus pneumonitis in HIV-infected patients with higher than average CD4 counts. *Thorax*, **47**, 301–304.
59. Studies of Ocular Complications of AIDS Research Group, in Collaboration with the AIDS Clinical Trials Group (1992). Mortality in patients with the acquired immunodeficiency syndrome treated with either foscarnet or ganciclovir for cytomegalovirus retinitis. *N. Engl. J. Med.*, **326**, 213–220.
60. Erice, Chou, S., Biron, K. K. *et al.* (1989). Progressive disease due to ganciclovir-resistant cytomegalovirus in immunocompromised patients. *N. Engl. J. Med.*, **320**, 289–293.
61. Drew, W. L., Miner, R. C., Busch, D. F. *et al.* (1991). Prevalence of resistance in patients receiving ganciclovir for serious cytomegalovirus infection. *J. Infect. Dis.*, **163**, 716–719.
62. Sullivan, V. and Coen, D. M. (1991). Isolation of foscarnet-resistant human cytomegalovirus patterns of resistance and sensitivity to other antiviral drugs. *J. Infect. Dis.*, **164**, 781–784.
63. Nelson, M. R., Barter, G., Hawkins, D. and Gazzard, B. G. (1991). Simultaneous treatment of cytomegalovirus retinitis with ganciclovir and foscarnet. *Lancet*, **338**, 250.
64. Knox, K. K., Drobyski, W. R. and Carrigan, D. R. (1991). Cytomegalovirus isolate resistant to ganciclovir and foscarnet from a marrow transplant patient. *Lancet*, **337**, 1292–1293.

Part C

RESPIRATORY VIRUSES

Basic Research

Clinical Treatment

10 Anti-picornaviral Agents

KOEN ANDRIES
Janssen Research Foundation, Beerse, Belgium

HISTORICAL PERSPECTIVE

The picornaviruses comprise one of the largest and most important families of human and animal pathogens. Enteroviruses such as poliovirus and human hepatitis A virus, and rhinoviruses, the single most important cause of the common cold, are all members of the picornavirus family. The diseases caused by picornaviruses range from life-threatening to mild and self-limiting. The important groups of enteroviruses, together with the infections attributed to them, are listed in reference 1. Because of their economic and medical importance, it is not surprising that the picornaviruses have been prominently involved in antiviral research. An almost complete picture (reviewed in reference 2) of their structure, molecular biology and replication has been constructed over the past twenty years. The targets in the replicative cycle of picornaviruses have been reviewed (2,3). The recent elucidation of the structures of prototype members of each of the four picornavirus genera to atomic detail, i.e. human rhinovirus (HRV) (4), human poliovirus (5), mengovirus (6) and foot and mouth disease virus (7), and the characterization of several receptors for picornaviral entry (8–11) have greatly enhanced the possible application of rational drug design and the development of protein-based inhibitors, such as soluble receptors, antireceptor antibodies, interferons and broad-spectrum antibodies. In this chapter, I will focus mainly on recently discovered synthetic antiviral agents.

THE SEARCH FOR ANTI-RHINOVIRAL DRUGS

STRATEGY TO FIND ACTIVE COMPOUNDS

Several approaches can be used to develop synthetic antiviral compounds. In the conventional medicinal chemical approach, a lead molecule is first identified by the screening of large series of possible candidates. Once a lead molecule has been identified, structure–activity relationships are investigated for a large series of related molecules, and chemists are able to

Antiviral Chemotherapy. Edited by D.J. Jeffries and E. De Clercq

synthesize compounds with improved activity profiles. The screening approach is considered not to be irrational, but to be rather empirical, if not serendipitous. Obviously, it is not an 'either–or' proposition and hence one can invoke the term rational serendipity or rational screening.

Rational drug design, defined as the directed synthesis of new compounds on the basis of an understanding of the interaction between a prototype drug and a structural or functional viral protein at the atomic level, has been made possible only in the past few years as a result of breakthroughs in the X-ray crystallography of animal viruses. Unfortunately, as of today no new anti-picornaviral drug has been developed by these modern techniques, but they have provided us with a better understanding of drug action, and enabled a more rational approach to drug modification. The problems that have to be tackled for the design of picornavirus capsid-binding compounds have been reviewed (12).

SELECTION OF REPRESENTATIVE SEROTYPES

One problem is particular to all anti-picornaviral agents. A multitude of serotypes must be inhibited by an agent before that agent is a potentially useful product clinically. The design or development of agents with maximal activity against one particular serotype does not necessarily result in activity against other serotypes (12,13). The choice of one or more particular test virus strains for either screening or rational drug design is therefore of paramount importance. This is especially true in the development of anti-rhinoviral compounds, because their antiviral activities often vary considerably according to the serotype tested.

The testing of a panel of 15 capsid-binding compounds belonging to structurally different chemical classes against all 100 typed rhinoviruses enabled the identification of two groups of rhinoviruses, designated antiviral group A and antiviral group B (or group A and group B rhinoviruses), with a differential susceptibility for capsid-binding compounds (14). Antiviral group B contains twice as many (67) serotypes as antiviral group A (33 serotypes) and consists of viruses having an above-average susceptibility to shorter capsid-binding compounds, whereas antiviral group A consists of viruses susceptible to structurally elongated antivirals (Figure 10.1).

The existence of two groups of rhinoviruses with contrasting susceptibilities for antivirals suggests that it is necessary to select at least one serotype from each antiviral group for the detection of a lead compound with weak but specific antiviral activity (13). Once a lead compound has been identified, it becomes increasingly important to discriminate between narrow-spectrum and broad-spectrum compounds. To this end, a panel of several rhinoviruses from each antiviral group has to be tested. We selected our own panel (Figure 10.2, Table 10.2) on the basis of the positions of the rhinoviruses within the spectral map derived from a multivariate analysis.

The calculation of a median IC_{50} from the IC_{50}s obtained for the serotypes of each antiviral group allows for a very simple but accurate comparison of a compound's potency and antiviral spectrum. When the panel of test viruses is carefully selected, the results obtained for the median antiviral inhibitory value will accurately predict the median value against 100 serotypes (13,15).

It is not yet known whether the proposed model is applicable to anti-rhinoviral compounds that do not share the same mechanism of action, i.e. binding to the hydrophobic pocket. However, as the antiviral grouping seems to be highly correlated to differences in amino acid sequences of several serotypes (14), it is possible that the model is indeed applicable to non-capsid-binding compounds as well. Additional studies using such compounds are needed to evaluate the potential of this approach. Similar studies, aimed to identify representative subsets of enterovirus serotypes, have not been reported.

TEST SYSTEMS

Most picornaviruses produce a distinct cytopathic effect (CPE) in either fibroblasts or certain HeLa cell lines. Fibroblasts may have the advantage of a more close resemblance to the natural host cell of some viruses, but HeLa cells are more convenient to use, particularly when many compounds have to be tested against many different serotypes.

The results obtained in HeLa cells are usually in accordance with results obtained with other cells, with the exception of 44081RP, a compound having cell-specific antiviral activity (see below). The nutritive status of the cells used can sometimes influence the development of enterovirus CPE (16).

The induction of a distinct CPE allows for a myriad of methods to be used for the assessment of the antiviral activity of compounds (reviewed in reference 17). Plaque methods and microscopic evaluation of microtitre plates have been gradually replaced by increasingly automated micromethods that allow for a computerized calculation of a drug's antiviral potency and cytotoxicity (15). The use of viral infectivity tests is preferable to the possible use of individual viral proteins (e.g. viral proteinase), as infectivity tests are designed to allow for several viral replicative cycles before the development of complete CPE, thus ensuring that an antiviral compound active at any of the possible steps of the replication will be detected.

Quantitative estimates of viral and toxic cytopathogenicity may be used to calculate the 50% inhibitory concentration *for a particular serotype*. The use of IC_{50} (or MIC) values is more appropriate than ID_{50} values, as the latter refer to the dose used in the test rather than to the antiviral concentration used. Similarly, CC_{50} values can be calculated to quantitate the 50% cytotoxic concentration of the same compound. The determination of the CC_{50} should preferably be performed with the same cells and the same conditions (e.g. incubation temperature) as the IC_{50} test. Toxicity should not be determined in already established cell monolayers, but in logarithmically growing cells (17). From the IC_{50} and the CC_{50} values, a selectivity index (a term preferable to 'therapeutic index', which should be reserved for *in vivo* studies), or SI, can be calculated for each individual serotype. Compounds with high selectivity indices may be less toxic for use in humans, although various side-effects such as organ-specific toxicity can of course not be predicted from the *in vitro* result.

The use of several serotypes to assess a compound's antiviral activity has

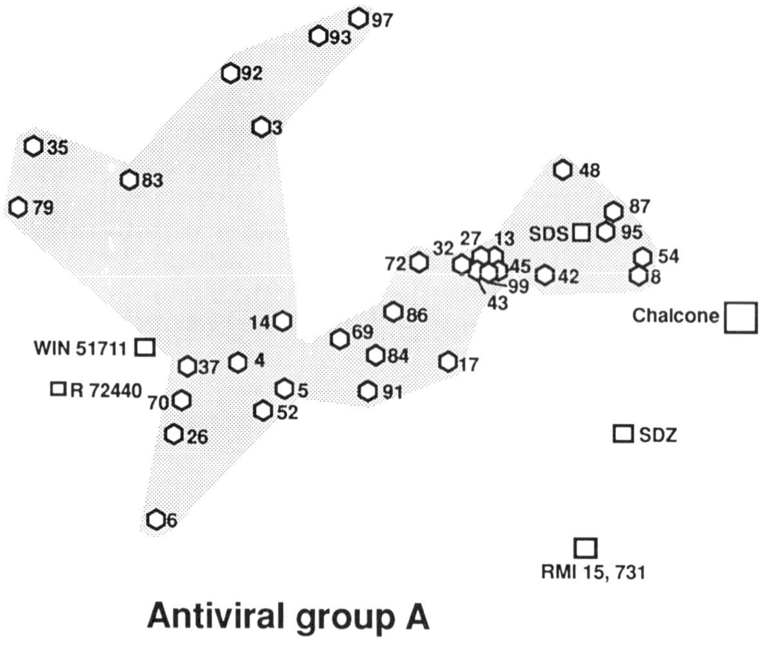

Figure 10.1. Spectral map obtained by multivariate analysis of antiviral tests. A panel of 15 capsid-binding compounds (for structures see reference 14) was tested against all rhinovirus serotypes. Hexagons represent serotypes; squares denote antiviral compounds. The positions of compounds are computed according to their specificities for the 100 rhinovirus serotypes, and irrespective of their potencies. (Potency is defined here as the median reciprocal IC_{50} of a compound against the various viruses). Viruses are located on the same map according to their specificities

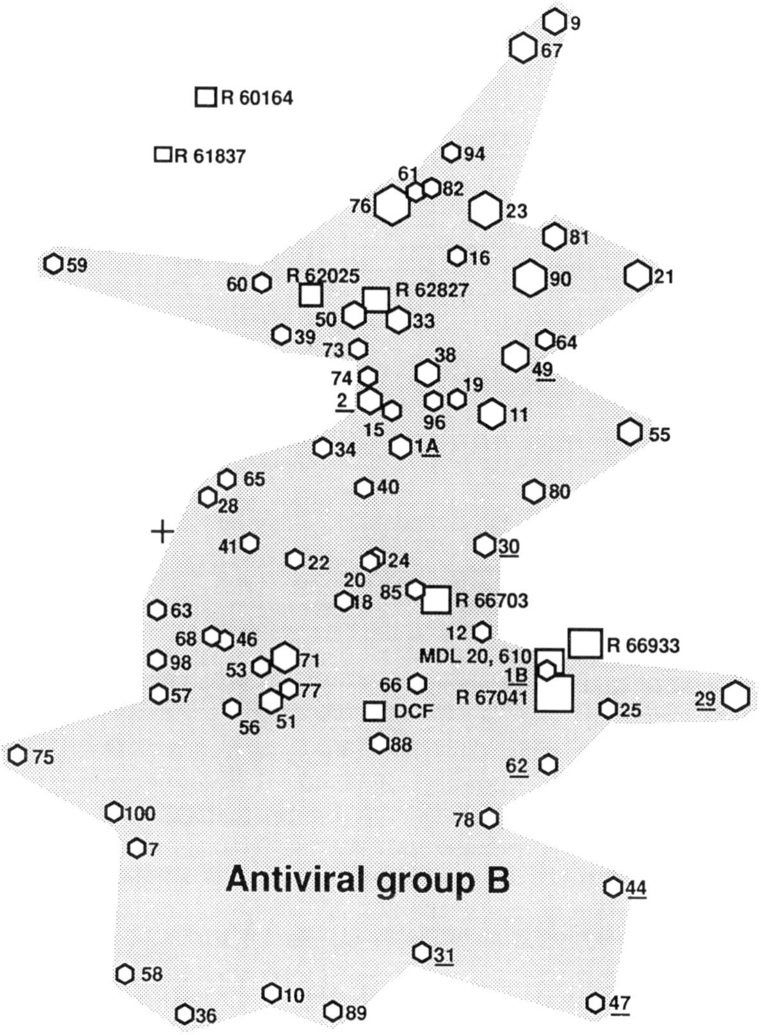

for the 15 compounds and irrespective of their sensitivities. (Sensitivity is defined here as the median reciprocal IC_{50} of a virus for the various compounds.) Median potencies of compounds and median sensitivities of serotypes are reflected by the sizes of hexagons and squares, respectively. The three-dimensional arrangement of compounds and serotypes has been rotated in order to show optimum separation of the two groups of serotypes (from Andries *et al.* (14); reproduced from the *Journal of Virology*, 1990, **64**: 1117–1123, by permission of the American Society for Microbiology)

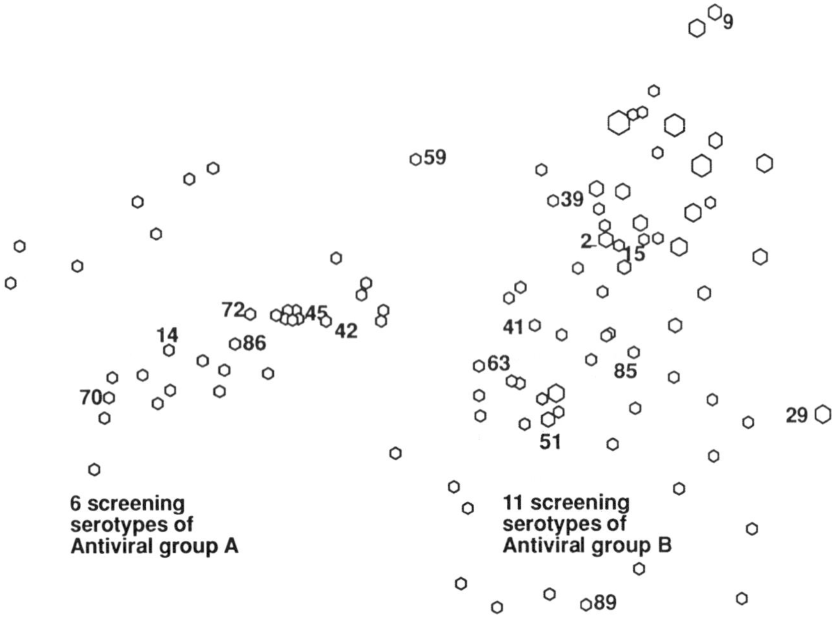

Figure 10.2. Panel of representative rhinovirus serotypes. Seventeen rhinovirus serotypes were selected from Figure 10.1. This set of serotypes was shown to be representative for all 100 (14), and was used to compare the potencies of anti-picornavirus agents (Table 10.2) (from Andries *et al.* (13); reproduced from *Antiviral Research*, **16**: 213–225, by permission of Elsevier Science Publishers BV)

the advantage that a specific antiviral activity of a lead compound can be more easily discriminated from aspecific cytotoxicity by a comparison of the selectivity indices obtained. Selectivity indices that are clearly different from serotype to serotype strongly indicate a specific antiviral effect.

The concentration effective in inhibiting a given percentage of serotypes tested is defined as the EC%, e.g. the EC_{50} and EC_{82} are the concentrations effective in inhibiting 50% and 82% *of the serotypes tested*, respectively. I will use the terms IC_{50}, CC_{50}, SI, EC_{50} and EC_{80} throughout this review.

MODE OF ACTION AND PHARMACOKINETICS

What are the preferential mode of action and pharmacokinetic profile of a potential anti-picornaviral agent?

If a drug is to be useful, it must act on the majority of serotypes and it is likely to do this if it acts on a target that is well conserved throughout rhinoviruses and enteroviruses. Although this preferential mode of action is very straightforward, it is very easy to jump to the wrong conclusions.

For instance, capsid-binding compounds affect capsid proteins which are clearly variable and they indeed generally affect serotypes to a very different extent. However, even very variable proteins may contain a few strongly conserved amino acids, and these may be sufficient to achieve broad-spectrum activity. The broad-spectrum activity of pirodavir (R 77975) was tentatively explained by its possible binding to two tyrosine residues within VP1, which seem to be conserved throughout several picornaviruses. Vice versa, if a molecule binds to the variable amino acids of a protein that bears 90% amino acid sequence homology with those of other serotypes, only a narrow spectrum will result. Generalizations concerning the preferential site of action are therefore difficult to draw.

The same reasoning goes for the preferential target of the viral replication cycle. Whether an antiviral agent acts at an early or a late stage makes little difference, since even inhibitors of an early stage, when administered in the middle of the cycle, will inhibit the replication of the virus at the start of the next cycle. The only small disadvantage of 'early' inhibitors is that it will take a few more hours before they will be able to completely arrest viral replication.

The reversibility of the antiviral effect might be the most important factor of all. Whether a drug is to be administered orally or topically, trough drug levels will be substantially lower than peak levels. If the trough level is a non-inhibitory concentration, and the interaction between the virus and the inhibitor is reversible, all inhibition will be lost. Viral replication can then resume if all elements essential for viral replication are still available. The necessity for an irreversible effect is especially high for drugs that are to be locally applied in the nose. The very short half-life for substances applied intranasally (approximately 20 min) (18) results in a difference between peak and trough concentrations that may amount to a factor of 4000 (2^{12}) for a drug that is applied every 4 h (12 half-lives).

The very rapid clearance of drugs from the nasal mucosa necessitates the administration of as many antiviral units as possible, preferably in an aqueous solution, as the drug has to penetrate the watery mucociliary layer that lies over the epithelial cells. This need for high concentrations in an aqueous solution is really a paradox, because most antivirals need to be hydrophobic in order to bind strongly to hydrophobic parts of viral proteins. The use of substituted cyclodextrins to resolve this dilemma (see discussion in reference 19) may be a significant advantage, but we may need to explore still better ways for delivering drugs to the affected mucosa.

Administration of antiviral compounds by the oral route may get round some of the problems. Upon oral administration, in a formulation that does not need to be an aqueous solution, a more constant amount of drug may reach the nasal mucosa. However, for at least some compounds the percentage of antiviral compound that reaches the nasal mucosa or mucosal cells is only a very small fraction of the total amount given orally, and this results in a greater risk of side-effects.

INHIBITORS OF VIRAL ENTRY

Rhodanine (**1**) (20) was probably the first of an impressive series of agents with selective anti-picornaviral properties, now commonly called the capsid-binding compounds: sodium dodecyl sulphate (SDS) (**2**) (21), S-7 (**3**) (22), RMI 15,731 (**4**) (23), arildone (**10**) (24), 4′,6-dichloroflavan (**5**) (25), chalcone (**8**) (26), phenoxypyridinecarbonitrile (**7**) (27), MDL 20,610 (**6**) (28), disoxaril or WIN 51711 (**11**) (29), R 61837 (**13**) (30), WIN 54954 (**12**) (31), isoflavans and isoflavenes (32), chalcone amides (**9**) (33), and R 77975 or pirodavir (**14**) (15). There is no doubt that more compounds will be added to this list in the near future. (Figures in bold refer to structural formulae below.)

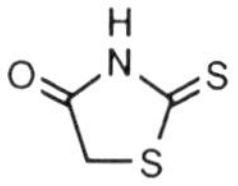

(1)

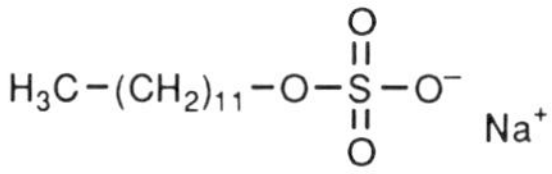

(2)

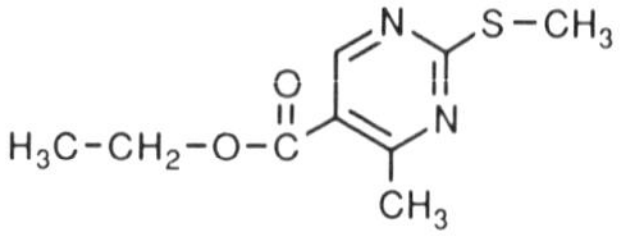

(3)

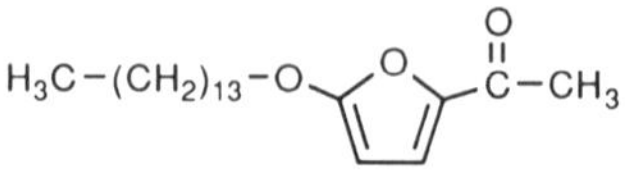

(4)

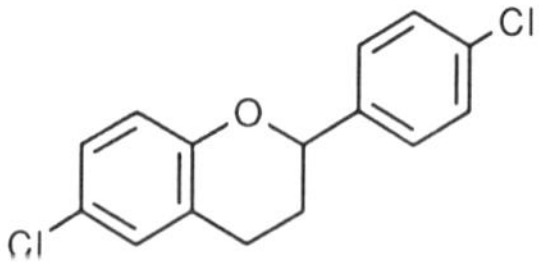

(5)

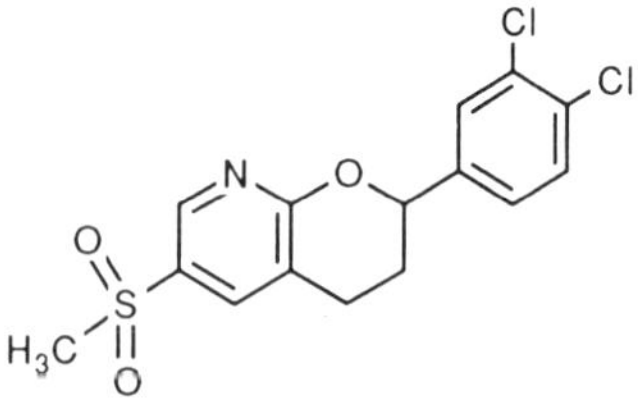

(6)

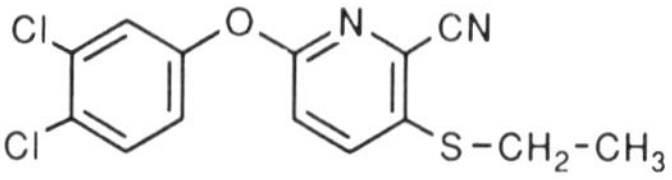

(7)

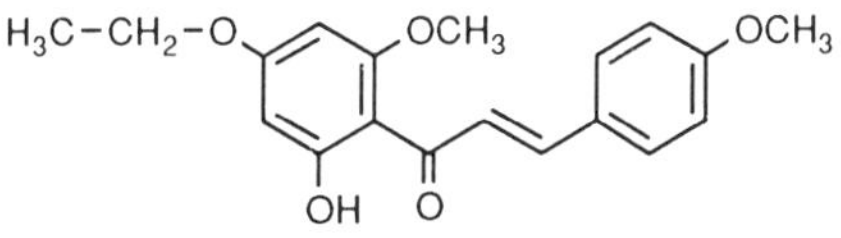

(8)

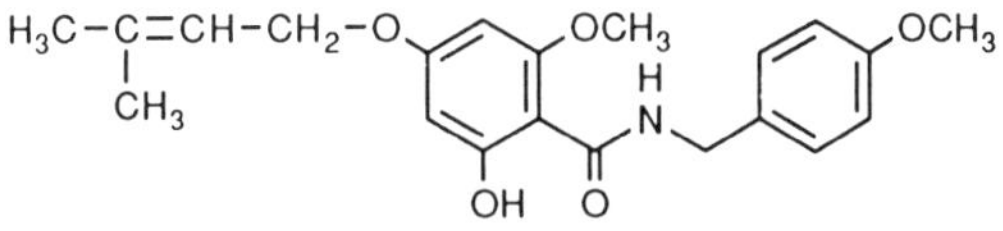

(9)

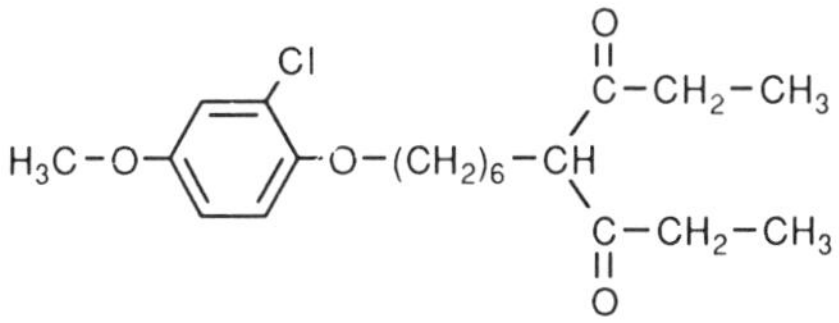

(10)

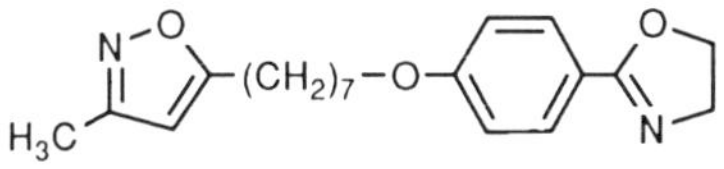

(11)

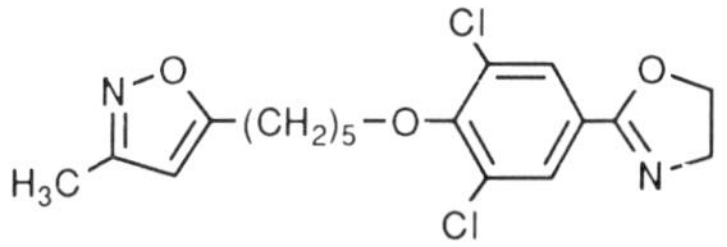

(12)

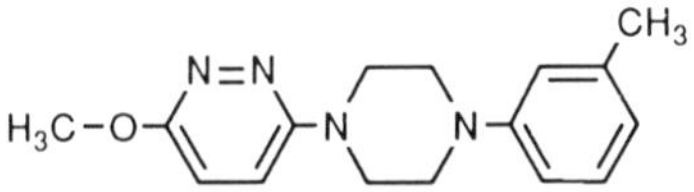

(13)

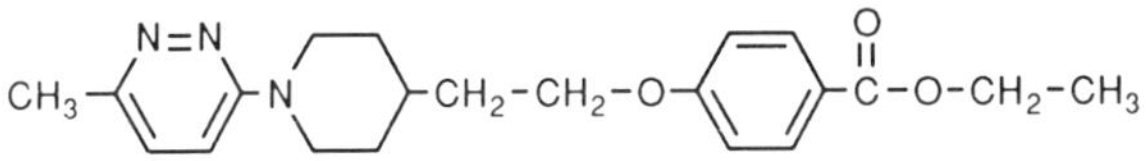

(14)

We will first review a few general properties of this group of compounds, before embarking on the specific discussion of each compound's antiviral spectrum and specific properties.

BINDING SITE

Capsid-binding compounds probably all bind to the same site on the virion since they are all affected to some extent by escape mutants selected against a specific compound. Cross-resistance was observed between dichloroflavan, chalcone, RMI 15,731 and MDL 20,610 for HRV-2 (34,35), between SDS, arildone, dichloroflavan and chalcone for HRV-1B (36), and between R 61837, MDL 20,610, Ro 09-410, dichloroflavan, RMI 15,731, SDS, and WIN 51711 for HRV-9 (37). Although the compounds thus probably bind to the same site, it does not necessarily mean that they bind to the same amino acids within that site. This is clear from the facts that (i) cross-resistance is not absolute, e.g. mutants of HRV-9 selected by chalcone were not cross-resistant to dichloroflavan (38), and (ii) the extent of cross-resistance is usually not the same for different compounds (33,34,37). Furthermore, the shape and the size of the hydrophobic pocket itself probably vary from one virus to another according to the particular amino acids that line the pocket.

A series of compounds developed by the Sterling Research Group (WIN compounds) has been studied structurally by X-ray diffraction while bound to HRV-14 (39,40). These are the first structural studies of antiviral agents complexed with a virion. All compounds were shown to bind into an interior hydrophobic pocket within VP1 underneath the canyon floor (Figures 10.3 and 10.4). In HRV-14 they cause conformational changes of up to 4 Å in main chain and 7.5 Å in side-chain positions. The changes induced by drug binding to HRV-14 in the internal hydrophobic pocket cause conformational changes to the virus exterior that are largely confined to the canyon (41). The largest changes are in the so-called FMDV loop where it crosses the canyon floor. It was therefore speculated that drug binding would also inhibit attachment. This was, indeed, demonstrated in a series of experiments measuring labelled virus attachment to membranes (42). A study of HRV-1A showed that the wild-type virus has a conformation similar to that of HRV-14 when complexed with WIN drugs. When WIN compounds are bound to HRV-1A no further conformational changes occur (43). A study using R 61837 in HRV-14 confirmed that capsid-binding compounds of a different chemical class also bind into the same pocket (44).

STABILIZATION

The binding of capsid-binding compounds to picornaviruses has been shown to prevent degradation of viral particles induced by heat or acidic pH (in the case of rhinoviruses) or alkaline pH (in the case of poliovirus or echovirus) (21,24,36,45–47). Since rhinoviruses require low pH for an event in the entry process (48), the ability of these compounds to stabilize the rhinovirus capsid against low pH by binding to the virion was initially thought to be causally related to inhibition of uncoating (21,35,47,49). The binding of the compounds to the virus capsid could make the protein shell less flexible (40) and could thereby inhibit disassembly of the virion *in vitro* as well as in the cell (35). The general feeling was therefore that the stabilization is directly (and thus quantitatively) related to the inhibition of replication. Attempts to prove the existence of such a correlation have produced controversial results. Indeed, it was established that there is a good correlation between the stabilizing properties of the analogues of one chemical family, the substituted isoxazoles, and the inhibition of replication of HRV-14 (50). On the other hand, when a pyridazinamine derivative was tested

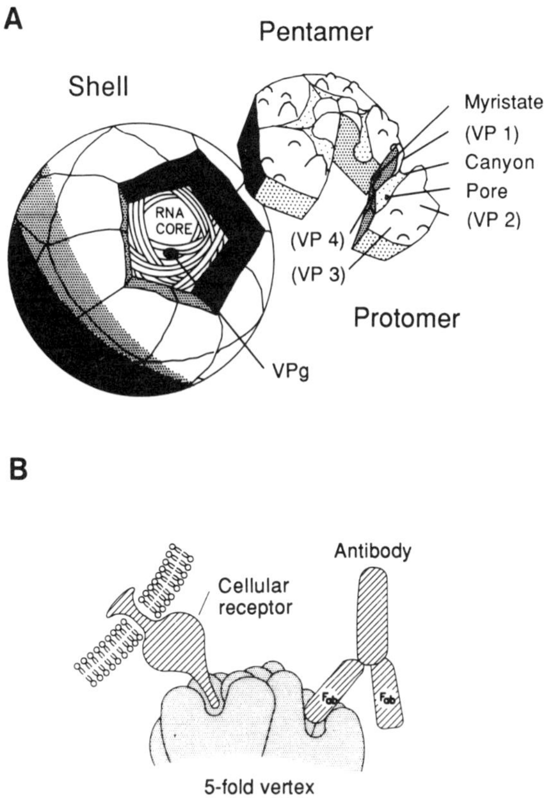

Figure 10.3. Key features in the function of a typical picornavirus. (A) Exploded diagram showing the RNA interior and the location of canyon structure. (B) Binding of cellular receptor to the floor of the canyon. The binding site of the cellular receptor, for the majority of rhinoviruses, has a diameter roughly half of that of an IgG antibody molecule (adapted from Rueckert, 1990, Picornaviridae and their replication, in *Virology*, ed. by Fields and Knipe, pp. 507–548; by permission of Raven Press)

against several serotypes (37), or when compounds belonging to different chemical classes were tested against one serotype (51), no such a correlation could be found. This indicates that the extent of stabilization is not predictive of the extent of inhibition of replication. Indeed, stabilization experiments themselves may not be relevant for the intracellular situation, and they are certainly not predictive of conformational changes or their effects on adsorption, penetration and uncoating. The isolation of drug-resistant variants that are stabilized by the compound to the same degree as the parenteral drug-sensitive virus further illustrates the absence of a strict correlation between inhibition of replication and protection against virion degradation (52,53).

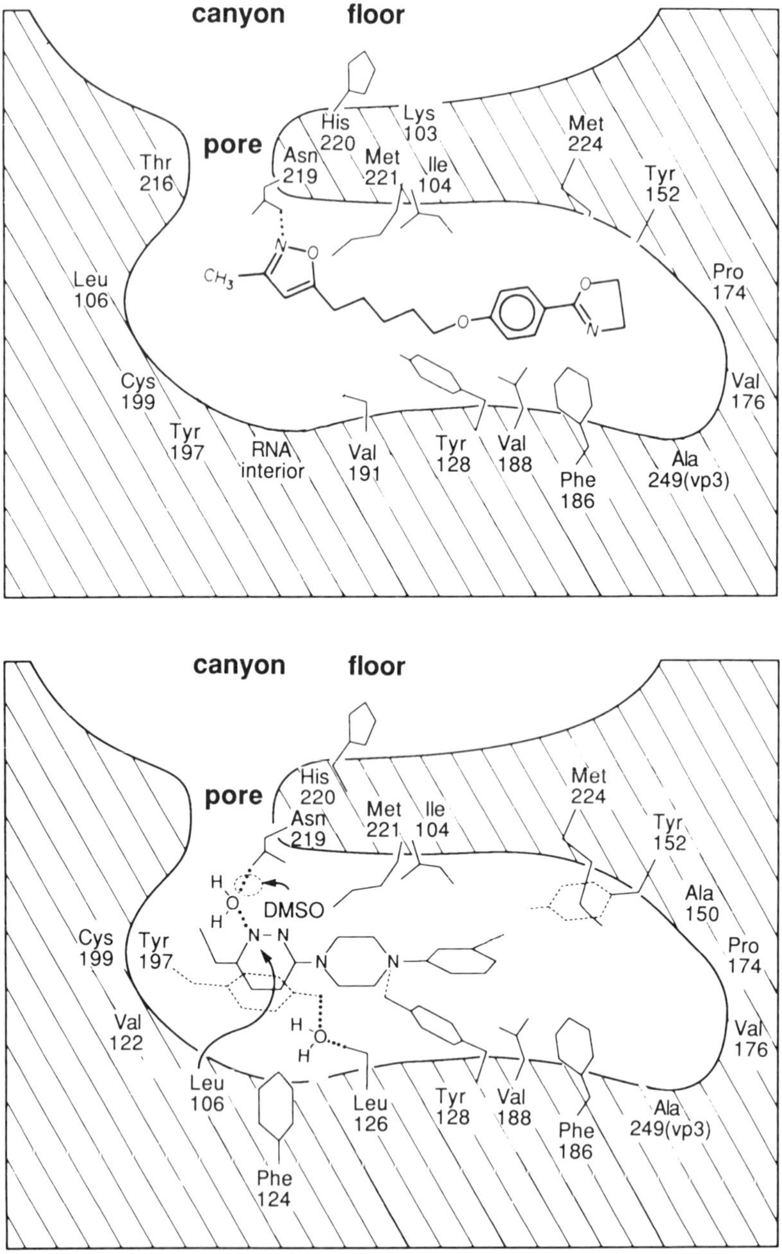

Figure 10.4. Location of the drug-binding site in VP1 of HRV-14 and identity of amino acid residues lining the wall. The drugs depicted here are WIN 52035 (top) and R 61837 (bottom) (adapted from Badger *et al.* (40) (top) and from Chapman *et al.* (44) (bottom), with permission)

Because of the stabilization phenomenon, capsid-binding compounds may be very useful stabilizers of poliovirus virions and procapsids. The antigenic composition of a virion is indeed conserved upon interaction with capsid binders (54).

MECHANISM OF ACTION

An appreciation of the mechanism of action of capsid-binding compounds requires a basic understanding of the early events in the replication cycle of picornaviruses. Polioviruses and rhinoviruses generally adsorb to a specific receptor (i.e. the adsorption step) on the surface of permissive cells and enter the host via receptor-mediated endocytosis (i.e. the penetration step) (reviewed in reference 2). Only two unique receptor groups have been identified for 99 out of the 100 known HRV serotypes (55,56). The major receptor has been identified as ICAM-1 (9,10). Once inside the cell, the virus is passed through endosomes and lysosomes at progressively lower pH. Native virions undergo conformational changes, resulting in antigenically different particles, the A particles. At an uncertain point in the progression of the viral particles, further conformational changes lead to the release of the viral RNA into the cell cytoplasm (i.e. the uncoating step) and the production of empty B particles.

Initially, most capsid-binding compounds have been thought to inhibit replication of picornaviruses by inhibition of the uncoating step (22,35,45,46,86). Evidence for the inhibition of the uncoating step was usually acquired by demonstration of inhibitory effects on the transition of neutral red encapsidated virus, which is light sensitive, into light-resistant virus. However, subsequent studies indicated that, at least for some compounds and in some rhinovirus serotypes, the adsorption step could be inhibited as well (15,42). Disoxaril was shown to have an effect on the penetration and uncoating of HRV-2 (45), and on the adsorption of HRV-14 (42). The minor receptor group serotypes HRV-1A (15), HRV-1B (57) and HRV-2 (41) cannot be inhibited in their attachment either by pirodavir, dichloroflavan or WIN, respectively. Structural studies enable us to correlate the presence or absence of conformational changes in the canyon with inhibition of viral attachment (41). However, as the extent of conformational changes can differ from serotype to serotype (41), and from compound to compound within the same serotype (51), a general rule for the mechanism of action of capsid-binding compounds is difficult to draw. Compounds can apparently have an effect on adsorption and/or penetration and/or uncoating, depending both on the serotype and the nature of the compound itself.

Rhodanine or 2-thio-4-oxothiazolidine (**1**) has been shown to inhibit selectively the multiplication of echovirus 12, and to stabilize the virus against heat inactivation (Figure 10.5). No activity was found against other picorna-

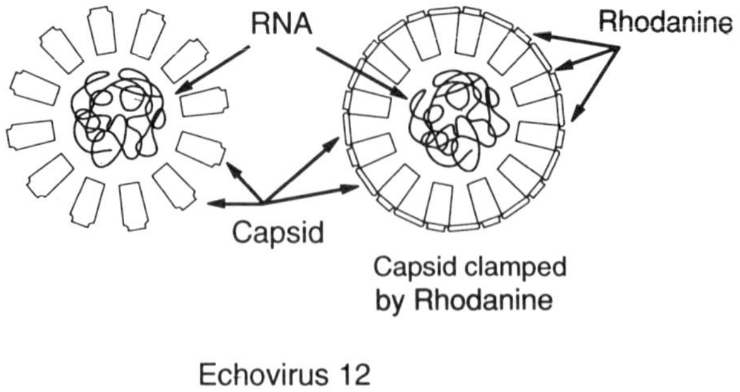

Figure 10.5. Stabilization of echovirus 12 by rhodanine according to a slide presented at a New York Academy meeting in 1969 by Prof. H. J. Eggers, a pioneer in the research on anti-picornaviral agents

viruses (Table 10.1). When tested against our panel of 17 representative rhinovirus serotypes (Figure 10.2), the compound displays a surprising specificity for rhinoviruses from antiviral group B (Table 10.2).

In the presence of rhodanine, penetration of intact virus into the cell takes place, but not uncoating (46). Upon removal of the reversible rhodanine block, uncoating occurs very fast (about 5 min). Combined autoradiography and electron microscopy indicated that, in the presence of the compound, fully infectious viruses become randomly localized in the cell cytoplasm (58).

SDS or sodium dodecyl sulphate (**2**) was originally described as an inhibitor of HRV-2 and HRV-1A, but not HRV-14. Antiviral activity paralleled the ability of SDS to inhibit *in vitro* acid-mediated eclipse, heat inactivation and also cell-mediated eclipse (21). Its capsid-stabilizing properties and its cross-resistance with other capsid-binding compounds (37) indicate that this compound is a true capsid-binding compound. Upon testing against all 100 rhinovirus serotypes, SDS was found to be specifically active against antiviral group B rhinoviruses (13). Its EC_{53} and EC_{82} against the set of 17 serotypes are 38 and > 170 μM, respectively (Table 10.2). SDS exerts weak activity (6 μM level) against echovirus 9 and enterovirus 70 (SI less than 5), but is not active against polioviruses or coxsackieviruses (Table 10.1).

The thiopyrimidines *2-thiouracil* and *S-7* (**3**) (22) specifically bind to polioviruses and stabilize them against heat inactivation. The major distinction between 2-thiouracil and S-7 appears to be the reversibility of the effect caused by the latter.

RMI 15,731 or (1,[5-tetradecycloxy-2-furanyl]ethanone) (**4**) was reported to be active against 77% of 52 rhinovirus serotypes, and to be inactive against poliovirus type 2 (23). RMI 15,731 directly neutralizes HRV-39 in a time- and temperature-dependent fashion (2 $\log_{10}$ after 1 h), and shows cross-resistance to other capsid-binding compounds (see above). Upon test-

Table 10.1. Anti-picornavirus spectrum of antiviral compounds

NR	Compound name	Polio	Echo	Coxsackie A	Coxsackie B	Other entero.	Ref.
1	Rhodanine	neg	*	neg	neg	?	20
2	SDS	neg	neg	neg	neg	neg	90
4	RMI 15,731	*	neg	**	neg	***	90
5	4′,6-Dichloroflavan	neg	*	*	neg	*	25,90
6	MDL 20,610	neg	*	neg	neg	*	28,90
8	Chalcone	***	*	***	neg	***	90
10	Arildone (WIN 38020)	**	?	*	?	*	65,66
11	Disoxaril (WIN 51711)	***	***	**	*	**	29,90
12	WIN 54954	**	***	***	***	?	31,73
13	R 61837	neg	neg	*	neg	*	30,90
14	Pirodavir (R 77975)	***	***	***	*	***	15
15	Guanidine hydrochloride	*	*	*	*	?	79
16	HBB	*	*	*	*	?	82
17	Bis-benzimidazolyl derivative	*	?	*	*	?	83
20	Ro 09-0179	***	***	***	***	?	88
21	4′-Hydroxy-3-methoxyflavone	***	?	?	?	?	89
22	44 081 R.P.	?	?	*	?	?	91
23	MDL 860	*	*	**	*	*	90

NR: compound numbers referring to the numbers used in the text. The antiviral activities are scored as follows: ?, no data; neg, selectivity index (SI) < 5; *SI > 5 and $IC_{50} > 1$ μM; **SI > 5 and $IC_{50} < 1$ μM; ***SI > 5 and $IC_{50} < 0.1$ μM. The scores given are based on the results obtained with the most susceptible serotypes of the group, e.g. if a compound is active against one poliovirus serotype (any serotype) with an SI > 5 and an IC_{50} of 0.5 μM, a score of ** is given in the column of polioviruses. The viruses tested in our own laboratory were: polioviruses type 1 Mahoney, type 2 Mefie and type 3 Leon, echovirus serotypes 9, 11 and 12, coxsackieviruses A13, A15, A18, A21, B1, B3 and B4, and enterovirus serotypes 68 and 70.

ing the compound against the set of 17 rhinovirus serotypes, an EC_{53} and EC_{82} of 1.1 and 50 μM was found, respectively (Table 10.2). Substantial activity was also found against coxsackie A viruses (serotypes 13 and 15), and enteroviruses (serotypes 68 and 70), weak activity against polio 2 (Mefie strain), and no activity against coxsackie B viruses or echoviruses (Table 10.1).

FLAVANS

4′,6-Dichloroflavan (BW683C) (**5**) was at the time (25) the most potent antiviral compound yet reported. Its activity is mainly confined to the rhinoviruses of antiviral group B (Figure 10.6). It is active against 53% and 82% of the 17 rhinoviruses at concentrations of 5 and > 70 μM, respectively (Table 10.2). Some serotypes are neutralized by 4′,6-dichloroflavan (about 0.5 $\log_{10}$ units). The infectivity of neutralized rhinoviruses can be reversed by chloroform extraction. In studies on the binding characteristics of 4′,6-dichloroflavan to the sensitive HRV-1B and the insensitive HRV-14, a small degree of binding was also observed with the insensitive HRV-14 (57). Flavans have been shown to be able to exert their antiviral activity in the vapour phase, and thus may have an advantage over non-volatile compounds (59).

Thiophene analogues of flavans have been described to have the same rhinovirus serotype specificity, but a significantly lesser antiviral potency (60). Halogenated isoflavans and, to a lesser extent, isoflavenes, have properties similar to those of 4′,6-dichloroflavan (32). Very little is known about their antiviral spectrum but, interestingly, both 4′,6-dichloroflavan and 4′,6-dichloroisoflavan have been reported to inhibit the replication of hepatitis A virus at fairly low concentrations (0.006 μM) and are postulated to interact with an early stage of hepatitis A infection (61).

Aza analogues of flavans such as *MDL 20,610* (**6**) (28) and other *2H*-pyrano[2,3-*b*]pyridines (62) are potent inhibitors of rhinoviruses, and also exert activity against enteroviruses and echoviruses. The compound of choice of this series, MDL 20,610, has an EC_{53} and EC_{82} of 2.9 and > 150 μM, respectively, against the 17 rhinovirus serotypes (Table 10.2), and is also active against some rotaviruses (28). MDL 20,610 does not neutralize the infectivity of HRV-1A, but does stabilize HRV 1B against inactivation by heat or low pH (35).

Some *phenoxypyridines* with moderate *in vitro* activity against rhinoviruses and coxsackievirus A21 have also been described (63). They are closely related to phenoxybenzenes such as MDL 860 (see below), but apparently have a different mode of action. The phenoxypyridinecarbonitrile 6-(3,4-dichlorophenoxy)-3-(ethylthio)-2-pyridinecarbonitrile (*DEPC*) (**7**) (27) was shown to inhibit the uncoating of poliovirus (64).

CHALCONES

Studies of various flavone analogues led to the discovery of 4′-ethoxy-2′-hydroxy-4,6′-dimethoxychalcone or Ro 09-410 (**8**), commonly described as *chalcone*. The neutralization of several rhinovirus serotypes (up to 2 $\log_{10}$ units) could be completely reversed by extraction of chalcone by chloroform. Radiolabelled chalcone was shown to bind to HRV-2, and to prevent the formation of 'A' particles upon exposure to pH 5 (47). The binding of radiolabelled chalcone to HRV-2 was inhibited by unlabelled compound, 4′,6-dichloroflavan and RMI 15,731, suggesting that the binding sites for these three agents are either the same or very close to each other (49).

The activity of chalcone is mainly but not strictly confined to the rhinoviruses of antiviral group B (Figure 10.6). The compound is active against 53% and 82% of the 17 rhinoviruses at concentrations of 0.82 and 4.1 μM, respectively. The CC_{50} is greater than 150 μM (Table 10.2). The compound was originally found to be inactive against poliovirus (type 1), coxsackievirus (types A21 and B1), echovirus (types 7, 11, 12 and 19) (26). In our hands, concentrations of chalcone as low as 0.1 μg/ml were inhibitory to coxsackieviruses A13 and A18, enterovirus types 68 and 70, and poliovirus type 2. Moderate activity was also found for some echoviruses (Table 10.1).

Amide analogues of chalcone such as Ro 09-0535, Ro 09-0881 and Ro 09-0696 (**9**) have been reported to be 5–10 times more active against a selection of 12 rhinoviruses (33), 10 of which belong to antiviral group B. The two serotypes from antiviral group A are less sensitive to the amide analogues than to chalcone itself. The CC_{50}s of the compounds range from 90 to 150 μM. The amide analogues disoxaril and 4′,6-dichloroflavan all competitively inhibit the binding of radiolabelled chalcone to HRV-2. Again, the neutralization of several rhinovirus serotypes (up to 3 $\log_{10}$ units) could be completely reversed by extraction of the compounds with chloroform (33).

ISOXAZOLES

The isoxazoles are a series of compounds developed over the past years by the Sterling Winthrop group. They are now usually referred to as the WIN compounds. The first compounds that were described of this series (reviewed in reference 65) were actually not isoxazoles but phenoxyalkyldiketones. The representative of this first group of compounds, *arildone* or WIN 38020 or 4-[6-(2-chloro-4-methoxyphenoxy)hexyl]-3,5-heptanedione (**10**), is active against equine rhinovirus, human poliovirus (IC_{50} 0.2 μM, $CC_{50} > 30$ μM) (65), enterovirus type 70 and coxsackievirus A24 (66). It is also active against most human rhinoviruses from antiviral group B (Table 10.2). Arildone was shown to inhibit the uncoating, but not the adsorption or penetration of poliovirus type 2 (67), and to stabilize the same virus against heat or alkali treatment (24). This observation led to its use in increasing the immunogenicity of inactivated poliovirus vaccine (68).

Table 10.2. Anti-rhinovirus spectrum of antiviral compounds

	NR	EC_{53}	EC_{82}	HRV-14	HRV-42	HRV-45	HRV-70	HRV-72	HRV-86	MedA
Rhodanine	1	80	>375	>375	>375	>375	>375	>375	>375	>375
SDS	2	38	>170	>170	>170	>170	94	>170	>170	>170
RMI 15,731	4	1.1	50	5	>160	>160	0.6	>160	50	74
4',6-Dichloroflavan	5	5	>70	>70	>70	>70	>70	>70	>70	>70
MDL 20,610	6	2.9	>150	>150	>150	>150	>150	>150	>150	>150
Chalcone	8	0.82	4.1	2	49	4	>150	4	49	26
Arildone (WIN 38020)	10	77	>140	>140	>140	0.3	>140	>140	>140	>140
Disoxaril (WIN 51711)	11	4.6	10	0.5	11	4	0.05	3	3	3
WIN 54954	12	0.48	6.2	6	>70	0.8	0.6	19	8	7
R 61837	13	20	>140	>140	>140	>140	>140	>140	>140	>140
Pirodavir (R 77975)	14	0.02	0.39	0.03	>130	4	0.006	0.4	0.03	0.21
Guanidine hydrochloride	15	2100	4000	300	>7900	420	340	280	120	320
HBB	16	570	>2500	110	130	85	>2500	180	90	120
Enviroxime	18	0.12	0.21	0.4	0.2	0.3	0.2	1.0	0.1	0.3
Ro 09-0179	20	0.52	0.64	0.7	0.6	0.6	0.6	3	0.5	0.6
4'-Hydroxy-3-methoxyflavone	21	0.62	0.64	0.6	0.6	0.6	0.7	5	0.5	0.6
MDL 860	23	2.6	26	26	26	26	3	100	3	26
3-Deazaguanine	24	>200	>200	>200	>200	>200	>200	>200	180	>200

NR: compound numbers referring to the numbers used in the text. The IC_{50}s (in μM) of 17 human rhinoviruses (HRV, followed by their serotype number) was assayed. Viruses are listed according to their antiviral group allocation (compare with Figure 10.2). IC_{50}: concentration required to reduce the inhibition of the formation of formazan from MTT by 50% (15). CC_{50}: concentration (in μM) required to reduce the

In the course of modifying the structure of arildone to achieve broad-spectrum anti-picornaviral activity, a series of isoxazoles was prepared, leading to the synthesis of *disoxaril* or WIN 51,711, or (5-[7-[4-(4,5-dihydro-2-oxazolyl)phenoxy]heptyl]-3-methylisoxazole (**11**) (69). The antiviral spectrum of disoxaril encompasses polioviruses, human rhinoviruses (Table 10.2), coxsackie A viruses and echoviruses (29), enteroviruses and, to a lesser extent, coxsackie B viruses (Table 10.1). Other RNA viruses and DNA viruses are unaffected by the compound. Soon after the structure of HRV-14 was resolved by X-ray crystallography (4), disoxaril and related compounds were shown to be inserted into the hydrophobic pocket in VP1 beneath the floor of the canyon (Figure 10.4) (39). Not all WIN compounds bind in the same orientation (40), but all active compounds seem to upheave the canyon floor, and in the case of HRV-14 this upheaval is correlated with loss of receptor-binding ability (42). In addition to its effect on adsorption for certain rhinovirus serotypes, disoxaril reportedly has an effect on the penetration of HRV-2, and on the uncoating of HRV-2 and poliovirus type 2 (45,70). The compound stabilizes HRV-2 (50) and the procapsids of poliovirus type 1, leading to an increased immunogenicity of both purified virions and procapsids in mice (71). The binding affinities and the rates of association and dissociation of several oxazolines have been described (72). Scatchard plots of each of four compounds for the binding data indicated that approximately 40–60 molecules were bound per HRV-14 virion. Hill plots showed no evidence of cooperativity in binding.

From the observation that phenyl-substituted analogues of disoxaril exhi-

MedB	HRV-2	HRV-9	HRV-15	HRV-29	HRV-39	HRV-41	HRV-51	HRV-59	HRV-63	HRV-85	HRV-89	CC_{50}
47	29	38	51	43	148	89	53	37	47	80	34	>375
33	6	2	11	39	73	35	38	37	18	32	33	>170
1.0	0.1	1	2	0.2	0.6	8	0.5	3	1	1.0	0.2	>160
0.8	0.5	0.4	0.6	0.01	0.8	0.7	20	7	5	0.9	2	70
0.4	0.004	0.087	0.4	0.019	3	8	0.3	17	2	0.7	0.2	>150
0.30	0.03	0.3	0.3	0.4	0.1	2.36	0.1	0.9	0.8	0.1	0.1	>150
19	13	19	3	21	9	>140	77	>140	97	5	12	>140
7	2	10	3	5	7	>150	7	>150	10	4	5	>150
0.10	0.03	0.1	0.1	0.07	0.3	1	0.07	0.6	0.5	0.03	0.005	70
6	0.2	0.04	0.9	0.2	4	7	24	20	20	6	9	140
0.01	0.005	0.07	0.08	0.007	0.02	0.8	0.01	0.02	0.007	0.006	0.005	>130
2500	700	2300	2800	>7900	1800	2500	4000	3300	>7900	2100	1900	7900
>2500	>2500	325	>2500	>2500	570	>2500	750	>2500	>2500	530	150	2500
0.1	0.1	0.1	0.1	0.1	0.2	0.1	0.2	0.1	0.1	0.1	0.1	18
0.5	0.5	0.5	0.5	0.5	0.5	0.5	0.7	0.5	0.4	0.4	0.5	>140
0.6	0.6	0.6	0.6	0.6	0.6	0.6	0.6	0.6	0.4	0.6	0.7	>160
1.9	0.9	0.7	5	1	6	2	0.8	2	0.6	2	6	>160
102	100	80	44	>200	90	190	>200	80	>200	>200	33	>200

formation of formazan from MTT by 50% after application of the compound to an HeLa cell suspension and subsequent incubation for 3 days at 33 °C. The concentrations needed to inhibit 9 or 14 out of the 17 serotypes (EC_{53} and EC_{82}) were calculated. MedA and MedB represent the median IC_{50}s of the viruses from antiviral groups A and B, respectively.

bited a broader spectrum and a greater degree of anti-rhinoviral activity than the unsubstituted analogues, Diana *et al.* prepared several 2,6-disubstituted compounds, of which *WIN 54954* or (5-[5-[2,6-dichloro-4-(4,5-dihydro-2-oxazolyl)phenoxy]pentyl]-3-methylisoxazole) (**12**) was the compound of choice (73).

In plaque-reduction assays, WIN 54954 reduced plaque formation of 50 of 52 rhinovirus serotypes (IC_{50}s ranged from 0.007 to 2.2 μg/ml). The EC_{80} for those 52 serotypes was 0.28 μg/ml (31). It is remarkable that WIN 51711 (disoxaril) is mainly active against antiviral group A rhinoviruses, whereas the reverse seems to be true for WIN 54954 (Table 10.2, Figure 10.6). WIN 54954 was also effective in inhibiting 15 echoviruses and coxsackieviruses (A and B), with an EC_{80} of 0.06 μg/ml (31), and 115 clinical isolates of echovirus and type B coxsackievirus (74).

PYRIDAZINAMINES

The pyridazinamines are a series of compounds developed by the Janssen Research Foundation. They are indicated by R (for research) numbers. The first compound to be described was *R 61837* or 3-methoxy-6-[4-(3-methylphenyl)-1-piperazinyl]pyridazine (**13**) (30). R 61837 was the first synthetic compound to be active in experimental rhinovirus infection in human volunteers (75). The spectrum of R 61837 is limited to the rhinoviruses, although some activity can be found against coxsackievirus A21 and enterovirus 70. The polioviruses, echoviruses (types 9, 11 and 12), and other

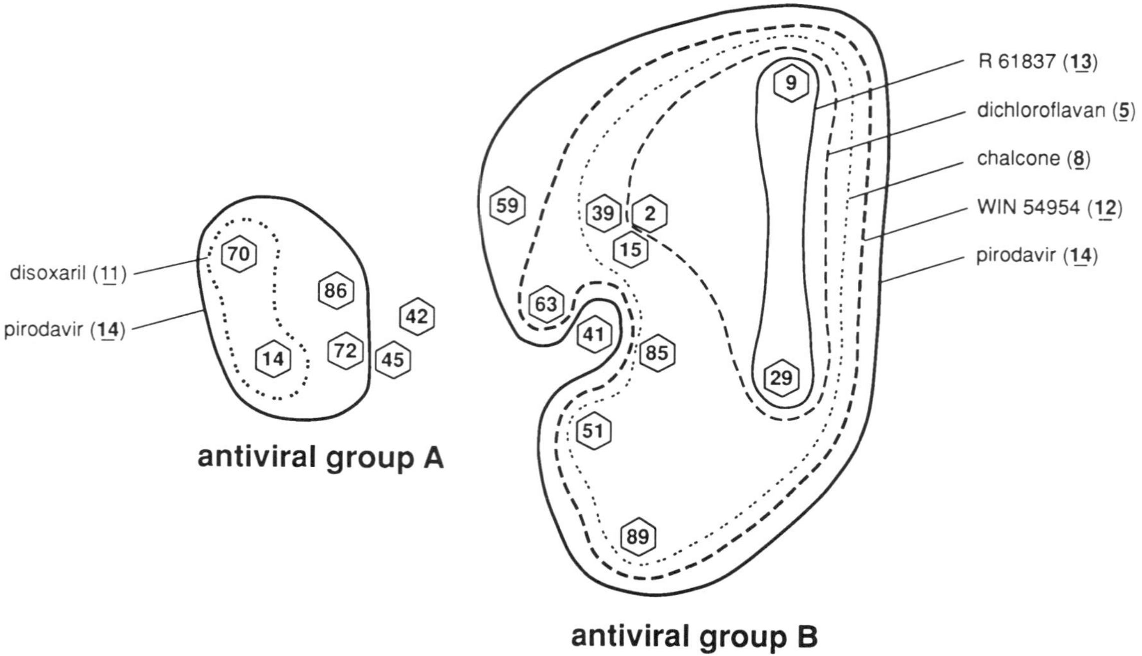

Figure 10.6. Anti-rhinovirus spectra of capsid-binding compounds. The susceptibility of 17 rhinovirus serotypes was assessed. The serotypes that are present within the circle representing a particular compound have IC_{50}s below 0.5 μM for that compound, while those outside the circle have higher IC_{50}s

coxsackieviruses (types A13, A15, A18, B1, B3 and B4) are insensitive. R 61837 is typically a compound that is almost exclusively active against rhinoviruses from antiviral group B (14). Even within this antiviral group, the different rhinovirus serotypes vary widely in their susceptibility to the antiviral agent. The IC_{50}s range from 0.004 to 15 μg/ml. R 61837 is active against 53% of the 17 rhinoviruses at a concentration of 20 μM. Susceptible serotypes all belong to antiviral group B (Table 10.2, Figure 10.6). The infectivity of several susceptible rhinoviruses is neutralized by R 61837 (up to about 1 $\log_{10}$ unit). The neutralizing effect of R 61837 appears to be stronger than the effects described for chalcone, RMI 15,731 and dichloroflavan, as the infectivity of viruses neutralized by R 61837 can often not be reversed by chloroform extraction (30,76).

R 61837 inhibits the adsorption of HRV-9, but not that of HRV-1B (51). Rate zonal centrifugation experiments and viral infectivity tests established that the compound stabilizes susceptible rhinoviruses against inactivation by acid or heat. This was confirmed immunochemically by use of a non-neutralizing and neutralizing monoclonal antibody. R 61837 prevented the switch from D to C antigenicity, which can be induced by exposure of rhinoviruses to mild denaturing conditions (76). No quantitative correlation between the concentrations needed to inhibit the replication of several rhinovirus serotypes and the concentrations needed to stabilize their capsids could be demonstrated (37). Hence, inhibition of replication and capsid stabilization are probably not causally linked but are more likely to be parallel events, independently resulting from the binding of the drug to the viral capsid.

The binding of R 61837 to HRV-9 was studied quantitatively and compared with binding to HRV-9H, a semi-resistant variant (76). For both strains, radiolabelled R 61387 bound to native particles only. The K_D values obtained by Scatchard analysis of saturation binding data were 37 nM for HRV-9 and 172 nM for HRV-9H, whereas the IC_{50} values were respectively 42 nM and 840 nM. Dissociation studies demonstrated that in the presence of excess unlabelled compound the $t_{1/2}$ values for HRV-9 and HRV-9H were 385 and 15 min, respectively.

In order to achieve a more broad-spectrum activity with pyridazinamines, the synthesis of compounds with activity against serotypes from antiviral group A was attempted. The use of such a compound with another one active against serotypes from antiviral group B (such as R 61837) would result in a mixture of compounds with broad-spectrum activity. By chemically combining substructures of R 61837 and WIN 51711, a lead compound with weak but specific activity against antiviral group A rhinoviruses was found. A screening programme involving the testing of about 600 compounds against the 17 representative serotypes was used to increase the potency and eventually led to the synthesis of pirodavir (15).

Pirodavir (R 77975) is a substituted phenoxy-pyridazinamine (**14**), distantly related to its predecessor R 61837, a substituted phenyl-pyridazinamine. While R 61837 was effective in inhibiting 80% of 100 rhinovirus serotypes tested at concentrations above 32 μg/ml, pirodavir inhibits the same percentage of viruses at 0.064 μg/ml. Whereas R 61837 was almost exclusively active against rhinovirus serotypes of antiviral group B, pirodavir is broad spectrum, in that it is highly active against serotypes of both group A and group B rhinovirus serotypes (Table 10.2, Figure 10.6). Pirodavir was also effective in inhibiting 16 enteroviruses, with an EC_{80} of 1.3 μg/ml (15) (Table 10.1).

Susceptible rhinovirus serotypes are rendered non-infectious by direct contact with pirodavir (up to 3 $\log_{10}$ units). Their infectivity can be regained by organic solvent extraction of the compound for most serotypes. The fact that neutralized viruses become stabilized to acid and heat strongly suggests a direct interaction of the compounds with viral capsid proteins. Mutants resistant to R 61837 (up to 85 times the IC_{50}) were shown to have some cross-resistance (up to 23 times the IC_{50}) with pirodavir. Pirodavir acts at an early stage of the viral replication cycle (up to 40 min after infection), but in a serotype-specific way, since the compound was able to inhibit the adsorption of HRV-9 but not that of HRV-1A.

INHIBITORS OF VIRAL REPLICATION (RNA SYNTHESIS)

Inhibitors of viral replication exhibit the greatest inhibition when the compound is added 1 h after viral adsorption or earlier. They prevent the formation of plus-stranded viral RNA (77) or of plus-stranded as well as minus-stranded viral RNA (78). Their spectrum differs considerably from compound to compound, but almost always includes various members of the genera Enterovirus and Poliovirus. Mengovirus is resistant to all compounds described so far. Resistant variants against low-potency compounds can easily be isolated. None of the compounds described below is in active clinical development. (Figures in bold refer to structural formulae.)

Guanidine hydrochloride (**15**) is one of the oldest and most extensively studied inhibitors of poliovirus replication, although its antiviral activity is very weak. At millimolar levels (100–2000 μM), it selectively blocks the growth of many picornaviruses (79) (Table 10.1) and rhinoviruses (Table 10.2). Although guanidine inhibits several virus-induced processes, its primary action is at the RNA synthesis step (80). Genetic and biochemical evidence suggests that the non-structural viral polypeptide 2C is responsible for the guanidine sensitivity of poliovirus (81).

2-(α-Hydroxybenzyl)-benzimidazole (*HBB*) (**16**) is similar but not identical to guanidine hydrochloride in its antiviral properties. The susceptibility of various viruses to HBB varies considerably. At concentrations of HBB nontoxic to cells (220 μM), many enteroviruses were found to be susceptible:

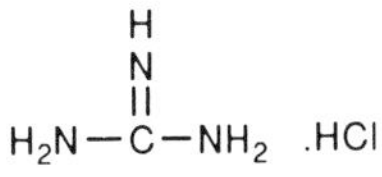

(**15**)

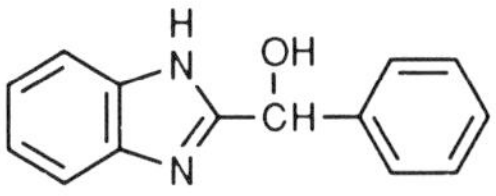

(**16**)

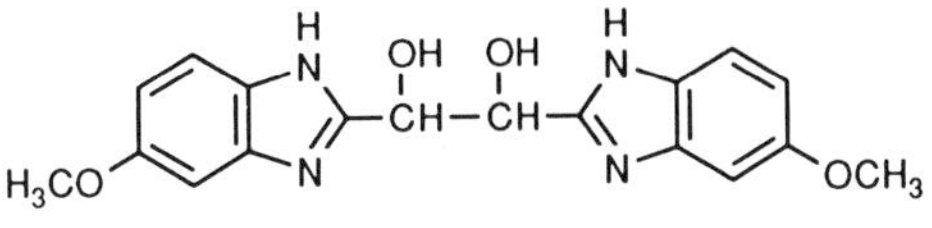

(**17**)

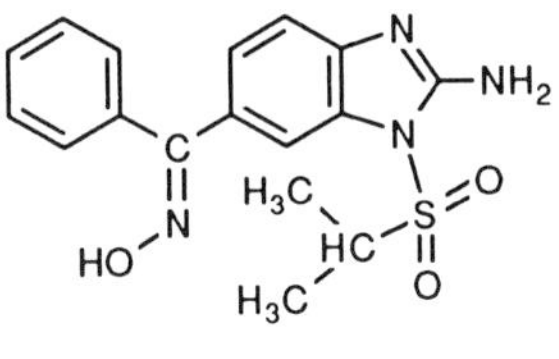

(**18**)

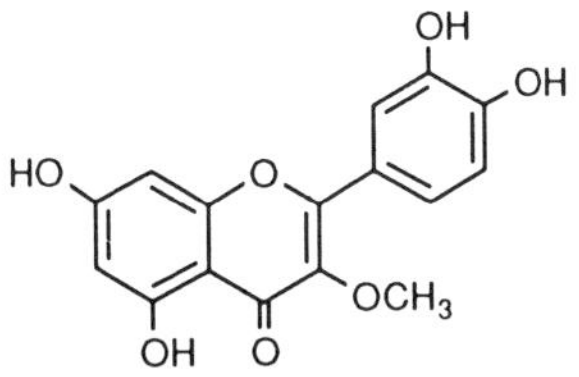

(**19**)

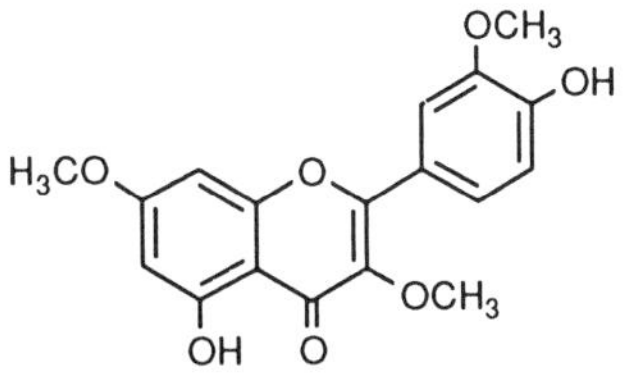

(**20**)

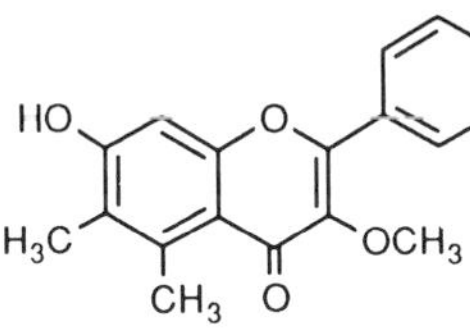

(**21**)

poliovirus 1–3, coxsackievirus B1–6, coxsackievirus A9, echovirus 1–11, 11–21 and 24–27. Echovirus 22 and 23, all coxsackie A viruses other than A9 and the majority of rhinoviruses tested were found to be insusceptible to HBB (82). Mutants of picornaviruses were isolated that were either resistant to or dependent on the drug. There is little cross-resistance between HBB and guanidine, and combined use of both compounds has synergistic effects both *in vitro* and *in vivo* (82).

Interestingly, a derivative of HBB, *S,S-1,2-bis-(5-methoxy-2-benzimidazolyl)-1,2-ethanediol* (**17**), has a different antiviral spectrum (active against 55 rhinoviruses) (83). Virus mutants against it are not cross-resistant to HBB (82).

The 2-amino-1-(isopropyl-sulphonyl)-6-benzimidazole phenyl ketone oxime or *enviroxime* (**18**) is active at non-cytotoxic concentrations against 83 serotypes (84), belonging to both antiviral group A and antiviral group B.

The IC_{50}s obtained against rhinoviruses range from < 0.01 to 0.12 μg/ml (85). Serotypes from both antiviral groups seem to have the same susceptibility (Table 10.2). The sensitivity of other picornaviruses to enviroxime has not been described. Due to lack of clinical efficacy, development of enviroxime has been discontinued (86).

Some naturally occurring flavonoids, such as *3-methylquercetin* (**19**) (isolated from *Euphorbia grantii*) (87) and *Ro 09-0179* (**20**) (isolated from *Agastache rugosa*) (88), show potent anti-picornaviral activity. Ro 09-0179 inhibited 20 rhinovirus serotypes with an EC_{50} and an EC_{90} of 0.1 and 0.3 μg/ml, respectively. The CC_{50} was about 15 μg/ml in a two-day culture of WI-38 cells (88). It was reported that 3-methylquercetin prevents the formation of plus-stranded as well as minus-stranded viral RNA (78), whereas Ro 09-0179 specifically blocks positive-strand RNA synthesis (77). Synthetic substituted flavones such as *4′-hydroxy-3-methoxyflavones* are potent inhibitors of poliovirus and several rhinoviruses (89). The 4′,7-dihydroxy-3-methoxy-5,6-dimethylflavone (**21**) has a potency that is similar to that of Ro 09-0179 (Table 10.2). Both compounds inhibit rhinoviruses from antiviral group A and B with equal efficiency (Table 10.2) (90).

OTHER TARGETS AND COMPOUNDS

The synthetic compound coded *44081 RP* or *S*-2-[(1,5,10,10*a*-tetrahydro-3*H*-thiazolo[3,4*b*]isoquinolin-3-ylidene)amino]-4-thiazoleacetic acid (**22**) (91) inhibits an early event in the replication of rhinoviruses, but cannot be considered to be a capsid-binding compound. This is suggested by the facts that (i) the antiviral activity is cell-type specific (44081 RP is active in MRC_5 cells, primary monkey kidney cells, and fetal tonsil fibroblasts, but not in Ohio HeLa cells); (ii) MRC_5 cells pre-treated with the compound acquire a state of resistance against further rhinovirus challenge; and (iii) the compound is water soluble. The protection of intracellular [5-^{3}H]uridine-labelled virions against the effects of RNase treatment indicates that the inhibition of virus uncoating is the mode of action (92). The antiviral spectrum of the compound appears to be limited to rhinoviruses, although coxsackie A21 was found to be susceptible too. The maximal non-toxic concentration is 362 μM, while the concentrations needed to inhibit cell destruction by rhinoviruses completely range between 0.43 and 362 μM.

The phenoxybenzene *MDL 860* or 2-(3,4-dichlorophenoxy)-5-nitrobenzonitrile (**23**) acts reportedly at an early step of the viral replication, but after uncoating (93). The absence of cross-resistance to capsid-binding agents (37) also suggests that this compound is not a capsid binder, although the closely related phenoxypyridines such as MDL 20,610 and DEPC (see above) apparently have a different mode of action. At 1 μg/ml, a non-cytotoxic concentration, MDL 860 inhibited 80% of 90 rhinovirus serotypes and 80% of 10 enteroviruses tested (94).

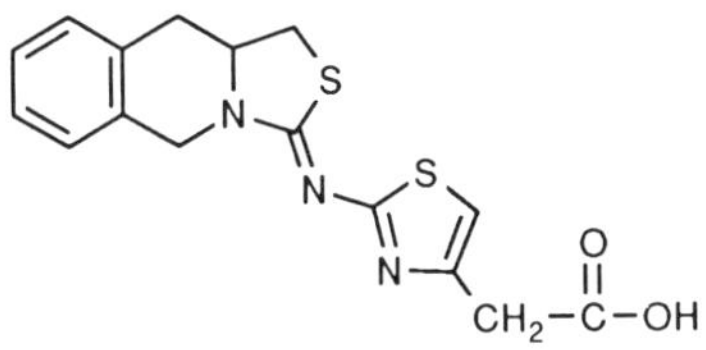

(**22**)

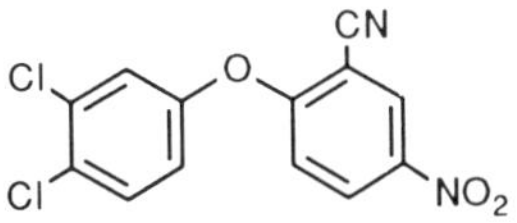

(**23**)

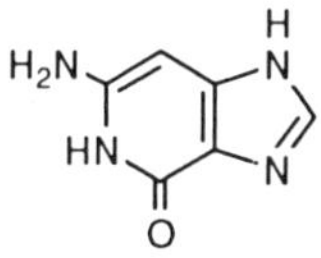

(**24**)

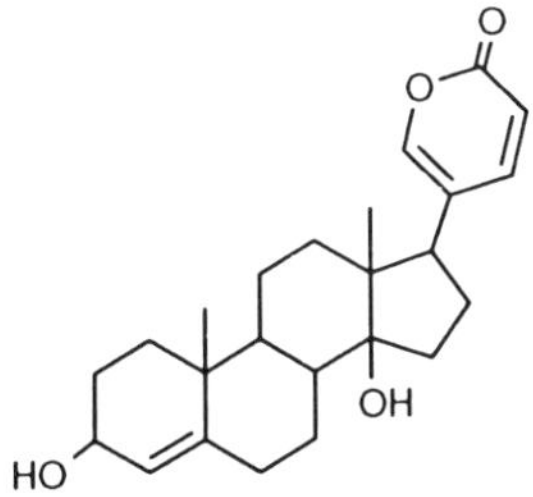

(**25**)

Among a wide variety of purine nucleoside (mainly tubercidin and adenosine) analogues, *3-deazaguanine* (**24**) was the most selective inhibitor of rhinovirus serotypes 1A, 1B and 9. The IC_{50}s ranged from 24 to 69 μM, with a selectivity index of 50 (95). Other rhinovirus serotypes seem to be less susceptible to the compound (Table 10.2).

The bufadienolide *Scillarenin* (**25**), prepared from a higher plant extract, was active against four rhinovirus serotypes (1A, 19, 30 and 63) and poliovirus 1 at fairly low concentrations (IC_{50} 0.010 μM) with a selectivity index of 32 (96).

Studies conducted in the mid-1970s revealed that relatively high concentrations of *zinc ions* inhibit the *in vitro* replication of several rhinovirus serotypes. This effect appears to be mediated through inhibition of post-translational cleavage of precursor polypeptides (97). More recent studies have shown that various zinc salts have very weak (IC_{50} 100 μM), non-selective anti-rhinoviral activity against HRV-1A and HRV-39 (98). The activity and toxicity of zinc complexes can be related to the amount of unbound zinc available to the cells and virus (99).

A lack of selective activity against rhinoviruses was also reported for *aspirin*, another controversial drug for the treatment of the common cold (100).

COMBINATIONS

Combinations of antiviral agents that act by different mechanisms against non-overlapping sites of viral replication theoretically offer several potential advantages. Combination of compounds with complementary spectra may result in a mixture that is active against a broader spectrum of viruses. If synergy is observed, the use of a mixture of substances may achieve greater therapeutic efficacy, the selection of drug-resistant mutants may be prevented and/or individual drugs may be used at lower concentrations *in vivo*.

It has been reported that the combination of synthetic anti-rhinoviral compounds (enviroxime, chalcone, Ro 09-410 and dichloroflavan) with other synthetic compounds or with interferons results in significantly synergistic interactions for HRV-2 and HRV-9 (101,102). However, the matter seems to be rather complicated. Indeed, (i) enviroxime, a non-capsid binder, was not consistent in producing synergistic effects with capsid-binding compounds, (ii) synergy that was observed in one serotype was not necessarily present in other serotypes tested, and (iii) capsid-binding compounds sometimes demonstrated significant synergy with each other. The difficulty of developing a formulation suitable for several antivirals and the possible differences in pharmacokinetics *in vivo* may further complicate the use of combinations.

RESISTANCE

A potential limitation in the development of anti-picornaviral agents is the selection of drug-resistant virus variants by these compounds. RNA viruses have been designated quasi-species, because of the genetic heterogeneity of their genome and the competitive replication of continuously arising variant genomes (103). Domingo and co-workers (103) showed that variation in the VP1 gene of poliovirus occurred with a frequency of 1×10^{-4} per nucleotide per infectious cycle, or roughly one substitution error for each genome. It is thus not surprising that drug-resistant virus variants against anti-picornaviral agents can be readily isolated under *in vitro* and *in vivo* conditions (34,37,38,52,104,106).

The frequency with which resistant variants can be isolated may vary from serotype to serotype and from compound to compound (34,38,106). This may be explained by the extent of conservation of the antiviral binding site involved. It has been suggested that resistant variants can be more easily selected by use of capsid-binding compounds than by use of inhibitors of the initiation of RNA replication such as Ro 09-0179 and enviroxime (34). On the other hand, polioviruses readily develop resistance towards guanidine and HBB (82). It is tempting to speculate that resistant variants arise more easily against compounds with limited antiviral spectra, as these are likely to bind to target sites that are less conserved. More research is needed for the full understanding of the potential limitations caused by viral resistance.

Picornaviruses made resistant to arildone (52), chalcone (34,38,104,107) and a WIN compound (106) have been characterized. A mutant of HRV-9, made resistant to chalcone, produced smaller plaques, grew to a lower titre than the wild-type virus, and was no longer stabilized by chalcone (38). A mutant of HRV-2 against the same antiviral had essentially the same changes in biological properties, and showed a reduced ability to be neutralized by both polyclonal and monoclonal antibodies (104). When given to human volunteers, this mutant could still produce colds, but at the same time had a reduced pathogenicity (107).

Two mutants of poliovirus type 2, made resistant to arildone, were stabilized against heat inactivation in the presence of the drug to the same degree as was the parental drug-sensitive virus. This suggested that arildone was still binding to the resistant virus, but that this interaction, *per se*, is not sufficient to inhibit its replication (52).

Heinz and collaborators analysed 69 escape mutants of HRV-14 that became resistant to one of the WIN compounds (WIN 52084) at the genetic and molecular level (106). High-resistance mutants were defined as those not susceptible to high concentrations of the drug, and these were observed with a frequency of 4×10^{-5}. When the regions of the RNA genome coding for the drug-binding pocket were sequenced, it was found that all these mutants mapped to only two of the 16 amino acid residues that form the wall of the drug-binding site (Cys-199 and Val-188). The side-chains of these two residues were invariably replaced by bulkier groups that point directly into the pocket. This led to the concept that high-resistance mutations hinder either the entry or the seating of drug within the pocket. The mutants had a normal plaque morphology. Some of them, although highly resistant to WIN 52084, were still sensitive to WIN 52035. Low-resistance mutants, defined as still being susceptible to high concentrations of the drug, invariably mapped to portions of the polypeptide chain near the canyon floor that move when the drug is inserted.

Continued research into the pathogenicity of mutant viruses of several serotypes and into the possible dominance of wild-type viruses over mutant viruses in mixed infections will be essential to ensure the future success of anti-picornaviral chemotherapy.

USE OF ANTI-PICORNAVIRAL AGENTS AS RESEARCH TOOLS

Antiviral agents can be used as an aid in the molecular analysis of viral functions, to identify targets for rational drug design, and as an aid in virus classification. Anti-picornaviral agents have been used for all these applications. Capsid-binding compounds have been used to identify a drug-binding pocket in VP1 (39), and subsequently led to the design of new compounds (12). Escape mutant analysis of this drug-binding site enabled the mapping of virus functions such as attachment and uncoating on the rhinovirus capsid (53). Similarly, the correlation between capsid stabilization and inhibition of replication was studied in different rhinovirus serotypes by use of capsid-binding compounds (21,37). The requirement of uncoating to early permeabilization of cell membranes by animal viruses has been studied with uncoating inhibitors (108).

Anti-picornaviral agents can be seen as small molecular probes that can be used to identify the presence or absence of specific amino acid fragments in a particular virus. They can thus be used as an aid in virus classification, provided the percentage of homology in the amino acid sequence of the drug-binding site is representative for the percentage of homology in the amino acid sequence of the whole virus (14,109).

ACKNOWLEDGEMENTS

The excellent assistance of Rudy Willebrords is gratefully acknowledged.

REFERENCES

1. Melnick, J. L. (1990). Enteroviruses: polioviruses, coxsackieviruses, echoviruses, and newer enteroviruses. In *Virology*, B. N. Fields and D. M. Knipe (eds), Raven Press, New York, pp. 549–606.
2. Rueckert, R. R. (1990). Picornaviridae and their replication. In *Virology*, B. N. Fields and D. M. Knipe (eds), Raven Press, New York, pp. 507–548.
3. Korant, B. D., Lonberg-Holm, K. and LaColla, P. (1983). Picornaviruses and togaviruses: targets for design of antivirals. In *Targets for the Design of Antiviral Agents*, E. De Clercq and R. T. Walker (eds), Plenum Press, New York, pp. 61–98.
4. Rossmann, M. G., Arnold, E., Erickson, J. W. *et al.* (1985). Structure of a human common cold virus and functional relationship to other picornaviruses. *Nature*, **317**, 143–153.
5. Hogle, J. M., Chow, M. and Filman, D. J. (1985). Three-dimensional structure of poliovirus at 2.9 Å resolution. *Science*, **229**, 1358–1365.
6. Luo, M., Vriend, G., Kamer, G., Minor, I. *et al.* (1988). The atomic structure of Mengovirus at 3.0 Å resolution. *Science*, **235**, 182–191.
7. Acharaya, R., Fry, E., Stuart, D. I. *et al.* (1989). The three-dimensional structure of foot and mouth disease virus at 2.9 Å. *Nature*, **337**, 709–716.
8. Mendelsohn, C. L., Wimmer, E. and Racienello, V. R. (1989). Cellular receptor for poliovirus: molecular cloning, nucleotide sequence and expression of a new member of the immunoglobulin superfamily. *Cell*, **56**, 855–865.
9. Staunton, D. E., Merluzzi, V. J., Rothlein, R. *et al.* (1989). A cell adhesion molecule, ICAM-1, is the major surface receptor for rhinoviruses, *Cell*, **56**, 849–853.
10. Greve, J. M., Davis, G., Meyer, A. M. *et al.* (1989). The major human rhinovirus receptor is ICAM-1. *Cell*, **56**, 839–847.
11. Colonno, R. J., Condra, J. H., Mitzutani, S. *et al.* (1988). Evidence for the direct involvement of the rhinoviruses canyon in receptor binding. *Proc. Natl Acad. Sci. USA*, **85**, 5449–5453.

12. McKinlay, M. A., Dutko, F. J., Pevear, D. C. *et al.* (1990). Rational design of anti-picornavirus agents. In *New Aspects of Positive-Strand RNA Viruses*, M. A. Brinton and F. X. Heinz (eds), American Society for Microbiology, Washington, pp. 366–372.
13. Andries, K., Dewindt, B., Snoeks, J. *et al.* (1991). A comparative test of 15 compounds against all rhinoviruses as a basis for a more rational screening. *Antiviral Res.*, **16**, 213–225.
14. Andries, K., Dewindt, B., Snoeks, J. *et al.* (1990). Two groups of rhinoviruses revealed by a panel of antiviral compounds present sequence divergence and differential pathogenicity. *J. Virol.*, **64**, 1117–1123.
15. Andries, K., Dewindt, B., Snoeks, J. *et al.* (1992). In vitro activity of pirodavir (R 77975), a substituted phenoxypyridazinamine with broad-spectrum anti-picornaviral activity. *Antimicrob. Agents Chemother.*, **36**, 100–107.
16. Koch, F. and Koch, G. (1985). The replication of polioviruses. In *The Molecular Biology of Polioviruses*, F. Koch and G. Koch (eds), Springer-Verlag, Vienna, pp. 203–266.
17. Eggers, H. J. (1987). Assay systems: testing of antiviral drugs in cell culture (in vitro). In *Antiviral Drug Development: A Multidisciplinary Approach*, E. De Clercq and R. T. Walker (eds), Plenum Press, New York, pp. 139–148.
18. Phillpotts, R. J., Davies, H. W., Willmann, J. *et al.* (1984). Pharmacokinetics of intranasally applied medication during a cold. *Antiviral Res.*, **4**, 71–74.
19. Barrow, G. I., Higgins, P. G., Tyrrell, D. A. J. and Andries, K. (1990). An appraisal of the efficacy of the antiviral R 61837 in rhinovirus infections in human volunteers. *Antiviral Chem. Chemother.*, **1**, 279–285.
20. Eggers, H. J., Koch, M. A., Furst, A. *et al.* (1970). Rhodanine: a selective inhibitor of the multiplication of echovirus 12. *Science*, **167**, 294–297.
21. Lonberg-Holm, K. and Noble-Harvey, J. (1973). Comparison of in vitro and cell-mediated alteration of a human rhinovirus and its inhibition by sodium dodecyl sulfate. *J. Virol.*, **12**, 819–826.
22. Lonberg-Holm, K., Gosser, L. B. and Kauer, L. C. (1975). Early alteration of poliovirus in infected cells and its specific inhibition. *J. Gen. Virol.*, **27**, 329–342.
23. Ash, R. J., Parker, R. A., Hagan, A. C. and Mayer, G. D. (1979). RMI 15,731 (1-[5-tetradecycloxy-2-furanyl]-ethanone), a new antirhinovirus compound, *Antimicrob. Agents Chemother.*, **16**, 301–305.
24. Caliguiri, L. A., McSharry, J. J. and Lawrence, G. W. (1980). Effect of arildone on modifications of poliovirus in vitro. *Virology*, **105**, 86–93.
25. Bauer, D. J., Selway, J. W. T., Batchelor, J. F. *et al.* (1981). 4′,6-dichloroflavan (BW683C), a new anti-rhinovirus compound. *Nature*, **292**, 369–370.
26. Ishitsuka, H., Ninomiya, Y. N., Ohsawa, C. *et al.* (1982). Direct and specific inactivation of rhinovirus by chalcone Ro 09-410. *Antimicrob. Agents Chemother.*, **22**, 617–621.
27. Kenny, M. T., Dulworth, J. K., and Torney, H. L. (1985). In vitro and in vivo antipicornavirus activity of some phenoxy pyridinecarbonitriles. *Antimicrob. Agents Chemother.*, **28**, 745–750.
28. Kenny, M. T., Dulworth, J. K., Bargar, T. M. *et al.* (1986). In vitro antiviral activity of the 6-substituted 2-(3′,4′-dichlorophenoxy)-2*H*-pyrano[2,3-*b*]pyridines MDL 20,610, MDL 20,646 and MDL 20, 957. *Antimicrob. Agents Chemother.*, **30**, 516–518.
29. Otto, M. J., Fox, M. P., Fancher, M. J. *et al.* (1985). In vitro activity of WIN 51711, a new broad-spectrum antipicornavirus drug. *Antimicrob. Agents Chemother.*, **27**, 883–886.
30. Andries, K., Dewindt, B., De Brabander, M. *et al.* (1988). In vitro activity of R 61837, a new antirhinovirus compound. *Arch. Virol.*, **101**, 155–167.

31. Woods, M. G., Diana, G. D., Rogge, M. C. *et al.* (1989). In vitro and in vivo activities of WIN 54954, a new broad-spectrum antipicornavirus drug. *Antimicrob. Agents Chemother.*, **33**, 2069–2074.
32. Conti, C., Orsi, N. and Stein, M. L. (1988). Effect of isoflavans and isoflavenes on rhinovirus 1B and its replication in HeLa cells. *Antiviral Res.*, **10**, 117–127.
33. Ninomiya, Y., Shimma, N. and Ishitsuka, H. (1990). Comparative studies on the antirhinovirus activity and the mode of action of the rhinovirus capsid binding agents, chalcone amides. *Antiviral Res.*, **13**, 61–74.
34. Ishitsuka, H., Ninomiya, Y. N. and Suhura, Y. (1986). Molecular basis of drug resistance to new antiviral agents. *J. Antimicrob. Chemother.*, **18** (Suppl. B), 11–18.
35. Kenny, M. T., Torney, H. L. and Dulworth, J. K. (1988). Mechanism of action of the antiviral compound MDL 20,610. *Antiviral Res.*, **9**, 249–261.
36. Tisdale, M. and Selway, J. W. T. (1984). Effect of dichloroflavan (BW683C) on the stability and uncoating of rhinovirus type 1B. *J. Antimicrob. Chemother.*, **14** (Suppl. A), 97–105.
37. Andries, K., Dewindt, B., Snoeks, J. and Willebrords, R. (1989). Lack of quantitative correlation between inhibition of replication of rhinoviruses by an antiviral drug and their stabilization. *Arch. Virol.*, **106**, 51–61.
38. Ahmad, A. L. M., Dowsett, A. B. and Tyrrell, D. A. J. (1987). Studies of rhinovirus resistant to an antiviral chalcone. *Antiviral Res.*, **8**, 27–39.
39. Smith, T. J., Kremer, M. J., Lou, M. *et al.* (1986). The site of attachment in human rhinovirus 14 for antiviral agents that inhibit uncoating. *Science*, **233**, 1286–1293.
40. Badger, G., Minor, I., Kremer, M. *et al.* (1988). Structural analysis of a series of antiviral agents complexed with human rhinovirus 14. *Proc. Natl Acad. Sci. USA*, **85**, 3304–3308.
41. Rossmann, M. G. (1990). Neutralizing rhinoviruses with antiviral agents that inhibit attachment and uncoating. In *Use of X-Ray Crystallography in the Design of Antiviral Agents*, W. G. Laver and G. M. Air (eds), Academic Press, New York, pp. 115–137.
42. Pevear, D. C., Fancher, M. J., Felock, P. J. *et al.* (1989). Conformational change in the floor of the human rhinovirus canyon blocks adsorption to HeLa cell receptors. *J. Virol.*, **63**, 2002–2007.
43. Kim, S., Smith, T. J., Chapman, M. S. *et al.* (1989). The crystal structure of human rhinovirus serotype 1A (HRV1A). *J. Mol. Biol.*, **210**, 91–111.
44. Chapman, M. S., Minor, I., Rossmann, M. G. *et al.* (1991). Human rhinovirus 14 complexed with antiviral compound R 61837. *J. Mol. Biol.*, **217**, 454–463.
45. Fox, M. P., Otto, M. J. and McKinlay, M. A. (1986). Prevention of rhinovirus and poliovirus uncoating by WIN 51711, a new antiviral drug. *Antimicrob. Agents Chemother.*, **30**, 110–116.
46. Rosenwirth, B. and Eggers, H. J. (1979). Early processes of echovirus 12-infection: elution, penetration and uncoating under the influence of rhodanine. *Virology*, **97**, 241–255.
47. Ninomiya, Y., Ohsawa, C., Aoyama, M. *et al.* (1984). Antivirus agent, Ro-09-410, binds to rhinovirus specifically and stabilizes the virus conformation. *Virology*, **134**, 269–276.
48. Madshus, I. G., Olsnes, S. and Sandvig, K. (1984). Different pH requirements for entry of two picornaviruses, human rhinovirus 2 and murine encephalomyocarditis virus. *Virology*, **139**, 346–357.
49. Ninomiya, Y., Aoyama, M., Umeda, I. *et al.* (1985). Comparative studies on the modes of action of the antirhinovirus agents, Ro 09-410, Ro 09-0179, RMI-15,731, 4′,6-dichloroflavan, and enviroxime. *Antimicrob. Agents Chemother.*, **34**, 595–599.
50. Gruenberger, M., Pevear, D., Diana, G. D. *et al.* (1991). Stabilization of human rhinovirus serotype 2 against pH-induced conformational change by antiviral compounds. *J. Gen. Virol.*, **72**, 431–433.

51. Andries, K., Dewindt, B., Van Eemeren, K. *et al.* (1992). Differential effects of capsid-binding antivirals on the adsorption of rhinoviruses. Abstr. International Conference on Antiviral Research, Vancouver, Canada, *Antiviral Res.*, **S** (1), 137.
52. Schrom, M., Laffin, J. A., Evans, B. *et al.* (1982). Isolation of poliovirus variants resistant and dependent on arildone. *Virology*, **122**, 492–497.
53. Heinz, A. H., Shepard, D. A. and Rueckert, R. R. (1990). Escape mutant analysis of a drug-binding site can be used to map functions in the rhinovirus capsid. In *Use of X-Ray Crystallography in the Design of Antiviral Agents*, W.G. Laver and G. M. Air (eds), Academic Press, New York, pp. 173–186.
54. Rombaut, B., Andries, K. and Boeyé, A. (1991). A comparison of WIN 51711 and R 78206 as stabilizers of poliovirus virions and procapsids. *J. Gen. Virol.*, **72**, 2153–2157.
55. Abraham, G. and Colonno, R. J. J. (1984). Many rhinovirus serotypes share the same cellular receptor. *Virology*, **51**, 340–345.
56. Unchapher, C. R., DeWitt, C. M. and Colonno, R. J. (1991). The major and minor receptor families contain all but one human rhinovirus serotype. *Virology*, **180**, 814–817.
57. Tisdale, M. and Selway, J. W. T. (1983). Inhibition of an early stage of rhinovirus replication by dichloroflavan (BW683C). *J. Gen. Virol.*, **64**, 795–803.
58. Eggers, H. J., Bode, D. and Brown, D. T. (1979). Cytoplasmic localization of the uncoating of picornaviruses. *Virology*, **92**, 211–218.
59. Bauer, D. J. and Selway, J. W. T. (1983). A novel method for detecting the antiviral activity of flavans in their vapour phase. *Antiviral Res.*, **3**, 235–239.
60. Binder, D., Noe, C. R. and Holzer, W. (1985). Thiophenanaloga antiviraler flavane. *Arch. Pharm. (Weinheim)*, **318**, 70–78.
61. Superti, F., Seganti, L., Orsi, N. *et al.* (1989). Effect of isoflavans and isoflavenes on the infection of Frp/3 cells by hepatitis A virus. *Antiviral Res.*, **11**, 247–254.
62. Bargar, T. M., Dulworth, J. K., Kenny, M. T. *et al.* (1986). 3,4-dihydro-2-phenyl-2*H*-pyrano[2,3-*b*]pyridines with potent antirhinovirus activity. *J. Med. Chem.*, **29**, 1590–1595.
63. Kenny, M. T., Dulworth, J. K., Bargar, T. M. and Daniel, J. K. (1987). Antipicornavirus activity of some diaryl methanes and aralkylaminopyridines. *Antiviral Res.*, **7**, 87–97.
64. Gonzales, M. E., Almena, M. J., Yacout, M. and Carrasco, L. (1990). 6-(3,4–Dichlorophenoxy)-3-(ethylthio)-2-pyridincarbonitrile inhibits poliovirus uncoating. *Antimicrob. Agents Chemother.*, **34**, 1259–1261.
65. Diana, G. D., Otto, M. J. and McKinlay, M. A. (1986). Inhibitors of picornavirus uncoating as antiviral agents. *Pharmacol. Ther.*, **29**, 287–297.
66. Langford, M. P., Carr, D. J. J. and Yin-Murphy, M. (1985). Activity of arildone with or without interferon against acute hemorrhagic conjunctivitis viruses in cell culture. *Antimicrob. Agents Chemother.*, **28**, 578–580.
67. McSharry, J. J., Caliguiri, L. A. and Eggers, H. J. (1979). Inhibition of uncoating of poliovirus by arildone, a new antiviral drug. *Virology*, **97**, 307–315.
68. Abe, S., Yamaki, A., Doi, Y. and Yoshioka, I. (1987). Effects of arildone on the immunogenicity of formalin-inactivated polioviruses. *Jpn. J. Med. Sci. Biol.*, **40**, 1–13.
69. Diana, G. D., McKinlay, M. A., Otto, M. J. *et al.* (1985). [[(4,5-Dihydro-2-oxazolyl)phenoxy]alkyl]isoxazoles: inhibitors of picornavirus uncoating. *J. Med. Chem.*, **28**, 1906–1910.
70. Zeichhardt, H., Otto, M. J., McKinlay, M. A. *et al.* (1987). Inhibition of poliovirus uncoating by disoxaril (WIN 51711). *Virology*, **160**, 281–285.
71. Rombaut, B., Brioen, P. and Boeyé, A. (1990). Disoxaril stabilization and immunogenicity of poliovirus procapsids. *J. Gen. Virol.*, **71**, 1081–1086.
72. Fox, M. P., McKinlay, M. A., Diana, G. D. and Dutko, F. J. (1991). Binding affin-

ities of structurally related human rhinovirus capsid-binding compounds are related to their activities against human rhinovirus type 14. *Antimicrob. Agents Chemother.*, **35**, 1040–1047.
73. Diana, G. D., Cutcliffe, D., Oglesby, R. C. *et al.* (1989). Synthesis and structure–activity studies of some disubstituted phenylisoxazoles against human picornaviruses. *J. Med. Chem.*, **32**, 450–455.
74. Baright, D. E., Dutko, F. J., Kernozek, T. H. *et al.* (1990). In vitro activity of WIN 54954 against 115 clinical isolates of echovirus and type B coxsackievirus. *Abstr. ICAAC*, 613.
75. Al-Nakib, W., Higgins, P. G., Barrow, G. I. *et al.* (1989). Suppression of colds in human volunteers challenged with rhinovirus by a new synthetic drug (R61837). *Antimicrob. Agents Chemother.*, **33**, 522–525.
76. Moeremans, M., De Raeymaeker, M., Daneels, G. *et al.* (1992). Study of the binding parameters of R 61837 to HRV9 and immunobiochemical evidence for a capsid stabilizing activity of the compound. *Antimicrob. Agents Chemother.*, **36**, 417–424.
77. González, M. E., Martínez-Abarca, F. and Carrasco, L. (1990). Flavonoids: potent inhibitors of poliovirus RNA synthesis. *Antiviral Chem. Chemother.*, **1**, 203–209.
78. Lopez Pila, J. M., Kopecka, H. and Vanden Berghe, D. (1989). Lack of evidence for strand-specific inhibition of poliovirus RNA synthesis by 3-methylquercetin. *Antiviral Res.*, **11**, 47–54.
79. Rightsel, W. A., Dice, J. R., McAlpine, R. J. *et al.* (1961). Antiviral effect of guanidine. *Science*, **134**, 558–559.
80. Tershak, D. R. (1982). Inhibition of poliovirus polymerase by guanidine in vitro. *J. Virol.*, **41**, 313–318.
81. Pincus, S. E. and Wimmer, E. (1986). Production of guanidine-resistant and -dependent poliovirus mutants from cloned cDNA: mutations in polypeptide 2C are directly responsible for altered guanidine sensitivity. *J. Virol.*, **60**, 793–796.
82. Eggers, H. J. (1982). Benzimidazoles. In *Chemotherapy of Viral Infections*, P. E. Came and L. A. Caliguiri (eds), Springer-Verlag, Berlin.
83. Schleider, J. B., Aquino, F., Rueter, A. *et al.* (1972). Antiviral activity in tissue culture systems of bis-benzimidazoles, potent inhibitors of rhinoviruses. *Appl. Microbiol.*, **23**, 113–116.
84. DeLong, D. C. (1984). Effect of enviroxime on rhinovirus infections in humans. In *Microbiology*, L. Leive and D. Schessinger (eds), American Society for Microbiology, Washington, DC.
85. Wikel, J. H., Paget, C. J., Delong, D. C. *et al.* (1980). Synthesis of syn and anti isomers of 6-[[(hydroxyimino)phenyl]methyl]-1-[(methylethyl)-sulfonyl]-1*H*-benzimidazol-2-amine. *J. Med. Chem.*, **23**, 363–372.
86. Anonymous (1984). Enviroxime. *Drugs of the Future*, **9**, 221–222.
87. Castrillo, J. L., Vanden Berghe, D. and Carrasco, L. (1986). 3-Methyl-quercetin is a potent and selective inhibitor of poliovirus RNA synthesis. *Virology*, **152**, 219–227.
88. Ishitsuka, H., Ohsawa, C., Ohiwa, T. *et al.* (1982). Antipicornavirus flavone Ro 09-0179. *Antimicrob. Agents Chemother.*, **22**, 611–616.
89. De Meyer, N., Haemers, A., Mishra, L. *et al.* (1991). 4′-Hydroxy-3-methoxyflavones with potent antipicornavirus activity. *J. Med. Chem.*, **34**, 736–746.
90. Andries, K. Unpublished observations.
91. Zerial, A., Werner, G. H., Phillpotts, R. J. *et al.* (1985). Studies on 44 081 R.P., a new antirhinovirus compound, in cell cultures and in volunteers. *Antimicrob. Agents Chemother.*, **27**, 846–850.
92. Alarcon, B., Zerial, A., Dupiol, C. and Carrasco, L. (1986). Antirhinovirus com-

pound 44 081 R.P. inhibits virus uncoating. *Antimicrob. Agents Chemother.*, **30**, 31–34.
93. Torney, H. L., Dulworth, J. K. and Steward, D. L. (1982). Antiviral activity and mechanism of action of 2-(3,4-dichlorophenoxy)-5-nitrobenzonitrile (MDL 860). *Antimicrob. Agents Chemother.*, **22**, 635–638.
94. Powers, R. D., Gwaltney, J. M. and Hayden, F. G. (1982). Activity of 2-(3,4-dichlorophenoxy)-5-nitrobenzonitrile (MDL-860) against picornaviruses in vitro. *Antimicrob. Agents Chemother.*, **22**, 639–642.
95. De Clercq, E., Bernaerts, R., Bergstrom, D. E. *et al.* (1986). Antirhinovirus activity of purine nucleoside analogs. *Antimicrob. Agents Chemother.*, **29**, 482–487.
96. Kamono, Y., Satoh, N., Nakayoshi, H. *et al.* (1988). Rhinovirus inhibition by bufadienolides. *Chem. Pharm. Bull.*, **36**, 326–332.
97. Korant, B. D. and Butterworth, B. E. (1976). Inhibition by zinc of rhinovirus protein cleavage: interaction of zinc with capsid polypeptides. *J. Virol.*, **18**, 298–306.
98. Geist, F. C., Bateman, J. A. and Hayden, F. (1987). In vitro activity of zinc salts against human rhinoviruses. *Antimicrob. Agents Chemother.*, **31**, 622–624.
99. Merluzzi, V. C., Cipriano, D., McNeil, D. *et al.* (1989). Evaluation of zinc complexes on the replication of rhinovirus 2 in vitro. *Res. Commun. Chem. Pathol. Pharmacol.*, **66**, 425–440.
100. Crump, C. E., Rollins, B. S. and Hayden, F. G. (1990). In vitro antiviral activity and cytotoxicity of aspirin: lack of selective activity against influenza A virus or rhinovirus. *Antiviral Chem. Chemother.*, **1**, 217–221.
101. Ahmad, A. L. M. and Tyrrell, D. A. J. (1986). Synergism between antirhinovirus antivirals: various human interferons and a number of synthetic compounds. *Antiviral Res.*, **6**, 241–252.
102. Al-Nakib, W. and Tyrrell, D. A. J. (1987). A 'new' generation of more potent synthetic antirhinovirus compounds: comparison of their MICs and their synergistic interactions. *Antiviral Res.*, **8**, 179–188.
103. Domingo, E., Martinez-Salas, E., Sobrino, F. *et al.* (1985). The quasi-species extremely heterogeneous nature of RNA genome populations: biological relevance: a review. *Gene*, **40**, 1–8.
104. Yasin, S. R., Al-Nakib, W. and Tyrrell, D. A. J. (1990). Isolation and preliminary characterization of chalcone Ro 09-410-resistant human rhinovirus type 2. *Antiviral Chem. Chemother.*, **1**, 149–154.
105. Dearden, C., Al-Nakib, W., Andries, K. *et al.* (1989). Drug resistant rhinoviruses from the nose of experimentally treated volunteers. *Arch. Virol.*, **109**, 71–81.
106. Heinz, B. A., Rueckert, R. R., Shepard, D. A. *et al.* (1989). Genetic and molecular analyses of spontaneous mutants of human rhinovirus 14 that are resistant to an antiviral compound. *J. Virol.*, **63**, 2476–2485.
107. Yasin, S. R., Al-Nakib, W. and Tyrrell, D. A. J. (1990). Pathogenicity for humans of human rhinovirus type 2 mutants resistant to and dependent on chalcone Ro 09-0410. *Antimicrob. Agents Chemother.*, **34**, 963–966.
108. Almela M. J., Gonzalez, M. E. and Carrasco, L. (1991). Inhibitors of poliovirus uncoating efficiently block the early membrane permeabilization induced by virus particles. *J. Virol.*, **65**, 2572–2577.
109. Eggers, H. J. and Tamm, I. (1961). 2-(α-Hydroxybenzyl)-benzimidazole (HBB) as an aid in virus classification. *Virology*, **13**, 545–546.

11 Clinical Studies of Antiviral Agents for Picornaviral Infections

EURICO ARRUDA and FREDERICK G. HAYDEN
University of Virginia Health Sciences Center, Charlottesville, Virginia, USA

INTRODUCTION

IMPACT OF PICORNAVIRAL INFECTIONS

Human rhinoviruses (HRV) and enteroviruses are among the most frequent causative agents of human infections. Rhinoviruses are the most frequent cause of common colds and probably the most common aetiological agent of acute infections in humans (1). Enteroviruses, which are also extremely frequent worldwide, can cause a broad spectrum of clinical syndromes, including severe ones, such as paralytic poliomyelitis, meningitis, encephalitis and myocarditis (2).

The term 'common cold' refers to a clinical syndrome of self-limited upper respiratory illness with symptoms of runny nose, nasal stuffiness, sneezing, sore throat and cough. Colds and their complications account for approximately one-fifth of all acute illnesses that are associated with restricted activity (3); they constitute the leading cause of acute morbidity and medical visits in the United States, where their incidence has not varied much in the past 60 years (4). Hundreds of millions of days of restricted activity, tens of millions of days absent from school or work, and the direct costs of physician visits, symptomatic medications and antibiotics contribute to the economic impact of colds (5). In the United Kingdom, approximately one-third of days taken off work are attributable to colds (4). Rhinoviruses, a genus of the Picornaviridae family, comprise over 100 different serotypes and account for 30–50% of colds in temperate climates. These viruses are also frequently documented as causes of acute respiratory illness in tropical areas of the non-developed world (6).

The enteroviruses comprise another genus of the family Picornaviridae, which includes polioviruses 1–3, coxsackieviruses A (23 types) and B (six types), echoviruses (31 types) and numbered enteroviruses 68–71. While the majority of enteroviral infections are asymptomatic, a proportion of the infections result in various clinical manifestations, which depend on the

Antiviral Chemotherapy. Edited by D.J. Jeffries and E. De Clercq

virus type and host susceptibility. The principal clinical syndromes caused by enteroviruses include poliomyelitis, meningitis, encephalitis, pleurodynia, herpangina, hand, foot and mouth disease, conjunctivitis, myopericarditis, neonatal diseases including fatal disseminated infection, upper respiratory illnesses and febrile illnesses with or without exanthems (2).

RATIONALE AND GOALS OF ANTIVIRAL USE

No specific antiviral agents are currently available for the control of rhinovirus infections. Early studies with intranasal administration of monotypic inactivated vaccine found that significantly fewer vaccinated individuals became ill after challenge with the homotypic virus (7). However, the large number of rhinovirus serotypes has been an obstacle for the development of a polyvalent vaccine. Two vaccines, each including 10 serotypes (8), failed to elicit response to more than 40% of the vaccinal serotypes, and heterotypic antibody responses were observed to a limited extent. This finding and the heterotypic antibody response elicited in animals immunized with synthetic peptides identical to rhinoviral epitopes (9,10) keep open the possibility of vaccine development.

Other possible methods for preventing HRV infection are by antiviral chemoprophylaxis, which has been achieved with intranasal application of interferons (reviewed in reference 11), and by interruption of HRV spread from person to person (reviewed in reference 12). The latter approach depends in part on the importance of the hand-contamination, self-inoculation mode of transmission, as contrasted with airborne spread, under natural conditions and on the development of practical ways of avoiding hand contamination (12). For example, virucidal hand treatments containing iodine have been used to reduce secondary illness in household contacts (12,13), and training of asthmatic children to reduce self-inoculatory behaviour has been associated with decreased frequency of respiratory illnesses (14).

The goals of chemotherapy as a means of reducing the impact of rhinovirus-induced colds include reduction of symptoms, improvement of the affected individual's functional activity, prevention of complications, such as otitis media, sinusitis, exacerbation of asthma or chronic lung disease, and reduction of spread of infection to contacts. Very few studies of symptomatic therapies or antiviral agents in natural colds have attempted to assess the effects of the intervention on complication rates or secondary illnesses in contacts (5). Importantly, it remains unclear how close is the linkage between ongoing viral replication, which can extend up to three weeks after onset of infection (15), and symptom expression. To the present none of the tested antiviral agents has been sufficiently potent to rapidly terminate viral replication in humans, so that the potential value of antiviral chemotherapy is uncertain in established rhinovirus colds.

In addition, important aspects of the pathogenesis of rhinovirus colds remain incompletely understood. The events that lead to the symptoms of cold upon infection of the upper respiratory tract, as well as the precise localization of the viral replication in the respiratory mucosa, are not defined. The modest evidence of nasal epithelial damage following infection of volunteers (16) suggests that the symptoms of colds are not solely a consequence of epithelial destruction. In addition, high concentrations of bradykinin and lysilbradykinin are found in the nasal secretions of persons with experimental (17) and natural colds (18). Upper respiratory symptoms occur in a dose-dependent manner following intranasal application of bradykinin (19) and other inflammatory substances like histamine and certain prostaglandins (20). These findings have led to the hypothesis that the symptoms of cold are not a direct consequence of epithelial destruction but rather of the release of host inflammatory mediators and sensitization of neurogenic reflexes triggered by the infection of a restricted number of cells. These responses lead to the vasodilation, tissue oedema, plasma transudation, sneezing and local discomfort associated with colds. This hypothesis provides part of the rationale for trials of combinations of antiviral compounds and anti-inflammatory agents (21).

Except for poliovirus vaccines, which have significantly reduced the impact of poliomyelitis worldwide, there are no general methods other than improved sanitation for the prevention of enteroviral infections (2). For these frequent infections, and particularly for their most serious manifestations, such as disseminated disease of the newborn, myocarditis and meningoencephalitis, chemoprophylaxis and chemotherapy have a great potential to impact on their morbidity and mortality. Studies of the more recently described capsid binders have produced encouraging results against enteroviral infections in animal models (22–25) and have culminated recently in a successful study of WIN 59954 in an experimental human model of coxsackievirus A21 infection (26). However, the theoretical issues discussed above for HRV infections, the requirements for systemic drug administration and effective delivery to sites of viral replication, and practical limitations including rapid identification of enteroviral infections need to be resolved before antiviral agents can be used effectively for these infections.

IN VIVO TESTING OF CANDIDATE COMPOUNDS

Picornaviruses have been included as part of empirical screening programmes for antiviral activity of newly discovered compounds since the early 1960s, and many compounds have been identified with *in vitro* antirhinoviral and/or anti-enteroviral activity (27). Since rational drug design became an alternative to empirical screening, with X-ray crystallographic studies of the virion and expression of virus-specific proteins (28), the search for new anti-picornaviral agents has intensified. Both this approach (29) and more traditional structure–biological activity studies (30,31) have led to the identification of capsid binders with potent anti-picornaviral activity.

One limitation in the development of anti-rhinoviral agents has been the paucity of relevant animal models. Chimpanzees possess receptors for the major receptor group of rhinoviruses described below, and their cells are able to support viral replication. Chimpanzees can be experimentally infected with human rhinoviruses after intranasal inoculation, but they do not develop measurable illness and are difficult to work with (32,33). Similar circumstances exist for experimental infections in gibbons (34). An immunosuppressed mouse model employing a highly adapted human rhinovirus has also been described (35). Fortunately, several experimental human models of rhinoviral infection involving direct intranasal or conjunctival (15,36,37) viral challenge or exposure methods that mimic natural routes of transmission have been described (38–40). These studies have used multiple different rhinovirus serotypes and result in reproducible rates of infection, determined by virus recovery from nasal secretions and by serology, and illness. In addition, the relative ease of confirming the rhinoviral aetiology of illnesses in studies of naturally acquired colds have provided favourable conditions for the testing of a number of candidate anti-rhinoviral agents in humans.

This contrasts with the circumstances in enteroviral infections. A number of animal models exist which employ different species and which include various enterovirus-induced syndromes like myocarditis, central nervous system disease and diabetes (41). These models have been used extensively in the testing of candidate antiviral agents (25,42–45). In addition, a rodent model of human poliovirus infection has recently been developed by expressing the cellular receptor in transgenic mice (46). However, aside from early studies with attenuated polioviruses, only few human models of enteroviral infection have been well characterized (26,47). One involves intranasal inoculation of coxsackievirus A21, which results in respiratory illness and shedding of virus in nasal secretions (26), and another employs oral administration of echovirus 12, which results in gastrointestinal shedding of virus but negligible illness (47). In addition, naturally occurring enteroviral infections are not usually promptly diagnosed owing to the protean array of clinical symptoms and practical difficulties associated with the identification of the causative agent. This has resulted in a virtual lack of clinical studies testing anti-picornaviral agents against enteroviral infections, despite the promise held by some more recently discovered compounds (48).

The remaining sections of this chapter review specific anti-picornaviral compounds that have been tested in clinical studies. As discussed in earlier reviews (5,11,21,27,49–51), many of these agents have been abandoned because of lack of efficacy or problems with toxicity. This chapter will summarize earlier findings and focus on compounds which have received recent testing. While the results of recent trials are encouraging, it is clear that new agents or combinations of agents and improved methods of drug delivery will be needed for management of these difficult infections.

AGENTS THAT INTERFERE WITH THE VIRUS–RECEPTOR INTERACTION

The initial interaction between virus and host cells takes place when a viral attachment protein binds to a molecule on the cell surface acting as a viral receptor. The specificity of this event makes it an ideal target for agents that prevent cell infection (52), and the identification of viral receptors has provided reagents which enable interference with the receptor–virus interaction. Some of the best-characterized viral receptors are molecules of the immunoglobulin superfamily, among which are the receptors for major group rhinoviruses and poliovirus (53,54).

The cell receptor for the major HRV receptor group, which contains approximately 90% of the serotypes, has been identified as the glycoprotein intercellular adhesion molecule 1 (ICAM-1) (55–57). The same molecule functions as cell receptor for some enteroviruses, such as coxsackieviruses A13, A18 and A21 (58). ICAM-1 is a member of the immunoglobulin superfamily, which functions as ligand for lymphocyte function-associated antigen 1 (LFA-1), and consists of five extracellular immunoglobulin-like domains, a transmembrane anchor and an intracytoplasmic domain. Computer modelling suggests that the N-terminal end of the more distal extracellular domain of ICAM-1 interacts with amino acids located at the bottom of the canyon which exists around the five-fold vertexes of the HRV capsid (59). The cell receptors for the minor HRV receptor group belong to the human low-density lipoprotein receptor (LDLR) family (60). Cell receptors have also been identified for poliovirus (61), echovirus 1 (62) and partially characterized for some B coxsackieviruses (54). Poliovirus receptor has been identified as another member of the immunoglobulin superfamily which is probably also important for cell–cell interaction (61). This receptor has only three extracellular domains. The receptor for echovirus 1 in HeLa cells has been recently identified as the integrin VLA-2 ($\alpha 2\beta 1$), a molecule which physiologically functions as an adhesion receptor promoting interaction between cells and with extracellular matrix (62).

ANTI-RECEPTOR ANTIBODY

Murine monoclonal antibody has been developed to HRV major group receptor which blocks the infection of susceptible cells *in vitro* (58,63). This murine antibody was found to be able to protect chimpanzees from infection by human rhinovirus (64). Chimpanzees treated with anti-HRV receptor monoclonal antibody (1.25 mg/ml) failed to develop an immune response upon challenge with HRV-15, while placebo-treated animals had the expected humoral immune response (64).

Two placebo-controlled pilot studies have assessed the prophylactic effectiveness of different dosages of rhinovirus receptor murine monoclonal antibody administered intranasally to volunteers (65). In the first study, a dose of 0.135 mg per subject over nine applications beginning 17 h before and continuing for 48 h after challenge was ineffective in altering viral replication or symptom production. In contrast, a dose of 1 mg per subject in 10 applications beginning 3 h before and extending up to 36 h after infection modified the virological and clinical course of HRV infection without adverse effects. Although there was no overall reduction in the frequency of infection or illness, significant delays in the appearance of nasal symptoms and in the peak of viral shedding were observed. No adverse effects associated with antibody administration were found. These results suggested that the blockade of host cell receptors may offer a realistic approach to ameliorating HRV infections.

SOLUBLE RECEPTOR

Another method to interfere with virus–receptor interaction is the use of agents, such as soluble forms of the cellular receptor, which compete with the host cell receptor for binding to the receptor-binding site on the virus surface. Soluble forms of ICAM-1 (sICAM-1) have been synthesized by transfection of eukaryotic cells with cDNA that contains a stop codon at the extracellular domain to yield a truncated form of ICAM-1 (66,67). One such sICAM-1 has been shown to inhibit infection of cell lines and primary cultures of human adenoid epithelium by a number of HRV serotypes (68,69), probably by inhibiting viral attachment and/or entry. However, clinical studies have not been conducted to date. Likewise, poliovirus cell receptor expressed in transfected insect cells has been shown to block the infection of susceptible cells with poliovirus (70), but no clinical studies have been described. The development of *in vitro* resistance to the inhibitory effects of such soluble receptors, which has been described for poliovirus (71) and rhinovirus (72), is another issue that requires study.

AGENTS THAT BIND TO THE VIRUS CAPSID

Early events in HRV replication include attachment, penetration of the host cell and viral uncoating. These constitute essential steps in viral replication and are attractive targets for antiviral therapy, because they are potentially virus-specific while sparing the host cell. Early studies by Eggers (73,74) showed that rhodamine inhibits echovirus replication by preventing uncoating and stabilizing the viral particle. A variety of chemically unrelated capsid-binding molecules which bind to the hydrophobic β-barrel of VP1 of diverse picornaviruses have been identified (5,27,29–31,48) (see also Chapter 10 in this volume). Depending on the drug and particular virus serotype, some agents cause conformational changes that inhibit viral attachment and others cause capsid stabilization and prevent virus uncoating. A number of such compounds have shown *in vitro* activity against different serotypes of rhinoviruses and some enteroviruses (30,44,75,76). However, considerable serotype-dependent variation in the inhibitory activity of such compounds has been observed (76). In addition, drug-resistant variants with high or low levels of resistance can be readily obtained *in vitro* for many agents and display varying levels of cross-resistance to other capsid binders (77,78). The clinical significance of resistant mutants has received limited study to date. Although resistant viruses may replicate less effectively *in vitro* (79), their pathogenicity and transmissibility have been assessed in only one clinical trial (78).

The following paragraphs consider only the capsid binders which have been tested topically or orally against HRV infection in humans. Table 11.1 summarizes efficacy data on capsid binders in the prevention of experimental HRV infections. The structures of the three capsid binders most recently tested in clinical studies are represented in Figure 11.1.

FLAVONOIDS

Flavonoids are among the most potent inhibitors of the replication of HRV and other picornaviruses *in vitro*. Some of the best-characterized flavonoids are 4′,6-dichloroflavan (BW683C) (88,89) and 4′,6-dicyanoflavan (90). Clinical studies have been conducted to assess the efficacy of BW683C in preventing experimentally induced colds (80,81). Prophylactic oral administration of BW683C, 1 mg/kg three times per day, did not protect volunteers against experimental infection with HRV-9 and resulted in no clinical or virological benefits (80). Plasma levels of BW683C were over four times the *in vitro* inhibitory concentration for the challenge virus 8 h after oral administration, but the drug was not detected in nasal washes. Because adequate antiviral levels were reportedly obtained after intranasal administration of BW683C (81), a subsequent study was conducted in which the compound was given intranasally 40 mg five times per day. However, topically applied BW683C also failed to reduce infection rates and did not protect volunteers, experimentally infected with HRV-9, against illness (81).

CHALCONES

The chalcones are synthetic compounds derived from a flavone originally isolated from a Chinese herb, *Agastasche folium*, which bind to the viral

Table 11.1. Summary of efficacy data on prevention of experimental picornavirus infection with capsid-binding agents

Compound (ref.) [virus serotype]	No. of subj.[a]	Route[b]	Dose (doses/day)	Duration[c]	Reduction relative to placebo[d] (%)[e]: Infection rate (% of subj.)	Virus shedding (% of days)	Colds (% of subj.)
4′,6-Dichloroflavan							
(80) [RV9]	63	PO	1 mg/kg (3)	−1/+4	0(−9)	0(NR)	0(21)
(81) [RV9]	49	IN	20 mg (5)	−1/+4	0(−7)	0(NR)	0(15)
Ro 09-0415 (82) [RV2]	57	PO	1.2 g (2)	−1/+5	0(13)	0(NR)	0(17)
Ro 09-0410 (83) [RV39]	50	IN	5 mg (5)	−1/+4	0(13)	0(NR)	0(−28)
RMI 15731 (84) [RV39]	24	IN	200 μg (5)	−1/+4	0(0)	0(16)	0(0)
WIN 54954 (85) [RV23]	25	PO	200 mg (3)	−1/+5	0(0)	0(NR)	0(−54)
[RV23]	45	PO	200 mg (3)	−1/+5	0(14)	0(NR)	+/0(53)
(26) [Cox A21]	50	PO	200 mg (3)	−1/+5	0(7)	+(22)[f]	+(83)
R61837 (86) [RV9]	55	IN	1 mg (6)	−1/+3	0(4)[g]	NR	0(3)
	50	IN	1 mg (6)	−4 h/+6	0(−7)	NR	+(71)
Pirodavir (87) [RV H]	25	IN	2 mg (6)	−3 h/+4	+(42)	+(65)	+(85)
	35	IN	2 mg (3)	−3 h/+6	0(16)	0(47)	0(−20)
	28	IN	2 mg (3)	−3 h/+5	0(2)	0(24)	0(−3)

[a] Total number in groups active and placebo challenged with virus.
[b] Route of administration: IN = intranasal spray, PO = oral.
[c] Timing of administration in days pre/post virus challenge.
[d] Symbols: +, statistically significant; +/0, trend; 0, not significant; NR = not reported.
[e] Percentage reduction was calculated as 100 × (frequency in the placebo group − frequency in the active group) + frequency in the placebo group. Negative value indicates higher proportion in the active group.
[f] Based on mean area under curve for virus positive days.
[g] In these studies only seroconversion was used as evidence of infection.

capsid (91,92) and have potent *in vitro* anti-rhinoviral activity (93–95). The first chalcone to be tested clinically was 5-ethoxy-3-methoxy-2-(*p*-methoxy-*trans*-cinnamoyl) phenylphosphate (Ro 09-0415), which functions as a prodrug for the original compound 4′-ethoxy-2′-hydroxy-4,6′-dimethoxychalcone (Ro 09-0410). Ro 09-0410 was poorly absorbed when given orally, while its derivative Ro 09-0415 was efficiently absorbed after oral administration and converted to Ro 09-0410 (82). Ro 09-0415 given orally (1200 mg twice daily for 15 h before and for an additional six days after challenge) was ineffective in preventing illness in humans experimentally infected with HRV-39 (82). Oral administration did not induce detectable drug levels in nasal washings despite adequate blood levels of both Ro 09-0415 (5–40 μg/ml) and Ro 09-0410 (0.51–1.43 μg/ml) (82). Intranasal administration of the parent compound Ro 09-0410 was also tested for prevention of experimentally induced colds with HRV-2 (83). In that study, intranasal administration of Ro 09-0410 2.5 mg per nostril five times per day during waking hours failed to protect against infection or illness and was associated with increased mucus production compared to placebo.

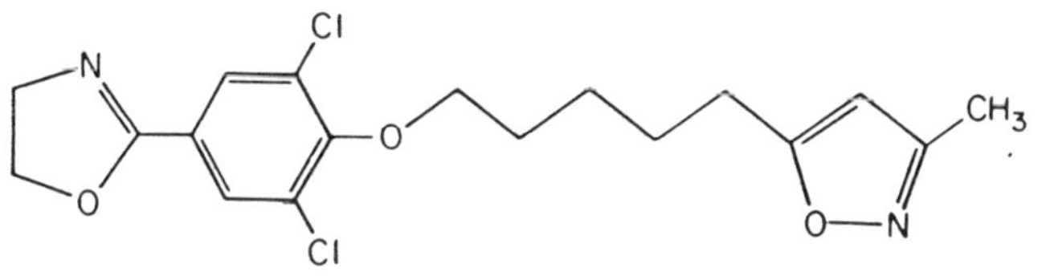

Win 54945

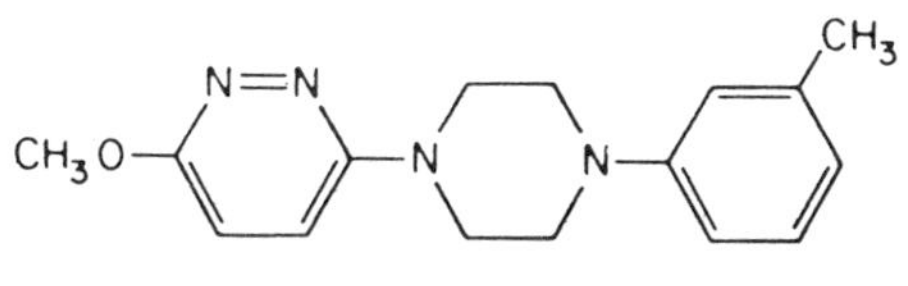

R61837

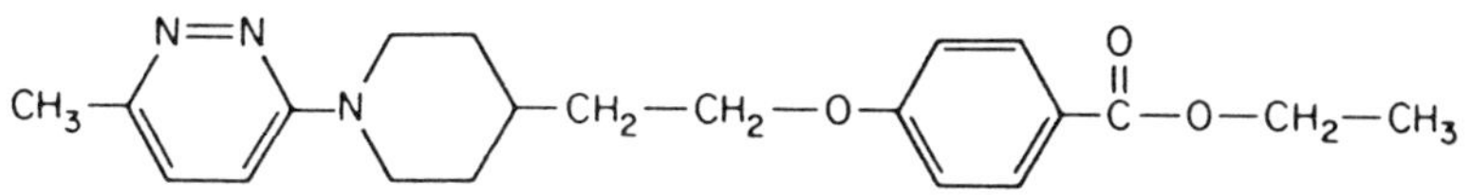

R77975

Figure 11.1. Structures of capsid binders

Clinical trials have compared the pathogenicity of HRV-2 selected for resistance with Ro 09-0410 *in vitro* with the parental wild-type virus (78). The minimal inhibitory concentration of the resistant strain was increased 16-fold after six *in vitro* passages. Volunteers were inoculated with approximately 2000 50% tissue culture infective doses ($TCID_{50}$) of wild-type, drug-resistant, or drug-dependent HRV-2. The proportion of volunteers developing laboratory evidence of infection was 92%, 27%, and 0, respectively. Although the resistant virus showed reduced infectivity for volunteers, the proportion of infected volunteers in the resistant group developing colds and the severity of the illnesses were not reduced compared to the group infected with wild-type virus. Also several isolates recovered from subjects infected with resistant virus remained resistant, a finding which suggested that the resistant phenotype was stable. Thus, the results of this study suggested that Ro 09-0410-resistant variants had reduced infectiousness without obvious loss of virulence compared with wild type.

RMI 15,731

RMI 15,731 (1-[5-tetradecycloxy-2-furanyl]-ethanone) is a rhinovirus-specific antiviral compound which inhibited 77% of 52 HRV serotypes tested *in vitro* (96). This compound administered intranasally (0.2 mg, five times per day) beginning 21 h before experimental rhinoviral infection failed to protect volunteers against illness (84).

WIN 54954

WIN 54954 is a methylisoxazole derivative with a broader anti-picornaviral spectrum than its predecessor disoxaril (WIN 51711) (25). In cell culture 80% of 52 HRV serotypes were inhibited at 0.28 μg/ml or less. When given orally to mice, the compound protected against lethal challenge with coxsackievirus A9 (50% protective dose, 2 mg/kg per day) or echovirus 9 (50% protective dose, 100 mg/kg per day) (25). This protection was associated with achieving trough blood concentrations of the compound that exceeded the *in vitro* inhibitory concentrations for the respective viruses.

In two randomized, double-blind, placebo-controlled studies, orally administered WIN 54954 was tested at a dose of 600 mg per day beginning one day before and continuing for five days after challenge. No significant antiviral or clinical effects were observed in the prevention of experimental infection with HRV-39 (85). In studies with RV23, a serotype which had 10-fold lower inhibitory concentrations *in vitro*, no significant antiviral effects but trends toward reduced illness frequency and severity were noted. On the last day of drug administration almost all WIN 54954 recipients had trough plasma levels of WIN 54954 greater than the minimal inhibitory concentration for the challenge virus. However, detectable levels of WIN 54954 were found in only a small fraction of the nasal wash samples collected at trough, and these levels were below the inhibitory concentration for either virus (85). These findings suggest that inability to reach sufficient drug levels in the nasal mucosa was the cause for the observed lack of efficacy.

Studies of the protective effect of disoxaril (24,42) and WIN 54954 (25,45) against infection with enteroviruses in mice found that these compounds possess a broad anti-picornaviral spectrum and therefore must be potentially useful in the therapy of human enteroviral infection. Efficacy studies in volunteers treated with WIN 54954 orally 600 mg three times per day beginning one day before and for five days after oral challenge with coxsackievirus A21 found that the compound reduced clinical illness attack rates with an efficacy of 83%, and that drug recipients experienced significantly milder disease and shed less virus compared with placebo recipients (26). The only drug-related adverse effects noted in these studies were morbilliform skin eruptions in a small number of subjects, possibly related to alcohol ingestion. This agent represents the first systemically administered synthetic antiviral which appears to provide protection in enteroviral infection in humans.

R 61837

R 61837 (3-methoxy-6[4-(methylphenyl)-1-piperazinyl]pyridazine) is a capsid binder which potently inhibits HRV replication *in vitro*. The minimal inhibitory concentrations ranged from 0.004 to 15 μg/ml against 43 different serotypes of HRV (97). R 61837 was the first capsid binder that was found to be effective in preventing the symptoms of experimental rhinovirus colds (86). In a prophylaxis study (86) R 61837 was administered by intranasal sprays in a hydroxy-β-cyclodextrin vehicle, beginning 4 h before challenge and continuing six times per day for a total of six days. R 61837 reduced the number of colds with an efficacy of 71%, and decreased both symptoms and nasal mucus production. However, it did not prevent laboratory evidence of infection following challenge with the highly sensitive HRV-9. A shorter duration of use for only four days was associated with breakthrough illness after cessation of drug administration.

Therapeutic administration starting shortly after the onset of symptoms and given up to 15 sprays per day for four days was ineffective and associated with increased nasal symptoms compared to placebo (86). Partial protection against illness was found in another study (98), in which R 61837 was initiated during the incubation period after viral challenge. This result suggests that it might be possible to use this approach for post-exposure prophylaxis of HRV infections.

This agent is also the first one for which *in vivo* emergence of resistant virus has been documented (99). Although of unknown clinical significance, approximately 30% of the 28 drug-exposed individuals in the first R 61837 study (86) shed resistant virus at some point during the study. Of the volunteers shedding resistant virus, most shed virus that showed low-level resistance (four- to eight-fold increase in inhibitory concentration), but at least one of the isolates recovered from one of the treated subjects was highly resistant to the compound, with a 100-fold increase in EC_{50} (99). This study did not directly address the ability of resistant virus to cause illness since all subjects were initially inoculated with sensitive virus. However, four of the volunteers had recovery of only resistant virus during the experiment. Interestingly, one volunteer initially shedding resistant virus later shed virus sensitive to R 61837, a finding which raises questions about the genetic stability of resistant variants and the ability of resistant virus to compete with wild type.

PIRODAVIR (R 77975)

Pirodavir is a substituted phenoxy-pyridazinamine with a broader antipicornaviral spectrum and approximately 500 times greater potency *in vitro* than its predecessor R 61837 (31). *In vitro* pirodavir inhibits the replication of 80% of the HRV serotypes at concentrations of 0.1 μg/ml or below (31). In one prophylaxis study with susceptible serotypes (50% inhibitory concentration < 0.01 μg/ml) pirodavir in a hydroxy-β-cyclodextrin vehicle administered intranasally six times per day reduced the frequency of clinical colds after experimental challenge with an efficacy of 85% and may have also reduced the frequency of infection (87). However, several volunteers with viral shedding after cessation of spray administration developed late-onset colds in the pirodavir group, and the optimal duration of administration remains to be determined. In contrast, two prophylaxis studies administering pirodavir in three daily doses did not find significant antiviral or clinical benefits (87). One small therapeutic study of pirodavir administered intranasally six times daily found no clinical evidence of benefit relative to placebo, despite a trend toward reduction of viral shedding in the treated group (87). Intranasal sprays of R 77975 were generally well tolerated but associated with a higher frequency of unpleasant taste probably related to clearance of the molecule through the posterior nasopharynx.

In summary, clinical trials have encountered differences between the *in vitro* and *in vivo* antiviral activities of capsid binders, and a number of capsid binders given topically or orally have been found to be ineffective in preventing experimental colds. This appears to relate to lack of potency and/or problems in drug delivery and achieving adequate levels in the respiratory epithelium and/or secretions (5,27,100). The fact that these agents exert antiviral activity through hydrophobic interactions with the virus capsid makes it difficult to administer adequate concentrations in an aqueous solution compatible with respiratory secretions. In the studies with R 61837 and R 77975, this was facilitated by using hydroxypropyl-β-cyclodextrin as a vehicle for these hydrophobic molecules and by frequent intranasal applications to overcome normal mucociliary clearance mechanisms. However, the use of such frequent intranasal applications is not practical for routine prophylaxis. This suggests that alternative formulations that may provide prolonged secretion concentrations need to be developed.

INTERFERON AND INTERFERON INDUCERS

In addition to stimulating local production of interferon (IFN) in the respiratory tract (101), HRV infection is associated with an activation of systemic cellular immune responses, with increased mitogen- and virus-stimulated *in vitro* production of interleukin 2 (IL-2) and interferon δ (IFN-δ) by peripheral mononuclear cells and with increased cytotoxicity mediated by natural killer cells (102). Spontaneous production of IFN by peripheral blood cells has not been observed (102), and only low titres of IFN have been detected in nasal washings of HRV-infected persons (101). Exogenously delivered natural and recombinant human IFNs have received comprehensive clinical testing for control of rhinovirus infections.

The first time exogenously administered IFN was used successfully to prevent experimental rhinovirus infection was in 1973 (103). A partially purified preparation of human leucocyte IFN-α was applied intranasally at a dose of 3.5 Mu per day in three daily doses, beginning one day before and continuing for three days after virus challenge. Significant reduction of symptoms and virus shedding was observed. Because sufficient quantities of purified human IFN were not readily available, efforts were then directed to the use of IFN inducers. A number of studies were conducted employing different compounds in the prophylaxis (104–110) and therapy (107) of experimental rhinoviral infections, but those studies in general met with little success as a consequence of different factors, including poor *in vivo* induction. The most convincing results were obtained with propanediamine, (*N*,*N*-dioctadecyl-*N'*,*N'*-bis(2-hydroxyethyl) which induced IFN in nasal washes and reduced viral shedding and illness occurrence after challenge with HRV-21 (105). It is unclear whether such molecules would have any clinical advantage with respect to efficacy or tolerability compared with exogenously administered IFN.

The subsequent availability of large amounts of natural and recombinant DNA-produced IFNs allowed for a large number of clinical studies of prophylaxis and therapy of rhinovirus infection employing different IFN preparations (reviewed in references 11,21,49–51). The results of representative clinical studies using IFN for prophylaxis and therapy of experimental and natural HRV infections are shown in Tables 11.2 and 11.3, respectively.

PROPHYLAXIS

Intranasally administered recombinant and leucocyte-derived IFN-α and recombinant IFN-β, but not IFN-γ, have been effective in the prophylaxis of experimental colds induced by HRVs. Efficacy is dependent on the IFN dose and duration of administration prior to challenge. Administration of high doses (over 20 Mu per day) of IFN-α beginning before challenge protects against laboratory evidence of infection and against illness, as determined by occurrence of colds in the volunteers and production of nasal mucus. Lower doses (2–10 Mu per day) of IFN-α were effective in preventing illness but allowed subclinical infection to occur (11,49). Consistent with the proposed induction of an antiviral state in host cells, the duration of the protection against HRV infection appears to be prolonged after topical IFN administration. This has allowed once-daily administration to be effective (50). In contrast, topical application of IFN-γ was associated with local intolerance and no significant protection (122).

The success obtained in the studies of prophylaxis of experimental HRV infection led to field studies designed to determine whether intranasal IFN would be effective in preventing natural HRV colds (Table 11.3). Intranasal rIFN-α2b was shown to be effective for seasonal prophylaxis of naturally acquired HRV infection. Protection against rhinovirus colds was observed at doses of 3–10 Mu per day, when administered as pre-exposure prophylaxis during peak periods of rhinovirus activity in the community. However, the prolonged periods of administration were not associated with reductions in overall respiratory illness occurrence, in part because of the high incidence of IFN-related nasal side-effects. Typically beginning during the second week of use, irritation was manifested by symptoms of nasal stuffiness, dryness, burning and bleeding, and signs of mucosal friability, erosion and sometimes overt ulcerations (11,49). Histopathological changes predominantly consisting of mononuclear cell infiltrates occurred early after initiating IFN exposure and appeared to precede the clinical manifestations (136,137). In general the side-effects were found to be dose and time dependent and resolved within days after stopping the administration (49). The minimal dose of IFN to prevent natural HRV infection (approximately 2–3 Mu per day) was also associated with an unacceptably high incidence of side-effects during long-term use (49,115). Another preparation, rIFN-β_{serine}, which appeared to be better tolerated at higher doses, was found to be less effective for prophylaxis of natural HRV infections (130).

Few studies have used IFN for the prevention of HRV colds in groups at increased risk of complications of common cold. Two studies using 2 Mu per day of rIFN-α2b for three four-week periods separated by one week in asthmatic individuals found no significant reductions in overall colds frequency or asthma symptoms (138,139), but the dose of IFN used in these trials may have been suboptimal.

One alternative to reduce the risk of nasal side-effects caused by prolonged administration has been short-term, post-exposure prophylaxis. This strategy was tested in household contacts of an index case with respiratory illness in several different trials (Table 11.3). Two studies found that intranasal IFN-α2b (5 Mu per day once daily for seven days) reduced the risk of rhinovirus colds by approximately 80–90% and total respiratory illnesses by about 40% in household contacts relative to placebo (132,133). The positive clinical and virological effects found in these studies demonstrated for the first time that intranasal delivery of antiviral agents could be used in the prevention of naturally occurring rhinovirus colds. In another study, lower doses (5 Mu once followed by 2.5 Mu once daily for four days) of IFN-α2b failed to prevent HRV-induced colds in a similar setting (135). This approach has not yet been tested in high-risk contacts.

Synergistic anti-rhinoviral effect has been demonstrated *in vitro* between human IFN-α and IFN-γ and various synthetic antiviral compounds (140). However, one clinical trial utilizing intranasal sprays of rIFN-α (0.72 Mu per day for four days) and of enviroxime (1.13 mg per day for six days) failed to demonstrate greater protection of volunteers from infection and illness induced by challenge with HRV-9 compared with the effects of IFN alone (141). Despite this negative result, the combined use of anti-picornaviral agents with different mechanisms of action offers the best likelihood of providing potent inhibition of rhinoviral replication *in vivo*. Possible advantages with regard to improved tolerance and reduced likelihood of resistance emergence also warrant study.

TREATMENT

Intranasal IFN has been generally ineffective in the therapy of established rhinovirus colds. Recombinant IFN-α2b (27 Mu per day) beginning 28 h after experimental rhinovirus infection or rIFN-β_{serine} (36 Mu per day) beginning 36 h after experimental infection reduced virus excretion but had only modest clinical benefits (49,50,123,124). In a placebo-controlled study, IFN-α2b (10 or 20 Mu per day for five days) also showed partial inhibition of viral replication but no clinical benefit or reductions in complications or secondary illness occurrence when used in the therapy of naturally occurring rhinovirus colds (142).

Based on the hypothesis that the symptoms of cold are induced by the release of inflammatory mediators triggered by rhinoviral infection of limited portions of the upper respiratory epithelium, a combination of IFN-α2 with drugs directed at the cold symptoms was tested in a double-blind, placebo-controlled study for therapy of experimental rhinovirus colds (143). In the active group, intranasal IFN-α2 (3 Mu three times per day) was administered in combination with an oral non-steroidal anti-inflammatory agent, naproxen (500 mg first dose, and 250 mg three times per day) and a

Table 11.2. Representative studies of intranasal IFNs for the prophylaxis and therapy of experimental rhinovirus infection

Virus serotype (ref.)	IFN type	No. of subj.[a]	Dose (Mu/day)	Doses/day (method)[b]	Duration[c]	Reduction relative to placebo[d] (%) [3]		
						Infection rate (% of subj.)	Virus shedding (% of days)	Colds (% of subj.)
Prophylaxis								
RV4 (103)	HuIFN-α (Le)	32	3.5	3(S)	−1/+3	+(76)	+(NR)	0(81)
RV9 (111)	HuIFN-α (Le)	19	22.5	3(S)	−1/+3	0(38)	+/0(40)	+(59)
(112)	rIFN-α2b	41	22.5	3(S)	−1/+3	+(51)	+(NR)	+(61)[f]
RV39 (113)	rIFN-α2b	24	45.5	4(D)	−1/+3	+(77)	+(82)	+/0(66)[f]
	rIFN-α2b	28	43	1(D)	−2/+3	+/0(46)	+(75)	+(75)
RV13 (114,115)	rIFN-α2a	26	10.0	2(S)	−0.5/+3	0(14)	+(42)	+(89)
	rIFN-α2a	32	2.4	2(S)	−0.5/+3	0(−1)	+/0(32)	+(60)
	rIFN-α2a	31	0.7	2(S)	−0.5/+3	0(1)	0(−8)	0(−6)
RV13 (116,117)	rIFN-α2b	21	10.0	2(S)	−1/+3	0(NR)	+/0(39)	+/0(−55)
	rIFN-α2b	21	2.0	2(S)	−1/+3	0(NR)	0(27)	0(−33)
	rIFN-α2b	28	2.0	2(S)	−7/+7	+(62)	+(87)	+(84)

RV9+14 (118)	rIFN-α2b	25	9.1	4(S)	−1/+3	0(22)	+(NR)	+(NR)[f]
	rIFN-α2b	20	2.3	1(S)	−1/+3	0(22)	+/0(NR)	+(NR)[f]
	rIFN-α2b	17	2.3	1(S)	−1.5/+2.5	0(0)	0(NR)	0(NR)
(119)	HuIFN-α(Ly)	42	8.1	3(S)	−1/+3	+(27)	+(NR)	+(NR)[f]
RV9+14 (120)	rIFN-βser	54	6	3(S)	−1/+3	0(24)	+(NR)	+/0(67)
(122)	rHuIFN-γ	34	2	3(S)	−1/+3	0(−7)	0(NR)	0(−29)
RVH+39 (121)	rIFN-βser	23	12	1(D)	−1.5/+5	0(9)	0(11)	+/0(61)
	rIFN-βser	22	3	1(D)	−1.5/+5	0(10)	0(4)	0(14)
Therapy								
RV39 (123)	rIFN-α2b	23	27	3(S)	+1/+5	0(17)	+(35)[g]	0(−14)
	rIFN-α2b	29	27	3(D)	+1/+5	0(14)	+(54)[g]	0(8)
(124)	2IFN-βser	40	36	3(D)	+1.5/+6	0(0)	+/0(26)	0(−8)
RV9 (125)	HuIFN-α	25	23	3(S)	+2/+6	0(NR)	0(NR)	0(NR)

[a] Total number in groups active and placebo challenged with virus.
[b] Method of administration: S = spray, D = drops.
[c] Timing of IFN administration in days pre/post virus challenge.
[d] Symbols: +, statistically significant; +/0, partial effect or trend; 0, not significant; NR = not reported. The determination of illness occurrence differed between studies.
[e] Percentage reduction was calculated as 100 × (frequency in the placebo group − frequency in the active group) + frequency in the placebo group. Negative value indicates higher proportion in the active group.
[f] This study found 100% efficacy in preventing definite colds.
[g] This study found significant reductions in nasal wash viral titres for active compared to placebo.

Table 11.3. Representative field studies of intranasal IFN spray for prophylaxis of naturally occurring respiratory illnesses in healthy adults

Year of study (ref.)	No. treated[a]	IFN				Reduction compared to placebo[b] (%)[c]		Nasal side-effects
		Type	Dosage (Mu/day)	Doses/day (method)[d]	Duration (weeks)	Rhinovirus colds	Respiratory illnesses	
Pre-exposure								
1982 (126)	304	rIFN-α2b	10.0	1(S)	3	+(100)	0(−47)[e]	++
1983 (127)	413	rIFN-α2b	2.0	2(S)	4	+(87)	0(−16)	+
1983 (128)	396	rIFN-α2b	3.0	2(S)	4	+(76)	0(0)	+
	150	rIFN-α2b	2.5	1(S)	4	+/0(59)	0(NR)	+
1984 (129)	300	rIFN-α2b	2.5	2(S)	4+4[f]	+(100)	0(NR)	+
	245	rIFN-α2b	1.7	2(S)	4+3[f]	+/0(29)	0(−57)[g]	+
1986 (130)	287	rIFN-βser	9.0	1(D)	4	+/0(52)	0(−7)	0
1987 (130)	363	rIFN-βser	24.0	1(D)	4	0(−19)	0(−3)	0
Post-exposure in families								
1983 (131)	337	rIFN-α2a	0.3 or 1.5	1(S)	5 days	0(37)	0(21)	0
1983 (132)	448	rIFN-α2b	5.0	1(S)	1	+(88)	+(39)	+
1984 (133)	644	rIFN-α2b	5.0	1(S)	1	+(68)[h]	+(41)	+
1983 (134)	419	rIFN-α2b	5.0	1(S)	1	+/0(52)	0(−2)	NR
1985 (135)	868	rIFN-α2b	5.0/2.5[i]	1(S)	5 days	0(−15)[j]	0(−37)	+/0

[a] Pre-exposure: total number in groups active and placebo. Post-exposure: total number of spraying episodes. [b] Symbols: +, statistically significant; +/0, trend; 0, not significant; ++, statistically significant including excess rate of nasal ulceration; NR = not reported. [c] Percentage was calculated as 100 × (frequency in the placebo group − frequency in the active group) + frequency in the placebo group. Negative value indicates higher attack rate in the IFN group. [d] S = spray, D = drops. [e] This study found decreased frequency of cough in IFN recipients compared to placebo. [f] In these studies, IFN was administered for one or two weeks, and administered again for three or four weeks. [g] Based on number of episodes which were cultured for virus. [h] Prophylactic efficacy of 78% for all rhinovirus-associated illnesses. [i] In this study, 5 Mu were administered on the first day followed by 2.5 Mu daily for four more days. [j] Prophylactic efficacy for all rhinovirus-associated episodes.

topical anticholinergic, ipratropium (80 μg intranasally three times per day), beginning 24 h after challenge with rhinovirus. In the group treated with the combination there was a reduction in viral shedding and the volunteers experienced reduced illness rates and less severe symptoms, but nasal mucus production was not significantly different from placebo recipients. In a second study, oral chlorpheniramine maleate (4 mg) and topical phenylephrine hydrochloride (0.25%) were added to the combination, and a reduction in the nasal mucus production was also observed. These studies showed that the addition of anti-inflammatory agents and/or drugs directed to host responses may improve symptom reduction in conjunction with the virological effects of antiviral agents. However, it remains to be determined whether such multi-ingredient interventions are well tolerated and safe in natural colds, what contribution is provided by individual components, and whether combinations of antiviral agents can improve antiviral activity.

OTHER AGENTS

A number of other agents with anti-HRV activity have been tested over the past two decades (Tables 11.4 and 11.5). Most of these have been abandoned because of lack of efficacy or unacceptable side-effects, but some remain under active investigation. The antiviral mechanisms of action of many of these agents are undefined.

ENVIROXIME

Enviroxime, (*E*)-6[(hydroxyimino)phenylmethyl]-1-[(-methylethyl)sulphonyl] -1*H*-benzimidazol-2-amine, is a benzimidazole derivative which has shown potent activity against 83 serotypes of HRV and against coxsackievirus A21, B4 and echovirus 7 (156). Its mechanism of action is not understood, but it has been reported to involve inhibition of viral RNA polymerase complex.

Studies which evaluated enviroxime for prophylaxis of experimentally induced HRV infections did not consistently show reductions in markers of illness or infection compared with placebo (Table 11.4) (125,145). One study (125) found a 33% reduction in illness rate and decreased virus shedding when enviroxime was given both orally (25 mg) and by intranasal spray (approximately 0.3 mg per nostril four times daily), beginning one day before and continuing for four days after challenge with HRV-9. However, rhinorrhoea was the only symptom significantly reduced relative to placebo. Enviroxime was also poorly tolerated when given orally (125,145) and caused side-effects of nausea, vomiting and abdominal pain with high frequency. In addition, oral administration was associated with low drug levels in blood and nasal secretions (145). When administered intranasally

Table 11.4. Summary of efficacy data of antiviral agents tested in clinical trials for the prophylaxis of experimental rhinovirus colds

Compound (ref.) [rhinovirus serotype]		No. of subj.[a]	Route[b]	Dose (doses/day)	Duration (days)	Reduction relative to placebo[c]		
						Infection rate (% of subj.)	Virus shedding (% of days)	Colds (% of subj.)
Enviroxime (144)	[RV9]	36	PO+IN	25 mg (4) +568 μg (4)	−1/+5	0(−22)[e]	0(NR)	0(33)
Enviroxime (145)	[RV39]	40	IN	568 μg (4)	−1/+4	0(11)	0(16)	0(2)
Enviroxime (152)	[RV4][d]	51	IN	568 μg (4)	−1h/+	0(1)	0(NR)	0(NR)
44081RP (146)	[RVEL][d]	46	IN	0.6 mg (6)	−1/+5	0(−5)	0(NR)	0(0)
Zinc gluconate (147)	[RV2]	57	PO	23 mg (12)	−1/+3.5	0(3)	0(NR)	0(31)
DIQA (148)	[RV24]	21	PO	500 mg (4)	−1/+6	0(−23)[e]	+/0(43)	0(1)
UK 2054 (149)	[RV9]	60	PO	375 mg (4)	−1/+5.5	0(−7)	0(NR)	0(6)
SKF 40491 (150)	[RV3]	19	IN	0.1 mg (10)	−1/+3.5	0(39)[e]	0(15)	0(−59)
GL R9-338 (150)	[RV9]	24	IN	3 mg (5)	−1/+4.5	0(29)[e]	0(28)[f]	0(20)
RP 19326 (150)	[RV9]	19	IN	0.5 mg (13)	−1/+3.5	0(10)[e]	0(8)[f]	0(−25)

[a]Total number of subjects in placebo and active groups challenged with virus.
[b]IN = intranasal, PO = oral.
[c]See footnotes in Tables 11.1 and 11.2 for description of symbols and calculation of effects.
[d]Untyped clinical isolate.
[e]Based on rates of seroconversion only.
[f]Significant reductions in virus titres in nasal washings were reported for active versus placebo.

Table 11.5. Summary of efficacy data of antiviral agents tested in clinical trials for the therapy of experimental rhinovirus colds

Treatment (ref.) [rhinovirus serotype]	No. of subj.[a]	Route[b]	Dose (doses/day)	Duration[c]	Reduction relative to placebo[d]		
					Infection rate (% of subjects)	Virus shedding (% of days)	Cold symptoms
Enviroxime (151) [RV9]	41	IN	568 μg(6)	+2/+7	0(0)	0(NR)[g]	0
Enviroxime (152) [RV4]	60	IN	568 μg(4)	+1 or +3/+7	0(4)	0(NR)	0
Zinc gluconate (153)							
[RV39]	32	PO	23 mg (8)	+1.5/+6.5	0(−6)	0(−24)	0
[RV13]	41	PO	23 mg (8)	+2h/+7	0(5)	0(12)[g]	0
Zinc gluconate (147)							
[RV2]	12	PO	23 mg (q2h)	–[f]/+6	NR	0(NR)[g]	+[e]
Local heat (154) [RV14]	87	IN	3 × 30 min	1	0(35)[h]	0(NR)	+(65)[i]
(155) [RVH]	20	IN	7 × 30 min	1/2	0(0)	0(NR)[g]	0

[a] Total number in groups active and placebo challenged with virus.
[b] IN = intranasal, PO = oral.
[c] Timing of administration in days (first dose/last dose) after virus challenge.
[d] Symbols: +, statistically significant; +/0, trend; 0, not significant; NR = not reported.
[e] Reduction of mean daily clinical scores relative to placebo.
[f] First dose administered when the first symptom appeared.
[g] No reduction in viral titres found in the active group versus placebo.
[h] Based on rates of seroconversion only.
[i] Proportion of volunteers who showed nasal symptoms improvement.

alone (568 μg five times daily) it did not produce significant reduction in illness or infection rates, mucus production or frequency of virus shedding compared to placebo (145).

A few studies have evaluated enviroxime in the therapy of experimentally induced HRV infections (Table 11.5) (151,152). In one trial (152), four sprays per day did not produce any clinical benefits, and with six sprays per day only modest clinical benefit was observed (151). In a family-based study (157) enviroxime (six sprays per day in the first two days, followed by four sprays per day for an additional five days) showed no significant benefits relative to placebo in the therapy of naturally acquired HRV infections.

The lack of efficacy observed in these studies has at least in part been attributed to difficulties with delivery of adequate doses of relatively water-insoluble enviroxime. Preliminary toxicity studies of aerosols of lysosome-encapsulated enviroxime (158) suggest that this may constitute an alternative method for the delivery of hydrophobic compounds into the respiratory tract. Efficacy studies utilizing this method have not been reported.

44081 RP

This compound, named 2-{(1,5,10,10*a*-tetrahydro-3*H*-thiazolo[3,4*b*]isoquinolin-3-ylidine)amino}-4-thiazolacetic acid (*S*), was shown to selectively inhibit HRV uncoating *in vitro*, with relatively high inhibitory concentrations (159). The compound was unable to directly inactivate infectivity of virions and did not affect adsorption or penetration of HRV in fibroblast cell cultures, but protected intracellular virions against RNase (159). Unlike capsid-binding agents, it is a water-soluble compound. 44081 RP was tested intranasally (0.6 mg six times daily) in human volunteers infected with HRV, beginning one day prior to infection and continuing for five days, and showed no clinical or virological benefit (Table 11.4) (146). Levels of 44081 RP in nasal secretions 2 h after administration were only equal to or several-fold higher than the minimal inhibitory concentration observed in cell culture for the serotype employed in the study. Therefore, insufficient concentration of drug in the nasal epithelium was probably the cause for lack of efficacy (146).

ZINC SALTS

Zinc chloride has been reported to inhibit the *in vitro* replication of HRV (160), with the proposed mechanism being inhibition of proteolytic cleavage of precursor polyprotein into individual viral peptides (161). More recently, a series of different zinc salts were tested *in vitro* against HRV in WI38 fibroblast and HeLa cells and only a weak, non-selective anti-rhinoviral effect was observed (162,163). Little difference existed between the zinc salt concentrations inhibiting virus replication and those causing cellular cytotoxicity (162), both of which relate to the amount of unbound zinc available (163).

Several studies have assessed the effect of zinc salt lozenges in the prophylaxis and therapy of experimentally induced HRV colds (147,153) and naturally acquired colds of non-specified aetiology (164–167). A high frequency of unpleasant side-effects, mainly unpalatable taste and mouth irritation, have been observed after oral zinc salt administration and seem to have been important confounders in some studies (168). In one prophylaxis study (147) volunteers received lozenges (23 mg zinc) for two days before and for several days after being experimentally inoculated with HRV-2. No significant reduction in symptoms or virus excretion was observed. One therapy study in which lozenges were given every 2 h while awake, beginning on the first day of infection, reported a significant reduction in the mean daily clinical score on days 4 and 5 (147). However, this apparent clinical effect was not associated with any reduction in viral excretion by the patients. Therapy with zinc gluconate (23 mg eight times per day) beginning 2 or 36 h after challenge did not show any clinical or antiviral effects, despite significant increase in serum zinc levels (153). Thus, these studies have provided no evidence that intraoral zinc salt administration is associated with antiviral effects or consistent clinical benefit.

Trials of zinc salts for the therapy of naturally occurring colds have also failed to demonstrate consistent clinical benefits (164–167). One study reported that zinc gluconate (23 mg zinc) every 2 h while patients were awake was associated with reductions in the duration of the symptoms of naturally acquired common colds of unspecified aetiology (164). However, this study was confounded by ineffective blinding and high dropout and side-effect rates. In another study (165), using a smaller dose (4.5 mg zinc) every 1–1.5 h, no significant positive effect was observed in patients with naturally acquired colds. Two other studies with zinc acetate (166) and zinc gluconate (167) also failed to document clinical benefits in the therapy of natural colds. In a more recent study a more palatable zinc gluconate–glycine was reported to reduce the duration of symptoms in natural colds (169).

DIQA

This compound, 3,4-dihydro-1-isoquinolineacetamide hydrochloride (DIQA), has been shown to protect mice against infection by coxsackievirus A23, and to be active in cell culture against coxsackievirus B1 (170). DIQA showed no significant clinical or virological effect when tested in prophylaxis of HRV experimentally induced colds (148).

UK2054

The isoquinoline UK2054, 1-(*p*-chlorophenoxymethyl)3,4-dihydroisoquinoline hydrochloride, has shown anti-rhinoviral activity *in vitro* in yield reduction assays (149). Although its mechanism of action is not determined, it does not involve direct inactivation of the virus (149). This compound given orally (375 mg four times daily) failed to demonstrate any clinical or antiviral benefit in the protection against experimentally induced HRV colds (149).

SKF 40491

A triazinoindole, 4-([8-amino-7-chloro-5-methyl-5*H*-*as*-triazino-(5,6-*b*)indol-3-yl]amino)-2 methyl-2-butanol (SKF 40491), at 4 μg/ml, showed *in vitro* inhibitory activity against a broad spectrum of picornaviruses (34,150). This compound provided antiviral activity when administered intranasally by aerosol to gibbons 3 h before and every 4 h for five days after infection with HRV-2 (34). SKF 40491 administered orally (16 mg/kg three times daily for five days) failed to protect gibbons against infection with HRV-1A (34). SKF 40491 was tested in the prophylaxis of experimentally induced colds, administered intranasally 0.1 mg 10 times daily beginning one day before and continuing for 3.5 days after challenge with HRV-3 (150). This study found no clinical or antiviral benefits of SKF 40491 and the symptoms were significantly worse in the active group relative to placebo.

GL R9-338

GL R9-338, 3-α-naphthyl-5-diethylcarbamoyl-1,2,4-oxadiazole, was tested *in vitro* against four different HRV serotypes, but only showed significant activity at 4 μg/ml against HRV-9 (150). This compound was tested in the prophylaxis of experimentally induced colds, administered intranasally 3 mg five times daily beginning one day before and continuing for 4.5 days after challenge with HRV-9 (150). No clinical benefits of GL R9-338 in protecting against HRV-9-induced colds were observed in that study, but a significant reduction in the proportion of specimens which yielded virus and in the mean daily virus titres was observed relative to placebo (150).

RP 19326

RP 19326, 2,6-diphenyl-3-methyl-2,3-dihydroimidazo[2,1-*b*]thiazole, at 4 μg/ml showed variable activity *in vitro* against four serotypes of rhinovirus (150). One study tested the ability of this compound to protect volunteers against experimentally induced HRV colds (150). The compound was intranasally administered in doses of 0.5 mg 13 times daily beginning one day before and continuing for 3.5 days after challenge with HRV-9. No significant clinical benefits were observed, but a significant reduction was observed in the mean virus titres recovered and in the proportion of specimens which yielded virus (150).

INTRANASAL HEAT

The fact that high temperatures are inhibitory of HRV replication *in vitro* has served in part as a rationale for studies employing inhalation of warm humidified air to treat rhinovirus colds. In one study a special device, called the Rhinotherm, was used to deliver 40 l/min of humidified air at 42–44 °C for 20 min in the nostrils of patients with natural colds of less than three days' duration (171). A significant reduction of cold symptoms was obtained with the treatment compared with placebo (inhalation of air at 20–24 °C) but results in this study may have been confounded by ineffective blinding. In similar studies by another group (172,173) no benefits were found.

One placebo-controlled study of warm steam inhalation for the treatment of experimentally induced colds used a different apparatus (154) and reported a significant reduction in nasal symptoms, but no effect was observed on virus excretion. Thus, these studies have failed to confirm that this type of intervention is associated with inhibition of rhinovirus replication or with consistent clinical benefits. Further trials are required to assess the usefulness of this approach. In a more recent study (155), inhalation of hot air had no effect on viral excretion and cold symptoms in volunteers experimentally infected with HRV.

IMMUNOTHERAPY

Meningitis and encephalitis caused by enteroviruses are the most common recognized viral infections of the central nervous system (CNS) (2,174). Although meningitis due to enteroviruses is usually benign, more serious diseases occur with perinatally acquired infection or in patients with deficient immunoglobulin synthesis. Most of the perinatal infections become apparent in the first week of life and cause a spectrum of illnesses that includes fatal disseminated disease (175). The occurrence of the most serious neonatal disease appears to correlate with the absence of specific neutralizing antibody (176). Anecdotal reports of improvement of disseminated neonatal enteroviral infection with intravenous immunoglobulin therapy (177) have been described, but controlled studies have not been published. Patients with agammaglobulinaemia are at an increased risk for persistent, sometimes fatal, infection of the CNS caused by enteroviruses (176). In some of the cases, chronic meningoencephalitis associated with persistent CNS viral replication and slowly progressive neurological deterioration may develop. Systemic administration of exogenous antibody therapy with commercially available immunoglobulin pools to these patients has shown little success (175). Although controlled studies have not been published, some positive clinical results have been obtained with combination of intravenous and intraventricular administration of immunoglobulin (178–180). This would be a potential target population for testing the antiviral effects of systemically administered anti-enteroviral agents that have shown efficacy in experimental human and animal model studies (24–26).

REFERENCES

1. Gwaltney, J. M., Jr (1989). Rhinoviruses. In *Viral Infections of Humans: Epidemiology and Control*, 3rd edn, A. S. Evans (ed.), Plenum, New York, pp. 593–615.
2. Melnick, J. L. (1989). Enteroviruses. In *Viral Infections of Humans: Epidemiology and Control*, 3rd edn, A. S. Evans (ed.), Plenum, New York, pp. 593–615.
3. National Center for Health Statistics (1986). *Current Estimates from the National Health Interview Survey, United States, 1985*. Vital and Health Statistics Series 10, no. 160. Public Health Service, Washington, DC.
4. Graham, N. M. H. (1990). The epidemiology of acute respiratory infections in children and adults: a global perspective. *Epidemiol. Rev.*, **12**, 149–178.
5. Sperber, S. J. and Hayden, F. G. (1988). Chemotherapy of rhinovirus colds. *Antimicrob. Agents Chemother.*, **32**, 409–419.
6. Arruda, E. N., Hayden, F. G., McAuliffe, J. F. *et al.* (1991). Acute respiratory viral infections in ambulatory children of Urban Northeast Brazil. *J. Infect. Dis.*, **164**, 252–258.
7. Perkins, J. C., Tucker, D. N., Knopf, H. L. S. *et al.* (1969). Evidence for protective effect of an inactivated rhinovirus vaccine administered by the nasal route. *Am. J. Epidemiol.*, **90**, 319–326.
8. Hamory, B. H., Hamparian, V. V., Conant, R. M. and Gwaltney, J. M. Jr (1975). Human responses to two decavalent rhinovirus vaccines. *J. Infect. Dis.*, **132**, 623–629.
9. McCray, J. and Werner, G. (1987). Different rhinovirus serotypes neutralized by antipeptide antibodies. *Nature*, **329**, 736–738.
10. Francis, M. J., Hastings, G. Z., Sangar, D. V. *et al.* (1987). A synthetic peptide which elicits neutralizing antibody against human rhinovirus type 2. *J. Gen. Virol.*, **68**, 2687–2691.
11. Hayden, F. G. (1988). Intranasal interferons for control of respiratory viral infections. In *Clinical Aspects of Interferons*, M. Revel (ed.), Kluwer, Boston, pp. 3–16.
12. Hendley, J. O. and Gwaltney, J. M., Jr (1988). Mechanisms of transmission of rhinovirus infections. *Epidemiol. Rev.*, **10**, 242–258.
13. Gwaltney, J. M., Jr, Moskalski, P. B. and Hendley, J. O. (1980). Interruption of experimental rhinovirus transmission. *J. Infect. Dis.*, **142**, 811–815.
14. Corley, D. L., Gevirtz, R., Nideffer, R. and Cummins, L. (1987). Prevention of postinfectious asthma in children by reducing self-inoculatory behavior. *J. Pediatr. Psychol.*, **12**, 519–531.
15. Winther, B., Gwaltney, J. M. Jr, Mygind, N. *et al.* (1986). Sites of rhinovirus recovery after point inoculation of the upper airway. *JAMA*, **256**, 1763–1767.

16. Winther, B., Farr, B., Turner, R. B. *et al.* (1984). Histopathologic examination and enumeration of polymorphonuclear leukocytes in the nasal mucosa during experimental rhinovirus colds. *Acta Otolaryngol.*, **413** (Suppl.), 19–24.
17. Naclerio, R. M., Proud, D., Lichtenstein, L. M. *et al.* (1988). Kinins are generated during experimental rhinovirus colds. *J. Infect. Dis.*, **157**, 133–142.
18. Proud, D., Naclerio, R. M., Gwaltney, J. M. Jr and Hendley, J. O. (1990). Kinins are generated in nasal secretions during natural rhinovirus colds. *J. Infect. Dis.*, **161**, 120–123.
19. Proud, D., Reynolds, C. J., LaCapra, S. *et al.* (1988). Nasal provocation with bradykinin induces symptoms of rhinitis and sore throat. *Am. Rev. Respir. Dis.*, **137**, 613–616.
20. Doyle, W. J., Boehm, S. and Skoner, D. P. (1990). Physiologic responses to intranasal dose–response challenges with histamine, methacholine, bradykinin, and prostaglandin in adult volunteers with and without nasal allergy. *J. Allergy Clin. Immunol.*, **86**, 924–935.
21. Sperber, S. J. and Hayden, F. H. (1988). Perspectives in the use of antiviral agents for prevention and treatment of respiratory virus infections. In *Clinical Use of Antiviral Drugs*, E. De Clercq (ed.), Martinus Nijhoff, Boston, pp. 317–340.
22. Kenny, M. T., Dulworth, J. K. and Torney, H. L. (1985). In vitro and in vivo antipicornavirus activity of some phenoxypyridine carbonitriles. *Antimicrob. Agents Chemother.*, **28**, 745–750.
23. Kenny, M. T., Dulworth, J. K. and Torney, H. L. (1986). In vitro and in vivo antipicornavirus activity of some *p*-benzoyl phenoxypyridines. *Antiviral Res.*, **6**, 355–367.
24. Jubelt, B., Wilson, A. K., Ropka, S. L. *et al.* (1989). Clearance of a persistent human enterovirus infection of the mouse central nervous system by the antiviral agent disoxaril. *J. Infect. Dis.*, **159**, 866–871.
25. Woods, M. G., Diana, G. D., Rogge, M. C. *et al.* (1989). In vitro and in vivo activities of WIN 54954, a new broad-spectrum antipicornavirus drug. *Antimicrob. Agents Chemother.*, **33**, 2069–2074.
26. Schiff, G. M., Sherwood, J. R., Young, E. C. and Mason, L. J. (1992). Prophylactic efficacy of WIN 54954 in prevention of experimental human Coxsackievirus A21 infection and illness. (Abstr. #92). Fifth International Conference on Antiviral Research, Vancouver, 1992. *Antiviral Res.*, **17** (Suppl. 1), 92.
27. Tyrrell, D. A. J. and Al-Nakib, W. (1988). Prophylaxis and treatment of rhinovirus infections. In *Clinical Use of Antiviral Drugs*, E. De Clercq (ed.), Martinus Nijhoff, Boston, pp. 241–276.
28. Knott, J. A., Orr, D. C., Montgomery, D. S. *et al.* (1989). The expression and purification of human rhinovirus protease 3C. *Eur. J. Biochem.*, **182**, 547–555.
29. McKinlay, M. A., Dutko, F. J., Pevear, D. C. *et al.* (1990). Rational design of antipicornavirus agents. In *New Aspects of Positive-strand RNA Viruses*, M. A. Brinton and F. X. Heinz (eds), American Society for Microbiology, Washington, DC, pp. 366–372.
30. Andries, K., Dewindt, B., Snoeks, J. *et al.* (1991). A comparative test of fifteen compounds against all known human rhinovirus serotypes as a basis for a more rational screening program. *Antiviral Res.*, **16**, 213–225.
31. Andries, K., Dewindt, B., Snoeks, J. *et al.* (1992). In vitro activity of pirodavir (R 77975), a substituted phenoxypyridazinamine with broad-spectrum antipicornaviral activity. *Antimicrob. Agents Chemother.*, **36**, 100–107.
32. Dick, E. C. (1968). Experimental infections of chimpanzees with human rhinovirus types 14 and 43. *Proc. Soc. Exp. Biol. Med.*, **127**, 1079–1081.
33. Shipkowitz, N. L., Bower, R. R., Schleicher, J. B. *et al.* (1972). Antiviral activity of

a bis-benzimidazole against experimental rhinovirus infections in chimpanzees. *Appl. Microbiol.*, **23**, 117–122.
34. Pinto, C. A., Bahnsen, H. P., Ravin, L. J. *et al.* (1972). The antiviral effect of a triazinoindole (SK&F 40491) in rhinovirus infected gibbons (36800). *Proc. Soc. Exp. Biol. Med.*, **141**, 467–474.
35. Yin, F. H. and Lomax, N. B. (1986). Establishment of a mouse model for human rhinovirus infection. *J. Gen. Virol.*, **67**, 2335–2340.
36. Douglas, R. G., Jr (1970). Pathogenesis of rhinovirus common colds in human volunteers. *Ann. Otol. Rhinol. Laryngol.*, **79**, 563–571.
37. Hendley, J. O., Edmondson, W. P. and Gwaltney, J. M., Jr (1972). Relation between naturally acquired immunity and infectivity of two rhinoviruses in volunteers. *J. Infect. Dis.*, **125**, 243–248.
38. Meschievitz, C. K., Schultz, S. B. and Dick, E. (1984). A model for obtaining predictable natural transmission of rhinovirus in human volunteers. *J. Infect. Dis.*, **150**, 195–201.
39. Couch, R. B., Cate, T. R., Douglas, R. C., Jr *et al.* (1966). Effect of route of inoculation on experimental respiratory viral disease in volunteers and evidence for airborne transmission. *Bacteriol. Rev.*, **30**, 517–529.
40. Gwaltney, J. M., Jr, Moskalski, P. B. and Hendley, J. O. (1978). Hand-to-hand transmission of rhinovirus colds. *Ann. Intern. Med.*, **88**, 463–467.
41. Khatib, R., Reyes, M. P. and Lerner, A. M. (1986). Animal models for coxsackievirus infections. In *Experimental Models in Antimicrobial Chemotherapy*, O. Zak and M. A. Sande (eds), Academic Press, London, pp. 175–193.
42. McKinlay, M. A. and Steinberg, B. A. (1986). Oral efficacy of WIN 51711 in mice infected with human poliovirus. *Antimicrob. Agents Chemother.*, **29**, 30–32.
43. Powers, R. D., Dotson, W. M., Jr and Hayden, F. G. (1983). Modification of encephalomyocarditis virus-induced diabetes in mice by antiviral agents. *Antiviral Res.*, **3**, 151–159.
44. Diana, G. D., Pevear, D. C., Otto, M. J. *et al.* (1989). Inhibitors of viral uncoating. *Pharmacol. Ther.*, **42**, 289–305.
45. See, D. M. and Tilles, J. G. (1992). Treatment of coxsackievirus A9 myocarditis in mice with WIN 54954. *Antimicrob. Agents Chemother.*, **36**, 425–428.
46. Koike, S., Taya, C., Kurata, T. *et al.* (1991). Transgenic mice susceptible to poliovirus. *Proc. Natl Acad. Sci. USA*, **88**, 951–955.
47. Schiff, G. M., Stefanovic, G. M., Young, E. C. *et al.* (1984). Studies of echovirus-12 in volunteers: determination of minimal infectious dose and the effect of previous infection on infectious dose. *J. Infect. Dis.*, **150**, 858–866.
48. Diana, G. D., Otto, M. J. and McKinlay, M. A. (1985). Inhibitors of picornavirus uncoating as antiviral agents. *Pharmacol. Ther.*, **29**, 287–297.
49. Hayden, F. G. (1989). Update on antiviral chemotherapy of respiratory infections. In *Antiviral Chemotherapy: New Directions for Clinical Application and Research*, Vol. 2, J. Mills and L. Corey (eds), Elsevier, New York, pp. 117–142.
50. Hayden, F. G. (1986). Use of interferons for prevention and treatment of respiratory viral infections. In *Antiviral Chemotherapy: New Directions for Clinical Application and Research*, J. Mills and L. Corey (eds), Elsevier, New York, pp. 28–39.
51. Greenberg, S. B. (1987). Human interferon in viral diseases. *Infect. Dis. Clin. North Am.*, **1**, 383–423.
52. Lentz, T. L. (1990). The recognition event between virus and host cell receptor: a target for antiviral agents. *J. Gen. Virol.*, **71**, 751–766.
53. White, J. M. and Littman, D. R. (1989). Viral receptors of the immunoglobulin superfamily. *Cell*, **56**, 725–728.

54. Racaniello, V. R. (1990). Cell receptors for picornaviruses. *Curr. Topics Microbiol. Immunol.*, **161**, 1–22.
55. Greve, J. M., Davis, G., Meyer, A. M. *et al.* (1989). The major human rhinovirus receptor is ICAM-1. *Cell*, **56**, 839–847.
56. Staunton, D. E., Merluzzi, V. J., Rothlein, R. *et al.* (1989). A cell adhesion molecule, ICAM-1, is the major surface receptor for rhinoviruses. *Cell*, **56**, 849–853.
57. Tomassini, J. E., Graham, D., DeWitt, C. M. *et al.* (1989). cDNA cloning reveals that the major group rhinovirus receptor on HeLa cells is intercellular adhesion molecule 1. *Proc. Natl Acad. Sci. USA*, **86**, 4907–4911.
58. Colonno, R. J., Callahan, P. L. and Long, W. J. (1986). Isolation of a monoclonal antibody that blocks attachment of the major group of human rhinoviruses. *J. Virol.*, **57**, 7–12.
59. Olson, N. H., Kolatkar, P. R., Oliveira, M. A. *et al.* (1993). Structure of a human rhinovirus complexed with its receptor molecule. *Proc. Natl Acad. Sci. USA*, **90**, 507–511.
60. Hofer, F., Gruenberger, M., Kowalski, H. *et al.* (1994). Members of the low density lipoprotein receptor family mediate cell entry of a minor-group common cold virus. *Proc. Natl Acad. Sci. USA*, **91**, 1839–1842.
61. Mendelsohn, C. L., Wimmer, E. and Racaniello, V. R. (1989). Cellular receptor for poliovirus: molecular cloning, nucleotide sequence, and expression of a new member of the immunoglobulin superfamily. *Cell*, **56**, 855–865.
62. Bergelson, J. M., Shepley, M. P., Chan, B. M. C. *et al.* (1992). Identification of the integrin VLA-2 as a receptor for Echovirus 1. *Science*, **255**, 1718–1720.
63. Sperber, S. J. and Hayden, F. G. (1989). Protective effect of rhinovirus receptor blocking antibody in human fibroblast cells. *Antiviral Res.*, **12**, 231–238.
64. Colonno, R. J., Tomassini, J. E. and Callahan, P. L. (1987). Isolation and characterization of a monoclonal antibody which blocks attachment of human rhinoviruses. In *Positive Strand RNA Viruses: Proceedings of a UCLA Symposium*, M. A. Brinton and R. L. Rueckert (eds), Liss, New York, pp. 93–102.
65. Hayden, F. G., Gwaltney, J. M., Jr and Colonno, R. J. (1988). Modification of experimental rhinovirus colds by receptor blockade. *Antiviral Res.*, **9**, 233–247.
66. Marlin, S. D., Staunton, D. E., Springer, T. A. *et al.* (1990). A soluble form intercellular adhesion molecule-1 inhibits rhinovirus infection. *Nature*, **334**, 70–72.
67. Greve, J. M., Forte, C. P., Marlor, C. W. *et al.* (1991). Mechanisms of receptor-mediated rhinovirus neutralization defined by two forms of ICAM-1. *J. Virol.*, **65**, 6015–6023.
68. Arruda, E., Crump, C., Marlin, S. D. *et al.* (1992). In vitro studies of the anti-rhinovirus activity of soluble ICAM-1. *Antimicrob. Agents Chemother.*, **36**, 1186–1191.
69. Crump, C. E., Arruda, E. and Hayden, F. G. (1993). In vitro inhibitory activity of soluble ICAM-1 for the numbered serotypes of human rhinovirus. *Antiviral Chem. Chemother.*, **4**, 323–327.
70. Kaplan, G., Freistadt, M. S. and Racaniello, V. R. (1990). Neutralization of poliovirus by cell receptors expressed in insect cells. *J. Virol.*, **64**, 4697–4702.
71. Kaplan, G., Peters, D. and Racaniello, V. (1990). Poliovirus mutants resistant to neutralization with soluble cell receptors. *Science*, **250**, 1596–1599.
72. Arruda, E., Crump, C. E. and Hayden, F. G. (1994). In vitro selection of human rhinovirus relatively resistant to soluble intercellular adhesion molecule-1. *Antimicrob. Agents Chemother.*, **38**, 66–70.
73. Eggers, H. J., Koch, M. A., Furst, A. *et al.* (1970). Rhodamine: a selective inhibitor of multiplication of echovirus 12. *Science*, **167**, 294–297.

74. Eggers, H. J. (1977). Selective inhibition of uncoating of echovirus 12 by rhodamine. *Virology*, **78**, 241–252.
75. McSharry, J. J., Caliguiri, L. A. and Eggers, H. J. (1979). Inhibition of uncoating of poliovirus by arildone, a new antiviral drug. *Virology*, **97**, 307–315.
76. Andries, K., Dewindt, B., Snoeks, J. *et al.* (1990). Two groups of rhinoviruses revealed by a panel of antiviral compounds present sequence divergence and differential pathogenicity. *J. Virol.*, **64**, 1117–1123.
77. Heinz, B. A., Rueckert, R. R., Shepard, D. A. *et al.* (1989). Genetic and molecular analyses of spontaneous mutants of human rhinovirus 14 that are resistant to an antiviral compound. *J. Virol.*, **63**, 2476–2485.
78. Yasin, S. R., Al-Nakib, W. and Tyrrell, D. A. J. (1990). Pathogenicity for humans of human rhinovirus type 2 mutants resistant to or dependent on chalcone Ro 09-0410. *Antimicrob. Agents Chemother.*, **34**, 963–966.
79. Ahmad, A. L. M., Dowsett, A. B. and Tyrrell, D. A. J. (1987). Studies of rhinovirus resistant to an antiviral chalcone. *Antiviral Res.*, **8**, 27–39.
80. Phillpotts, R. J., Wallace, J., Tyrrell, D. A. J. *et al.* (1983). Failure of an oral 4′,6-dichloroflavan to protect against rhinovirus infection in man. *Arch. Virol.*, **75**, 115–121.
81. Al-Nakib, W., Willman, J., Higgins, P. G. *et al.* (1987). Failure of intranasally administered 4′,6-dichloroflavan to protect against rhinovirus in man. *Arch. Virol.*, **92**, 255–260.
82. Phillpotts, R. J., Higgins, P. G., Willman, J. S. *et al.* (1984). Evaluation of the anti-rhinovirus chalcone Ro 09-0415 given orally to volunteers, *J. Antimicrob. Chemother.*, **14**, 403–409.
83. Al-Nakib, W., Higgins, P. G., Barrow, I. *et al.* (1987). Intranasal chalcone, Ro 09-0410, as prophylaxis against rhinovirus infection in human volunteers. *J. Antimicrob. Chemother.*, **20**, 887–892.
84. Gwaltney, J. M., Jr and Hayden, F. G. (1983). Prophylactic efficacy of intranasal RMI 15731 in experimental rhinovirus infection. (Abstr.) *23rd Interscience Conference on Antimicrobial Agents and Chemotherapy*, No. 931, Las Vegas.
85. Turner, R. B., Dutko, F. J., Goldstein, N. H. *et al.* (1993). Efficacy of oral WIN 54954 for the prophylaxis of experimental rhinovirus infection. *Antimicrob. Agents Chemother.*, **37**, 297–300.
86. Al-Nakib, W., Higgins, P. G., Barrow, G. I. *et al.* (1989). Suppression of colds in human volunteers challenged with rhinovirus by a new synthetic drug (R 61837). *Antimicrob. Agents Chemother.*, **33**, 522–525.
87. Hayden, F. G., Andries, K. and Janssen, P. A. J. (1992). Safety and efficacy of intranasal pirodavir (R77975) in experimental rhinovirus infection. *Antimicrob. Agents Chemother.*, **36**, 727–732.
88. Bauer, D. J., Selway, J. W. T., Batchelor, J. F. *et al.* (1981). 4′,6-Dichloroflavan (BW683C), a new anti-rhinovirus compound. *Nature*, **292**, 369–370.
89. Tisdale, M. and Selway, J. W. T. (1984). Effect of dichloroflavan (BW683C) on the stability and uncoating of rhinovirus type 1B. *J. Antimicrob. Chemother.*, **14** (Suppl. A), 97–105.
90. Conti, C., Tomao, P., Genovese, D. *et al.* (1992). Mechanism of action of the antirhinovirus flavanoid 4′,6-dicyanoflavan. *Antimicrob. Agents Chemother.*, **36**, 95–99.
91. Ninomiya, Y., Ohsawa, C., Aoyama, M. *et al.* (1984). Antivirus agent Ro 09-0410 binds to rhinovirus specifically and stabilizes the virus conformation. *Virology*, **134**, 269–276.
92. Ninomiya, Y., Shimma, N. and Ishitsuka, H. (1990). Comparative studies on the

antirhinovirus activity and the mode of action of the rhinovirus capsid binding agents, chalcone amides. *Antiviral Res.*, **13**, 61–74.
93. Ishitsuka, H., Ohsawa, C., Ohiwa, T. *et al.* (1982). Antipicornavirus flavone Ro 09-0179m. *Antimicrob. Agents Chemother.*, **22**, 611–616.
94. Ishitsuka, H., Ninomiya, Y. T., Ohsawa, C. *et al.* (1982). Direct and specific inactivation of rhinovirus by Chalcone Ro 09-0410. *Antimicrob. Agents Chemother.*, **22**, 617–621.
95. De Meyer, N., Haemers, A., Mishra, L. *et al.* (1991). 4′-Hydroxy-3-methoxyflavones with potent antipicornavirus activity. *J. Med. Chem.*, **34**, 737–746.
96. Ash, R. J., Parker, R. A., Hagan, A. C. and Mayer, G. L. (1979). RMI 15,731 (1-[tetradecycloxy-2-furanyl]-ethanone), a new antirhinovirus compound. *Antimicrob. Agents Chemother.*, **16**, 301–305.
97. Andries, K., Dewindt, B., De Brabander, M. *et al.* (1988). In vitro activity of R 61837, a new antirhinovirus compound. *Arch. Virol.*, **101**, 155–167.
98. Barrow, G. I., Higgins, P. G., Tyrrell, D. A. J. and Andries, K. (1990). An appraisal of the efficacy of the antiviral R 61837 in rhinovirus infections in human volunteers. *Antiviral Chem. Chemother.*, **1**, 279–283.
99. Dearden, C., Al-Nakib, W., Andries, K. *et al.* (1989). Drug resistant rhinoviruses from the nose of experimentally treated volunteers. *Arch. Virol.*, **109**, 71–81.
100. Tyrrell, D. A. J. (1988). Hot news on the common cold. *Ann. Rev. Microbiol.*, **42**, 35–47.
101. Cate, T. R., Douglas, R. G., Jr and Couch, R. B. (1969). Interferon and resistance to upper respiratory virus illness (33941). *Proc. Soc. Exp. Biol. Med.*, **131**, 631–636.
102. Hsia, J., Goldstein, A. L., Simon, G. L. *et al.* (1990). Peripheral blood mononuclear cell interleukin-2 and interferon-δ production, cytotoxicity, and antigen-stimulated blastogenesis during experimental rhinovirus infection. *J. Infect. Dis.*, **162**, 591–597.
103. Merrigan, T. C., Hall, T. S., Reed, S. E. and Tyrrell, D. A. J. (1973). Inhibition of respiratory virus infection by locally applied interferon. *Lancet*, **i**, 563–567.
104. Hill, D. A., Baron, S., Perkins, J. C. *et al.* (1972). Evaluation of an interferon inducer in viral respiratory disease. *JAMA*, **219**, 1179–1184.
105. Panusarn, C., Stanley, E. D., Dirda, V. *et al.* (1974). Prevention of illness from rhinovirus infection by topical interferon inducer. *N. Engl. J. Med.*, **291**, 57–61.
106. Douglas, R. G., Jr and Betts, R. F. (1974). Effect of interferon in experimental rhinovirus infection in volunteers. *Infect. Immun.*, **9**, 506–510.
107. Waldman, R. H. and Ganguly, R. (1978). Effect of CP-20,961, and interferon inducer, on upper respiratory infections due to rhinovirus type 21 in volunteers. *J. Infect. Dis.*, **138**, 531–535.
108. Stanley, E. D., Jackson, G. G., Dirda, V. A. and Rubenis, M. (1976). Effect of topical interferon inducer on rhinovirus infections in volunteers. *J. Infect. Dis.*, **133** (Suppl.), A121–A127.
109. Aoki, F. Y., Reed, S. E., Craig, J. W. *et al.* (1978). Effect of a polynucleotide interferon inducer of fungal origin on experimental rhinovirus infection in humans. *J. Infect. Dis.*, **137**, 82–86.
110. Douglas, R. G., Jr, Waldman, R. H., Betts, R. F. and Ganguly, R. (1979). Lack of effect of an interferon inducer, *N,N*-dihexadecyl-*m*-xylylenediamine, on rhinovirus challenge in humans. *Antimicrob. Agents Chemother.*, **15**, 269–272.
111. Scott, G. M., Phillpotts, R. J., Wallace, J. *et al.* (1982). Purified interferon as protection against rhinovirus infection. *Br. Med. J.*, **284**, 1822–1825.
112. Scott, G. M., Wallace, J., Greiner, J. *et al.* (1982). Prevention of rhinovirus colds by human interferon alpha-2 from *Escherichia coli*. *Lancet*, **ii**, 186–188.

113. Hayden, F. G. and Gwaltney, J. M., Jr (1983) Intranasal interferon α2 for prevention of rhinovirus infection and illness. *J. Infect. Dis.*, **148**, 543–550.

114. Samo, T. C., Greenberg, S. B., Couch, R. B. *et al.* (1983). Efficacy and tolerance of intranasally applied recombinant leukocyte A interferon in normal volunteers. *J. Infect. Dis.*, **148**, 535–542.

115. Samo, T. C., Greenberg, S. B., Palmer, J. M. *et al.* (1984). Intranasally applied recombinant leukocyte A interferon in normal volunteers. II. Determination of minimal effective and tolerable dose. *J. Infect. Dis.*, **150**, 181–188.

116. Treanor, J. J., Betts, R. F., Reichman, R. C. and Dolin, R. (1983). Comparison of two doses of intranasal interferon in experimental rhinovirus infection in humans. (Abstr.) *23rd Interscience Conference on Antimicrobial Agents and Chemotherapy*, No. 386, Las Vegas, Nevada.

117. Treanor, J. J., Betts, R. F., Reichman, R. C. and Dolin, R. (1984). Prolonged pretreatment with low dose intranasal interferon-α2 in experimental rhinovirus infection in humans. (Abstr.) *24th Interscience Conference on Antimicrobial Agents and Chemotherapy*, No. 920, Washington, D.C.

118. Phillpotts, R. J., Scott, G. M., Higgins, P. G. *et al.* (1983). An effective dosage regimen for prophylaxis against rhinovirus infection by intranasal administration of HuIFN-α2. *Antiviral Res.*, **3**, 121–136.

119. Phillpotts, R. J., Higgins, P. G., Willman, J. S. *et al.* (1984). Intranasal lymphoblastoid interferon ('Wellferon') prophylaxis against rhinovirus and influenza virus in volunteers. *J. Interferon Res.*, **4**, 535–541.

120. Higgins, P. G., Al-Nakib, W., Willman, J. and Tyrrell, D. A. J. (1986). Interferon-β_{ser} as prophylaxis against experimental rhinovirus infection in volunteers. *J. Interferon Res.*, **6**, 153–159.

121. Sperber, S. J., Levine, P. A., Innes, D. J. *et al.* (1988). Tolerance and efficacy of intranasal administration of recombinant β_{serine} interferon in healthy adults. *J. Infect. Dis.*, **158**, 166–175.

122. Higgins, P. G., Al-Nakib, W., Barrow, G. I. and Tyrrell, D. A. J. (1988). Recombinant human interferon-δ as prophylaxis against rhinovirus colds in volunteers. *J. Interferon Res.*, **8**, 591–596.

123. Hayden, F. G. and Gwaltney, J. M., Jr (1984). Intranasal interferon-α2 treatment of experimental rhinoviral colds. *J. Infect. Dis.*, **150**, 174–180.

124. Sperber, S. J., Doyle, W. J., McBride, T. P. *et al.* (1992). Otologic effects of interferon beta serine in experimental rhinovirus colds. *Arch. Otolaryngol. Head Neck Surg.*, **118**, 933–936.

125. Phillpotts, R. J. and Tyrrell, D. A. J. (1985). Rhinovirus Colds. *Br. Med. Bull.*, **41**, 386–390.

126. Farr, B. M., Gwaltney, J. M., Jr, Adams, K. F. and Hayden, F. G. (1984). Intranasal interferon-α2 for prevention of natural rhinovirus colds. *Antimicrob. Agents Chemother.*, **26**, 31–34.

127. Douglas, R. M., Albrecht, J. K., Miles, H. B. *et al.* (1985). Intranasal interferon-α2 prophylaxis of natural respiratory virus infection. *J. Infect. Dis.*, **151**, 731–736.

128. Monto, A. S., Shope, T. C., Schwartz, S. A. and Albrecht, J. K. (1986). Intranasal interferon-α2b for seasonal prophylaxis of respiratory infection. *J. Infect. Dis.*, **154**, 128–133.

129. Monto, A., Albrecht, J. K. and Schwartz, S. A. (1988). Demonstration of dose–response relationship in seasonal prophylaxis of respiratory infections with alpha-2b interferon. *Antimicrob. Agents Chemother.*, **32**, 47–50.

130. Sperber, S. J., Levine, P. A., Sorrentino, J. V. *et al.* (1989). Ineffectiveness of recombinant interferon-β_{serine} nasal drops for prophylaxis of natural colds. *J. Infect. Dis.*, **160**, 700–705.

131. Herzog, C., Berger, R., Fernex, M. *et al.* (1986). Intranasal interferon (rIFN-αA,

Ro 22-8181) for contact prophylaxis against common cold: a randomized, double-blind and placebo-controlled field study. *Antiviral Res.*, **6**, 171–176.
132. Hayden, F. G., Albrecht, J. K., Kaiser, D. L. and Gwaltney, J. M., Jr (1986). Prevention of natural colds by contact prophylaxis with intranasal alpha2-interferon. *N. Engl. J. Med.*, **314**, 71–75.
133. Douglas, R. M., Moore, B. W., Miles, H. B. *et al.* (1986). Prophylactic efficacy of intranasal alpha2-interferon against rhinovirus infections in the family setting. *N. Engl. J. Med.*, **314**, 65–70.
134. Foy, H. M., Fox, J. P. and Cooney, M. K. (1986). Efficacy of alpha2-interferon against the common cold. *N. Engl. J. Med.*, **315**, 513–514.
135. Monto, A. S., Schwartz, S. A. and Albrecht, J. K. (1989). Ineffectiveness of post-exposure prophylaxis of rhinovirus infection with low-dose intranasal alpha 2b interferon in families. *Antimicrob. Agents Chemother.*, **33**, 387–390.
136. Hayden, F. G., Winther, B., Donowitz, G. R. *et al.* (1987). Human nasal mucosal responses to topically applied recombinant leukocyte A interferon. *J. Infect. Dis.*, **156**, 64–72.
137. Hayden, F. G., Innes, D. J., Mills, S. E. and Levine, P. A. (1988). Intranasal tolerance and histopathologic effects of a novel synthetic interferon, rIFN-αCon$_1$. *Antiviral Res.*, **10**, 225–234.
138. Geha, R., Maguire, J., McIntosh, K. and Meschievitz, C. (1986). A trial of intranasal alpha interferon in asthmatic children. *J. Allergy Clin. Immunol.*, **77** (Suppl.), 160A, Abstr. 157.
139. Michaels, D., Foy, H., Krouse, H. *et al.* (1986). Intranasal interferon prophylaxis of viral infections in adult and pediatric asthmatic patients. *J. Allergy Clin. Immunol.*, **77** (Suppl.), 160A, Abstr. 158.
140. Ahmad, A. L. M. and Tyrrell, D. A. J. (1986). Synergism between anti-rhinovirus antivirals: various human interferons and a number of synthetic compounds. *Antiviral Res.*, **6**, 241–252.
141. Higgins, P. G., Barrow, G. I., Al-Nakib, W. *et al.* (1988). Failure to demonstrate synergy between interferon-α and a synthetic antiviral, enviroxime, in rhinovirus infections in volunteers. *Antiviral Res.*, **10**, 141–149.
142. Hayden, F. G., Kaiser, D. L. and Albrecht, J. K. (1988). Intranasal recombinant alfa-2b interferon treatment of naturally occurring common colds. *Antimicrob. Agents Chemother.*, **32**, 224–230.
143. Gwaltney, J. M., Jr (1992). Combined antiviral and antimediator treatment of rhinovirus colds. *J. Infect. Dis.*, **166**, 776–782.
144. Phillpotts, R. J., Delong, D. C., Wallace, J. *et al.* (1981). The activity of enviroxime against rhinovirus infection in man. *Lancet*, **i**, 1342–1344.
145. Hayden, F. G. and Gwaltney, J. M., Jr (1982). Prophylactic activity of intranasal enviroxime against experimentally induced rhinovirus type 39 infection. *Antimicrob. Agents Chemother.*, **21**, 892–897.
146. Zerial, A., Werner, G. H., Phillpotts, R. J. *et al.* (1985). Studies on 44081 RP, a new antirhinovirus compound, in cell cultures and in human volunteers. *Antimicrob. Agents Chemother.*, **27**, 846–850.
147. Al-Nakib, W., Higgins, P. G., Barrow, I. *et al.* (1987). Prophylaxis and treatment of rhinovirus colds with zinc gluconate lozenges. *J. Antimicrob. Chemother.*, **20**, 893–901.
148. Togo, Y., Schwartz, A. R. and Hornick, R. B. (1973). Antiviral effect of 3,4-dihydro-1-isoquinolineacetamide hydrochloride in experimental human rhinovirus infection. *Antimicrob. Agents Chemother.*, **4**, 612–616.
149. Reed, S. E. and Bynoe, M. L. (1970). The antiviral activity of isoquinoline drugs for rhinoviruses in vitro and in vivo. *J. Med. Microbiol.*, **3**, 346–352.
150. Reed, S. E., Craig, J. W. and Tyrrell, D. A. J. (1976). Four compounds active

against rhinovirus: comparison in vitro and in volunteers. *J. Infect. Dis.*, **133**, A128–A135.
151. Phillpotts, R. J., Wallace, J., Tyrrell, D. A. J. *et al.* (1983). Therapeutic activity of enviroxime against rhinovirus infection in volunteers. *Antimicrob. Agents Chemother.*, **23**, 671–675.
152. Levandowski, R. A., Pachucki, C. T., Rubenis, M. and Jackson, G. G. (1982). Topical enviroxime against rhinovirus infection. *Antimicrob. Agents Chemother.*, **22**, 1004–1007.
153. Farr, B. M., Conner, E. M., Betts, R.F. *et al.* (1987). Two randomized controlled trials of zinc gluconate lozenge therapy of experimentally induced rhinovirus colds. *Antimicrob. Agents Chemother.*, **31**, 1183–1187.
154. Tyrrell, D., Barrow, I. and Arthur, J. (1989). Local hyperthermia benefits natural and experimental common colds. *Br. Med. J.*, **298**, 1280–1283.
155. Hendley, J. O., Abbott, R. D., Beasley, P. P. and Gwaltney, J. M. (1994). Effect of inhalation of hot humidified air on experimental rhinovirus infection. *JAMA*, **271**, 1112–1113.
156. DeLong, D. C. (1984). Effect of enviroxime on rhinovirus in humans. In *Microbiology*, L. Leive and D. Schlessinger (eds), American Society for Microbiology, Washington, DC, pp. 431–434.
157. Miller, F. D., Monto, A. S., DeLong, D. C. *et al.* (1985). Controlled trial of enviroxime against rhinovirus infections in a community. *Antimicrob. Agents Chemother.*, **27**, 102–106.
158. Gilbert, B. E., Six, H. R., Wilson, S. Z. *et al.* (1988). Small particle aerosols of enviroxime containing liposomes. *Antiviral Res.* **9**, 355–365.
159. Alarcon, B., Zerial, A., Dupiol, C. and Carrascom, L. (1986). Anti-rhinovirus compound 44081 R P inhibits virus uncoating. *Antimicrob. Agents Chemother.*, **30**, 31–34.
160. Korant, B. D., Kauer, J. C. and Butterworth, B. E. (1974). Zinc ions inhibit replication of rhinoviruses. *Nature*, **248**, 588–590.
161. Korant, D. D. and Butterworth, B. E. (1976). Inhibition by zinc of rhinovirus protein cleavage: interaction of zinc with capsid polypeptides. *J. Virol.*, **18**, 298–306.
162. Geist, F. C., Bateman, J. A. and Hayden, F. G. (1987). In vitro activity of zinc salts against human rhinoviruses. *Antimicrob. Agents Chemother.*, **31**, 622–624.
163. Merluzzi, V. J., Cipriano, D., McNeil, D. *et al.* (1989). Evaluation of zinc complexes on the replication of rhinovirus 2 in vitro. *Res. Commun. Chem. Pathol. Pharmacol.*, **66**, 425–440.
164. Eby, G. A., Davis, D. R. and Halcomb, W. W. (1984). Reduction in duration of common colds by zinc gluconate lozenges in a double-blind study. *Antimicrob. Agents Chemother.*, **25**, 20–24.
165. Weismann, K., Jakobsen, J. P., Weismann, J. E. *et al.* (1990). Zinc gluconate lozenges for common cold. *Danish Med. Bull.*, **37**, 279–281.
166. Douglas, R. M., Miles, H. B., Moore, B. W. *et al.* (1987). Failure of effervescent zinc acetate lozenges to alter the course of upper respiratory infections in Australian adults. *Antimicrob. Agents Chemother.*, **31**, 1263–1265.
167. Smith, D. S., Nuttall, C. E., Helzner, E. C. *et al.* (1987). Zinc gluconate in the treatment of the common cold. (Abstr.) Meeting of the Society for General Internal Medicine, San Diego. *Clin. Res.*, **35**, 761A.
168. Farr, B. M. and Gwaltney, J. M., Jr (1987). The problems of taste in placebo matching: an evaluation of zinc gluconate for the common cold. *J. Chronic Dis.*, **40**, 875–879.
169. Godfrey, J. C., Sloane, B. C., Turco, J. H. *et al.* (1991). Zinc and common cold:

positive findings in controlled clinical study of a new formulation. *31st Interscience Conference on Antimicrobial Agents and Chemotherapy*, p. 329 (Abstr. 1381), Chicago, Illinois.
170. Grunberg, E. and Prince, H. N. (1968). The antiviral activity of 3,4-dihydro-1-isoquinolineacetamide hydrochloride in vitro, in vivo and in small laboratory animals. *Proc. Soc. Exp. Biol. Med.*, **129**, 422–430.
171. Ophir, D. and Elad, Y. (1987). Effects of steam inhalation on nasal patency and nasal symptoms in patients with the common cold. *Am. J. Otolaryngol.*, **3**, 149–153.
172. MacKinin, M. L., Mathew, S. and Medendorp, S. V. (1990). Effects of inhaling heated vapor on symptoms of the common cold. *JAMA*, **264**, 989–991.
173. Forstall, G. J., Mackinin, M. L., Yen-Lieberman, B. R. and Medendorp, S. V. (1994). Effect of inhaling heated vapor on symptoms of the common cold. *JAMA*, **271**, 1109–1111.
174. Griffin, D. E. (1991). Therapy of viral infections of the central nervous system. *Antiviral Res.*, **15**, 1–10.
175. Wilfert, C. M. and McKinney, R. E. (1986). Immunotherapy of enterovirus infections. In *Antiviral Chemotherapy: New Directions for Clinical Applications and Research*, J. Mills and L. Corey (eds), Elsevier, New York, pp. 90–96.
176. Modlin, J. F. (1990). Coxsackieviruses, echoviruses and newer enteroviruses. In *Principles and Practice of Infectious Diseases*, G. L. Mandell, R. G. Douglas and J. E. Bennett (eds), Churchill Livingstone, New York, pp. 1367–1383.
177. Johnston, J. M. and Overall, J. C. (1989). Intravenous immunoglobulin in disseminated neonatal echovirus 11 infection. *Pediatr. Infect. Dis. J.*, **8**, 254–256.
178. McKinney, R. E., Jr, Katz, S. L. and Wilfert, C. M. (1987). Chronic enteroviral meningoencephalitis in agammaglobulinemic patients. *Rev. Infect. Dis.*, **9**, 334–356.
179. Dwyer, J. M. and Erlendsson, K. (1988). Intraventricular gamma-globulin for the management of enterovirus encephalitis. *Pediatr. Infect. Dis. J.*, **7**, S30–S33.
180. Erlendsson, K., Swartz, T. and Dwyer, J. M. (1985). Successful reversal of echovirus encephalitis in X-linked hypogammaglobulinemia by intraventricular administration of immunoglobulin. *N. Engl. J. Med.*, **312**, 351–353.

12 Respiratory Syncytial Virus: Antiviral Therapy

MARY ANN CARMACK and CHARLES G. PROBER
Division of Infectious Diseases, Stanford University School of Medicine, Stanford, California, USA

RESPIRATORY SYNCYTIAL VIRUS

HISTORY

> During October, 1955, a respiratory illness characterized by coughing, sneezing and mucopurulent nasal discharge occurred in a colony of 20 'normal' chimpanzees at the Walter Reed Army Institute of Research. (1)

Thus, Morris, Blount and Savage (1) began their seminal description of the isolation of a virus collected by throat swab from one of the chimpanzees named Sue. They named this virus chimpanzee coryza agent (CCA). Subsequently, using intranasal instillation of tissue culture-adapted CCA, they reproduced similar clinical illnesses in another group of six chimpanzees. Sera containing antibodies to CCA were recovered from the infected chimpanzees as well as from a laboratory worker who developed a clinical upper respiratory infection while working with CCA cultures and the infected chimpanzees. However, viral isolation from either the infected chimpanzees or laboratory worker was unsuccessful.

The following year, Chanock and colleagues (2) reported the recovery of two similar viruses from throat swabs of two infants with severe lower respiratory illnesses (patient Long with bronchopneumonia and patient Snyder with laryngotracheobronchitis). These agents, which they named Long virus and Snyder virus, demonstrated the striking property of producing large syncytial areas in tissue cultures. This cytopathogenic effect was identical to that seen with CCA virus.

In epidemiological studies the same year, Chanock and Finberg (3) found that 80% of children by age 4 years demonstrated antisera to Long virus. These investigators therefore proposed the name 'respiratory syncytial virus', acknowledging the respiratory nature of the illness and the tissue culture properties of the virus.

In the ensuing 1958–9 winter season, using improved culture techniques,

Antiviral Chemotherapy. Edited by D.J. Jeffries and E. De Clercq

Beem and co-workers (4) successfully isolated from 41 patients an agent having similar cytopathic characteristics in tissue culture: formation of giant cells and extensive syncytial areas. Complement fixation tests suggested antigenic similarity among the viruses they had isolated, the Long strain, and CCA. In their report, the investigators described the clinical illness they observed, well known today as respiratory syncytial virus (RSV) infection:

> The illnesses of patients from whom this virus was isolated ranged from mild coryzal symptoms to fatal bronchiolitis. However, some degree of involvement of the lower respiratory tract was present in almost every patient from whom the virus was isolated. In the youngest age groups this frequently presented as bronchiolitis or bronchopneumonia . . .
>
> The rate of virus isolation varied inversely with age and was particularly high among infants less than six months of age (46 per cent) as compared to older patients (10 per cent). However, it was observed that there was a history of concomitant acute respiratory illness among older members of the family of 12 of 13 virus-positive patients less than six months of age . . . In general, the clinical illness of infants was more severe and protracted . . .
>
> This agent appears to have been prevalent in the community for a relatively brief period . . . Isolations of chimpanzee coryza agent were made from December, 1958, through April, 1959, but the great majority (70 per cent) were made during January and February, 1959. No isolations were made during May or June. (4)

EPIDEMIOLOGY AND SIGNIFICANCE OF RSV AS PATHOGEN

In subsequent years, major epidemiological studies have substantiated and elaborated upon the prescient observations recorded by Beem and co-workers over three decades ago (4). These studies have established RSV as the major respiratory pathogen causing acute lower respiratory illness in infants and young children (5–12).

Remarkable constancy in the characteristics of RSV infection is evident in the variety of studies reflecting markedly disparate geographies and populations. Unlike other viral respiratory agents which cause epidemics at irregular intervals, RSV is unique in its ability to cause yearly predictable epidemics of respiratory disease (8). The epidemics last approximately five months spanning autumn, winter, and spring, with alternating short (7- to 12-month) and long (13- to 16-month) intervals between successive epidemic peaks (8). In some areas, the mid-winter epidemics which occur after the short intervals have been noted to be more severe than are the epidemics which follow the long intervals (13).

During extensive epidemiological studies conducted from 1957 to 1970 in the Washington, DC area, Parrott and colleagues (5,8,10,14) analysed respiratory tract illnesses in over 17 000 infants and children. Their work established that approximately one-half of infants were infected with the RSV during their first RSV epidemic, and almost all infants had been infected after two epidemics. From their data, these researchers estimated that 1% of primary RSV infections during infancy resulted in hospitalization (8).

Based on data collected over a five-year period (1975–1979) in Houston, Texas, Glezen and co-workers (15) estimated that the risk of hospitalization due to RSV infection during the first year of life was five per 1000 live births per year among low-income families. Over 80% of those hospitalized were less than six months of age. In an 11-year study conducted in a paediatric outpatient setting in Chapel Hill, North Carolina (1964–1974), Murphy and colleagues collected throat cultures for isolation of viruses and mycoplasmas from over 1400 children (from birth to 15 years of age) who were diagnosed with pneumonia. RSV alone accounted for one-third of all isolates from children less than seven years of age (9).

A collaborative study conducted at 10 centres in Britain between 1973 and 1975 also confirmed that RSV was the major cause of acute lower respiratory infection in infancy. Hospital admission rates as high as one in 40 in industrial areas were observed for infants one to three months of age (11).

The severity of infection and risk for hospitalization due to RSV infection is higher among younger infants. In a four-year study in Houston of children hospitalized with RSV infection, 95% were less than one year of age, and 81% were less than six months of age (15). In another study of 87 previously well infants hospitalized for RSV infection, those under six weeks of age were at greatest risk for a prolonged and complicated hospital course (16).

Infants and young children who are compromised by underlying disease, such as bronchopulmonary dysplasia, congenital heart disease, cystic fibrosis and immunodeficiency, also are at especially high risk of severe infection caused by RSV (17–20). In a prospective study of 30 young children with bronchopulmonary dysplasia, RSV infection was found to be the most frequent reason for rehospitalization during the winter months. During the four-month study period, 59% of the children with bronchopulmonary dysplasia developed RSV infection, and 11 of 15 hospitalizations were due to this agent. Morbidity in this population was high: although no fatalities occurred, seven patients were hospitalized more than seven days and four required admission to the intensive care unit (18).

Similarly, in a four-year prospective study of infants hospitalized during RSV seasons, MacDonald and co-workers (20) found that RSV-infected infants with congenital heart disease had significantly more severe or fatal illness than did those who were not so compromised. Intensive care unit support was four times more likely to be required by the 27 infants with congenital heart disease. Furthermore, 37% of those with congenital heart disease died in contrast with 1.5% of the previously normal infants.

Hall and co-workers (19) prospectively evaluated the severity of RSV infection in patients with compromised immune function in comparison with normal children. Whereas 15% of patients with normal immunity required intensive care, 60% of patients undergoing chemotherapy and 80% of those with immunodeficiency disease required intensive care. Fifteen per cent of patients undergoing chemotherapy and 40% of patients with immunodeficiency disease died compared with a mortality rate of 0.5% in patients with normal immunity.

In summary, RSV is the most important respiratory pathogen in infants and young children, accounting for significant morbidity, occasional mortality, and considerable health care expense. The virus is ubiquitous, causes predictable yearly outbreaks, and poses greatest risk to the very young and those who are compromised by underlying disease.

RSV: THE PATHOGEN

RSV is classified as a member of the family Paramyxoviridae, genus Pneumovirus (21). It is a fragile, medium-sized virus (120–300 nm in diameter) containing single-stranded RNA within a spiked helical nucleocapsid (22). Because the virus is heat labile, predominantly cell associated, and easily distorted during purification procedures, attempts to elucidate its proteins have been complicated (22,23).

Identification of two distinct subtypes (1 and 2 or A and B) of RSV was reported in 1985 by Anderson and colleagues (24) and by Mufson and colleagues (25) using monoclonal antibody analysis. Subsequently, cloning and sequencing studies showed that the two subtypes have greatest divergence in the structure of the G (attachment) protein; in contrast, the other major surface glycoprotein, the F (fusion) protein, is more highly conserved (26,27). Studies have shown that the two strain types can co-circulate within the same community during the same RSV season and that the relative frequency of isolation of the two strains can vary in different years and even between communities during the same season (28). Although the epidemiological and clinical significance of these antigenic differences remains to be fully clarified, they may help to explain certain features of RSV disease: variation in disease severity, susceptibility to disease in spite of the presence of maternal antibodies, failure of vaccines to provide protection, and lifelong susceptibility to recurrent infections (25,28,29).

Hall and co-workers studied 1209 RSV isolates collected over a 15-year period from hospitalized and ambulatory children. Although the distribution pattern of strain groups was not related to more severe outbreaks of RSV disease and infection with one strain did not more frequently result in hospitalization, the proportion of hospitalized children who required intensive care correlated with strain group. Specifically, 15.4% of children with group A infections required intensive care in contrast to 8.3% of those with group B infections. The investigators proposed that these findings may suggest greater pathogenicity for group A strains (30).

CLINICAL SPECTRUM OF DISEASE

Signs and symptoms of RSV infection can range in severity from mild upper respiratory infection to severe life-threatening bronchiolitis or pneumonia. In most cases, the disease resolves without difficulty within one to two weeks, but some infants require hospitalization. As detailed above, estimates of the proportion of infants who are hospitalized for an RSV infection during the first year of life range from 5 to 20 in 1000 (8,11,15). Among hospitalized patients, frequent clinical manifestations include rhinitis, wheezing, tachypnoea, cough, retractions, hyperinflation, hypoxia and apnoea (31).

Most hospitalized patients improve rapidly with supportive care alone. For example, in a study of 87 previously well infants, the mean duration of hospitalization was 3.4 ± 2.6 days (16). Nevertheless, 11% of the infants were admitted to the intensive care unit and 7% required mechanical ventilation. Other studies have reported similar results for previously normal infants (19,20). As previously discussed, infants with underlying cardiorespiratory and immunological problems are at substantially greater risk for severe and prolonged illness (18–20).

RSV can cause acute respiratory illness in individuals of any age. Indeed, immunity to RSV is short lived, and infections can recur throughout life (7). However, with increased age and subsequent reinfection, severity of illness progressively diminishes for normal individuals. It is the primary infection occurring in almost all children by two years of age which is potentially most serious, and specifically it is the infant under six months of age who is at greatest risk to require hospitalization for RSV infection (7,15).

PATHOGENESIS OF LOWER RESPIRATORY ILLNESS DUE TO RSV

Delineation of the pathogenic mechanisms of RSV infection has been the subject of intense study over the past 30 years. Such understanding is important in guiding the development and use of therapeutic interventions as well as immunoprophylactic strategies.

The very small terminal airways of infants presumably are a major factor increasing the infant's susceptibility to respiratory infections (32). A number of observations also have focused on the role of the immune system in augmenting or ameliorating the severity of the infection (32,33). Initial speculation concentrated on the role of serum antibodies. Following the administration of formalin-inactivated vaccine to children aged six months to five years, it was noted that the younger subjects experienced a more severe illness following natural infection than did the unvaccinated controls. This result, combined with the observation that RSV infections tend to be more severe in infants less than six months of age (a time when passively transferred maternal antibody is present) led to the suggestion that serum antibody might contribute to the pathogenesis of RSV disease (34). However, when Bruhn and Yeager evaluated the severity of clinical illness due to RSV in 41 infants less than six months of age, no relationship was demonstrated between severity of illness and the complement fixation titre to RSV in cord sera, acute sera or convalescent sera (35). In fact, data from more recent prospective studies indicate that infants born to mothers with high titres of IgG antibody to RSV are better protected against RSV infection during the first months of life (15,36). Moreover, animal models of RSV infection have demonstrated that treatment with human immunoglobulin results in significant reduction in the quantity of virus recovered from lung specimens and no adverse histopathological effects (37,38). Overall, studies show that IgG, IgM and IgA isotypes do not appear to exacerbate the disease process and, in fact, ameliorate primary infection and provide partial protection against reinfection (32).

Various theories focusing on the immune mediation of RSV disease have been advanced. Welliver (32) has reviewed these theories of pathogenesis, which include immune complex reactions, cell-mediated cytotoxicity and IgE mediation. The role of cell-mediated immune hyper-responsiveness in the pathogenesis of RSV infection is particularly interesting. It has been demonstrated that infants with bronchiolitis or asthma at the time of RSV infection have significantly greater cell-mediated immune responses than those with mild upper respiratory illness or pneumonia without wheezing (39,40). These observations suggest that excessive RSV-specific cell-mediated immune responsiveness leads to increased airway reactivity.

RSV infection during infancy has been associated with continuing airway hyper-reactivity in childhood (41–44). However, an unequivocal causal link has not been shown (45). Welliver and co-workers have found that titres of RSV-specific IgE in nasopharyngeal secretions are higher in individuals who manifest wheezing with their RSV infections (46). Prospective studies by these investigators also suggest that the magnitude of the RSV IgE response at the time of primary RSV bronchiolitis has predictive value for the development of recurrent wheezing through 48 months of age (47,48). Whether RSV bronchiolitis predisposes an individual to subsequent reactive airway disease and pulmonary dysfunction or identifies those who have a genetic proclivity for airway hyper-reactivity is an important question. The answer has potential implications regarding the role of antiviral therapy at the time of acute illness in mitigating subsequent immunologically mediated airway hyper-reactivity (47).

ANTIVIRAL THERAPY

Until recently, therapy for severe RSV infection was limited to supportive measures such as supplemental oxygen, hydration and assisted ventilation.

With approval of ribavirin, by the Food and Drug Administration (FDA) in 1986, for the treatment of RSV infection, a new controversial and costly antiviral chemotherapeutic intervention became available. Few drugs have evoked more discussion or debate.

In this section, discussion will focus primarily on aerosolized ribavirin and to a lesser extent on intravenous immunoglobulin therapy for the treatment of RSV infection. The published evidence for the efficacy of each modality will be carefully considered. The role of adjunctive therapies such as β-agonists, theophylline, physiotherapy, mist treatment, supplemental oxygen, antibiotics and corticosteroids is beyond the scope of this review.

RIBAVIRIN

History of drug development

Ribavirin (1-β-D-ribofuranosyl-1,2,4-triazole-3-carboxamide) is a synthetic nucleoside analogue. The synthesis of this antiviral was first described in 1972 by researchers at the ICN Nucleic Acid Research Institute (49). In early studies, the developers demonstrated a broad spectrum of antiviral activity *in vitro* and in animal studies against at least 16 RNA and DNA viruses (49–51).

Initially, ribavirin was administered orally to humans for the treatment of influenza A and B infections. These studies yielded inconclusive and generally unimpressive results; some trials failed to show any effect while others demonstrated mild to moderate symptomatic improvement (52–54). However, when administered by aerosol, ribavirin was shown to be effective in mitigating severity and duration of illness and viral shedding in adults with influenza A and B infections (55,56). In West Africa, oral and intravenous ribavirin decreased mortality in adults with Lassa fever, an often fatal disease caused by infection with an arenavirus (57). Favourable results have also been reported with the use of oral ribavirin in the treatment of measles, acute viral hepatitis and herpes simplex virus infections (58–61).

Antiviral activity of ribavirin was first demonstrated against RSV *in vitro* in 1980 (62) and in the cotton rat model in 1982 (63). In cotton rats, treatment with ribavirin reduced the quantity of RSV in nasal turbinates and in lung tissue by over 90% in comparison with untreated rats. Although ribavirin was equally effective when administered intraperitoneally or by aerosol, the drug was effective at lower dosage following aerosol delivery (63).

In 1983, Hall and colleagues (64) first demonstrated the efficacy of aerosolized ribavirin in the treatment of experimentally infected adult human volunteers. Beginning on the third day following intranasal inoculation with RSV, drug or placebo was administered by aerosol for a total of 12 h per day for three days. Although the drug appeared to have no effect on minor upper respiratory symptoms, the frequency of systemic complaints and fever was reduced in the treated group. No adverse effects were noted. The first report of aerosolized ribavirin in the treatment of RSV-infected hospitalized infants soon followed (65).

In 1986, aerosolized ribavirin was approved by the FDA for use in non-mechanically ventilated patients with moderately severe disease caused by RSV. This approval was based on three double-blind placebo-controlled trials which demonstrated clinical improvement in infants who were treated with aerosolized ribavirin for RSV infection (64–66). Subsequent studies have continued to examine the efficacy of aerosolized ribavirin in infants with RSV infection (18,67–70).

In 1986, the Canadian Paediatric Society (71) published indications for the use of aerosolized ribavirin in infants and young children with RSV infection. In 1987, the American Academy of Pediatrics (72) published similar recommendations. These guidelines enumerated the indications for *consideration* for treatment with ribavirin, as follows: (a) infants at high risk for severe or complicated RSV infection; (b) infants judged to be severely

Table 12.1. Recommendations of the American Academy of Pediatrics Committee on Infectious Diseases: candidates for ribavirin treatment (73)

I. Ribavirin treatment is *recommended* for the following patients hospitalized with lower respiratory tract disease caused by RSV.

A. Infants at high risk for severe or complicated RSV infection, including those with
   1. Congenital heart disease
   2. Bronchopulmonary dysplasia
   3. Cystic fibrosis
   4. Other chronic lung conditions
   5. Premature infants
   6. Immunodeficiency (e.g., chemotherapy, recent transplant, immunodeficiency disease)

B. Infants hospitalized with RSV lower respiratory tract disease who are severely ill, as judged by
   1. $PaO_2 < 65$ mmHg
   2. Increasing $PaCO_2$

C. All patients mechanically ventilated for RSV infection

II. Ribavirin treatment should be *considered* for the following patients hospitalized with RSV lower respiratory tract disease which is not initially severe, but who may be at some increased risk of progressing to a more complicated course, by virtue of
   A. Young age (less than 6 weeks)
   B. Underlying condition (e.g., multiple congenital anomalies, neurologic disease, metabolic disease)

From American Academy of Pediatrics, *Report of the Committee on Infectious Diseases*, 23rd edn. Elk Grove Village, IL: American Academy of Pediatrics, 1994, 570–574.

ill with RSV lower respiratory tract disease; and (c) infants whose lower respiratory tract disease is not initially severe but who are at risk for progression to a complicated course due to young age or underlying condition. However, in 1994, the guidelines of the American Academy of Pediatrics (73) were revised as follows: ribavirin is *recommended* for (a) infants at high risk for severe or complicated RSV infection; (b) infants who are severely ill with RSV infection; and (c) all patients mechanically ventilated for RSV infection. The 1994 guidelines continue to recommend that ribavirin treatment be *considered* for infants who may be at risk for progressing from a mild to more complicated course due to young age or underlying condition. These 1994 guidelines are detailed in Table 12.1. Of note, the Committee's change from wording that suggested *consideration* to treat with ribavirin to an unequivocal *recommendation* to treat with ribavirin has been controversial and has been criticized as a premature endorsement of the drug based on insufficient and unconvincing evidence of therapeutic efficacy (74–76).

Pharmacology and drug delivery

X-ray crystallography has shown that ribavirin most closely resembles guanosine in structure (77), and *in vitro* interference with ribavirin antiviral activity has been demonstrated by adding guanosine to the system (78,79). These findings suggest that ribavirin may act as an analogue of this metabolite (77).

The exact mechanism of action by ribavirin has not been fully elucidated; proposed mechanisms are based primarily on studies with the influenza viruses. After rapid absorption across cell membranes, ribavirin is enzymatically converted into its 5′-phosphate derivatives and the deribosylated base (80,81). These metabolites appear to inhibit the expression of messenger RNA by interfering with the capping and elongation of messenger RNA; additionally, ribavirin may reduce guanine nucleosides via feedback inhibition (82,83). The potential for multi-site inhibition may help explain why viral resistance to ribavirin has not been observed (84).

Although the pharmacokinetic properties of ribavirin have been studied extensively in rats, only limited data are available for non-human primates and humans (85,86). Data derived from rat studies should not be extrapolated to humans because of major differences in distribution and metabolism between the species (85).

In humans, orally administered ribavirin is eliminated primarily by the renal route and has an elimination half-life of approximately 9 h in plasma (87). Ribavirin and ribavirin metabolites concentrate in red blood cells and other tissues; in humans, the erythrocyte levels decline with a half-life of approximately 40 days (85). Following intravenous administration of [^{14}C]ribavirin to monkeys, less than 1% of the drug was found in the lungs 8 h later; 45–60% was excreted in urine within 72 h (85,86).

Aerosolized delivery of ribavirin has been accomplished with a small particle aerosol generator (SPAG) which continuously delivers a flow of small particles with a mass medium diameter of about 1.3 μm (55,88). This device can be used to deliver the aerosol by mask, oxygen tent, oxygen hood or endotracheal tube. With a ribavirin concentration of 20 mg/ml in the delivery system reservoir and a constant aerosol flow rate, an estimated 0.82 mg/kg per hour of ribavirin is deposited in the respiratory tract (56). This estimate assumes that 70% of the inhaled aerosol is deposited in the respiratory tract; the actual dose will be dependent on the patient's ventilation and lung pathology.

Ribavirin is absorbed systemically following delivery by aerosol, but the concentration of drug in the respiratory tract is much higher than in plasma. In non-intubated children receiving aerosolized ribavirin, plasma concentrations increase with duration of treatment from a mean plasma concentration of 0.19 μg/ml after 2.5 h of aerosolized ribavirin to 1.10 μg/ml after 8 h (87). In an intubated four-month-old infant who was treated with continuously aerosolized ribavirin for 16 h per day for seven days, daily peak plasma concentrations of ribavirin ranged from 0.2 to 1.6 μg/ml (mean peak concentration 1.0 μg/ml); in contrast, the peak concentration in endotracheal secretions ranged from 31.5 to 412.4 μg/ml (mean peak concentration 197.4 μg/ml). Maximum peak plasma and secretion concentrations were attained on day 2 of therapy (Prober, unpublished observations). In another report, the elimination half-life of ribavirin in tracheal secretions was approximately 1.5–2.5 h (87).

In North America, ribavirin is licensed only for aerosolized delivery, and the product package insert carries a warning stating that the use of aerosolized ribavirin in patients receiving mechanical ventilation should be undertaken only when personnel are familiar with the ventilator being used and this mode of administration of the drug (89). This warning was required by the FDA due to problems encountered with precipitation of the drug in mechanical ventilation equipment leading to increased positive inspiratory and end-expiratory pressures. However, delivery systems have been developed for use in mechanically ventilated patients (90,91). In centres with personnel who are experienced in its use, safe administration has been demonstrated provided the equipment is vigilantly monitored to detect drug precipitation and filters, valves and tubing are changed frequently (70,90,91).

Immunoregulatory effects

Although the mechanism has not been established, ribavirin has been reported to have immunosuppressive effects. *In vitro* antigen- and mitogen-induced human lymphocyte proliferation is suppressed when ribavirin is added to lymphocyte cultures (92). Similarly, antigen-stimulated release of mast cell mediators (β-hexosaminidase and leukotriene C_4) is inhibited when ribavirin is added to mast cell cultures (42). In studies conducted in infants receiving either ribavirin or placebo aerosol, serum-neutralizing antibody (66) and RSV-specific IgA and IgE responses in nasopharyngeal secretions (93) are suppressed in those receiving ribavirin. The potential significance of these immunological phenomena on the short-term and long-term consequences of RSV infection needs to be evaluated in prospectively conducted studies.

Adverse effects and toxicity

In general, ribavirin is well tolerated. Although oral and intravenous ribavirin have been associated with transient decreases in red blood cell counts and increases in serum bilirubin (52,54,57,81,94), no such effects have been reported with the use of aerosolized ribavirin (64–69,95). Aerosolized ribavirin occasionally has been associated with bronchospasm, but whether this effect is due to the treatment or the viral respiratory infection is difficult to determine (90,96).

Ribavirin is a teratogen, carcinogen and mutagen in animals and cell culture (97,98). When administered to pregnant hamsters in relatively small, single doses, ribavirin caused fetal absorption and malformations (98). Although there are no pertinent human data, teratogenicity and/or embryolethality have been demonstrated in virtually all animal species in which ribavirin has been tested. Based on these data, ribavirin is contraindicated in women who are or may become pregnant during exposure to the drug (89).

Aerosolization of ribavirin into the atmosphere exposes health care providers, visitors and other patients to the drug. In studies evaluating environmental exposure to ribavirin, analysis of air samples indicates that exposure to health care workers is greatest when ribavirin is delivered by oxygen tent and least when delivered by mechanical ventilation (99). In one study, ribavirin was not detected in erythrocytes, plasma or urine from any of 19 nurses caring for infants who received ribavirin by ventilator, oxygen tent and oxygen hood (100). In another study conducted by the California Department of Health Services, multiple blood and urine specimens were analysed for 10 health care workers who cared for patients receiving ribavirin. No ribavirin was detected in any urine or serum samples; however, the drug was detected at a concentration of 0.44 μg/ml in one erythrocyte sample which was collected from a nurse five days after she first cared for a patient receiving ribavirin by oxygen tent (99).

The potential health risks thus posed have caused considerable controversy and concern among health care workers, especially those who are of reproductive age. As a result of the findings regarding teratogenicity and environmental exposure of health care providers, a task force at the University of California recommended restriction of ribavirin aerosol to administration only via endotracheal tube in mechanically ventilated patients (101). In 1990 the Children's Hospital in Boston established stringent precautions for administration of ribavirin, including (a) use of an exhausted containment chamber around the oxygen hood and patient, (b) use of an isolation room with negative air pressure, (c) required use of disposable full-body coverings for all who enter the patient's room, and (d) provision of air-purifying respirator or disposable particulate respirator to health care workers when exposure is prolonged (102). In response to concerns about environmental exposure, the drug manufacturer now markets an aerosol delivery hood scavenger system for use in aerosolized ribavirin delivery. However, due to size restrictions of the hood, this system is practical only in infants weighing less than 5 kg (96).

In 1991 the American Academy of Pediatrics Committee on Infectious Diseases (73) and the Canadian Paediatric Society of Infectious Diseases and Immunization Committee (103) concluded that the collective evidence regarding ribavirin's teratogenicity and risk of exposure for health care workers does not support the need for extensive precautions. Noting that the absorption of ribavirin from the lung into the circulation appears to be minimal and that no adverse effects in human fetuses have been reported after five years of clinical use in the United States, the American committee concluded that 'the teratogenicity of ribavirin in humans remains highly questionable' (73); similarly, the Canadian committee concluded that 'the risk to hospital personnel caring for children treated with ribavirin aerosol appears to be negligible' (103).

Cost of ribavirin

Ribavirin is an expensive drug. The wholesale cost to the pharmacy per 6.0 g vial of drug in 1994 was about $1300. Wholesale hospital acquisition cost is not substantially less for this drug which has a single vendor. Thus, the cost of the drug alone for a five-day course of therapy is approximately $6500. The expense of ancillary services required to administer the drug adds significantly to the total cost; these services include respiratory therapist time and respiratory therapy equipment. Therefore, the total charges attributable to the use of this drug (in excess of those resulting from the hospitalization itself) are many thousands of dollars.

Clinical trials: paediatric patients

In 1986, the FDA approved the licensure of aerosolized ribavirin for treatment of RSV infection in spontaneously breathing infants. This approval was based on treatment efficacy demonstrated in three controlled clinical trials (64–66). Subsequent to the drug's licensure, an additional five controlled clinical studies have been published (67–70,104). Although each trial demonstrates some measure of therapeutic benefit from ribavirin, critical review of many of these studies has raised important unresolved questions, including the clinical meaning and significance of reported therapeutic benefits, cost-effectiveness and appropriate guidelines for patient selection for treatment (105–111).

Thus, despite eight major clinical trials involving collectively over 170 patients treated with ribavirin since 1983, the clinical efficacy of ribavirin across a variety of patient populations is not unequivocally established and debate continues. In 1988, Wald and colleagues published a detailed and carefully considered critical review of five of these eight clinical trials (111). Many others have contributed articles, editorials and letters debating the role of ribavirin therapy for RSV infections as well as the need for further studies. In sum, considerable controversy continues to surround the use of ribavirin for the treatment of RSV infection in infants. Therefore, it is important to review these studies critically in some detail. The therapeutic effects demonstrated by these trials published before and after the licensure of ribavirin are summarized in Tables 12.2 and 12.3, respectively.

Hall et al., *1983 (65)*

The first published prospective, randomized, double-blind study enrolled previously normal infants hospitalized because of documented RSV lower respiratory tract infection. Patients were randomized to receive aerosol treatment with either ribavirin ($n = 16$) or water placebo ($n = 17$) for an average of 20 h per day for three to six days. Daily clinical signs were recorded using a rating scale of 0 (normal) to 3+ (severe); in addition, an overall assessment ('severity of illness' score) was assigned based on a visual scale ranging from 0 (normal) to 4+ (severe). Of note, by the time therapy was initiated, patients in the placebo group had improved so much that their illness score was significantly lower than that of the ribavirin group. In addition, determinations of arterial oxygen tension or saturation and quantitative viral cultures were performed upon enrolment and daily during treatment.

The results indicated the following statistically significant improvements for the ribavirin group compared with the placebo group: (a) lower illness severity score by the fourth day of treatment; (b) greater mean increment of improvement in illness score between day 1 and the end of therapy; (c) greater degree of improvement in scored lower respiratory tract signs (cough, rales, retractions) and lethargy from start to end of therapy; (d) greater mean increment in improvement in oxygen tension from start to end of therapy; and (e) decreased quantity of viral shedding by the end of therapy and shorter duration of viral shedding from the start of therapy. The authors concluded that the ribavirin-treated infants had 'significant

Table 12.2. Demonstrated therapeutic effects of ribavirin: clinical trials prior to drug licensure

Ref.	Patient population	Illness score[a]	Oxygenation[b]	Antiviral effect[c]	Other parameters
(65)	16 R 17 P	Scale: 0 to 4+ 0.9 (R) vs 1.6 (P)[d]	62.4 mmHg (R) vs 56 mmHg (P)	Viral shedding (days): 2.9 (R) vs 4.3 (P) Viral titres at end of therapy: 0.3 (R) vs 1.3 (P)	Improved cough, rales, retractions; lethargy No significant difference in fever, nasal congestion, wheezing
(66)	12 R 14 P	Scale: 0 to 3+ 0.6 (R) vs 1.3 (P)	Not reported	Viral shedding and viral titres not significantly different	No significant difference in rhinitis, respiratory rate, length of treatment, length of hospitalization
(94)	14 R (6 with BPD/CHD) 12 P (7 with BPD/CHD)	Scale: 0 to 10+ 2.6 (R) vs 3.2 (P)[d]	72.5 mmHg (R) vs 58.2 mmHg (P)	Fewer patients shedding on day 5; Viral titres on day 5: 0.8 (R) vs 2.9 (P)	Not reported

R = ribavirin group; P = placebo group; BPD = bronchopulmonary dysplasia; CHD = congenital heart disease.
[a] Normal (0) to most severe illness; expressed as absolute scores at end of treatment period.
[b] Expressed as PaO_2 (mmHg) at end of treatment period.
[c] Measured by reduction in duration of viral shedding and/or decrease in titres of virus shed ($\log_{10}TCID_{50}$/ml).
[d] Estimated from figure in article; actual values not reported.
From Carmack and Prober (1992), *Infectious Agents and Diseases* **1**, 99–107; reproduced by permission of Raven Press.

Table 12.3. Demonstrated therapeutic effects of ribavirin: clinical trials after drug licensure

Ref.	Patient population	Illness score[a]	Oxygenation[b]	Antiviral effect[c]	Other parameters
(67)	14 R 12 P	Not used	Not reported	Viral shedding not significantly different; Viral titres not reported	Improved cough, crepitations, respiratory rate, heart rate No significant difference in nasal discharge, feeding, nasal flare, wheeze, retractions, rhonchi
(68)	33 R[d] 97 supportive care	Not used	Not reported	Not reported	More rapid decline in 'therapeutic intervention score'
(69)	20 R (2 with BPD) 10 P (2 with BPD)	Scale: 0 to 4+ 0.6 (R) vs 1.2 (P)[e]	95.5% (R) vs 94.5% (P)[e]	No significant difference in viral shedding and titres	No difference in days of fever, respiratory rate, wheezing, rhonchi, duration of treatment, length of hospitalization
(104)	20 R 27 P (all with BPD or CHD)	Scale: 0 to 10+ 1.7 (R) vs 2.3 (P)[e]	90.5% (R) vs 88% (P)	Not reported	Improved oxygen requirement (l/min) after day 3: 0.25 (R) vs 0.75 (P) No difference in respiratory score, treatment failures, duration of hospitalization
(70)	14 R (3 with underlying disease) 14 P (4 with underlying disease)	Not used	Not reported	Not reported	Fewer days of mechanical ventilation: 4.9 (R) vs 9.9 (P); fewer days of oxygen supplementation: 8.7 (R) vs 13.5 (P); fewer days of hospitalization: 13.3 (R) vs 15.0 (P); lower cost of hospitalization for patients without underlying disease: $50 738 (R) vs $77 693 (P)

R = ribavirin group; P = placebo group; BPD = bronchopulmonary dysplasia; CHD = congenital heart disease.
[a] Normal (0) to most severe illness; expressed as absolute scores at end of treatment period.
[b] Expressed as oxygen saturation (%) at end of treatment period.
[c] Measured by reduction in duration of viral shedding and/or decrease in titres of virus shed.
[d] All patients had one or more 'predisposing condition' and/or severe RSV disease (progressive pulmonary insufficiency or imminent pulmonary failure).
[e] Estimated from figure in article; actual values not reported.
From Carmack and Prober (1992), *Infectious Agents and Diseases* **1**, 99–107; reproduced by permission of Raven Press.

improvement in lower-respiratory tract signs . . . associated with better levels of arterial oxygen saturation and diminished viral shedding'. However, although the difference between groups was statistically significant for each of these parameters, the actual numerical differences were relatively small, as demonstrated in Table 12.2 (e.g., the difference in oxygen tension at the end of therapy was only 6.4 mmHg between groups).

This study has been criticized for several flaws (111), including: (a) vague entry criteria; (b) unspecified criteria for determining duration of treatment; (c) lack of stratification according to illness severity prior to randomization; (d) incompletely described criteria for rating of 'signs and symptoms'; (e) incompletely described and subjective 'severity of illness' scoring system; (f) unspecified clinical importance and correlations of the illness scores (differences between groups, although significant, were small and never greater than one point); and (g) spontaneous improvement in the placebo group prior to initiation of treatment which may have left less potential for improvement in the placebo group compared with the ribavirin group. In sum, although small but statistically significant improvements were demonstrated for the ribavirin treatment group, the practical clinical significance of these differences was less clear. Although the ribavirin recipients had greater improvement in oxygen tension, the mean oxygen tension at the end of ribavirin therapy was only 62.4 mmHg. As noted by Wald and colleagues (111), this value corresponds to an oxygen saturation of approximately 92%, which would not obviate the need for supplemental oxygen. Moreover, the trial did not demonstrate measurable differences in objective outcomes such as length of treatment, need for supportive care or cost of hospitalization.

Taber et al., *1983 (66)*

Published approximately five months after the first study by Hall and colleagues (65), this prospective, randomized, partially blinded placebo-controlled trial enrolled full-term previously normal infants with bronchiolitis caused by RSV infection. Patients were randomized, without stratification, to receive either ribavirin aerosol ($n = 12$) or saline aerosol placebo ($n = 14$). Treatment was given for 12 h per day for five days. Clinical course was evaluated using a check-list of 70 items to estimate severity of illness score on a scale of 0 (normal) to 3+ (most severe). In addition, nasal wash specimens from virus isolation and quantification were collected on admission and daily during hospitalization. Based on the illness score assigned by a blinded observer, the authors concluded that patients treated with ribavirin aerosol showed more rapid improvement than did control patients; the difference between groups was not significant until day 3, at which time only 17 patients continued to receive treatment (seven ribavirin patients and 10 placebo patients).

This study has several of the same types of flaws identified in the first study (111). The poorly described and subjectively scored rating system is the most substantial problem with this study. Moreover, the demonstrated 'therapeutic effect' of ribavirin therapy occurred late in the treatment course and was based on a small but statistically significant difference in the illness score (Table 12.2). The clinical significance of this difference is unclear. Differences in viral shedding, viral titres, length of treatment or length of hospitalization were not significant.

Hall et al., *1985 (95)*

The second prospective, randomized, placebo-controlled, double-blind study conducted by Hall and co-workers included patients with and without underlying disease. Patients with lower respiratory tract illness caused by RSV were randomized, without stratification, to receive aerosolized ribavirin ($n = 14$, six with bronchopulmonary dysplasia and/or congenital heart disease) or water placebo ($n = 12$, seven with bronchopulmonary dysplasia and/or congenital heart disease). The drug or placebo was given for approximately 20 h per day for an average of five days. The clinical status of the infants in each group was compared by the assignment of an overall 'severity of illness' score which was recorded daily using a 'visual analogue scale' ranging from 0 (normal) to 10 (more severe). Specific details regarding the derivation and reproducibility of this scale were not provided.

Comparison of the severity of illness scores from beginning to end of therapy showed a higher mean percentage improvement for patients treated with ribavirin than with placebo, both as a total group and for the subset of patients with underlying disease. Much of the improvement occurred over the first 24 h of treatment with ribavirin. In addition, the increment of improvement in mean oxygen tension by the end of treatment was significantly greater for the ribavirin treatment group. The quantity of virus shed in nasal washings also was favourably and significantly impacted by the fifth day of ribavirin treatment. The authors concluded that 'ribavirin aerosol therapy is beneficial and well-tolerated in infants with underlying cardiac and pulmonary diseases' and suggested that such treatment 'may be particularly important in preventing the cascade of complications that are more likely to ensue because of the underlying disease'.

Once again, as demonstrated in Table 12.2, the actual numerical differences between groups were relatively small. Although the reported mean percentage improvement for the ribavirin-treated patients was significantly greater than for the placebo recipients, the absolute difference in illness severity score (calculated from the reported percentage data) was approximately only 0.6 on the 10-point scale. Moreover, mean duration of therapy for the patients with underlying disease was six days for the ribavirin group and five days for the placebo group. In addition, the study is flawed by the previously discussed problems of subjective scoring, vague entry criteria and lack of stratification. Finally, as Wald and colleagues have noted, manipulation of ordinal data to calculate percentage improvement is not methodologically appropriate (111). In sum, as with the previous studies, this clinical trial did not demonstrate dramatic benefits in outcomes attributable to ribavirin therapy. Reductions in length of treatment, length of hospitalization or hospital cost were not shown.

Barry et al., *1986 (67)*

The first published clinical trial following ribavirin licensure was a randomized, double-blind, placebo-controlled study of 26 infants with clinically diagnosed bronchiolitis and no underlying disease (Table 12.3). Patients were stratified (according to age, capillary carbon dioxide tension, respiratory rate and interval since onset of respiratory symptoms) and randomized to receive either aerosolized ribavirin ($n = 14$) or saline placebo ($n = 12$) for 18 h per day for at least three days. Nasopharyngeal aspirates for immunofluorescent assay and viral culture were collected upon trial entry and daily during therapy. RSV was identified in nasal secretions of 10 patients in each group. Patients were evaluated according to eight clinical variables using a three-point scale as well as heart rate and respiratory rate.

The median time from beginning of treatment with ribavirin to 'sustained improvement' was significantly less than that in placebo recipients for the variables 'cough' and 'crepitations'. The definition of 'sustained improvement' was not provided. In addition, a decrease in respiratory rate from pre-treatment values was significantly greater at 24 and 30 h in the ribavirin group compared with the placebo group. The absolute difference in respiratory rate was approximately five breaths per minute. The authors concluded that 'infants with bronchiolitis who were treated with ribavirin aerosol showed a more rapid rate of improvement than those given saline aerosol'. However, based upon these data and noting that ribavirin aerosol treatment is both inconvenient and expensive, the authors concluded that they did not support the routine use of ribavirin for treatment of acute bronchiolitis in otherwise healthy infants.

Conrad et al., *1987 (68)*

This clinical trial involved 33 infants with lower respiratory tract disease caused by RSV who were either severely ill or had one or more risk factors associated with increased morbidity from this infection. Because the authors considered randomization to placebo treatment to be unethical, the study was neither randomized nor blinded. Infants with documented respiratory syncytial virus infection who received only supportive care at the same hospital during the same epidemic served as controls ($n = 97$). Ribavirin aerosol treatment was administered for 12–20 h per day for a minimum of three days; mean treatment duration was 4.5 days. Thirteen patients in the ribavirin group required mechanical ventilation versus eight patients in the control group. Comparisons between the two groups were based on a retrospective chart review which focused on the relative utilization of 57 types of 'therapeutic interventions'. Linear regression analysis of mean therapeutic intervention score on each hospital day for the two groups showed more rapid decline in scores for the ribavirin recipients than for the controls (Table 12.3). The authors regarded this as evidence for 'prompter resolution of illness with therapy'.

This study has been criticized for the non-randomly applied entry criteria used to assign patients to ribavirin therapy (including undescribed cardiac lesions and uncomplicated prematurity) and the inclusion of 17 control patients who had apnoea at presentation (111). Wald and colleagues (111) note that most investigators do not consider uncomplicated prematurity to be a risk factor for progression to severe RSV disease. Yet at least 11 of the 33 ribavirin treatment patients had uncomplicated prematurity as their single entry criterion. Conversely, 17 control patients had apnoea on presentation; and eight progressed to require mechanical ventilation, three during the first day. These characteristics of the control group raise questions about the assignment of patients to high- and low-risk groups and about the ultimate conclusions reached by the investigators (111).

Rodriguez et al., *1987 (69)*

This prospective, placebo-controlled, double-blind trial was modelled after the first Hall study (65). Infants with lower respiratory tract disease caused by RSV who were expected to require at least three days of hospitalization were enrolled. Patients were randomly assigned in a non-stratified fashion in a ratio of 2 : 1 to treatment with ribavirin aerosol ($n = 20$) or water aerosol placebo ($n = 10$). Twenty-six of the 30 (87%) patients were previously normal, and four had bronchopulmonary dysplasia (two patients in each group). Aerosol was administered for approximately 20 h per day for a minimum of 36 h; mean treatment duration was 55.7 h. Severity of illness was evaluated daily using a scale of 0 (normal) to 4+ (most severe) to rate clinical signs.

The rate of improvement in oxygen saturation from the first to the final day of treatment was significantly better for the ribavirin recipients, but the magnitude of the effect was small. For ribavirin recipients saturation rose from approximately 91% to 95.5%, whereas for placebo recipients it rose from about 93% to 94.5% (a final difference of only 1% between groups at the end of therapy). The rate of improvement in the subjectively scored severity of illness variable was significantly greater for ribavirin patients on days 2 and 3. The absolute scores from admission to day 3 dropped from approximately 2.9 to 0.6 in the ribavirin group and from 2.4 to 1.2 in the control group. Thus, the difference between groups at the conclusion of therapy was only about 0.6 on a four-point scale. As with previous studies, this trial also has been criticized for lack of stratification and use of a subjective scoring system with unknown clinical significance (111). Again, as shown in Table 12.3, although statistically significant differences were reported in rates of improvement in oxygen saturation and subjective severity of illness scores, the actual differences were small and of unknown clinical significance. No differences were demonstrated in duration of treatment or length and cost of hospitalization.

Groothuis et al., *1990 (104)*

This three-year, prospective, multi-centre trial was designed to evaluate the efficacy of early ribavirin therapy in mild RSV illness in infants with bronchopulmonary dysplasia or congenital heart disease. Patients were excluded if acute symptoms had been present for greater than 72 h or if symptoms were moderate or severe. Patients were stratified according to severity of underlying disease and randomized to receive either ribavirin aerosol ($n = 20$) or water aerosol ($n = 27$) for 18–20 h per day. Total treatment ranged from 72 to 120 h; at one of the three centres, treatment was administered in patients' homes under supervision of a home respiratory therapy company. Illness severity measurements included a global clinical assessment score (rated 0–10) and a respiratory score ranging from 0 (well or baseline) to 5 (respiratory failure); the respiratory score was based on oxygen saturation, respiratory rate, retractions and adventitious sounds. For patients treated at home, the observations were recorded by the respiratory therapist, who was aware of the treatment given. Additional outcome measures included room air oxygen saturation, supplemental oxygen required to maintain an oxygen saturation greater than or equal to 91%, duration of hospitalization, need for admission to an intensive care unit and need for mechanical ventilation.

Statistically significant improvements observed among patients receiving ribavirin treatment included the following: (a) greater rate of improvement in global clinical assessment score from hospital admission to day 3 of treatment; (b) improvement in oxygen saturation from hospital admission to day 3 of treatment; and (c) lower supplemental oxygen required to maintain oxygen saturation greater than or equal to 91% at the end of the three-day treatment period. However, the number of treatment failures and total hospital days were not significantly different between groups. As demonstrated in Table 12.3, the actual numerical differences between groups after three days of therapy were relatively small (i.e., the difference in clinical assessment score was only approximately 0.6 on a 10-point scale, and the difference in oxygen saturation was only 2.5%).

There are several criticisms of this study. Although treatment was continued beyond 72 h if clinical assessment score or oxygen saturation worsened beyond this time and treatment failure criteria were not met, analysis was based solely on the first three days of therapy. No data are provided concerning the number of patients in each group who required additional therapy. Also, although the patients who were treated with ribavirin had a lower supplemental oxygen requirement at the end of the treatment period, no data are provided regarding the baseline supplemental oxygen requirements for patients in each group. As before, the small but statistically significant reported improvements beg the question of clinical significance and cost-effectiveness. Cost and duration of treatment were not analysed.

Smith et al., *1991 (70)*

This randomized, double-blind, placebo-controlled trial evaluated the efficacy of aerosolized ribavirin administered continuously to infants receiving mechanical ventilation for respiratory failure due to RSV infection. The average duration of treatment was 19.9 h per day for placebo patients and 18.0 h per day for ribavirin patients. Patients were stratified according to presence of underlying disease (five with bronchopulmonary dysplasia, one with congenital heart disease, and one with neuromuscular disease) and then randomized to receive aerosolized ribavirin ($n = 14$, three with underlying disease) or aerosolized water ($n = 14$, four with underlying disease). Entry criteria were clearly specified.

Outcome variables were entirely objective and included the following statistically significant favourable results for ribavirin-treated patients (Figure 12.1): (a) shorter mean duration of mechanical ventilation (4.9 versus 9.9 days); (b) shorter mean length of supplemental oxygen use (8.7 versus 13.5 days); and (c) shorter mean length of hospital stay (13.3 versus 15.0 days). Even more dramatic differences in all three endpoints favouring the ribavirin recipients were evident when only the 21 previously normal infants were considered. Mean cost of hospitalization was not significantly different between groups when all patients were considered; however, when only the previously normal infants were considered, the mean cost of hospitalization was significantly less for the ribavirin recipients ($50 738 versus $77 693). No mechanical problems were encountered in the administration of ribavirin during the course of the study. On the basis of these findings, the authors recommended 'that infants with severe respiratory syncytial virus infection who require mechanical ventilatory support be treated with ribavirin'. However, they emphasized that 'further study of ribavirin should involve large numbers of infants, including those with underlying cardiopulmonary, neuromuscular, and immunologic diseases'.

Unlike all previously published clinical trials, this study analysed only

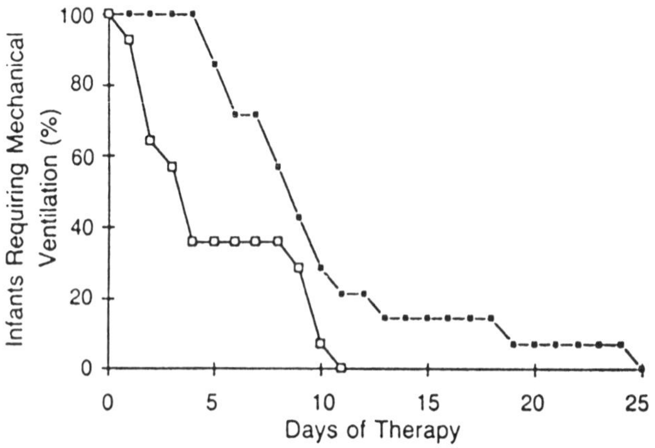

Percentage of Infants in the Ribavirin (□) and Control (■) Groups Requiring Mechanical Ventilation after Aerosol Therapy Began.

The difference between the groups was significant (P = 0.01 by the Mann–Whitney rank-sum test).

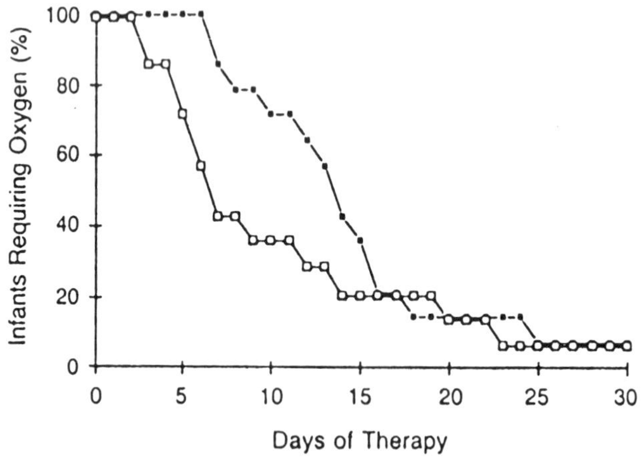

Percentage of Infants in the Ribavirin (□) and Control (■) Groups Requiring Supplemental Oxygen after Aerosol Therapy Began.

The difference between the groups was significant (P = 0.01 by the Mann–Whitney rank-sum test).

Figure 12.1. Therapeutic effects of ribavirin in severely ill infants. (From Smith *et al.* (70); reprinted by permission of the *New England Journal of Medicine,* **325**: 24–29, 1991)

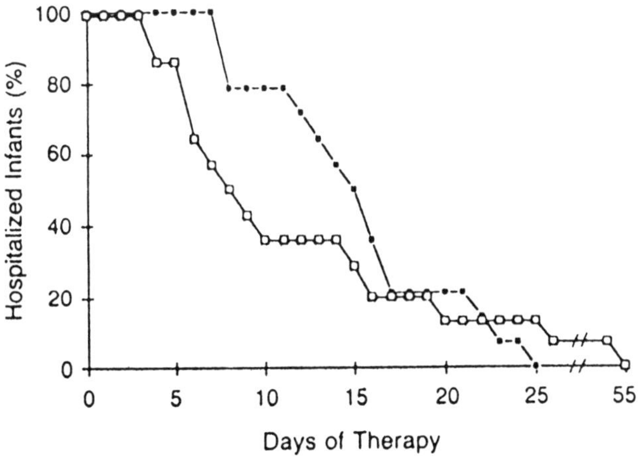

Percentage of Infants in the Ribavirin (□) and Control (■) Groups Remaining in the Hospital after Aerosol Therapy Began.

The difference between the groups was significant (P = 0.04 by the Mann–Whitney rank-sum test).

Figure 12.1. Continued.

objective outcome variables. Ribavirin treatment resulted in significant benefits as reflected in reduced duration of mechanical ventilation, length of supplemental oxygen requirement, length of hospital stay and cost of hospitalization.

IMMUNOGLOBULIN THERAPY

The role of immunoglobulin both for prophylaxis and for therapy of RSV infection has been investigated in animal models and to a limited extent in humans. For many years, investigators hypothesized that serum antibody might contribute to the pathogenesis of lower respiratory tract infections caused by RSV. This speculation arose after the observation that natural infection following the administration of formalin-inactivated vaccine was more severe than natural infection in unimmunized hosts (33,34). Much later, this unexpected outcome was shown to be caused by the imbalanced immune response evoked by the vaccine itself, due to the effect of formalin on the virus (112). Moreover, accumulated epidemiological and prospectively collected data suggest that passively acquired maternal antibody is protective against RSV infection during the first months of life (10,36).

Prince and colleagues (113) investigated the role of passively acquired immunity to RSV in cotton rats. Following parabiotic linkage (i.e., surgical connection which permits development of cross-circulation) of control non-immune animals with immune animals that had been intranasally inoculated with virus 21 days earlier, the two animals acquired equivalent serum antibody titres. After subsequent intranasal inoculation with RSV, the immune animals were completely resistant to nasal and pulmonary infection, whereas control animals exhibited only pulmonary resistance. Thus, the immunity passively acquired through parabiotic linkage protected the lungs but not the nose of the animals.

In an effort to determine which component of the immune system was more critical for the observed immunity, the investigators compared the effect of immune serum or immune lymphocytes administered intraperitoneally to susceptible rats. Following intranasal inoculation with RSV, complete or near-complete pulmonary resistance was observed among animals who received immune serum, but only minimal resistance was seen among those who received immune lymphocytes. These investigators also demonstrated that infant cotton rats can acquire varying degrees of passive immunity to RSV either transplacentally or by suckling from immune foster mothers (113).

Prince and co-workers (38) also studied the effect of human immunoglobulin given one day before or two days after intranasal RSV inoculation of cotton rats. The titre of RSV measured in nasal and lung tissue homogenate was inversely correlated with the titres of serum antibodies against RSV. No histological changes compatible with antibody-potentiated pulmonary disease were observed in the animals. In a subgroup of cotton rats first immunized with formalin-inactivated RSV, striking histopathological changes were seen, including neutrophilic infiltration of bronchiolar epithelium and alveolar septae.

In an owl monkey primate model (37), human immunoglobulin was administered five days after experimental infection with RSV. Seven days after infection, virus was detected in lung washes of all untreated animals ($n = 8$) compared with only three of 12 monkeys that had received immunoglobulin. No adverse effects were noted clinically or in histopathological examination of lung specimens.

The efficacy of topically administered immunoglobulin also has been investigated in cotton rats (114). When immunoglobulin (0.025 g/kg) was dripped into the respiratory tract of RSV-infected animals, a 2.2-fold log reduction in viral titres in lung tissue was observed. Complete clearance of virus occurred in 92% of the treated animals within 24 h. To achieve a similar effect following parenteral administration of immunoglobulin, a much higher dosage (4 g/kg) was required. Similar results have been reported in studies with the owl monkey (115). The fact that the serum level of immunoglobulin in the animals treated topically was considerably lower than that in animals treated parenterally implied that the therapeutic effect reflected the concentration of immunoglobulin attained at the site of infection. No adverse effects were noted. The investigators proposed that the same enhanced therapeutic effect might be achieved in high-risk infants by administering immunoglobulin as small-particle aerosol (114).

Gruber and colleagues (116) studied the effects of combined treatment with intraperitoneal immunoglobulin and ribavirin aerosol in cotton rats experimentally infected with RSV. In one set of experiments, the immunoglobulin was given prophylactically 24 h prior to intranasal inoculation with RSV. In another set of experiments, the immunoglobulin was given three days after inoculation. In all cases, ribavirin was administered three days after inoculation. In the first set of experiments, the geometric mean titres (GMT) of virus isolated from the lungs of animals treated with either ribavirin alone (GMT, $\log_{10} = 1.9$) or prophylactic immunoglobulin alone (GMT, $\log_{10} = 1.8$) were not significantly different. However, these titres were significantly lower than the titres in untreated animals (GMT, $\log_{10} = 3.7$). Viral titres for animals that received both ribavirin and prophylactic immunoglobulin (GMT, $\log_{10} = 0.14$) were significantly lower than titres in the untreated animals as well as in the animals who received either agent alone. Similar but less striking results were observed when the immunoglobulin administration was delayed until day 3 after inoculation. The animals that received both immunoglobulin and ribavirin had the least amount of lung histopathology. The investigators suggested that administration of intravenous immunoglobulin may be beneficial for high-risk infants when given either prophylactically in hopes of preventing infection or in combination with ribavirin when treating established RSV infections.

Hemming and co-workers (117) conducted a double-blind placebo-controlled trial of intravenous immunoglobulin in non-critically ill hospitalized infants with lower respiratory tract disease caused by RSV. Patients were randomized to receive a single 2 g/kg dose of intravenous immunoglobulin ($n = 17$) or albumin ($n = 18$) infused over 12–24 h. The following significant differences were found: (a) reduced titres of virus recovered from nasal washes two days after treatment; (b) rise in immunoglobulin titre and rise in RSV neutralization antibody titres one day after completion of therapy; and (c) increased pO_2 measured by transcutaneous oximetry one day after treatment. However, a significant difference in oxygen tension was not observed beyond this initial improvement. Duration of clinical symptoms such as wheezing, rhonchi, retractions, supplemental oxygen requirements and length of hospitalization were not significantly different between the immunoglobulin- and placebo-treated subjects. No adverse effects were observed.

In conclusion, although these studies suggest that immunoglobulin is involved in the termination of viral shedding, the implications for the treatment of natural infection in humans are far from clear (32). In sum, data regarding the efficacy of immunoglobulin therapy for RSV infection are limited. Reported benefits are modest and of unknown clinical significance in terms of duration of hospitalization, morbidity and need for supportive therapy. Results of a phase I trial demonstrated that monthly intravenous immunoglobulin therapy is feasible and safe in high-risk infants (118). Recently, a multi-centre clinical trial evaluated monthly prophylactic intravenous administration of an RSV-enriched immunoglobulin preparation (RSV immune globulin) to infants and young children at high risk for RSV disease (119). Although the investigations concluded that a high dose (750 mg/kg) was a safe and effective means of preventing lower respiratory tract infection in these high risk patients, an FDA advisory committee determined that the data were insufficient to clearly establish efficacy and safety of the product (120). Thus these results remain preliminary and have not resulted in FDA licensure of RSV immune globulin.

THE RIBAVIRIN CONTROVERSY: CONCLUSIONS

The use of ribavirin for RSV infection has been embroiled in controversy. Major issues include weaknesses in the design and methodology of the studies which have claimed treatment efficacy, the cost-effectiveness of this intervention, and potential teratogenicity to exposed health care providers (99–102,106,108,111). In consideration of all these issues, a consensus regarding which patients should be treated has not been developed.

How can the collective data from clinical trials guide decisions regarding ribavirin therapy for RSV infections? Proponents and detractors of ribavirin hold widely disparate views regarding guidelines for ribavirin usage and the need for further studies. On the one hand, proponents have argued that ribavirin treatment is indicated for 'essentially all infants with documented respiratory syncytial virus infection who require hospitalization' (65) and have contended that the demonstrated therapeutic benefits of ribavirin render 'further double-blinded placebo-controlled clinical trials unethical, especially for patients at higher risk during respiratory syncytial virus infection' (68). Meanwhile, detractors have lamented that 'physicians are in a position in which they must use an agent with a potential, yet unclear, efficacy in the treatment of an infection with no alternative pharmacologic treatment' (106) and have expressed regret that 'the Committee's statement on the use of ribavirin espouses a policy that, de facto, establishes a standard of case whereas a careful consideration of the pertinent data available at this time will lead thoughtful clinicians to use ribavirin, if at all, in a very limited number of highly selected cases' (74).

Only the 1991 study of severely ill intubated patients by Smith and colleagues (70) based conclusions on completely objective outcome variables such as number of days of intubation and length and cost of hospitalization. However, sample size was small, and results can be generalized only to severely ill infants without underlying disease. Although all other studies have demonstrated modest improvement based primarily on a variety of subjective scoring systems of illness severity, careful review reveals that none has shown significant effects on measurable outcomes such as mortality, length and cost of hospitalization or requirements for supportive therapy. Moreover, meaningful clinical correlations and significance of the demonstrated improvements in the subjective scores are entirely unknown.

At issue is not whether therapeutic benefits have been demonstrated, but whether the benefits demonstrated are clinically meaningful. Numerous critics have contended that most of the differences demonstrated to date do not make a meaningful difference. Thus, the decision to prescribe ribavirin therapy to an individual patient is difficult. There is greater concurrence about the treatment of RSV-infected children who are severely ill or who have underlying problems which place them at risk for severe disease. Most agree that these children should be treated with ribavirin. Much less clear is whether any patient who is ill enough to be hospitalized with RSV infection is ill enough to be treated with ribavirin (as implied by aggressive product advertisements). The usual course of ribavirin therapy is three to seven days; yet in one study, the mean duration of hospitalization for previously well infants hospitalized with RSV infection was only 3.4 days (16). However, if treatment with ribavirin is shown to reduce long-term morbidity due to impaired respiratory function, such an effect might outweigh cost considerations even if duration of hospitalization is not shortened.

To answer these questions, more well-designed trials are needed to evaluate the effectiveness of ribavirin treatment of RSV infection in the noncritically ill, previously healthy infant. These trials must evaluate objective outcomes such as length and cost of hospitalization and need for supportive therapies. In addition, optimum duration of treatment and guidelines for discontinuation of therapy are yet to be established. Longitudinal prospective studies are required to evaluate potential late adverse effects of treatment as well as whether treatment can reduce the possible long-term sequelae which have been ascribed to lower respiratory tract infection with RSV.

REFERENCES

1. Morris, J. A., Blount, R. E., Jr and Savage, R. E. (1956). Recovery of cytopathogenic agent from chimpanzees with coryza. *Proc. Soc. Exp. Biol. Med.*, **92**, 544–549.
2. Chanock, R., Roizman, B. and Myers, R. (1957). Recovery from infants with respiratory illness of a virus related to chimpanzee coryza agent (CCA) Part I. Isolation, properties and characterization. *Am. J. Hyg.*, **66**, 281–290.
3. Chanock, R. M. and Finberg, L. (1957). Recovery from infants with respiratory illness of a virus related to chimpanzee coryza agent (CCA) Part II. Epidemiologic aspects of infection in infants and small children. *Am. J. Hyg.*, **66**, 291–300.

4. Beem, M., Wright, F. H., Hamre, D. *et al.* (1960). Association of the chimpanzee coryza agent with acute respiratory disease in children. *N. Engl. J. Med.*, **263**, 523–530.
5. Brandt, C. D., Kim, H. W., Arrobio, J. O. *et al.* (1973). Epidemiology of respiratory syncytial virus infection in Washington, D.C.: III. Composite analysis of eleven consecutive yearly epidemics. *Am. J. Epidemiol.*, **98**, 355–364.
6. Glezen, W. P. and Denny, F. W. (1973). Epidemiology of acute lower respiratory disease in children. *N. Engl. J. Med.*, **288**, 498–505.
7. Henderson, F. W., Collier, A. M., Clyde, W. A. and Denny, F. W. (1979). Respiratory-syncytial-virus infections, reinfections and immunity. *N. Engl. J. Med.*, **300**, 530–534.
8. Kim, H. W., Arrobio, J. O., Brandt, C. D. *et al.* (1973). Epidemiology of respiratory syncytial virus infection in Washington, D.C.: I. Importance of the virus in different respiratory tract disease syndromes and temporal distribution of infection. *Am. J. Epidemiol.*, **98**, 216–225.
9. Murphy, T. F., Henderson, F. W., Clyde, W. A., Jr *et al.* (1981). Pneumonia: an eleven-year study in a pediatric practice. *Am. J. Epidemiol.*, **113**, 12–21.
10. Parrott, R. H., Kim, H. W., Arrobio, J. O. *et al.* (1973). Epidemiology of respiratory syncytial virus infection in Washington, D.C.: II. Infection and disease with respect to age, immunologic status, race and sex. *Am. J. Epidemiol.*, **98**, 289–300.
11. Report to the Medical Research Council Subcommittee on Respiratory Syncytial Virus Vaccines (1978). Respiratory syncytial virus infection: admissions to hospitals in industrial, urban, and rural areas. *Br. Med. J.*, **2**, 796–798.
12. Wright, A. L., Taussig, L. M., Ray, C. G. *et al.* (1989). The Tucson children's respiratory study: II. Lower respiratory tract illness in the first year of life. *Am. J. Epidemiol.*, **129**, 1232–1246.
13. Glezen, W. P. (1977). Pathogenesis of bronchiolitis: epidemiologic considerations. *Pediatr. Res.*, **11**, 239–243.
14. Parrott, R. H., Kim, H. W., Brandt, C. D. and Chanock, R. M. (1974). Respiratory syncytial virus in infants and children. *Prev. Med.*, **3**, 473–480.
15. Glezen, W. P., Paredes, A., Allison, J. E. *et al.* (1981). Risk of respiratory syncytial virus infection for infants from low-income families in relationship to age, sex, ethnic group, and maternal antibody level. *J. Pediatr.*, **98**, 708–715.
16. Green, M., Brayer, A. F., Schenkman, K. A. and Wald, E. R. (1989). Duration of hospitalization in previously well infants with respiratory syncytial virus infection. *Pediatr. Infect. Dis. J.*, **8**, 601–605.
17. Abman, S. H., Ogle, J. W., Butler-Simon, N. *et al.* (1988). Role of respiratory syncytial virus in early hospitalizations for respiratory distress of young infants with cystic fibrosis. *J. Pediatr.*, **113**, 826–830.
18. Groothuis, J. R., Gutierrez, K. M. and Lauer, B. A. (1988). Respiratory syncytial virus infection in children with bronchopulmonary dysplasia. *Pediatrics*, **82**, 199–203.
19. Hall, C. B., Powell, K. R., MacDonald, N. E. *et al.* (1986). Respiratory syncytial viral infection in children with compromised immune function. *N. Engl. J. Med.*, **315**, 77–81.
20. MacDonald, N. E., Hall, C. B., Suffin, S. C. *et al.* (1982). Respiratory syncytial viral infection in infants with congenital heart disease. *N. Engl. J. Med.*, **307**, 397–400.
21. Kingsbury, D. W., Bratt, M. A., Choppin, P. W. *et al.* (1978). Paramyxoviridae. *Intervirology*, **10**, 137–152.
22. Bernstein, J. M. and Hruska, J. F. (1981). Respiratory syncytial virus proteins: identification by immunoprecipitation. *J. Virol.*, **38**, 278–285.

23. Katz, S. L. (1985). *New Vaccine Development: Establishing Priorities*, Vol. I. National Academy Press, Washington, DC, pp. 397–409.
24. Anderson, L. J., Hierholzer, J. C., Tsou, C. *et al.* (1985). Antigenic characterization of respiratory syncytial virus strains with monoclonal antibodies. *J. Infect. Dis.*, **151**, 626–633.
25. Mufson, M. A., Örvell, C., Rafnar, B. and Norrby, E. (1985). Two distinct subtypes of human respiratory syncytial virus. *J. Gen. Virol.*, **66**, 2111–2124.
26. Johnson, P. R. and Collins, P. L. (1988). The fusion glycoproteins of human respiratory syncytial virus of subgroups A and B: sequence conservation provides a structural basis for antigenic relatedness. *J. Gen. Virol.*, **69**, 2623–2628.
27. Johnson, P. R., Spriggs, M. K., Olmsted, R. A. and Collins, P. L. (1987). The G glycoprotein of human respiratory syncytial viruses of subgroups A and B: extensive sequence divergence between antigenically related proteins. *Proc. Natl Acad. Sci. USA*, **84**, 5625–5629.
28. Anderson, L. J., Hendry, R. M., Pierik, L. T. *et al.* (1991). Multicenter study of strains of respiratory syncytial virus. *J. Infect. Dis.*, **163**, 687–692.
29. McConnochie, K. M., Hall, C. B., Walsh, E. E. and Roghmann, K. J. (1990). Variation in severity of respiratory syncytial virus infections with subtype. *J. Pediatr.*, **117**, 52–62.
30. Hall, C. B., Walsh, E. E., Schnabel, K. C. *et al.* (1990). Occurrence of groups A and B of respiratory syncytial virus over 15 years: associated epidemiologic and clinical characteristics in hospitalized and ambulatory children. *J. Infect. Dis.*, **162**, 1283–1290.
31. Hall, C. B. (1987). Respiratory syncytial virus. In *Textbook of Pediatric Infectious Diseases*, R. D. Feigin and J. D. Cherry (eds), Saunders, Philadelphia, pp. 1653–1676.
32. Welliver, R. C. (1988). Detection, pathogenesis, and therapy of respiratory syncytial virus infections. *Clin. Microbiol. Rev.*, **1**, 27–39.
33. Chanock, R. M., Kapikian, A. Z., Mills, J. *et al.* (1970). Influence of immunological factors in respiratory syncytial virus disease of the lower respiratory tract. *Arch. Environ. Health*, **21**, 347–355.
34. Kapikian, A. Z., Mitchell, R. H., Chanock, R. M. *et al.* (1969). An epidemiologic study of altered clinical reactivity to respiratory syncytial (RS) virus infection in children previously vaccinated with an inactivated RS virus vaccine. *Am. J. Epidemiol.*, **89**, 405–421.
35. Bruhn, F. W. and Yeager, A. S. (1977). Respiratory syncytial virus in early infancy: circulating antibody and the severity of infection. *Am. J. Dis. Child.*, **131**, 145–148.
36. Ogilvie, M. M., Vathenen, A. S., Radford, M. *et al.* (1981). Maternal antibody and respiratory syncytial virus infection in infancy. *J. Med. Virol.*, **7**, 263–271.
37. Hemming, V. G., Prince, G. A., Horswood, R. L. *et al.* (1985). Studies of passive immunotherapy for infections of respiratory syncytial virus in the respiratory tract of a primate model. *J. Infect. Dis.*, **152**, 1083–1087.
38. Prince, G. A., Hemming, V. G., Horswood, R. L. and Chanock, R. M. (1985). Immunoprophylaxis and immunotherapy of respiratory syncytial virus infection in the cotton rat. *Virus Res.*, **3**, 193–206.
39. Mito, K., Chiba, Y., Suga, K. and Nakao, T. (1984). Cellular immune response to infection with respiratory syncytial virus and influence of breast-feeding on the response. *J. Med. Virol.*, **14**, 323–332.
40. Welliver, R. C., Kaul, A. and Ogra, P. L. (1979). Cell-mediated immune response to respiratory syncytial virus infection: relationship to the development of reactive airway disease. *J. Pediatr.*, **94**, 370–375.

41. Hall, C. B., Hall, W. J., Gala, C. L. *et al.* (1984). Long-term prospective study in children after respiratory syncytial virus infection. *J. Pediatr.*, **105**, 358–364.
42. McConnochie, K. M. and Roghmann, K. J. (1984). Bronchiolitis as a possible cause of wheezing in childhood: new evidence. *Pediatrics*, **74**, 1–10.
43. Rooney, J. C. and Williams, H. E. (1971). The relationship between proved viral bronchiolitis and subsequent wheezing. *J. Pediatr.*, **79**, 744–747.
44. Webb, M. S. C., Henry, R. L., Milner, A. D. *et al.* (1985) Continuing respiratory problems three and a half years after acute viral bronchiolitis. *Arch. Dis. Child.*, **60**, 1064–1067.
45. Sims, D. G., Downham, M. A. P. S., Gardner, P. S. *et al.* (1978). Study of 8-year-old children with a history of respiratory syncytial virus bronchiolitis in infancy. *Br. Med. J.*, **1**, 11–14.
46. Welliver, R. C., Wong, D. T., Sun, M. *et al.* (1981). The development of respiratory syncytial virus-specific IgE and the release of histamine in nasopharyngeal secretions after infections. *N. Engl. J. Med.*, **305**, 841–846.
47. Welliver, R. C. and Ogra, P. L. (1987). Respiratory syncytial virus-specific IgE antibody responses at the mucosal surface: predictive value for recurrent wheezing and suppression by ribavirin therapy. *Adv. Exp. Med. Biol.*, **216B**, 1701–1708.
48. Welliver, R. C., Sun, M., Rinaldo, D. and Ogra, P. L. (1986). Predictive value of respiratory syncytial virus-specific IgE responses for recurrent wheezing following bronchiolitis. *J. Pediatr.*, **109**, 776–780.
49. Witkowski, J. T., Robins, R. K., Sidwell, R. W. and Simon, L. N. (1972). Design, synthesis, and broad spectrum antiviral activity of 1-β-D-ribofuranosyl-1,2,4-triazole-3-carboxamide and related nucleosides. *J. Med. Chem.*, **15**, 1150–1154.
50. Huffman, J. H., Sidwell, R. W., Khare, G. P. *et al.* (1973). In vitro effect of 1-β-D-ribofuranosyl-1,2,4-triazole-3-carboxamide (Virazole, ICN 1229) on deoxyribonucleic acid and ribonucleic acid viruses. *Antimicrob. Agents Chemother.*, **3**, 235–241.
51. Sidwell, R. W., Huffman, J. H., Khare, G. P. *et al.* (1972). Broad-spectrum antiviral activity of Virazole: 1-β-D-ribofuranosyl-1,2,4-triazole-3-carboxamide. *Science*, **177**, 705–706.
52. Cohen, A., Togo, Y., Khakoo, R. *et al.* (1976). Comparative clinical and laboratory evaluation of the prophylactic capacity of ribavirin, amantadine hydrochloride, and placebo in induced human influenza type A. *J. Infect. Dis.*, **133** (Suppl.), A114–A120.
53. Smith, C. B., Charette, R. P., Fox, J. P. *et al.* (1980). Lack of effect of oral ribavirin in naturally occurring influenze A virus (H1N1) infection. *J. Infect. Dis.*, **141**, 548–554.
54. Togo, Y. and McCracken, E. A. (1976). Double-blind clinical assessment of ribavirin (Virazole) in the prevention of induced infection with type B influenza virus. *J. Infect. Dis.*, **133** (Suppl.), A109–A113.
55. Knight, V., McClung, H. W., Wilson, S. Z. *et al.* (1981). Ribavirin small-particle aerosol treatment of influenza. *Lancet*, **ii**, 945–949.
56. McClung, H. W., Knight, V., Gilbert, B. E. *et al.* (1983). Ribavirin aerosol treatment of influenza B virus infection. *JAMA*, **249**, 2671–2674.
57. McCormick, J. B., King, I. J., Webb, P. A. *et al.* (1986). Lassa fever: effective therapy with ribavirin. *N. Engl. J. Med.*, **314**, 20–26.
58. Ayrosa-Galvão, P. A. and Castro, I. O. (1977). The effect of 1-β-D-ribofuranosyl-1,2,4-triazole-3-carboxamide on acute viral hepatitis. *Ann. NY Acad. Sci.*, **284**, 278–283.
59. Banks, G. and Fernandez, H. (1984). Clinical use of ribavirin in measles: a sum-

marized review. In *Clinical Applications of Ribavirin*, R. A. Smith, V. Knight and J. A. D. Smith (eds), Academic Press, New York, pp. 203–209.
60. Fernandez, H. (1980). Ribavirin: a summary of clinical trials—herpes genitalis and measles. In *Ribavirin: A Broad Spectrum Antiviral Agent*, R. A. Smith and W. Kirkpatrick (eds), Academic Press, New York, pp. 215–230.
61. Sidwell, R. W. (1984). In vitro and in vivo inhibition of DNA viruses by ribavirin. In *Clinical Applications of Ribavirin*, R. A. Smith, V. Knight and J. A. D. Smith (eds), Academic Press, New York, pp. 19–32.
62. Hruska, J.F., Bernstein, J. M., Douglas, R. G., Jr and Hall, C. B. (1980). Effects of ribavirin on respiratory syncytial virus in vitro. *Antimicrob. Agents Chemother.*, **17**, 770–775.
63. Hruska, J. F., Morrow, P. E., Suffin, S. C. and Douglas, R. G. Jr (1982). In vivo inhibition of respiratory syncytial virus by ribavirin. *Antimicrob. Agents Chemother.*, **21**, 125–130.
64. Hall, C. B., Walsh, E. E., Hruska, J. F. *et al.* (1983). Ribavirin treatment of experimental respiratory syncytial viral infection: a controlled double-blind study in young adults. *JAMA*, **249**, 2666–2670.
65. Hall, C. B., McBride, J. T., Walsh, E. E. *et al.* (1983). Aerosolized ribavirin treatment of infants with respiratory syncytial viral infection. *N. Engl. J. Med.*, **308**, 1443–1447.
66. Taber, L. H., Knight, V., Gilbert, B. E. *et al.* (1983). Ribavirin aerosol treatment of bronchiolitis associated with respiratory syncytial virus infection in infants. *Pediatrics*, **72**, 613–618.
67. Barry, W., Cockburn, F., Cornall, R. *et al.* (1986). Ribavirin aerosol for acute bronchiolitis. *Arch. Dis. Child.*, **61**, 593–597.
68. Conrad, D. A., Christenson, J. C., Waner, J. L. and Marks, M. I. (1987). Aerosolized ribavirin treatment of respiratory syncytial virus infection in infants hospitalized during an epidemic. *Pediatr. Infect. Dis. J.*, **6**, 152–158.
69. Rodriguez, W. J., Kim, H. W., Brandt, C. D. *et al.* (1987). Aerosolized ribavirin in the treatment of patients with respiratory syncytial virus disease. *Pediatr. Infect. Dis. J.*, **6**, 159–163.
70. Smith, D. W., Frankel, L. R., Mathers, L. H. *et al.* (1991). A controlled trial of aerosolized ribavirin in infants receiving mechanical ventilation for severe respiratory syncytial virus infection. *N. Engl. J. Med.*, **325**, 24–29.
71. Infectious Diseases and Immunization Committee, Canadian Paediatric Society (1986). Ribavirin: indications for use in pediatrics. *Can. Med. Assoc. J.*, **135**, 1351–1352.
72. Committee on Infectious Diseases, 1986–1987, American Academy of Pediatrics (1987). Ribavirin therapy of respiratory syncytial virus. *Pediatrics*, **79**, 475–478.
73. Committee on Infectious Diseases, American Academy of Pediatrics (1994). Use of ribavirin in the treatment of respiratory syncytial virus infection. In Report of the Committee on Infectious Diseases 23rd edn. G. Peter (ed.), American Academy of Pediatrics, Elk Grove Village, IL, pp. 570–574.
74. Wald, E. R. and Dashefsky, B. (1994). Ribavirin. Red Book Committee recommendations questioned. *Pediatrics*, **93**, 672–673.
75. Zucker, A. R. (1994). Red Book recommendations on ribavirin challenged. *Pediatrics*, **93**, 872–873.
76. Turner, R. B. (1994). Red Book recommendations on ribavirin challenged. *Pediatrics*, **93**, 873.
77. Prusiner, P. and Sundaralingam, M. (1973). A new class of synthetic nucleoside analogues with broad-spectrum antiviral properties. *Nat. New Biol.*, **244**, 116–118.

78. Smith, R. A. (1980). Mechanisms of action of ribavirin. In *Ribavirin: A Broad Spectrum Antiviral Agent*, R. A. Smith and W. Kirkpatrick (eds), Academic Press, New York, pp. 99–118.
79. Streeter, D. G., Witkowski, J. T., Khare, G. P. *et al.* (1973). Mechanism of action of 1-β-D-ribofuranosyl-1,2,4-triazole-3-carboxamide (Virazole), a new broad-spectrum antiviral agent. *Proc. Natl Acad. Sci. USA*, **70**, 1174–1178.
80. Miller, J. P., Kigwana, L. J., Streeter, D. G. *et al.* (1977). The relationship between the metabolism of ribavirin and its proposed mechanism of action. *Ann. NY Acad. Sci.*, **284**, 211–229.
81. Sidwell, R. W., Robins, R. K. and Hillyard, I. W. (1979). Ribavirin: an antiviral agent. *Pharmacol. Ther.*, **6**, 123–146.
82. Wray, S. K., Gilbert, B. E. and Knight, V. (1985). Effect of ribavirin triphosphate on primer generation and elongation during influenza virus transcription in vitro. *Antiviral Res.*, **5**, 39–48.
83. Wray, S. K., Gilbert, B. E., Noall, M. W. and Knight, V. (1985). Mode of action of ribavirin: effect of nucleotide pool alterations on influenza virus ribonucleoprotein synthesis. *Antiviral Res.*, **5**, 29–37.
84. Gilbert, B. E. and Knight, V. (1986). Biochemistry and clinical applications of ribavirin. *Antimicrob. Agents Chemother.*, **30**, 201–205.
85. Catlin, D. H., Smith, R. A. and Samuels, A. I. (1980). ^{14}C-ribavirin: distribution and pharmacokinetic studies in rats, baboons and man. In *Ribavirin: A Broad Spectrum Antiviral Agent*, R. A. Smith and W. Kirkpatrick (eds), Academic Press, New York, pp. 83–98.
86. Ferrara, E. A., Oishi, J. S., Wannemacher, R. W., Jr and Stephen, E. L. (1981). Plasma disappearance, urine excretion, and tissue distribution of ribavirin in rats and rhesus monkeys. *Antimicrob. Agents Chemother.*, **19**, 1042–1049.
87. Connor, J. D., Hintz, M., Van Dyke, R. *et al.* (1984). Ribavirin pharmacokinetics in children and adults during therapeutic trials. In *Clinical Applications of Ribavirin*, R. A. Smith, V. Knight and J. A. D. Smith (eds), Academic Press, New York, pp. 107–123.
88. Wilson, S. Z., Knight, V., Moore, R. and Larson, E. W. (1979). Amantadine small-particle aerosol: generation and delivery to man. *Proc. Soc. Exp. Biol. Med.*, **161**, 350–354.
89. ICN Pharmaceuticals, Inc. (1993). *Virazole (Ribavirin for Inhalation Solution): Prescribing Information*. ICN Pharmaceuticals, Inc., Costa Mesa, CA.
90. Frankel, L. R., Wilson, C. W., Demers, R. R. *et al.* (1987). A technique for the administration of ribavirin to mechanically ventilated infants with severe respiratory syncytial virus infection. *Crit. Care Med.*, **15**, 1051–1054.
91. Outwater, K. M., Meissner, H. C. and Peterson, M. B. (1988). Ribavirin administration to infants receiving mechanical ventilation. *Am. J. Dis. Child.*, **142**, 512–515.
92. Jolley, W. B. and Suchil, C. (1984). Effects of ribavirin on the immune system (second report). In *Clinical Applications of Ribavirin*, R. A. Smith, V. Knight and J. A. D. Smith (eds), Academic Press, New York, pp. 93–96.
93. Rosner, I. K., Welliver, R. C., Edelson, P. J. *et al.* (1987). Effect of ribavirin therapy on respiratory syncytial virus-specific IgE and IgA responses after infection. *J. Infect. Dis.*, **155**, 1043–1046.
94. Magnussen, C. R., Douglas, R. G., Jr, Betts, R. F. *et al.* (1977). Double-blind evaluation of oral ribavirin (Virazole) in experimental influenza A virus infection in volunteers. *Antimicrob. Agents Chemother.*, **12**, 498–502.
95. Hall, C. B., McBride, J. T., Gala, C. L. *et al.* (1985). Ribavirin treatment of respir-

atory syncytial viral infection in infants with underlying cardiopulmonary disease. *JAMA*, **254**, 3047–3051.
96. Cosgrove, M., Jenkins, H. R., Rowlandson, P. H. and Gray, O. P. (1989). Idiosyncratic reaction to nebulized ribavirin in an artificially ventilated neonate. *J. Infect.*, **19**, 85–87.
97. ICN Pharmaceuticals, Inc. (1988). *Aerosol Delivery Hood: Instructions for Use.* ICN Pharmaceuticals, Inc., Costa Mesa, CA.
98. Kilham, L. and Ferm, V. H. (1977). Congenital anomalies induced in hamster embryos with ribavirin. *Science*, **195**, 413–414.
99. Harrison, R., Bellows, J., Rempel, D. *et al.* (1988). Assessing exposures of health-care personnel to aerosols of ribavirin—California. *MMWR*, **37**, 560–563.
100. Rodriguez, W. J., Dang Bui, R. H., Connor, J. D. *et al.* (1987). Environmental exposure of primary care personnel to ribavirin aerosol when supervising treatment of infants with respiratory syncytial virus infections. *Antimicrob. Agents Chemother.*, **31**, 1143–1146.
101. Guglielmo, B. J., Jacobs, R. A. and Locksley, R. M. (1989). The exposure of health care workers to ribavirin aerosol. *JAMA*, **261**, 1880–1881.
102. Fackler, J. C., Flannery, K., Zipkin, M. and McIntosh, K. (1990). Precautions in the use of ribavirin at the Children's Hospital. *N. Engl. J. Med.*, **322**, 634.
103. Infectious Diseases and Immunization Committee, Canadian Paediatric Society (1991). Ribavirin: is there a risk to hospital personnel? *Can. Med. Assoc. J.*, **144**, 285–286.
104. Groothuis, J. R., Woodin, K. A., Katz, R. *et al.* (1990). Early ribavirin treatment of respiratory syncytial viral infection in high-risk children. *J. Pediatr.*, **117**, 792–798.
105. Grant, A. (1988). Randomised trials and ribavirin. *Arch. Dis. Child.*, **63**, 989.
106. Hebert, M. F. and Guglielmo, B. J. (1990). What is the clinical role of aerosolized ribavirin? *DICP*, **24**, 735–738.
107. Isaacs, D., Moxon, E. R., Harvey, D. *et al.* (1988). Ribavirin in respiratory syncytial virus infection: a double blind placebo controlled trial is needed. *Arch. Dis. Child..*, **63**, 986–987, 989–990.
108. Milner, A. D. (1988). Ribavirin and acute bronchiolitis in infancy: not needed for those who were previously well. *Br. Med. J.*, **297**, 998–999.
109. Ray, C. G. (1988). Ribavirin: ambivalence about an antiviral agent. *Am. J. Dis. Child.*, **142**, 488–489.
110. Sullivan, B. J. and Treuhaft, M. W. (1987). Ribavirin for respiratory syncytial virus infection. *Pediatr. Infect. Dis. J.*, **6**, 697.
111. Wald, E. R., Dashefsky, B. and Green, M. (1988). In re ribavirin: a case of premature adjudication? *J. Pediatr.*, **112**, 154–158.
112. Prince, G. A., Jenson, A. B., Hemming, V. G. *et al.* (1986). Enhancement of respiratory syncytial virus pulmonary pathology in cotton rats by prior intramuscular inoculation of formalin-inactivated virus. *J. Virol.*, **57**, 721–728.
113. Prince, G. A., Horswood, R. L., Camargo, E. *et al.* (1983). Mechanisms of immunity to respiratory syncytial virus in cotton rats. *Infect. Immun.*, **42**, 81–87.
114. Prince, G. A., Hemming, V. G., Horswood, R. L. *et al.* (1987). Effectiveness of topically administered neutralizing antibodies in experimental immunotherapy of respiratory syncytial virus infection in cotton rats. *J. Virol.*, **61**, 1851–1854.
115. Hemming, V. G., Prince, G. A., London, W. T. *et al.* (1988). Topically administered immunoglobulin reduces pulmonary respiratory syncytial virus shedding in owl monkeys. *Antimicrob. Agents Chemother.*, **32**, 1269–1270.

116. Gruber, W. C., Wilson, S. Z., Throop, B. J. and Wyde, P. R. (1987). Immunoglobulin administration and ribavirin therapy: efficacy in respiratory syncytial virus infection of the cotton rat. *Pediatr. Res.*, **21**, 270–274.
117. Hemming, V. G., Rodriguez, W., Kim, H. W. *et al.* (1987). Intravenous immunoglobulin treatment of respiratory syncytial virus infections in infants and young children. *Antimicrob. Agents Chemother.*, **31**, 1882–1886.
118. Groothuis, J. R., Levin, M. J., Rodriguez, W. *et al.* (1991). Use of intravenous gamma globulin to passively immunize high-risk children against respiratory syncytial virus: safety and pharmacokinetics. *Antimicrob. Agents Chemother.*, **35**, 1469–1473.
119. Groothuis, J. R., Simoes, E. A. F., Levin, M. J. *et al.* (1993). Prophylactic administration of respiratory syncytial virus immune globulin to high risk infants and young children. *N. Engl. J. Med.*, **329**, 1524–1530.
120. Ellenberg, S. S., Epstein, J. S., Fratanoni, J. C. *et al.* (1994). A trial of RSV immune globulin in infants and young children: the FDA's view. *N. Engl. J. Med.*, **331**, 203–204.

Part D

EXOTIC VIRUSES

Clinical Treatment

13 Exotic Viruses

SUSAN FISHER-HOCH
Centers for Disease Control, Atlanta, Georgia, USA

INTRODUCTION

The term 'exotic' has been applied to a heterogeneous group of RNA viruses, loosely connected by their occurrence mainly, though not always, in tropical climes (Table 13.1). In some instances the term 'exotic' belies the nature and epidemiology of viruses which are locally commonplace, sometimes widespread, and thus cause a considerable burden of disease. In others the diseases, though uncommon, are so terrible and mortality so high that they incite justifiable dread.

Exotic viruses most certainly share one characteristic. Most are infections of extreme poverty, with the result that there is little data on treatment. They affect populations living at or little above subsistence, who have minimal access to medical care even of the most limited nature, and little or no economic or political 'clout'. Vaccines or specific drug development is unlikely to be profitable and thus unlikely to drive research. Furthermore, in many instances the diseases are difficult and expensive to study because of the inaccessibility of patients to modern science, or simply the rarity of human cases. Demands for development of treatment have arisen primarily because of the importation of patients to countries where they threaten medical or civilian populations or where military intervention might place troops at risk.

There are some notable exceptions. In some cases excellent animal models, particularly primates, have allowed progress to be made. Successful clinical trials in endemic areas have shown that fatal Lassa fever is treatable with ribavirin, and Argentine haemorrhagic fever with immune plasma. The efficacy of post-exposure prophylaxis for rabies infection is proven. Other arenaviruses and some bunyaviruses may also be amenable to treatment with ribavirin, but clinical studies are lacking. Data on the treatment of haemorrhagic fever with renal syndrome (HFRS) with ribavirin is marginal; most patients make an uneventful recovery with supportive care. There is no treatment, however, for the most lethal exotic viruses—rabies, Ebola and Marburg, or yellow fever—nor is any remotely in sight.

Antiviral Chemotherapy. Edited by D.J. Jeffries and E. De Clercq

Table 13.1. Table of the exotic viruses showing their geographic distribution, ecology and disease patterns with current established therapy

Virus	Geographic distribution	Vector/host	Est. incubation period (days)	Disease	Estimates of mortality (%)	Treatment	Post-exposure prophylaxis
Arenaviridae							
Lassa fever	W. Africa	Rodent	7–22	Haemorrhagic fever	17	Ribavirin	Ribavirin
Junin	Argentina	Rodent	7–14	Haemorrhagic fever	17	Immune plasma	?Ribavirin
Machupo	Bolivia	Rodent	7–14	Haemorrhagic fever	15	?Ribavirin	?Ribavirin
Guanarito	Venezuela/Brazil	Rodent	?	Haemorrhagic fever	60	?Ribavirin	?Ribavirin
Bunyaviridae							
CCHF	Africa/Asia	Tick/small mammal	2–9	Haemorrhagic fever	15–30	Ribavirin	Ribavirin
RVF	Africa	Mosquito/mammal	3–6	Encephalitis/ haemorrhagic fever	30–50	None	None
HFRS	N. Hemisphere	Rodent	10–35	Haemorrhagic fever/ renal failure	2–10	Ribavirin	None
Flaviviridae							
Yellow fever	Africa/S. America	Mosquito/primate	3–7	Haemorrhagic fever	10–50	None	None
DHF/DSS	Africa/Asia	Mosquito/human	5–8	Haemorrhagic fever	2–10	Supportive	None
JE	S. & S.E. Asia	Mosquito/bird	3–7	Encephalitis	20–30	None	None
TBE	Asia/E. Europe	Tick	3–7	Encephalitis	20	None	None
SLE	N. America	Mosquito/bird	3–7	Encephalitis	0–8		
Togaviridae							
WEE/EEE/VEE	Americas	Mosquito/bird	3–7	Encephalitis	0–10	None	None
Filoviridae							
Ebola	Africa (?Asia)	?Monkey	3–10	Haemorrhagic fever	60–90	None	None
Marburg	Africa	?Monkey	2–21	Haemorrhagic fever	20–30	None	None
Rhabdoviridae							
Rabies	Worldwide	Dog/fox, etc.	14–600	Encephalitis	100	None	Vaccine/ immune globulin

THE VIRUSES

Any generalized discussion of these viruses is difficult because their geographic distribution and genetic and pathological properties are disparate (Table 13.1). However, the clinical syndromes divide roughly into haemorrhagic fevers or encephalitis. There is some overlap; for example, Rift Valley fever (RVF) can manifest with haemorrhage, and encephalopathy and post-infectious encephalitis are not uncommon in arenavirus infections. Though most of the viruses are acquired directly from animal hosts (usually rodents) or via insect vectors, human to human transmission has been a major feature of some of the most lethal of the exotic infections, usually by means of blood contact or contamination, or common use of needles.

The viruses discussed belong to six different families, among which arenaviruses are the most important in causing haemorrhagic fever. Arenaviruses persistently infect rodents, and include Lassa virus in West Africa (1). Junin, Machupo and Guanarito viruses (2–4) are from South America, and are the causes of Argentine haemorrhagic fever (AHF), Bolivian haemorrhagic fever (BHF) and Venezuelan haemorrhagic fever (VHF) respectively. Lassa virus is transmitted to humans from *Mastomys natalensis*, a rodent which commonly infests homes in secondary forest and savannah areas. Lassa fever probably results in over 100 000 infections per year with 1000–3000 deaths. Prospective studies in Sierra Leone villages have demonstrated disease to infection ratios of 10–25%. In the same studies 5–14% of all febrile illnesses were shown to be associated with Lassa virus (1).

Arthropod-borne virus (Arbovirus) is a generic term for viruses which are spread by insect vectors—specifically mosquitoes or ticks. Many are considered 'exotic' viruses, and they include members of several different families; bunyaviruses, flaviviruses and togaviruses. There are several bunyaviruses important in human disease. Crimean–Congo haemorrhagic fever (CCHF) is a rare tick-borne disease, though the virus is widely distributed in arid regions of Africa and Asia; RVF is chiefly a veterinary problem, but large epizootics have resulted in epidemics of encephalitis in humans.

Though not transmitted by an insect vector and therefore not arboviruses, hantaviruses are also members of the Bunyaviridae. They chronically infect rodents, much in the same way as arenaviruses, and in humans cause HFRS. Though usually a much milder disease than arenavirus haemorrhagic fever, HFRS is common in the Northern Hemisphere of the Old World, accounting for considerable morbidity and mortality.

Flaviruses include yellow fever virus, which is still responsible, despite effective vaccines, for massive epidemics and uncounted deaths in West Africa (5). The mosquito-borne dengue viruses remain endemic and epidemic throughout southeast Asia and parts of Central America and Africa, with recurrent epidemics of the severe disease mainly in children—dengue haemorrhagic fever (DHF) and dengue shock syndrome (DSS). Flaviruses spread by mosquitoes also cause encephalitis. Japanese encephalitis (JE) is endemic and epidemic in southeast and southern Asia, and may be severe and often fatal. Vaccines are available for human use for this infection. St Louis encephalitis (SLE) causes epidemics in the United States. Both are spread by mosquitoes from the natural hosts, which are birds.

Among the important togaviruses are Venezuelan equine encephalitis (VEE), and Eastern (EEE) and Western (WEE) equine encephalitis viruses. These are seasonal in the Americas, and cause periodic epidemics of severe disease in humans and in equines, though they are principally viruses of rodents and birds.

Marburg and Ebola viruses are related but serologically distinct filoviruses of uncertain ecology and unknown natural reservoir, but mortality is high (30–90%). In 1976, simultaneous outbreaks of Ebola virus infections in Zaire and Sudan, and again in 1979 in Sudan (mortality 53–91%) (6,7), were associated with needle sharing in remote clinics and hospitals (6,8). Since then only a handful of sporadic cases have been seen, though a closely related virus, apparently non-pathogenic for humans, has been the cause of epidemics and deaths in cynomolgus monkeys from the Philippines. Finally, rabies, a rhabdovirus, which is now provisionally classified with the filoviruses and the paramyxoviruses in the order Mononegavirales, shares with Marburg and Ebola a reputation for devastating mortality and may be the most lethal virus known to man.

GENERAL TREATMENT CONSIDERATIONS

Early diagnosis and institution of appropriate supportive care are critical, since specific treatment for many of these infections is not available. With haemorrhagic fevers, fluid, electrolyte and osmotic imbalances and respiratory failure must be managed carefully. The characteristic leaky capillary syndrome of the haemorrhagic fevers make fluid overload a real hazard. Indeed, even without fluid replacement, patients develop pulmonary oedema despite hypovolaemic shock, and may die with full-blown adult respiratory distress syndrome (ARDS) (1,9). Full intensive care support, including mechanical ventilation and blood, plasma or platelet replacement may be necessary. Medical personnel may avoid hazards of infection to themselves by adhering strictly to procedures appropriate for prevention of transmission of blood-borne pathogens, such as HIV (10,11). Every effort is justified since the crisis is short lived, and for many infections with exotic viruses complete recovery can be expected in survivors. Although much has been written about disseminated intravascular coagulation (DIC), particularly concerning the use of heparin, there is little objective evidence for the role of DIC in the pathogenesis of viral haemorrhagic fevers, and use of heparin remains controversial and potentially dangerous. Corticosteroids have not been found to be useful. Pregnant patients present a particular challenge, since they often present with absent fetal movements, and their survival may depend on aggressive obstetric intervention. However, even vigorous support may be insufficient to prevent fatal progression of advanced disease and specific therapy, where it is available, needs to be instituted as soon as the diagnosis is suspected.

Supportive therapy for DHF/DSS, essentially a paediatric disease, is very successful (12). In accordance with the guidelines developed by the WHO expert committee, emphasis is on early diagnosis, management of fluid balance, and careful monitoring of haematocrit, acid–base balance and urinary output. Indeed, many patients are successfully managed on an outpatient basis, since recovery is usually rapid. Corticosteroids have been shown to have no benefit, and there seems little urgency to develop antiviral chemotherapy. Uncomplicated dengue infection in adults, though painful, is generally mild and self-limiting, as are most infections caused by the other arboviruses which cause febrile disease in humans. Analgesia, antipyretics and bedrest usually suffice.

Unfortunately there is no specific treatment for any of the exotic viral encephalitides or for the most devastating haemorrhagic fevers. Yellow fever remains untreatable. Early hopes from *in vitro* studies that ribavirin might be effective have not been borne out. No antiviral therapy, including convalescent plasma, interferon, ribavirin or related compounds, has been shown to be effective against either Marburg or Ebola virus infection in patients or in experimentally infected non-human primates. The viral encephalitides are of necessity treated symptomatically; that is, appropriate use of anticonvulsants and control of intracranial pressure. Fluid balance and respiratory support may be necessary.

INTERFERONS AND OTHER CYTOKINES

Non-specific therapeutic approaches such as use of interferons (IFNs) and IFN inducers or macrophage activators have been shown to be able to inhibit the replication of many viruses *in vitro*, and to protect animals in some instances, but none have yet been proved clinically useful (13). The best prospects so far are with bunyaviruses, which are sensitive to IFNs *in vitro* (Table 13.2) (13). Animal protection studies using IFN inducers (poly-ICLC) have been successful in treatment and prophylaxis of experimental RVF infections (14,15). If treatment was initiated within 24 h of infection, protection against death could be achieved with 20 μg of poly-ICLC per mouse. If treatment was delayed until 48 h after infection, the best that could be achieved was 40% survivors (14). Ribavirin added to this regimen improved survival. Similar results have been obtained with treatment of tick-borne encephalitis virus (TBE), using combination therapy and lower

Table 13.2. Review of published *in vitro* data of inhibition of various exotic viruses in a number of cell systems with ribavirin

Virus	Cell lines used	Range of MIC (μg/ml)	Range of ED_{50} (μg/ml)	Refs
Arenaviridae				
Pichinde	Vero E6		60–61	(47,49)
Lassa	Vero, RAM	10–50		(48)
Junin	Vero		22	(50)
Machupo	Vero		32	(50)
Bunyaviridae				
RVF	MRC-5, Vero, Vero 76	25–200	80–>250	(15,46,47,50)
Hantaviruses	Vero E6		15–16	(47,49)
CCHF	Vero, SW13, CEF			(46,50,62)
SFV	Vero 76	40–80	77	(49,77)
Flaviviridae				
Yellow fever	LLC-MK, Vero		8–450	(47,49,50)
JE	Vero 76		42–65	(47,49)
Togaviridae				
VEE	Vero 76		25–190	(47,49)
Filoviridae				
Ebola	Vero		>500	(50)

RVF, Rift Valley fever; CCHF, Congo–Crimean haemorrhagic fever; SFV, sandfly fever; JE, Japanese encephalitis; VEE, Venezuelan equine encephalitis; Vero, African green monkey kidney; RAM, rhesus alveolar macrophages; CEF, chick embryo fibroblasts; LLC-MK, rhesus monkey kidney; SW13, human adrenal adenocarcinoma cells.

doses of poly-ICLC (16). Poly-ICLC is too toxic for use in man, and the regimen is, in any event, essentially only effective as post-exposure prophylaxis. Pathogenesis studies of RVF virus infection in rhesus monkeys have shown a significant correlation between a delayed endogenous IFN response and mortality (17). Reduction in duration of viraemia and viral titres were dose related in monkeys, given recombinant IFN or human leucocyte IFN pre-inoculation, all of which survived (18). Similar results were obtained with 'treatment' regimens (5×10^4 U/kg rIFN-α); however, the latest treatment was instituted 6 h after inoculation of virus, which must again be considered post-exposure prophylaxis. The medical relevance of such regimens, except in cases of known laboratory exposure, is doubtful, but would be worth further evaluation in primate models. IFN has been given to patients with CCHF infection, a tick-borne bunyavirus, but no conclusions could be reached as to efficacy (19).

IFNs have not yet been successfully used in animals or in humans for the treatment of exotic diseases. An attempt to treat rabies encephalitis with large doses of intravenous and intrathecal IFN was unsuccessful (20). Flaviruses are relatively insensitive to IFNs with the exception of JE, against which poly-ICLC and other IFN inducers have again shown efficacy in experimental mice and monkeys (13,21). Arenaviruses are also relatively insensitive to IFNs (21). Indeed, in AHF, severity is related to the serum levels of endogenous IFN naturally produced by patients in response to the infection (22,23). These are high: between 2000 and 64 000 IU/ml (22). Filoviruses are insensitive to IFN *in vitro* and in infected primates. The single case report of Ebola fever treated with human IFN remains anecdotal; the patient was also given immune plasma and supportive care (24).

Cytokines becoming available for therapy of malignancies and other conditions have not yet been applied to haemorrhagic fevers or viral encephalitides. This is not to say that some form of generic cytokine-based therapy may not become clinically available for these patients in due course—the magic bullet. A generic approach designed to counter some common, critical pathological pathway would certainly offer the best solution in view of the difficulty of rapid and accurate aetiological diagnosis of many of these infections.

IMMUNE GLOBULIN

A common approach to therapy has been the use of immune plasma, which has had a long history in the treatment of viral haemorrhagic fevers. Its success depends on the immunological potential of each virus and the family to which it belongs. Most work has been done with arenaviruses, even though there is some suggestion that an enhancement phenomenon in macrophages may be associated with high titres of virus-specific antibody in an *in vitro* system (25). The most striking demonstration of the use of immune plasma and the first effective treatment for any haemorrhagic fever is for AHF, reported by Maiztegui *et al.* in 1979 (26). Junin virus infections are geographically and epidemiologically circumscribed, so that collection, screening and storage of adequate plasma supplies is possible. Convalescent-phase plasma has been shown to be highly efficacious, reducing mortality from 16% to 1% in patients treated in the first eight days of illness. Late initiation of therapy is, however, less successful. In treated patients, viraemia is reduced within 24 h, and clinical symptoms and haematological alterations are less severe than in control cases receiving non-immune plasma. Efficacy is directly related to a dose of neutralizing antibodies of no less than 3000 therapeutic units total dose (27). In patients, a late neurological syndrome consisting of fever and cerebellar signs two to three weeks following recovery has been associated with successful treatment with immune plasma (26). However, the syndrome correlated with very high titres of neutralizing antibody in the immune plasma the patient received (27,28). There is thus a therapeutic 'window'.

A similar, but not identical, late neurological syndrome has been associated with successful immune plasma therapy of experimental Junin virus infection in marmosets. The syndrome comprised hind-limb paralyses, but no meningoencephalitis or meningitis, as was seen in untreated animals dying of acute infection (29). Similar effects, particularly hind-limb paralyses, were seen in treated guinea-pigs (30). Immune globulin has also been shown to be effective in protecting monkeys against experimental infection with the closely related Bolivian haemorrhagic fever virus (31).

Immune plasma has not been successful in treatment of Lassa fever, despite early anecdotal reports of success (32,33). Passive protection with antibody to Lassa virus has been demonstrated in animals given selected immune plasma at the time of, or soon after, inoculation with virus (34–37). However, unlike Junin infections, the immunological response to Lassa virus infection is complex. There is a substantial macrophage response in tissues, but little if any lymphocytic infiltrate. A brisk B cell response, with a classical primary IgG and IgM antibody response to Lassa virus early in the illness, does not coincide with virus clearance (38,39). Indeed virus may persist in the serum and urine of humans for several months after infection. Neutralizing antibodies to Lassa virus are absent in the serum of patients at the beginning of convalescence. In a minority of patients some low-titre serum neutralizing activity may be observed several months after resolution of the disease and clearance of the virus. The biological significance of this observation is not understood. There is also evidence from primate vaccine studies in which immunofluorescent antibody (IFA) did not correlate with protection. Animals vaccinated with a vaccinia recombinant vaccine expressing the Lassa glycoproteins survived challenge with Lassa virus. None of the pre-challenge specimens from vaccinated animals demonstrating protection had any neutralizing activity measurable *in vitro*. In fact, neutralizing antibody could only be demonstrated by a fixed serum, varying virus dilution technique in a few samples between 21 and 97 days post challenge, at a time when the IFA antibody was as much as 1 : 250 000, and when all animals had long cleared challenge virus from their serum (39). Antibodies to all viral proteins could be detected by IFA in unprotected animals which died following challenge, and to the nucleoprotein in animals vaccinated with a recombinant vaccine expressing the nucleoprotein which also died. Neutralizing antibody does not play any role in clearance of virus from serum in acute infection, and it seems unlikely to be playing a major role in protection from challenge. Though at present unavailable, purified hyperimmune globulin, with specific anti-Lassa virus titres comparable to those recommended for treatment of Junin infection, may have a place in treatment, particularly for patients presenting late in disease, and thus less likely to respond to a single chemotherapeutic agent, or in pregnancy, where problems of potential teratogenicity make use of ribavirin controversial. Its cost is likely to be prohibitive for those who need it most.

There has been some success with immune plasma in treatment of bunyavirus infections. Immune plasma has been shown to be effective in protecting six- to eight-week-old mice from RVF virus infection when given within 4 h of infection (15), and hyperimmune globulin or immune plasma has been used for CCHF infections in Bulgaria and in South Africa, apparently with some success, though numbers are very small (19,40,41). Unfortunately, the most severe of the haemorrhagic fevers, such as Ebola and Marburg, come from parts of the world with high endemicity for persistent blood-borne pathogens such as hepatitis viruses and HIV, and where laboratory facilities are limited. Purified fractionated hyperimmune globulin could be prepared for these viruses, but again efficacy would need to be established, and there is considerable evidence that this will be difficult. Once again, the cost of production and quality control of such material, and its storage, distribution and safe administration to those most at need of it (and of necessity least able to afford it), appear insurmountable problems.

CHEMOTHERAPY OF EXOTIC VIRUSES—RIBAVIRIN

A cheap, non-toxic, broadly effective chemotherapeutic agent would be the ideal solution. Many candidates have been assayed in *in vitro* and in animal model systems in an effort to find effective therapy for the more serious of the exotic pathogens. With the exception of ribavirin these compounds have not reached clinical trials (13). Indeed, the major advance in treatment of viral haemorrhagic fevers has been ribavirin, firstly for the treatment of Lassa fever and subsequently for HFRS (33,42). The treatment of Lassa fever with ribavirin, reported by McCormick *et al.* in 1986, was in fact the first demonstration of an effective antiviral treatment of a disseminated, life-threatening viral disease (33). Ribavirin is also, in theory at least, sufficiently cheap, stable and non-toxic for use in developing countries.

Ribavirin closely resembles guanosine in structure (Figure 13.1). Its antiviral activity may be via inhibition of IMP dehydrogenase and consequent effect on the guanine nucleotide pools, but it is likely that it also affects the formation of the 5′ 'cap' common to many mRNAs (43). Reversible toxicity has been associated with the development of a normochromic normocytic anaemia, mild with low doses and severe with high doses. This is accompanied by thrombocytosis, with dose-related erythroid hypoplasia and megakaryocytic hyperplasia (44). Anaemia is due to decreased red blood cell survival as well as decreased red blood cell production. Ribavirin has been shown to be teratogenic or to have embryocidal effects in rats and in rabbits when given during the first trimester of pregnancy, and is therefore not recommended for pregnant women (45).

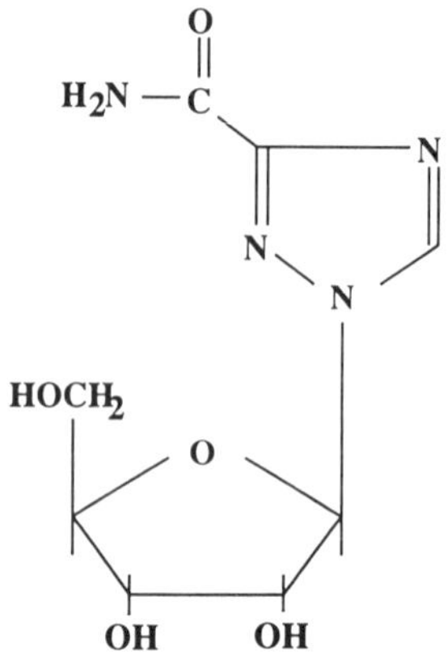

Figure 13.1. The ribavirin molecule

Ribavirin and its analogues inhibit the replication of many RNA viruses *in vitro* and *in vivo*, including rhabdoviruses, arboviruses, arenaviruses, respiratory syncytial viruses and other para-, ortho- and myxoviruses, hepatitis viruses, retroviruses and a variety of members of all four genera of the family Bunyaviridae that have been tested, including RVF virus, CCHF, Sicilian sandfly fever (SFV) virus, and Hantaan virus (13,46). There are problems with extrapolation of *in vitro* data since there are marked cell system differences depending on the ability of the cell line used to absorb, metabolize or retain drugs, and the different receptor properties and susceptibility of the cell line to infection by a particular virus. This leads to inconsistent and sometimes conflicting data (Table 13.2). However, bunyaviruses, arenaviruses and some togaviruses are inhibited in *in vitro* systems (15,46–49). The only truly resistant family is, unfortunately, that of the filoviruses (50).

The greatest success of ribavirin has been with arenaviruses, particularly Lassa fever. Studies with rhesus monkeys show that ribavirin administered early in the course of Lassa fever infection prevents death and decreases viraemia levels and biochemical abnormalities (37,48,51). No deaths and no sequelae were observed in four monkeys treated with 50 mg/kg per day loading dose followed by 30 mg/kg per day i.m. for 10 days on the day of virus inoculation and in four others treated five days after receiving an inoculation of Lassa fever virus. This was the first demonstration of the possibility of effective treatment as opposed to post-exposure prophylaxis.

Trials of the effectiveness of ribavirin against Lassa fever have been conducted over a number of years in Sierra Leone (33,52). Initially, orally administered ribavirin was compared with convalescent-phase plasma. Patients with a clinical diagnosis of Lassa fever were randomly assigned and treated with either convalescent plasma (250–300 ml) with an IFA titre

> 128 or oral ribavirin for 10 days. For analysis, patients were grouped by two risk factors: the levels of AST and viraemia on admission. Patients treated with ribavirin at any time in illness had significantly lower case fatality than untreated patients with the same risk factors (33). (Untreated patients were those studied three or four years earlier at the same hospitals prior to the availability of ribavirin.) Survival was significantly higher following oral ribavirin therapy than in untreated patients or in patients treated with plasma. Survival after convalescent plasma therapy was no higher than in those who were untreated.

Subsequently, patients were further selected for therapy if they had in addition to the diagnosis of Lassa fever an AST of > 150 IU/l at the time of admission. The patients received either intravenous ribavirin for 10 days or intravenous ribavirin and a unit of convalescent-phase plasma at the time of admission (33). Ribavirin was given intravenously as a 2 g loading dose followed by 1 g every 6 h for four days then 0.5 g every 8 h for six more days. Survival was significantly improved in patients treated with intravenous ribavirin. A five- to ten-fold decrease in the case–fatality ratio was demonstrated in patients treated with ribavirin compared with untreated patients when therapy was given within the first six days of illness. Patients with high AST and viraemia, risk factors for unfavourable outcome, who were treated within the first six days of illness experienced a 5–9% case fatality. Those with the same risk factors receiving treatment more than six days after the onset of illness had a 26–47% fatality, compared with 52–78% in untreated patients. Furthermore, patients treated with ribavirin had a significant reduction in viraemia regardless of outcome compared with untreated patients. Subsequent studies have suggested that reduction of the ribavirin dose by half is still effective (52). Ribavirin is contraindicated in early pregnancy because of potential teratogenicity, but the fetus rarely survives the infection. It has been used in Lassa fever in late pregnancy but its efficacy in these patients has not yet been determined.

Ribavirin is also effective in animal models against South American haemorrhagic fever viruses, but data are conflicting because of late neurological complications. Treatment of marmosets experimentally infected with Junin virus improved survival from the acute infection, but five of the seven survivors died of neurological complications 24 days post infection, much as was seen with treatment with immune plasma (53,54). Similar results have been observed in rhesus monkeys with both AHF and BHF viruses (55,56). Paradoxically, ribavirin protected 40% of intracerebrally infected 10-day-old rats from encephalitis, administered 2 h before infection (57). Several factors should be considered. The pathophysiology of the late neurological syndrome is not understood. Failure of ribavirin to cross the blood–brain barrier has been cited, but it is not at all clear whether the syndrome is due to direct virus replication or immunological phenomena. That it may be immunologically determined is supported by the clear species differences. Unlike monkeys and guinea-pigs, the late neurological syndrome appears to be confined to mild ataxia in humans. Ataxia may be seen also in recovered Lassa fever patients, and is self-limiting. Lack of efficacy of ribavirin in Junin-infected guinea-pigs further emphasizes that rodents are not good models for human arenavirus disease. Ribavirin only delayed viraemia and death, and ribavirin-treated animals had higher-titre virus in their brains than untreated animals (58). In a limited study of patients with AHF of more than seven days duration ribavirin reduced viraemia, but there was no obvious effect on mortality (59).

Efficacy data from some animal studies are shown in Table 13.3. Ribavirin has been shown to be effective in animals infected with RVF virus (60,61). Death was prevented in all rats and rhesus monkeys given ribavirin in a dose of 100 mg/kg per day beginning immediately after viral inoculation. In rhesus monkeys viraemia was significantly reduced when ribavirin was given i.m. in an initial dose of 50 mg/kg, followed by 10 mg/kg three times daily, beginning 2 h after viral inoculation (15). Ribavirin administered up to 48 h post infection has also been shown to be effective in prophylaxis of another bunyavirus, CCHF virus, in the only animal model available, the suckling mouse (62). Preliminary data from a clinical trial of ribavirin for treatment of CCHF in South Africa are promising. Again, treatment is most effective when given early in disease (63).

Hantaviruses have also been the target of ribavirin therapy. Ribavirin has been shown to be effective prophylactically in a SCID mouse model (64). In suckling mice infected with Hantaan virus, ribavirin in a dose of 25 mg/kg on day 10 post inoculation increased survival to 30% ($p < 0.05$), while 50 mg/kg increased survival to 55% ($p < 0.001$). Neutralizing antibodies appeared at the same time as in controls (65). Clinical trials have been conducted in the People's Republic of China (PRC) using ribavirin produced in China, and reporting efficacy (66–69). A collaborative, multicentre, placebo-controlled trial of intravenous ribavirin therapy of HFRS was conducted in nine study sites in Hubei Province, PRC, during two epidemic seasons (42). Two hundred and forty-four enrolled patients met the study criteria for analysis, and the treatment group were given 33 mg/kg loading dose, 16 mg/kg every 6 h for four days and 8 mg/kg every 8 h for three days. Treatment reduced mortality from 10 of 118 in the placebo group to three of 126 in the ribavirin-treated group ($p = 0.041$, one-tailed, by Fisher's exact test). However, the numbers are small, and the study centres were tertiary care hospitals. There may also have been multiple confounding factors due to non-uniformity of patient selection and clinical practice in different centres. It would be interesting to know if use of oral ribavirin at the time of first presentation with symptoms, presumably at primary health care clinics, is effective in preventing progression to disease necessitating hospitalization. Mortality is low in HFRS, but

Table 13.3. Review of published *in vivo* animal studies of protection against various exotic viruses with ribavirin

	Species	Initiation of therapy	Loading dose	Schedule	Outcome	Refs
Arenaviruses						
Pichinde virus	Hamsters, guinea-pigs				Survival increased from 11% to 100%	(13)
Junin virus	Guinea-pigs	Day −1		45 mg/kg per day	Survived haemorrhagic disease but died of late neurological syndrome	(30)
Junin virus	Marmosets	Day 6		15 mg/kg b.i.d.	Survival increased from 0 to 29% but 5/6 died of late neurological syndrome	(53,54)
Junin virus	Rats i.c.	−2 h		60–90 mg/kg	40% protection	(57)
	Rats i.p.	Day 0		30 mg/kg per day, 5 days	>70% protection	(57)
Junin virus	Rhesus monkeys	Day 0	60 mg/kg days 0–3	30 mg/kg days 4–7	4/4 survived	(55)
		Day 6	60 mg/kg	15 mg/kg days 7–20	1/4 survived	(55)
Machupo virus	Rhesus monkeys			10–20 mg/kg per day	Survived haemorrhagic disease but died of late neurological syndrome	(56)
Lassa virus	Cynomolgus monkeys	Days 0–4	75 mg/kg	15 mg/kg b.i.d.	All survived	(48)
		Day 7	75 mg/kg	15 mg/kg b.i.d.	4/8 survived	(48)
Bunyaviruses						
Hantaan virus	Suckling mice	Day 10		50 mg/kg per day	50% increase in survival	(65)
Hantaan virus	SCID mice	2 h			90% survival	(64)
RVF	Mice	8 h	75 mg/kg	25 mg/kg b.i.d.	18/24	(15)
RVF	Hamsters	Day 0	60 mg/kg b.i.d.	20 mg/kg b.i.d.	8/10	(15)
RVF	Rhesus monkeys	Day 0		50 mg/kg t.i.d.	Day 3 mean viraemia reduced by 50%	(15)
RVF	Mice	Days 0–4		60–100 mg/kg	>90% protection	(56)
RVF	Rhesus monkeys		50 mg/kg	30 mg/kg b.i.d.	Eliminates viraemia	(56)

RVF, Rift Valley fever; SCID, severe combined immunodeficient.

morbidity is a major problem, and a cheap and effective early therapy would have considerable economic as well as public health benefits.

Treatment for established rabies encephalomyelitis remains essentially hopeless. There are reports of two cases of documented survival (one had been pre-immunized) following supposed inhalation of rabies virus aerosol in laboratories, and two patients who had been exposed to bats in caves have survived with severe neurological sequelae (70). Two patients who developed severe neurological manifestations but who had received post-exposure prophylaxis recovered after intensive care (71,72). Attempted treatment with intravenous and intrathecal ribavirin and IFN, rabies immune plasma and corticosteroids has been equally unsuccessful (73). Similarly, attempts to treat experimentally infected monkeys with intrathecal attenuated rabies vaccine strain were inconclusive (20). Intensive care may prolong survival by correcting cardiac arrhythmias, cardiac and respiratory failure, raised intracranial pressure, convulsions, fluid and electrolyte disturbances and hyperpyrexia. Unfortunately, sedation and analgesia remain the only relief that can currently be offered for this terrifying disease.

POST-EXPOSURE PROPHYLAXIS

Post-exposure prophylaxis for rabies has a long history of success provided it is administered promptly and the appropriate schedule completed (74). Tissue culture vaccines are preferred, but the cheaper duck embryo and mouse brain vaccines are more readily available throughout the developing world, and are certainly effective. Vaccine should be given by intramuscular injection on days 0, 3, 7, 14 and 30. Immune plasma should be given at the time of the first injection, with half of the dose infiltrated around the bite wound. This schedule can reduce the risk of developing rabies to approaching zero with tissue culture vaccines. If prophylaxis is delayed beyond 48 h after the bite, or if the patient is in any way debilitated or immunosuppressed, the initial vaccine dose should be doubled or tripled. If pre-exposure vaccination has been completed, passive immunization with immune globulin is not necessary, and a booster course of vaccine may be given on days 0, 3 and 7.

Though data on efficacy for post-exposure prophylaxis for viral haemorrhagic fevers are lacking and unlikely to become available in the foreseeable future, anecdotal experience and animal studies suggest that for arenaviruses this approach is likely to be effective, and carries negligible risk of toxicity. On present evidence, oral ribavirin is recommended as post-exposure prophylaxis as soon as possible after exposure, provided there is a good history of potential parenteral or mucosal contamination with blood or other material containing live virus (high-risk contacts) (10). Currently, ribavirin, 600 mg orally four times a day for 10 days, may be offered (75). The same approach may be taken with bunyaviruses though in one study intravenous ribavirin was given to six of nine high-risk contacts who had needle stick exposure, three of whom also received a short course of IFN. One of the contacts who received ribavirin but no IFN developed mild CCHF; all three untreated contacts developed severe CCHF (76). Oral ribavirin is probably also effective. Ribavirin has also been evaluated for its prophylactic efficacy in the prevention of SFV (Sicilian) infection in human volunteers (77). Six individuals each received ribavirin (1200 mg per day orally) or placebo beginning one day prior to receiving undiluted human plasma containing SFV (Sicilian) virus, and continuing for a total of eight days. Illness was prevented in all individuals receiving ribavirin, whereas four of six placebo-treated controls became sick. However, sandfly fever is a mild, self-limiting disease, and use of potentially toxic therapeutic agents may be of less interest.

PROSPECTS FOR THE FUTURE

Most of the 'exotic' viruses are essentially orphans. The lack of investment and interest in developing therapy is unfortunate since many of them are clearly amenable to one if not more approaches to treatment. Realistically, however, it is unlikely that a range of agents will be developed for these diseases. Those that are available and cheap and safe, such as ribavirin, clearly need further trials and further development, and the expense involved would be justified. An issue that demands urgent attention is the treatment of pregnant women. In the case of Lassa fever, merely getting ribavirin to the hospitals in West Africa where the disease is so common would save countless lives. As so often happens in developing countries, the logistics are formidable and have so far thwarted efforts. Unless some generic approach to acute viral disease can be found that is cheap, broad spectrum and has a long shelf-life at room temperature (?ribavirin), the best hopes currently lie with prevention, by vaccination or by protection of the individual from the vector or source of virus.

REFERENCES

1. McCormick, J.B., Webb, P. A., Krebs, J. W. *et al.* (1987). A prospective study of the epidemiology and ecology of lassa fever. *J. Inject. Dis.*, **155**, 437–444.
2. McCormick, J. B. and Fisher-Hoch, S. P. (1990). Viral hemorrhagic fevers. In *Tropical and Geographical Medicine*, 2nd edn, K. S. Warren and A. A. F. Mahmoud (eds), McGraw-Hill, New York, pp. 700–727.
3. Maiztegui, J. I. (1975). Clinical and epidemiological patterns of Argentine haemorrhagic fever. *Bull. World Health Organ.*, **52**, 567–575.

4. Salas, R., Manzione, N. de, Tesh, R. B. *et al.* (1991). Venezuelan haemorrhagic fever. *Lancet*, **338**, 1033–1036.
5. De Cock, K. M., Monath, T. P., Nasidi, A. *et al.* (1988). Epidemic yellow fever in eastern Nigeria, 1986. *Lancet*, **i**, 630–632.
6. World Health Organization (1978). Ebola haemorrhagic fever in Sudan, 1976. Report of a WHO/International Study Team. *Bull. World Health Organ.*, **56**, 247–270.
7. Baron, R. C., McCormick, J. B. and Zubeir, O. A. (1983). Ebola virus disease in southern Sudan: hospital dissemination and intrafamilial spread. *Bull. World Health Organ.*, **61**, 997–1003.
8. World Health Organization (1978). Ebola haemorrhagic fever in Zaire, 1976: report of an international commission. *Bull. World Health Organ.*, **56**, 271–293.
9. Fisher-Hoch, S. P., Price, M. E., Craven, R. B. *et al.* (1985). Safe intensive-care management of a severe case of lassa fever with simple barrier nursing techniques. *Lancet*, **ii**, 1227–1229.
10. Centers for Disease Control (1988). Management of patients with suspected viral hemorrhagic fever. *MMWR*, **37** (Suppl. 3), 1–16.
11. Centers for Disease Control (1988). Update: universal precautions for prevention of transmission of human immunodeficiency virus, hepatitis B virus and other bloodborne pathogens in health-care settings. *MMWR*, **37**, 377–388.
12. World Health Organization (1986). *Dengue Haemorrhagic Fever*, WHO, Geneva.
13. Canonico, P. G., Kende, M., Luscri, B. J. and Huggins, J. W. (1984). In-vivo activity of antivirals against exotic RNA viral infections. *J. Antimicrob. Chemother.*, **14** (Suppl. A), 27–41.
14. Kende, M., Lupton, H. W., Rill, W. L. *et al.* (1987). Enhanced therapeutic efficacy of poly(ICLC) and ribavirin combinations against Rift Valley fever virus infection in mice. *Antimicrob. Agents Chemother.*, **31**, 986–990.
15. Peters, C. J., Reynolds, J. A., Slone, T. W. *et al.* (1986). Prophylaxis of Rift Valley fever with antiviral drugs, immune serum, an interferon inducer, and a macrophage activator. *Antiviral Res.*, **6**, 285–297.
16. Vilner, L. M. and Lashkevich, V. A. (1984). Virazole effect on antiviral activity of poly(G):poly(C) and other polyribonucleotide interferogens. *Antibiotiki (Moscow)*, **29**, 450–453.
17. Morrill, J. C., Jennings, G. B., Johnson, A. J. *et al.* (1990). Pathogenesis of Rift Valley fever in rhesus monkeys: role of interferon response. *Arch. Virol.*, **110**, 195–212.
18. Morrill, J. C., Jennings, G. B., Cosgriff, T. M. *et al.* (1989). Prevention of Rift Valley fever in rhesus monkeys with interferon-alpha. *Rev. Infect. Dis.*, **11** (Suppl. 4), S815–S825.
19. van Eeden, P. J., van Eeden, S. F., Joubert, J. R. *et al.* (1985). A nosocomial outbreak of Crimean–Congo haemorrhagic fever at Tygerberg Hospital. Part II. Management of patients. *S. Afr. Med. J.*, **68**, 718–721.
20. Warrell, M. J., Ward, G. S., Elwell, M. R. and Tingpalapong, M. (1987). An attempt to treat rabies encephalitis in monkeys with intrathecal live rabies virus RV675. *Arch. Virol.*, **96**, 271–273.
21. Stephen, E. L., Scott, S. K., Eddy, G. A. and Levy, H. B. (1977). Effect of interferon on togavirus and arenavirus infections of animals. *Texas Rep. Biol. Med.*, **35**, 449–454.
22. Levis, S. C., Saavedra, M. C., Ceccoli, C. *et al.* (1985). Correlation between endogenous interferon and the clinical evolution of patients with Argentine hemorrhagic fever. *J. Interferon Res.*, **5**, 383–389.
23. Levis, S. C., Saavedra, M. C., Ceccoli, C. *et al.* (1984). Endogenous interferon in Argentine hemorrhagic fever. *J. Infect. Dis.*, **149**, 428–433.

24. Emond, R. T. D., Evans, B., Bowen, E. T. W. and Lloyd, G. (1977). A case of ebola virus infection. *Br. Med. J.*, **2**, 541–544.
25. Lewis, R. M., Cosgriff, T. M., Griffin, B. Y. *et al.* (1988). Immune serum increases arenavirus replication in monocytes. *J. Gen. Virol.*, **69**, 1735–1739.
26. Maiztegui, J. I., Fernandez, N. J. and de Damilano, A. J. (1979). Efficacy of immune plasma in treatment of Argentine haemorrhagic fever and association between treatment and a late neurological syndrome. *Lancet*, **ii**, 1216–1217.
27. Enria, D. A., Briggiler, A. M., Fernandez, N. J. *et al.* (1984). Importance of dose of neutralising antibodies in treatment of Argentine haemorrhagic fever with immune plasma. *Lancet*, **ii**, 255–256.
28. Enria, D. A., de Damilano, A. J., Briggiler, A. M. *et al.* (1985). Late neurologic syndrome in patients with Argentinian hemorrhagic fever treated with immune plasma. *Medicina* (*B. Aires*), **45**, 615–620.
29. Avila, M. M., Samoilovich, S. R., Laguens, R. P. *et al.* (1987). Protection of Junin virus-infected marmosets by passive administration of immune serum: association with late neurologic signs. *J. Med. Virol.*, **21**, 67–74.
30. Kenyon, R. H., Green, D. E., Eddy, G. A. and Peters, C. J. (1986). Treatment of Junin virus-infected guinea pigs with immune serum: development of late neurological disease. *J. Med. Virol.*, **20**, 207–218.
31. Eddy, G. A., Wagner, F. S., Scott, S. K. and Mahlandt, B. J. (1975). Protection of monkeys against Machupo virus by the passive administration of Bolivian haemorrhagic fever immunoglobulin (human origin). *Bull. World Health Organ.*, **52**, 723–727.
32. Monath, T. P., Maher, M., Casals, J. *et al.* (1974). Lassa fever in the Eastern Province of Sierra Leone, 1970–1972. II. Clinical observations and virological studies on selected hospital cases. *Am. J. Trop. Med. Hyg.*, **23**, 1140–1149.
33. McCormick, J. B., King, I. J., Webb, P. A. *et al.* (1986). Lassa fever: effective therapy with ribavirin. *N. Engl. J. Med.*, **314**, 20–26.
34. Jahrling, P. B., Smith, S., Hesse, R. A. and Rhoderick, J. B. (1982). Pathogenesis of Lassa virus infection in guinea pigs. *Infect. Immun.*, **37**, 771–778.
35. Peters, C. J., Jahrling, P. B., Liu, C. T. *et al.* (1987). Experimental studies of arenaviral hemorrhagic fevers. *Curr. Top. Microbiol. Immunol.*, **134**, 5–68.
36. Jahrling, P. B. and Peters, C. J. (1984). Passive antibody therapy of Lassa fever in cynomolgus monkeys: importance of neutralizing antibody and Lassa virus strain. *Infect. Immun.*, **44**, 528–533.
37. Jahrling, P. B., Peters, C. J. and Stephen, E. L. (1984). Enhanced treatment of Lassa fever by immune plasma combined with ribavirin in cynomolgus monkeys. *J. Infect. Dis.*, **149**, 420–427.
38. Walker, D. H., McCormick, J. B., Johnson, K. M. *et al.* (1982). Pathologic and virologic study of fatal Lassa fever in man. *Am. J. Pathol.*, **107**, 349–356.
39. Fisher-Hoch, S. P., McCormick, J. B., Auperin, D. *et al.* (1989). Protection of rhesus monkeys from fatal Lassa fever by vaccination with a recombinant vaccinia virus containing the Lassa virus glycoprotein gene. *Proc. Natl Acad. Sci. USA*, **86**, 317–321.
40. Shepherd, A. J., Swanepoel, R., Shepherd, S. P. *et al.* (1985). A nosocomial outbreak of Crimean–Congo haemorrhagic fever at Tygerberg Hospital. Part V. Virological and serological observations. *S. Afr. Med. J.*, **68**, 733–736.
41. Vassilenko, S. M., Vassilev, T. L., Bozadjiev, L. G. *et al.* (1990). Specific intravenous immunoglobulin for Crimean–Congo haemorrhagic fever [letter]. *Lancet*, **335**, 791–792.
42. Huggins, J. W., Hsiang, C. M., Cosgriff, T. M. *et al.* (1991). Prospective, double-blind, concurrent, placebo-controlled, clinical trial of intravenous ribavirin therapy of hemorrhagic fever with renal syndrome (HFRS). *J. Infect. Dis.*, **164**, 1119–1127.

43. Smith, R. A. (1980). Mechanisms of action of ribavirin. In *Ribavirin: A Broad Spectrum Antiviral Agent,* R. A. Smith and W. Kirkpatrick (eds), Academic Press, New York, pp. 99–118.
44. Canonico, P. G., Kende, M. and Huggins, J. (1984). The toxicology and pharmacology of ribavirin in experimental animals. In *Clinical Applications of Ribavirin,* R. A. Smith, V. Knight and J. A. Smith (eds), Academic Press, New York, p. 77.
45. Hillyard, I. W. (1980). The preclinical toxicological safety of ribavirin. In *Ribavirin: A Broad Spectrum Antiviral Agent,* R. A. Smith and W. Kirkpatrick (eds), Academic Press, New York, pp. 58–71.
46. Watts, D. M., Ussery, M. A., Nash, D. and Peters, C. J. (1989). Inhibition of Crimean–Congo hemorrhagic fever viral infectivity yields in vitro by ribavirin. *Am. J. Trop. Med. Hyg.*, **41**, 581–585.
47. Huggins, J. W., Robins, R. K. and Canonico, P. G. (1984). Synergistic antiviral effects of ribavirin and the C-nucleoside analogs tiazofurin and selenazofurin against togaviruses, bunyaviruses, and arenaviruses. *Antimicrob. Agents Chemother.*, **26**, 476–480.
48. Jahrling, P. B., Hesse, R. A., Eddy, G. A. *et al.* (1980). Lassa virus infection of rhesus monkeys: pathogenesis and treatment with ribavirin. *J. Infect. Dis.*, **141**, 580–589.
49. Kirsi, J. J., North, J. A., McKernan, P. A. *et al.* (1983). Broad-spectrum antiviral activity of 2-beta-D-ribofuranosylselenazole-4-carboxamide, a new antiviral agent. *Antimicrob. Agents Chemother.*, **24**, 353–361.
50. Huggins, J. W. (1989). Prospects for treatment of viral hemorrhagic fevers with ribavirin, a broad-spectrum antiviral drug. *Rev. Infect. Dis.*, **11** (Suppl. 4), S750–S761.
51. Wannarka, G. L., Stephen, E. L. and Canonico, P. G. (1982). Preclinical evaluation of monkeys of a ribavirin regimen proposed for use in lassa fever patients. *Toxicol. Appl. Pharmacol.*, **64**, 155–159.
52. McCormick, J. B., Parker, L., Bennett, D. *et al.* (1991). Therapy of lassa fever with the nucleoside ribavirin. *40th Annual Meeting of the American Society of Tropical Medicine and Hygiene,* Boston (abstract).
53. Weissenbacher, M. C., Calello, M. A., Merani, M. S. *et al.* (1986). Therapeutic effect of the antiviral agent ribavirin in Junin virus infection of primates. *J. Med. Virol.*, **20**, 261–267.
54. Weissenbacher, M. C., Avila, M. M., Calello, M. A. *et al.* (1986). Effect of ribavirin and immune serum on Junin virus-infected primates. *Med. Microbiol. Immunol.*, **175**, 183–186.
55. McKee, K. T. Jr, Huggins, J. W., Trahan, C. J. and Mahlandt, B. G. (1988). Ribavirin prophylaxis and therapy for experimental Argentine hemorrhagic fever. *Antimicrob. Agents Chemother.*, **32**, 1304–1309.
56. Stephen, E. L., Jones, D. E., Peters, C. J. *et al.* (1980). Ribavirin treatment of toga-, arena-, and bunyavirus infections in subhuman primates and other animal species. In *Ribavirin: A Broad Spectrum Antiviral Agent,* R. A. Smith and W. Kirkpatrick (eds), Academic Press, New York, p. 183.
57. Remesar, M. C., Blejer, J. L., Weissenbacher, M. C. and Nejamkis, M. R. (1988). Ribavirin effect on experimental Junin virus-induced encephalitis. *J. Med. Virol.*, **26**, 79–84.
58. Kenyon, R. H., Canonico, P. G., Green, D. E. and Peters, C. J. (1986). Effect of ribavirin and tributylribavirin on Argentine hemorrhagic fever (Junin virus) in guinea pigs. *Antimicrob. Agents Chemother.*, **29**, 521–523.
59. Maiztegui, J. I. (1988). Progress in the treatment and prevention of Argentine hemorrhagic fever. *Proceedings of the 37th annual meeting of the American Society of Tropical Medicine and Hygiene,* Washington, DC (abstract).
60. Kende, M., Lupton, H. W., Rill, W. L. *et al.* (1987). Enhanced therapeutic efficacy

of poly(ICLC) and ribavirin combinations against Rift Valley fever virus infection in mice. *Antimicrob. Agents Chemother.*, **31**, 986–990.
61. Kende, M., Alving, C. R., Rill, W. L. *et al.* (1985). Enhanced efficacy of liposome-encapsulated ribavirin against Rift Valley fever virus infection in mice. *Antimicrob. Agents Chemother.*, **27**, 903–907.
62. Berezina, L. K., Leont'eva, N. A., Kondrashina, N. G. *et al.* (1983). Influence of ribavirin on the reproduction of bunyaviruses in cell culture and in experiments on white mice. *Vopr. Virusol.*, **5**, 627–629.
63. Swanepoel, R., Leman, P., Abbott, J. C. *et al.* (1990). Epidemiology, diagnosis, clinical pathology and treatment of Crimean–Congo hemorrhagic fever (CCHF) in South Africa. *Abstracts of the VIIth International Congress of Virology*, Berlin, P70–003 (abstract).
64. Zhang, Z. X. and Huggins, J. W. (1990). Comparison of ribavirin analogues in Hantaan-infected SCID mice. *Abstracts of the Third International Conference on Antiviral Research*, Brussels.
65. Huggins, J. W., Kim, G. R., Brand, O. M. and McKee, K. T. Jr. (1986). Ribavirin therapy for Hantaan virus infection in suckling mice. *J. Infect. Dis.*, **153**, 489–497.
66. Yang, Z. Q., Zhang, T. M., Zhang, M. V. *et al.* (1991). Interruption study of viremia of patients with hemorrhagic fever with renal syndrome in the febrile phase. *Chin. Med. J.*, **104**, 149–153.
67. Luo, D. D., Wang, X. H. and Cia, S. Q. (1988). Studies on antiviral therapy of epidemic hemorrhagic fever. *Virol. Sinica*, **3**, 290–292.
68. Huang, Q. T., Pong, L. K., Wu, Z. O. *et al.* (1988). Observations of clinical treatment of EHC by interferon and ribavirin. *Chin. J. Clin. Med.*, **5**, 18–19.
69. Markin, V. A., Pashanin, Iu. G., Markov, V. I. *et al.* (1990). The antiviral efficacy of ribamidil in an experimental infection of animals with the Venezuelan equine encephalomyelitis virus. *Vopr. Virusol.*, **35**, 237–240.
70. Tillotson, J. R., Axelrod, D. and Lyman, D. O. (1977). Follow-up on rabies—New York. *MMWR*, **26**, 249–250.
71. Wattwick, M. A. W., Weis, T. T., Stechschulte, C. J. *et al.* (1972). Recovery from rabies: a case report. *Ann. Intern. Med.*, **76**, 931–942.
72. Porras, C., Barboza, J. J., Fuenzahda, E. *et al.* (1976). Recovery from rabies in man. *Ann. Intern. Med.*, **85**, 44–48.
73. Warrell, M. J., White, N. J., Looareesuwan, S. *et al.* (1989). Failure of interferon alfa and tribavirin in rabies encephalitis. *Br. Med. J.*, **299**, 830–833.
74. Centers for Disease Control (1984). Rabies prevention—United States 1984. *MMWR*, **33**, 393–408.
75. Holmes, G. P., McCormick, J. B., Trock, S. C. *et al.* (1990). Lassa fever in the United States: investigation of a case and new guidelines for management. *N. Engl. J. Med.*, **323**, 1120–1123.
76. van de Wal, B. W., Joubert, J. R., van Eeden, P. J. and King, J. B. (1985). A nosocomial outbreak of Crimean–Congo haemorrhagic fever at Tygerberg Hospital. Part IV. Preventive and prophylactic measures. *S. Afr. Med. J.*, **68**, 729–732.
77. Canonico, P. G., Gibbs, P. H., Huggins, J. W. *et al.* (1986). Ribavirin prophylaxis of sandfly fever Sicilian infection in human volunteers. *US Army Scientific Conference*, West Point (abstract).

Part E

VIRAL HEPATITIS

14 Viral Hepatitis

TIM J. HARRISON and ARIE J. ZUCKERMAN
The Royal Free Hospital School of Medicine, London, UK

INTRODUCTION

Since the agents of the two major forms of viral hepatitis, 'infectious hepatitis' (hepatitis A) and 'serum hepatitis' (hepatitis B), were recognized and distinguished more than two decades ago, the inventory of viruses which cause hepatitis in humans has been growing steadily. Originally identified as a new antigen/antibody system in carriers of hepatitis B, the delta agent (hepatitis D virus, HDV) is a defective virus which requires a coat of the envelope protein of hepatitis B virus (HBV) for transmission. Cases of viral hepatitis which were not hepatitis A or B (or attributable to other agents such as those herpesviruses which occasionally cause hepatitis) were diagnosed by exclusion as 'non-A, non-B hepatitis'. The virus responsible for the majority of cases of parenterally transmitted non-A, non-B hepatitis has recently been identified and designated hepatitis C virus (HCV) and diagnostic tests developed. Another virus which, like hepatitis A virus (HAV), causes acute hepatitis and is transmitted by the faecal–oral route—enterically transmitted non-A, non-B hepatitis (ET–NANBH)—has been named hepatitis E virus (HEV). Other viruses which may be responsible for a minority of cases of parenterally transmitted and for sporadic non-A, non-B hepatitis remain to be identified.

HEPATITIS A

Outbreaks of jaundice were frequently described during recent centuries and the term infectious hepatitis was coined in 1912 to describe the epidemic form of the disease. HAV is known now to be spread by the faecal–oral route and continues to be endemic throughout the world and hyperendemic in areas with poor standards of sanitation and hygiene. The seroprevalence of antibodies to HAV has declined during recent decades in most of the developed world. Individuals are at risk of infection when travelling or during occasional outbreaks, for example, an outbreak of hepatitis A associated with the consumption of clams in Shanghai in 1988 claimed almost 300 000 victims (1).

Antiviral Chemotherapy. Edited by D.J. Jeffries and E. De Clercq

Hepatitis A has a relatively short incubation period of around four weeks. The initial site of virus replication may be extrahepatic (in the gut or associated tissues), although this has not been proven. Relatively large quantities of virus are shed in the stools before the onset of clinical symptoms. A brief viraemia occurs prior to the start of acute infection and accounts for the spread of the virus from the gut to the liver. The severity of illness ranges from the asymptomatic through anicteric to icteric hepatitis. The virus is non-cytopathic when grown in cell culture. Its pathogenicity *in vivo*, which involves necrosis of parenchymal cells and histiocytic periportal inflammation, may be mediated via the cellular immune response. By the time of onset of symptoms, excretion of virus in the faeces has declined and may have ceased and anti-HAV IgM (diagnostic of acute infection) is rising in titre. Anti-HAV IgG may be detected one to two weeks later and persists for years.

CLASSIFICATION

Electron microscopical examination of concentrates of filtered stool extracts from patients in the early stages of infection reveals 27 nm icosahedral particles typical of the Picornaviridae. These particles may be aggregated by incubation with sera positive for anti-HAV antibodies (immune electron microscopy). HAV was classified in 1983 in the genus Enterovirus (as enterovirus 72) of the family Picornaviridae, on the basis of its biophysical and biochemical characteristics, including stability at low pH (2). However, this decision pre-empted the isolation and analysis of complementary DNA (cDNA) clones leading to the determination of the entire nucleotide sequence of the viral genome (3–5). Comparison with other picornavirus sequences revealed limited homology to the enteroviruses or, indeed, the rhinoviruses; although the structure and genome organization is typical of the Picornaviridae. HAV has now been reclassified in its own genus as a Hepatovirus (6).

ORGANIZATION OF THE HAV GENOME

The HAV genome comprises around 7500 nucleotides (nt) of positive sense RNA which is polyadenylated at the 3′ end and has a polypeptide (VPg) attached to the 5′ end. A single, large open reading frame (ORF) occupies most of the genome and encodes a polyprotein with a theoretical molecular mass of M_r 252 000. An untranslated region of around 735 nt precedes the ORF. Secondary structure within this region of the genome may be important for efficient translation of the RNA (7). There is also a short untranslated region at the 3′ end of the HAV genome.

In common with other picornaviruses, the HAV polyprotein is processed to yield the structural (located at the amino-terminal end) and non-structural viral polypeptides. Many of the features of replication of the picornaviruses have been deduced from studies of prototype enteroviruses and rhinoviruses, in particular poliovirus type 1. Figure 14.1 shows the predicted products of processing of the HAV polyprotein. Such studies have shown that, during translation of the precursor polypeptide, a proteinase activity encoded within the 2A domain autocatalyses cleavage of its amino terminus from the structural region. Most of the other cleavages which occur during processing are catalysed by a second proteinase located in the 3C domain (8).

The three-dimensional structures of a number of picornaviruses have been solved by high-resolution crystallography: polypeptides VP1 (1D), VP2 (1B) and VP3 (1C) are exposed on the surface of the virion whilst VP4 (1A) is located internally. Following release of the structural domain from the polyprotein, the 3C proteinase cleaves the 1B/1C and 1C/1D junctions to yield VP0 (VP4 plus VP2), VP3 and VP1. The three polypeptides remain associated as a protomer and five protomers assemble to form a pentamer, so that the five copies of VP1 form the apex. Finally, 12 pentamers assemble around a molecule of viral RNA to form the icosahedral capsid. As the structure locks into place, most copies of VP0 cleave (presumably autocatalytically) to yield VP2 and VP4. However, in the case of HAV, it has not been possible to demonstrate VP4, which is predicted to comprise only 23 amino acids.

The functions of some of the other cleavage products of the polyprotein, such as 2B, 2C and 3A, are less well understood. Product 3B corresponds to the genome-linked polypeptide VPg which in other picornaviruses is the primer for the synthesis of both genome sense RNA and the negative sense RNA found in replicative intermediates. Polypeptide 3AB may be the precursor of VPg. Finally, the 3D product seems to be the viral replicase and contains the Gly-Asp-Asp motif common to viral RNA-dependent RNA polymerases.

PREVENTION OF HEPATITIS A

In areas of high prevalence, most children have antibodies to HAV by the age of three years and such infections usually are asymptomatic. Infections acquired later in life are of increasing clinical severity. Less than 10% of cases of acute hepatitis A in children up to the age of six years are icteric

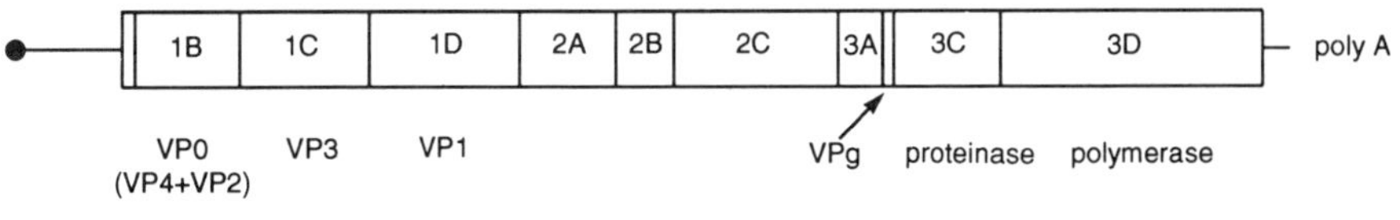

Figure 14.1. Organization of the HAV genome. See text for details

but this rises to between 40% and 50% for the 6–14-year age group and to 70–80% for adults. Of 115 551 cases of hepatitis A in the USA between 1983 and 1987, only 9% of the cases, but more than 70% of the fatalities, were in the over 49-year age group. Therefore, it is desirable to protect those at risk through contact with infected individuals or because of travel to a highly endemic area. In some developing countries, the incidence of clinical hepatitis A is increasing as improvements in hygiene result in some individuals acquiring infection later in life.

Passive protection may be gained through the administration of immunoglobulin, containing at least 100 IU/ml of anti-HAV, given intramuscularly at a dose of at least 2 IU/kg body weight. Post-exposure prophylaxis, if given early enough, may prevent or attenuate a clinical illness. Infection of a partially protected individual may be subclinical but lead to seroconversion and life-long immunity. Although the precise level of antibody required for protection has not been established, the decreasing prevalence of antibody in blood donors in developed countries may lead to problems in maintaining the titre of pooled material, necessitating the selection of appropriate pools (9) and, perhaps in the future, donations from vaccinee volunteers.

There has been considerable interest in the development of hepatitis A vaccines over the past decade (10) and an inactivated vaccine is now licensed in some European countries. The virus grows poorly in cell culture but yields have been improved by adaptation and are sufficient to permit gradient purification. This virus is inactivated with formaldehyde and the antigen adsorbed to aluminium hydroxide and given intramuscularly. The preparation is safe and immunogenic in man and has been shown to induce a protective immune response in marmosets. Such inactivated vaccines will be useful for the protection of travellers from prosperous countries but are likely to be too costly for use in the developing world.

Attenuated strains of HAV have been developed and potentially may be useful as vaccines. This approach is attractive because live vaccines may be cheaper to produce (the attenuated virus grows more efficiently in cell culture), can be given orally and induce a local antibody response. As with vaccine strains of polioviruses, attenuation may be associated with mutations in the 5′ non-coding region of the genome which affect secondary structure. There is also evidence that mutations in the region of the genome encoding the non-structural polypeptides may be important for adaptation to cell culture and attenuation (11,12). However, the markers of attenuation of HAV are not so well defined as those for the polioviruses and reversion to virulence may also be a problem. There is also concern that 'over-attenuated' viruses may not be very immunogenic.

Although there is some sequence variation between different isolates of HAV and evidence for different strains infecting non-human primates (for example, New World owl monkeys) (13), there is only one serotype of the virus and immunity gives effective cross-protection against all strains. Considerable efforts have been made to define the epitope(s) involved. The immunodominant epitope may be highly conformational and involve alignment of domains from VP1 to VP3 (14), posing problems to those who wish to express immunogenic proteins using recombinant DNA technology. A recombinant vaccinia virus expressing most of the HAV capsid coding region has been shown to protect tamarin monkeys from subsequent challenge (15). Expression of the entire HAV polyprotein using a recombinant vaccinia virus led to assembly of virus-like particles in cells infected in culture (16). HAV cDNA and its RNA transcripts, like those of other picornaviruses, are infectious when transfected into permissive cells in culture (17), permitting recovery of virus following site-directed mutagenesis and other manipulations *in vitro*.

HEPATITIS E

Retrospective testing of serum samples from patients involved in various epidemics of hepatitis associated with contamination of water supplies with human faeces led to the conclusion that an agent other than HAV (or hepatitis B) was involved. Epidemics of ET-NANBH in the Indian subcontinent were the first to be reported (18) but outbreaks involving up to tens of thousands of cases have also been documented in the USSR, southeast Asia, northern Africa and Mexico. The average incubation period is slightly longer than for hepatitis A, with a mean of six weeks. The highest attack rates are found in young adults and high mortality rates (up to 20%) have been reported in women in the third trimester of pregnancy.

Virus-like particles have been detected in the stools of infected individuals by immune electron microscopy using convalescent serum. However, such studies often have proved inconclusive and a large proportion of the excreted virus may be degraded during passage through the gut. The particles are slightly larger than those of HAV, with a mean diameter of 32–34 nm. Cross-reaction studies between sera and virus in stools associated with a variety of epidemics in several different countries suggest that a single serotype of virus is involved.

Research into the viral agent of ET-NANBH, now known as hepatitis E virus (HEV), has advanced following the development of animal models. HEV was first transmitted to cynomolgus macaques (19) and a number of other species of monkeys and chimpanzees also have been infected. Reports of transmission to pigs (20) and rodents await confirmation. Attempts to amplify the virus by replication in cell culture have thus far proved unsuccessful.

The problem of degradation of HEV in the gut was circumvented when the bile of infected monkeys was found to be a rich source of virus. This material enabled the molecular cloning of DNA complementary to the HEV (RNA) genome (21) and the entire 7.5 kb sequence was determined (22). The organization of the genome is distinct from the Picornaviridae and the non-structural and structural polypeptides are encoded respectively at the 5′ and 3′ ends. HEV resembles the caliciviruses (23) in the size and organization of its genome as well as the size and morphology of the virion.

ORGANIZATION OF THE HEV GENOME

The HEV genome is a polyadenylated, positive sense RNA of around 7500 nt. The genome of another calicivirus, vesicular exanthema of swine virus (VESV), has a polypeptide, VpG, attached to the 5′ end which (unlike the Picornaviridae) is required for infectivity (24). Whether this holds true for HEV is not known. Hybridization of HEV cDNA probes to RNA isolated from infected liver reveals species of 7.5, 3.7 and 2.0 kg (22) and it is likely that the smaller transcripts are subgenomic messenger RNAs for the capsid and other viral polypeptides.

Analysis of the sequence of the HEV genome reveals three ORFs (Figure 14.2) (22). The first, of approximately 5 kb, begins 28 nt from the 5′ end of the genome and encodes motifs associated with NTP binding, helicase and RNA-dependent RNA polymerase activity. A second ORF of around 2 kb begins 37 nt downstream of the first, terminates 68 nt from the polyA tail and is believed to encode the structural polypeptides. The third ORF is very short (369 nt) and overlaps the other two. The subgenomic RNAs are required presumably for translation of the second and third ORFs and the products may be subject to proteolytic processing.

Sequencing of the HEV genome has enabled the development of a number of specific diagnostic tests. For example, HEV RNA was detected, using the polymerase chain reaction (PCR), in stool samples obtained during a recent epidemic in Kanpur (north India) (25). An ELISA assay, which detects both IgG and IgM anti-HEV, has been developed using a recombinant HEV-glutathione-S-transferase fusion protein and used to detect antibodies in sporadic cases of ET-NANBH in children in Egypt (26).

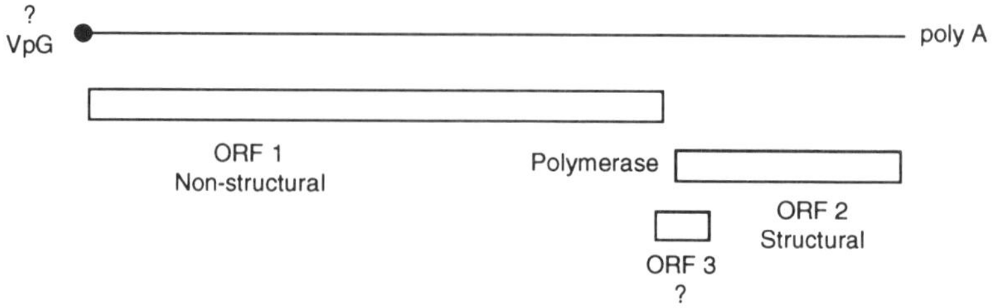

Figure 14.2. Organization of the HEV genome. See text for details

HEPATITIS B

HBV originally was recognized as the agent responsible for 'serum hepatitis', the most common form of parenterally transmitted viral hepatitis, and may cause acute and chronic infection of the liver. The incubation period of hepatitis B is variable and averages around six months, and the clinical features of acute infection resemble those of the other viral hepatitides. Frequently, acute hepatitis B is anicteric and asymptomatic although a severe icteric illness can occur and occasionally acute liver failure may develop. In up to 10% of immunocompetent adults, but in as many as 90% of infants infected perinatally, the infection persists. Chronic hepatitis B, defined by the presence of hepatitis B surface antigen (HBsAg) in serum for more than six months, has been estimated to affect around 300 million people worldwide. The pathology is mediated by the responses of the cellular immune response of the host to the infected hepatocytes. Long-term continuing virus replication may lead to progression to cirrhosis and hepatocellular carcinoma (HCC).

In the first phase of chronicity, virus replication is ongoing in the liver and replicative intermediates of the viral genome may be detected in DNA extracted from biopsies. Markers of virus replication in serum include HBV DNA, the pre-S1 proteins (see below) and a soluble antigen, hepatitis B *e* antigen (HBeAg), which is secreted by productively infected hepatocytes. In those infected at a very young age this phase may persist for life but, more usually, virus levels decline over time. Eventually, in most individuals, there is immune clearance of infected hepatocytes associated with seroconversion from HBeAg to anti-HBe positivity. Antiviral therapy seeks to facilitate this process. During the period of replication, the viral genome may integrate into the chromosomal DNA of some hepatocytes and these cells may persist and expand clonally. Rarely, seroconversion to anti-HBs follows clearance of virus replication but, more frequently, HBsAg persists during a second phase of chronicity as a result of the expression of integrated viral DNA.

STRUCTURE OF THE VIRUS

The hepatitis B virion is a 42 nm particle comprising an electron-dense core (nucleocapsid) 27 nm in diameter surrounded by an outer envelope of the surface protein (HBsAg) embedded in membraneous lipid derived from the host cell. The surface antigen is produced in excess by the infected hepatocytes and is secreted in the form of 22 nm particles and tubular structures of the same diameter. These subviral particles are produced in vast excess over the virions and may prevent an effective humoral immune response to the surface protein in those who become chronically infected.

The 22 nm particles are composed of the major surface protein in both non-glycosylated (p24) and glycosylated (gp27) form in approximately equimolar amounts, along with a minority component of the so-called middle proteins (gp33 and gp36) which contain the pre-S2 domain, a glycosylated 55 amino acid N-terminal extension. The surface of the virion has a similar composition but also contains the large surface proteins (p39 and gp42) which include both the pre-S1 and pre-S2 regions. These large surface proteins are not found in the 22 nm spherical particles (but may be present in the tubular forms in highly viraemic individuals) and their detection in serum correlates with viraemia. The domain which binds to the specific HBV receptor on the hepatocyte seems to reside within the pre-S1 region (27). Further details of the structure and synthesis of the pre-S proteins are given below.

The nucleocapsid of the virion consists of the viral genome surrounded by the core antigen (HBcAg). The carboxyl-terminus of the core protein is arginine rich and this highly basic domain is believed to interact with the genome. The genome, which is approximately 3.2 kb in length, has an unusual structure and is composed of two linear strands of DNA held in a circular configuration by base-pairing at the 5′ ends (cohesive end region). One of the strands is incomplete and the 3′ end is associated with a DNA polymerase molecule which is able to complete that strand when supplied with deoxynucleoside triphosphates. In the past, this endogenous DNA polymerase reaction was used as a serological assay for the hepatitis B virion but this has now been superseded by DNA–DNA hybridization and the polymerase chain reaction (PCR). The 5′ ends of both strands of the genome are modified. The 5′ end of the complete strand is covalently linked to a protein and the 5′ end of the incomplete strand is an oligoribonucleotide. In both cases, these moieties seem to be primers for the synthesis of the respective strands during the genome replication, as described below. A motif of 12 base pairs is directly repeated in the genome near to the 5′ ends of the two strands (DR1 and DR2 respectively) and these sequences play an important role in the replication of the genome.

ORGANIZATION OF THE HBV GENOME

To date, the genomes of more than a dozen isolates of hepatitis B virus have been cloned and the complete nucleotide sequences determined. Analysis of the coding potential of the genome reveals four ORFs which are conserved between all of these isolates (Figure 14.3). These have the same polarity as the incomplete strand of genomic DNA which therefore has been designated the plus strand.

The first ORF encodes the various forms of the surface protein and contains three in-frame methionine codons which are used for initiation of translation. Both the middle (gp33 and gp36) and major (p24 and gp27) proteins are translated from a family of 2.1 kb mRNAs transcribed from a

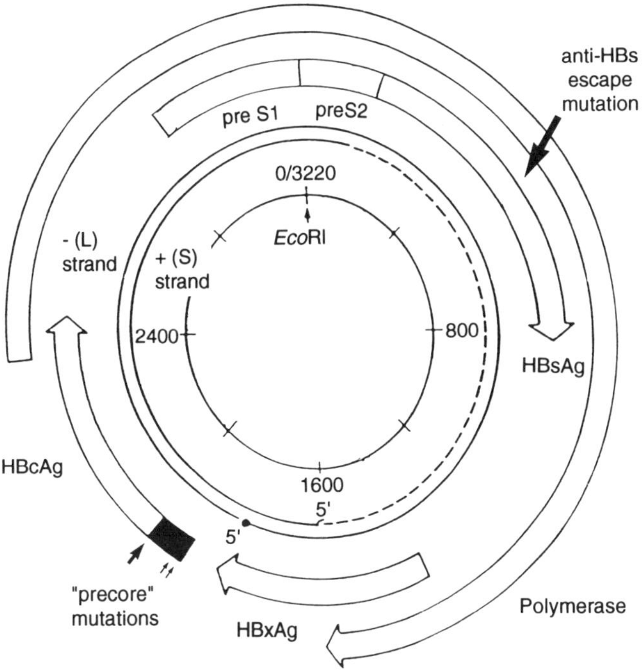

Figure 14.3. Organization of the HBV genome. See text for details

promoter located in the pre-S1 region and polyadenylated in response to a signal sequence located just downstream from the start of the core ORF. This promoter lacks the TATA box which normally determines the cap site of eukaryotic mRNAs. In consequence, the 5′ ends of this family of mRNAs are heterogeneous and span the pre-S2 initiation codon. The absence of this signal from many of the transcripts, perhaps coupled with the fact that it seems to be in a poor context for recognition by the scanning ribosome, leads to the synthesis of a vast excess of the major (p24 and gp27), over the middle, proteins.

A second promoter, which contains an extended TATA box (TATATAA), is located upstream of the pre-S1 initiation codon. This directs the synthesis of a 2.4 kb mRNA which is co-terminal with the other surface messages and is translated to yield the large (pre-S1) surface proteins. This promoter seems to be weak (or may be downregulated) so that the message is of low abundance and relatively few of the larger surface proteins are synthesized. Unlike the middle and major surface proteins, the large surface proteins are not secreted from the cell. In fact, its synthesis inhibits the secretion of the smaller proteins and may be a signal for virus assembly.

The core open reading frame also has two in-phase initiation codons (Figure 14.3). The 'precore' region is highly conserved, has the properties of a signal sequence and is responsible for the secretion of HBeAg (27). A family of greater-than-genome length (3.5 kb) RNAs are generated by a promoter upstream of the precore region and are 3′ co-terminal with the surface mRNAs. Again, the promoter has no TATA box and the 5′ ends are heterogeneous. A subspecies of this family, with 5′ ends most distal from the promoter, is an intermediate in the replication of the genome (pregenomic RNA, see below). Translation of mRNA lacking the precore initiation codon yields the structural core antigen (21 kDa). Translation of the longer mRNA from the precore AUG yields a 25 kDa precursor to HBeAg which is processed by proteolytic removal of the protamine-like carboxyl-terminus and secreted with cleavage of the signal sequence as the 17 kDa *e* antigen. Proteolysis of the precursor reveals two antigenic epitopes, characteristic of HBeAg, which are masked in HBcAg.

The third ORF, which is the largest and overlaps the other three, encodes the viral polymerase. This protein seems to be another translation product of the 3.5 kb RNA, and is synthesized apparently following internal initiation of the ribosome (29). Recent evidence suggests that this large protein has four domains (30). The amino terminal domain is believed to be the protein primer for minus strand synthesis. There is then a spacer region followed by the (RNA- and DNA-dependent) DNA polymerase. The carboxyl-terminal domain has an RNase H-like activity.

The fourth ORF was designated 'x' for the unknown function of its small gene product. However, recently this has been demonstrated to be a transcriptional transactivator and may be an 'early' gene product which functions to upregulate the viral promoters. The x protein is active on a wide range of promoters and seems to function by acting upon cellular factors which are DNA binding rather than by binding directly to DNA. Recently it has been shown to have a protein serine/threonine kinase activity (31). The x gene has its own promoter which is located adjacent to a transcriptional enhancer and which transcribes an RNA of around 1.0 kb which is also polyadenylated in response to the signal in the core ORF.

REPLICATION OF THE HBV GENOME

Following infection of a hepatocyte, the single-stranded region of the virion DNA is repaired (presumably by the endogenous polymerase) and the genome appears in a covalently closed, circular form in the nucleus. This DNA is the template for the transcription of all of the viral RNAs. As mentioned above, a subset of the 3.5 kb RNA is destined to become pregenomes and these are encapsidated in immature core particles in the cytoplasm. Synthesis of minus strand DNA is primed by a protein, now believed to be the amino-terminal domain of the polymerase, and proceeds with the concomitant degradation of the RNA template by the RNase H activity. Whether one or two copies of the polymerase molecule are involved and whether the primer domain is cleaved from the remainder of the polymerase remain unclear.

The pregenomic RNA contains two copies of DR1 and minus strand synthesis is primed at the copy nearest the 3′ end so that the completed strand has a short terminal redundancy. Degradation of the pregenome by the RNase H activity leaves a short, capped oligoribonucleotide which contains a copy of DR1 and this is now translocated to the copy of DR2 on the minus strand, where it primes plus strand synthesis. If the primer for minus strand synthesis and the polymerase are the same molecule, the two ends of the minus strand will be held in close proximity. This may facilitate the translocation of the primer for the other strand. Plus strand synthesis proceeds to the 5′ end of the minus strand and a second template switch is required as the molecule is circularized via the redundancy in the minus strand. Completion of the core during plus strand synthesis starves the polymerase of deoxynucleoside triphosphate precursors and leaves the single-stranded region characteristic of genomic DNA.

There is no semi-conservative replication of the covalently closed circular DNA in the nucleus and a pool of up to 30 copies of template DNA initially is built up by transfer of some of the progeny DNA from the cytoplasm to the nucleus. The mode of replication of the viral genome resembles those of the phylogenetically related retroviruses and, more closely, a family of plant viruses (the caulimoviruses). The HBV polymerase has homology with the polymerases of these viruses at the amino acid level. (A more detailed account of HBV genome replication is given in reference 32.)

ANIMAL MODELS

A number of animal species have been found to be susceptible to infection by viruses related to HBV and the human virus is now considered the prototype of a group of viruses known as hepadnaviruses (*hepa*tropic DNA viruses). These viruses share the same genome structure and organization and all replicate through an RNA intermediate. Woodchucks were found to have a high incidence of chronic active hepatitis and hepatocellular carcinoma. In their circulation particles resembling hepatitis B virions were detected which exhibited an endogenous DNA polymerase activity. The high rate of progression of woodchuck hepatitis virus (WHV)-infected woodchucks to tumour made them an attractive model for the study of hepadnavirus-associated hepatocellular carcinoma. WHV-infected woodchucks have been superinfected with hepatitis delta virus (HDV) and provide a model for the study of that agent. Beechey ground squirrels also may be infected naturally by a hepadnavirus, ground squirrel hepatitis virus (GSHV), although in this model the virus seems to be less pathogenic with a low rate of progression to primary liver cancer. The viral genome has approximately 90% nucleotide homology to WHV, while both rodent viruses are approximately 70% homologous to HBV.

Duck hepatitis B virus (DHBV) naturally infects Pekin ducks and the virus is endemic in many domestic flocks. Transmission is vertical through the egg and hatchlings have a high level of viraemia, which later declines. Similar viruses have been described in wild ducks and herons. Not surprisingly, the avian viruses have diverged from those infecting mammals; there is a smaller genome (around 3.0 kb) and the x gene is absent. The Pekin duck has also proved useful for the study of hepadnavirology and it was with this model that Summers and Mason (33) elucidated the mechanism of genome replication. DHBV-infected ducks are used in many laboratories for the evaluation of potential antiviral drugs.

EXPRESSION OF HBV *IN VITRO*

Over the years, many unsuccessful attempts have been made to propagate HBV in cells in culture both using primary hepatocytes and using established cell lines. Following the molecular cloning of the viral DNA, the various gene products have been expressed using both prokaryotic and eukaryotic systems. The production of complete virions has also been achieved following transfection of cloned DNA into cell lines, usually tumour cells of hepatic origin which do not have integrated HBV DNA. Because the pregenomic RNA is greater than genome length, head-to-tail dimers or recircularized molecules are used for transfection in order to provide a suitable template for transcription. The success of this approach implies that the block to infection with virus is at an early stage in the replicative cycle. The duck hepatitis B virus may be produced in human cells transfected with DHBV DNA, suggesting that the species specificity of the hepadnaviruses may be attributed to the cellular receptor. There is interest in using virus-producing cell lines for the testing *in vitro* of potential anti-HBV therapeutics (34).

PROTECTION AGAINST HEPATITIS B

The discovery of variation in the epitopes presented on the surface of the virions and subviral particles enabled the definition of subtypes of HBV which differ in their geographical distribution. All isolates of the virus share a common epitope, *a*, which is a domain of the major surface protein and seems to protrude as a double loop from the surface of the particle (35). Two other pairs of mutually exclusive antigenic determinants, *d* or *y* and *w* or *r*, are also present on the major surface protein. These variations have been correlated with single nucleotide changes in the surface ORF which lead to variation in single amino acids in the protein (36). Four principal subtypes of HBV are recognized: *adw*, *adr*, *ayw* and *ayr*. Subtype *adw* predominates in northern Europe, the Americas and Australasia and also is found in Africa and Asia. Subtype *ayw* is found in the Mediterranean region, eastern Europe, northern and western Africa, the Near East and the Indian subcontinent. In the Far East, *adr* predominates but the rarer *ayr* occasionally may be found in Japan and Papua New Guinea.

The major response of recipients of hepatitis B vaccine seems to be to the common *a* epitope with consequent protection against all subtypes of the virus. First-generation vaccines were prepared from 22 nm HBsAg particles purified from plasma donations from chronic carriers. These preparations were safe and immunogenic but have been superseded largely by recombinant vaccines produced by the expression of HBsAg in yeast cells. The expression plasmid contains only the 3′ portion of the HBV surface ORF and only the major surface protein, without pre-S epitopes, is produced. Vaccines containing pre-S2 as well as the major surface proteins expressed in yeast currently are undergoing clinical trial.

In many areas of the world with a high prevalence of HBsAg carriage, such as China and southeast Asia, the predominant route of transmission is perinatal. Although HBV does not usually cross the placenta, the infants of viraemic mothers have a very high risk of infection at the time of birth. Administration of a course of vaccine with the first dose immediately after birth is effective in preventing transmission from an HBeAg-positive mother in approximately 70% of cases (37) and this protective efficacy rate may be increased to greater than 90% if the vaccine is accompanied by the simultaneous administration of hepatitis B immune globulin (HBIG) (38,39).

The emergence of mutants of HBV resistant to vaccine-induced antibody has not been a problem so far. However, two independent incidents in Italy (40) and in Singapore (41) have recently been described. In each case, the neonate of an infectious carrier mother became chronically infected despite circulating anti-surface antibody (anti-HBs) following combined immunoprophylaxis with HBIG and vaccine. Nucleotide sequence analysis of the region of the HBV genome encoding the major antigenic domain of the surface protein revealed a point mutation (guanine to adenine) which specifies a coding change from glycine to arginine in the surface antigen. The amino acid residue involved is located in the second loop of the *a* determinant. Although it has not been possible to detect the variant in the mothers' sera, it is likely that their infecting dose of virus may have included the variant. It is possible then that the anti-HBs antibody present in HBIG neutralized wild-type virus, leaving the variant to become established in the neonate despite vaccination. This hypothesis is supported by a report from the United States (42) of the identical mutation in an HBV variant isolated from an adult following transplantation for HBV-related liver disease. The human monoclonal anti-HBs which was given in an unsuccessful attempt to prevent reinfection of the graft seems to have selected the mutant.

HBV PRECORE MUTANTS

When DNA–DNA hybridization replaced the less sensitive assay of the endogenous DNA polymerase activity as a method for detecting hepatitis B virions in serum, it became clear that some patients with anti-HBe were viraemic (43,44). These and other early reports suggested that this finding was more common in Greece and other Mediterranean regions than elsewhere, raising the possibility of the involvement of a variant form(s) of HBV.

In 1988 we reported the nucleotide sequence of the genome of a strain of HBV cloned from the serum of a naturally infected chimpanzee (45). A surprising feature was a point mutation in the penultimate codon of the precore region which changed the tryptophan codon (TGG) to an amber termination codon (TAG). The nucleotide sequence of the HBV precore region from a number of anti-HBe-positive Greek patients was investigated by direct sequencing of PCR-amplified HBV DNA from serum (46). An identical mutation of the penultimate codon of the precore region to a termination codon was found in seven of eight anti-HBe-positive patients who were positive for HBV DNA in serum by hybridization. In most cases there was an additional mutation in the preceding codon.

Similar variants were found in an Italian study by amplification of HBV DNA from serum from a further seven anti-HBe-positive patients, one of whom seemed to be co-infected with wild-type virus (47). These variants are not confined to the Mediterranean region; the same nonsense mutation (without a second mutation in the adjacent codon) has been observed in patients from Japan and elsewhere along with rarer examples of defective precore regions caused by frameshifts or loss of the initiation codon for the precore region (48).

HBeAg-negative patients with high levels of HBV replication from various geographical areas frequently may be infected by viruses with variant precore regions. Presumably, these can replicate without secretion of HBeAg. The majority of patients who are infected with these variants are anti-HBe positive, implying past infection with non-defective HBV. It is not clear whether these individuals originally were infected with a mixture of wild-type and mutant viruses or whether the variants arose throughout the course of natural infection. The process of seroconversion from HBeAg to anti-HBe positivity seems to select the variant viruses and this may be related to the expression of HBeAg on the surface of hepatocytes infected by the wild-type virus (49).

In many cases, precore variants have been described in patients with severe chronic liver disease and who may have failed to respond to therapy with interferon (47). This observation raises the question of whether they are more pathogenic than the wild-type virus. Several recent publications support this hypothesis. In one such study (50), patients infected with mutant alone, or with a predominantly mutant virus population, were found to have more severe liver disease than those in whom the wild type was the sole or predominant virus. Furthermore, infection with precore mutants *ab initio* may lead to fulminant hepatitis B. In a Japanese study, precore mutants were found in all three patients with fulminant hepatitis B from whom serum HBV DNA could be amplified by PCR, as well as in a further four patients with severe exacerbations of chronic hepatitis (51). In other studies in Japan, precore mutants were associated with nine of 10 cases of fulminant hepatitis B (52) and in a further eight cases of post-transfusion fulminant hepatitis B where HBsAg was not detected on routine screening of the donations (53). In the latter study, the course of infection was traceable in one case, the implicated donation being positive for anti-HBe and for HBV DNA following PCR and dot blot hybridization. A nosocomial outbreak of fatal fulminant hepatitis B in Israel was associated with transmission of mutant HBV from a common source to five individuals (54). In a study of British patients with fulminant hepatitis B, precore mutants were found in eight of nine HBeAg-negative patients but in none of six who were HBeAg positive on presentation (55).

HBV AND HEPATOCELLULAR CARCINOMA

When tests for HBsAg became widely available, regions of the world where the chronic carrier state is common were found to be coincident with those where there is a high prevalence of HCC. Furthermore, in these areas, patients with tumour almost invariably are seropositive for HBsAg. In an elegant prospective study, Beasley and colleagues (56) investigated the incidence of this tumour in male HBsAg carriers and controls in Taiwan. After more than 11 years of follow-up, 184 cases of HCC occurred in the 3454 individuals who were HBsAg positive at the start of the study but only 10 such tumours arose in the 19 253 individuals who were HBsAg negative (57).

Southern hybridization of tumour DNA yields evidence of chromosomal integration of viral sequences in at least 80% of HCCs from HBsAg carriers. There is no similarity in the pattern of integration between different tumours, and variation is seen both in the integration site(s) and in the number of copies or partial copies of the viral genome. Sequence analysis of the integrants reveals that the direct repeats in the viral genome often lie close to the virus/cell junctions, suggesting that sequences around the ends of the viral genome may be involved in recombination with host DNA (58). Integration seems to involve microdeletion of host sequences, and rearrangements and deletions of part of the viral genome also may occur. When an intact surface gene is present, the tumour cells may produce and secrete HBsAg in the form of 22 nm particles. Production of HBcAg by tumours is rare, however, and the core ORF is often incomplete and modifications such as methylation may also modulate its expression. Cytotoxic T cells targeted against core gene products on the hepatocyte surface seem to be the major mechanism of clearance of infected cells from the liver, and cells with integrated viral DNA which are capable of expressing these proteins also may be lysed. Thus, there may be immune selection of cells with integrated viral DNA which are incapable of expressing HBcAg.

Despite considerable efforts by many research groups, the mechanisms of oncogenesis by HBV remain obscure. HBV may act non-specifically by stimulating active regeneration and cirrhosis which may be associated with long-term chronicity. However, HBV-associated tumours occasionally arise in the absence of cirrhosis and such hypotheses do not explain the frequent finding of integrated viral DNA in tumours. In rare instances, the viral genome has been found to be integrated into cellular genes such as cyclin A (59) and a retinoic acid receptor (60). Translocations and other chromosomal rearrangements also have been observed. Although insertional mutagenesis of HBV remains an attractive hypothesis to explain its oncogenicity, supportive evidence has not been very forthcoming. In contrast with these findings for human HCC, WHV-associated liver cancer in woodchucks frequently involves integration of the viral genome in or near to cellular *myc* genes (61).

An alternative possibility is that tumour formation is associated with the action of a viral gene product. The product of the x gene is known to be a transactivator of transcription and so may cause inappropriate upregulation of cellular genes. Truncated forms of HBsAg, which may be produced from incomplete surface ORFs integrated in tumour cells, also can have transactivating activity (62), perhaps through interaction with receptors in the cell membrane. Like many other cancers, development of HCC is likely to be a multi-step process involving a number of factors. The clonal expansion of cells with integrated viral DNA seems to be an early stage in this process and such clones may accumulate in the liver throughout the period of active virus replication. In areas where the prevalence of HCC is high, virus infection usually occurs at an early age and virus replication may be prolonged, although the peak incidence of tumour is some decades after the initial infection.

HEPATITIS D

Delta hepatitis was first recognized following detection of a novel protein, delta antigen (HDAg), by immunofluorescent staining in the nuclei of hepatocytes from patients with hepatitis B (63). Hepatitis delta virus (HDV) is now known to require a helper function of HBV for its transmission. HDV is coated with HBsAg, which is needed for release from the host hepatocyte and for entry in the next round of infection.

Two forms of delta hepatitis infection are known. In the first, a susceptible individual is co-infected with HBV and HDV, often leading to aggravation of the acute hepatitis caused by HBV. Vaccination against HBV also prevents co-infection. In the alternative, an individual chronically infected with HBV becomes superinfected with HDV. This may accelerate the course of the chronic liver disease and bring about overt disease in 'healthy' HBsAg carriers. HDV itself seems to be cytopathic and HDAg may be directly cytotoxic.

An interesting phenomenon has been observed in delta-positive patients without HBV replication who proceed to liver transplantation. HDV in the circulation is able to infect the graft and replicate but progeny virus is not released from the infected hepatocytes. In this situation, HDV remains latent and may reactivate following subsequent infection of the graft with HBV.

Delta hepatitis is a problem primarily in some areas of the world with a high prevalence of HBV infection, particularly the Mediterranean region, the Middle East, Africa and South America. It has been estimated that 5% of HBsAg carriers worldwide (approximately 15 million people) are infected with HDV. In areas of low prevalence of HBV, those at risk of hepatitis B, particularly intravenous drug abusers, also are at risk of HDV infection.

STRUCTURE AND REPLICATION OF HDV

The HDV particle is approximately 36 nm in diameter and composed of an RNA genome associated with HDAg, surrounded by an envelope of HBsAg. The virus reaches higher concentrations in the circulation than HBV: up to 10^{12} particles per millilitre have been recorded. The precise constitution of the envelope depends on the level of HBV replication. Thus, in patients who are highly viraemic for HBV, pre-S1 and pre-S2 proteins will be present on the surface of the HDV particle, whilst in HBsAg carriers without HBV replication there will be no pre-S1 and relatively little of the pre-S2 proteins. That HDV can infect HBsAg carriers who are no longer replicating HBV suggests that further helper functions are not required and recently it has been shown that the major form of HBsAg alone (without pre-S proteins) is sufficient for assembly of hepatitis D virions (64).

The HDV genome is a closed circular RNA molecule of 1679 nucleotides with extensive sequence complementarity that permits pairing of approximately 70% of the bases to form an unbranched rod structure. The genome thus resembles those of the satellite viroids and virusoids of plants (65) and similarly seems to be replicated by the host RNA polymerase II with autocatalytic cleavage and circularization of the progeny genomes via *trans*-esterification reactions (ribozyme activity) (66). Consensus sequences of viroids which are believed to be involved in these processes also are conserved in HDV. Further details of the replication of the hepatitis delta virus genome may be found in a review by Taylor (67).

Unlike the plant viroids, HDV codes for a protein, HDAg. This is encoded in an ORF in the antigenomic RNA but four other ORFs which are also present in the genome do not appear to be utilized. Around 600 copies of a polyadenylated mRNA, approximately 800 nt in length, may be detected in the cytoplasm of infected hepatocytes. The antigen, which contains a nuclear localization signal, was originally detected in the nuclei of infected hepatocytes and may be detected in serum only after stripping off the outer envelope of the virus with detergent. HDAg is phosphorylated at serine residues. Two species, 22–24 and 24–27 kDa, may be detected in the infected liver following polyacrylamide gel electrophoresis. The precise mechanism of their synthesis remains to be determined but seems to involve mutation of an amber termination codon in the ORF (68), allowing translation of the larger protein. The small form of HDAg is required for RNA replication, whilst the large form binds to the RNA rod structure and is involved in virion assembly (69).

HEPATITIS C

Prior to the description of hepatitis C virus (HCV), transmission studies in chimpanzees helped establish that the main agent of parenterally acquired non-A, non-B hepatitis was likely to be an enveloped virus some 30–60 nm in diameter (70,71). These studies made available a pool of plasma that contained a relatively high titre of the agent. In order to clone the genome, the virus was pelleted from the plasma. Because it was not known whether the genome was DNA or RNA, a denaturation step was included prior to the synthesis of complementary DNA so that either DNA or RNA could serve as a template (72). The resultant cDNA was then inserted into the bacteriophage expression vector lambda gt11 and the libraries screened using serum from a patient with chronic non-A, non-B hepatitis.

This approach led to the detection of a clone (designated 5-1-1) which was found to bind to antibodies present in the sera of several individuals infected with non-A, non-B hepatitis. This clone was used as a probe to detect a larger, overlapping clone in the same library. It was possible to demonstrate that these sequences hybridized to a positive sense RNA molecule of around 10 000 nt which was present in the livers of infected chimpanzees but not in uninfected controls. No homologous sequences could be detected in the chimpanzee or human genomes. By employing a 'walking' technique, it was possible to use newly detected overlapping clones as hybridization probes in turn to detect further virus-specific clones in the library. Thus, clones covering the entire viral genome were assembled and the complete nucleotide sequence determined. The organization of the genome closely resembles those of the enveloped RNA viruses, the pestiviruses and flaviviruses, as discussed below.

DETECTION OF HCV INFECTION

The advances described above made possible the development of new diagnostic tests for infection by the virus. Since the 5-1-1 antigen was originally detected by antibodies in the serum of an infected patient it was an obvious candidate for the basis of an enzyme-linked immunosorbent assay (ELISA) test to detect anti-HCV antibodies. A larger clone, C100, was assembled from a number of overlapping clones and expressed in yeast as a fusion protein using human superoxide dismutase sequences to facilitate expression (73). This fusion protein formed the basis of first-generation tests for HCV infection. The 5-1-1 and C100 antigens comprise amino acid sequences from the non-structural, NS4, region of the genome (Figure 14.4). It is now known that antibodies to C100 are detected relatively late following an acute infection. Furthermore, the first-generation ELISAs were associated with a high rate of false positivity when applied to low-incidence populations and there were further problems with some retrospective studies on stored sera. Data based on this test alone should, therefore, be interpreted with caution.

Second-generation tests include antigens from the nucleocapsid and further non-structural regions of the genome. The former (C22) is particularly useful and antibodies to the HCV core protein seem to appear relatively early in infection. These second-generation tests confirm that HCV is the major cause of parenterally transmitted non-A, non-B hepatitis. Routine testing of blood donations is now in place in many countries and prevalence rates vary from 0.2–0.5% in northern Europe to 1.2–1.5% in southern Europe and Japan. Most of those who are found to be antibody positive have a history of parenteral risk such as a history of transfusion or administration of blood products or of intravenous drug abuse. There is minimal evidence for sexual or perinatal transmission of HCV and it is not clear what are the natural routes of transmission.

The availability of the nucleotide sequence of HCV made possible the use of the PCR as a direct test for the (genome of the) virus itself. The first step is the synthesis of a complementary DNA copy of the target region of the RNA genome using reverse transcriptase (primed by the antigenomic

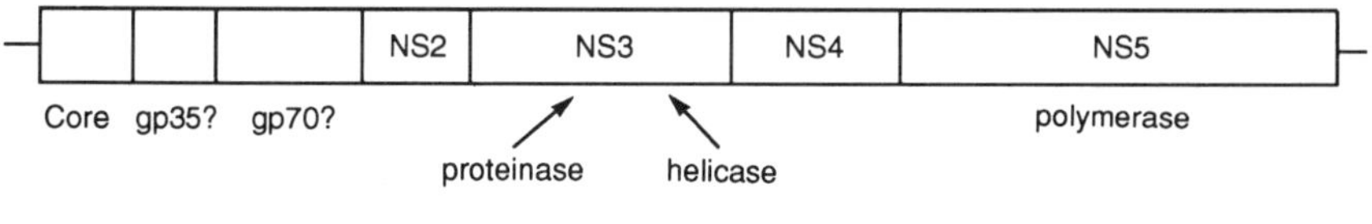

Figure 14.4. Organization of the HCV genome. See text for details

PCR primer or, better, by random hexamers) and the product of this reaction is then a suitable target for amplification. The concentration of virus in serum samples is often very low, so that the mass of product from the PCR reaction is insufficient for visualization on a stained gel. Thus, either a second round of amplification (with nested primers) or detection of the primary product by Southern hybridization is required. There is considerable variation in nucleotide sequences among different isolates of HCV and the 5′ non-coding region, which seems to be highly conserved, is the preferred target for the PCR (74).

Current data suggest that at least 50% of infections with HCV progress to chronicity. Histological examination of liver biopsies from 'healthy' HCV carriers (blood donors) reveals that none has normal histology and that up to 70% have chronic active hepatitis and/or cirrhosis. Whether the virus is cytopathic or whether there is an immunopathological element remains unclear. HCV infection also is associated with progression to HCC. For example, in Japan, where the incidence of HCC has been increasing despite a decrease in the prevalence of HBsAg, HCV is the major risk factor. There is no DNA intermediate in the replication of the HCV genome or integration of viral nucleic acid, and viral pathology may contribute to oncogenesis through cirrhosis and regeneration of liver cells. HCV rarely seems to cause fulminant hepatitis.

THE ORGANIZATION OF THE HCV GENOME

The genome of HCV (Figure 14.4) resembles those of the pestiviruses and flaviviruses (75) in that it comprises around 10 000 nt of positive sense RNA, lacks a 3′ polyA tract and has a similar gene organization. It has been proposed that HCV should be the prototype of a third genus in the family Flaviviridae. All of these genomes contain a single large ORF which is translated to yield a polyprotein (of around 3000 amino acids in the case of HCV) from which the viral proteins are derived by post-translational cleavage and other modifications.

There is a short, untranslated region at the 5′ end of the genomic RNA and a further untranslated region at the 3′ end, the large ORF accounting for over 95% of the sequence. The structural proteins are located towards the 5′ end and the non-structural proteins towards the 3′ end. The first product of the polyprotein is the non-glycosylated capsid protein, C, which complexes with the genomic RNA to form the nucleocapsid. As with the flaviviruses, a hydrophobic domain may anchor the growing polypeptide in the endoplasmic reticulum and facilitate cleavage by a cellular signalase (76) releasing a nucleocapsid precursor (anchored C). The amino acid sequence of the nucleocapsid protein seems to be highly conserved among different isolates of HCV.

The next domain in the polyprotein also has a signal sequence at its carboxyl-terminus and may be processed in a similar fashion. The product is a glycoprotein which is probably found in the viral envelope and is variably termed E1/S or gp35. The third domain may be cleaved by a proteinase within the viral polyprotein to yield what is probably a second surface glycoprotein, E2/NS1 or gp70. These glycoproteins have not been visualized *in vivo* and the molecular sizes are estimated from sequence data and expression studies *in vitro* (77). Other post-translational modifications, including further proteolytic cleavages, are possible. These proteins are the focus of considerable interest because of their potential use in tests for the direct detection of viral proteins and for anti-HCV vaccines. Nucleotide sequencing studies reveal that both domains contain hypervariable regions. It is possible that this divergence has been driven by antibody pressure and that these regions specify important immunogenic epitopes.

The non-structural region of the HCV genome is divided into regions NS2 to NS5 (Figure 14.4). In the flaviviruses, NS3 has two functional domains: a proteinase which is involved in cleavage of the non-structural region of the polyprotein, and a helicase which is presumably involved in RNA replication. Motifs within this region of the HCV genome have homology to the appropriate consensus sequences, suggesting similar functions. NS5 seems to be the replicase and contains the Gly-Asp-Asp motif common to viral RNA-dependent RNA polymerases.

OTHER HEPATITIS VIRUSES

It is likely that other human hepatitis viruses will be identified in the future. Whilst HCV is clearly the major cause of parenterally transmitted non-A, non-B hepatitis, data from some of the original transmission experiments suggest that at least one other agent might be involved (77). A number of candidates are already emerging. Togavirus-like particles (candidate HFV?) have been observed in the livers of patients with fulminant, sporadic (community acquired) non-A, non-B hepatitis (78). A number of these patients proceeded to transplantation with apparent reinfection of the graft with haemorrhagic manifestations. A severe form of sporadic hepatitis, characterized histologically by large syncytial giant hepatocytes and perhaps caused by a paramyxovirus (candidate HGV?), has been described recently (79).

REFERENCES

1. Halliday, M. L., Kang, L.-Y., Zhou, T.-K. *et al.* (1991). An epidemic of hepatitis A attributable to the ingestion of raw clams in Shanghai, China. *J. Infect. Dis.*, **164**, 852–859.

2. Gust, I. D., Coulepis, A. G., Feinstone, S. M. *et al.* (1983). Taxonomic classification of hepatitis A virus. *Intervirology*, **20**, 1–7.
3. Ticehurst, J. R., Racaniello, V. R., Baroudy, B. M. *et al.* (1983). Molecular cloning and characterization of hepatitis A virus cDNA. *Proc. Natl Acad. Sci. USA*, **80**, 5885–5889.
4. Najarian, R., Caput, D., Gee, W. *et al.* (1985). Primary structure and gene organization of human hepatitis A virus. *Proc. Natl Acad. Sci. USA*, **82**, 2627–2631.
5. Cohen, J. I., Ticehurst, J. R., Purcell, R. H. *et. al.* (1987). Complete nucleotide sequence of wild-type hepatitis A virus: comparison with different strains of hepatitis A virus and other picornaviruses. *J. Virol.*, **61**, 50–59.
6. Melnick, J. L. (1992). Properties and classification of hepatitis-A virus. *Vaccine*, **10**, 524–526.
7. Brown, E. A., Day, S. P., Jansen, R. W. and Lemon, S. M. (1991). The 5′ nontranslated region of hepatitis A virus RNA: secondary structure and elements required for translation in vitro. *J. Virol.*, **65**, 5828–5838.
8. Jia, X.-Y., Ehrenfeld, E. and Summers, D. F. (1991). Proteolytic activity of hepatitis A virus 3C protein. *J. Virol.*, **65**, 2595–2600.
9. Thorpe, R., Minor, P. and Wood, D. (1991). Hepatitis-A virus concentrations in immunoglobulin preparations. *Lancet*, **337**, 497.
10. Gust, I. D. (1990). Design of hepatitis-A vaccines. *Br. Med. Bull.*, **46**, 319–328.
11. Cohen, J. I., Rosenblum, B., Feinstone, S. M. *et al.* (1989). Attenuation and cell culture adaptation of hepatitis A virus (HAV): a genetic analysis with HAV cDNA. *J. Virol*, **63**, 5364–5370.
12. Emerson, S. U., Huang, Y. K., McRill, C. *et al.* (1992). Mutations in both the 2B-gene and 2C-gene of hepatitis-A virus are involved in adaptation to growth in cell culture. *J. Virol.*, **66**, 650–654.
13. Brown, E. A., Jansen, R. W. and Lemon, S. M. (1989). Characterization of a simian hepatitis A virus (HAV): antigenic and genetic comparison with human HAV. *J. Virol.*, **63**, 4932–4937.
14. Ping, L. H., Jansen, R. W., Stapleton, J. T. *et al.* (1988). Identification of an immunodominant antigenic site involving the capsid protein VP3 of hepatitis A virus. *Proc. Natl Acad. Sci. USA*, **85**, 8281–8285.
15. Karayiannis, P., O'Rourke, S., McGarvey, M. J. *et al.* (1991). A recombinant vaccinia virus expressing hepatitis A virus structural polypeptides: characterization and demonstration of protective immunogenicity. *J. Gen. Virol.*, **72**, 2167–2172.
16. Winokur, P. L., McLinden, J. H. and Stapleton, J. T. (1991). The hepatitis-A virus polyprotein expressed by a recombinant vaccinia virus undergoes proteolytic processing and assembly into viruslike particles. *J. Virol.*, **65**, 5029–5036.
17. Cohen, J. I., Ticehurst, J. R., Feinstone, S. M. *et al.* (1987). Hepatitis A virus cDNA and its RNA transcripts are infectious in cell culture. *J. Virol.*, **61**, 3035–3039.
18. Khuroo, M. S. (1980). Study of an epidemic of non-A, non-B hepatitis: possibility of another human hepatitis virus distinct from post-transfusion non-A, non-B type. *Am. J. Med.*, **68**, 818–824.
19. Balayan, M. S., Andjaparidze, A. G., Savinskaya, S. S. *et al.* (1983). Evidence for a virus in non-A, non-B hepatitis transmitted via the fecal–oral route. *Intervirology*, **20**, 23–31.
20. Balayan, M. S., Usmanov, R. K., Zamyatina, N. A. *et al.* (1990). Experimental hepatitis-E infection in domestic pigs. *J. Med. Virol.*, **32**, 58–59.
21. Reyes, G. R., Purdy, M. A., Kim, J. P. *et al.* (1990). Isolation of a cDNA from the virus responsible for enterically transmitted non-A, non-B hepatitis. *Science*, **247**, 1335–1339.

22. Tam, A. W., Smith, M. M., Guerra, M. E. *et al.* (1991). Hepatitis-E virus (HEV): molecular cloning and sequencing of the full-length viral genome. *Virology*, **185**, 120–131.
23. Carter, M. J., Milton, I. D. and Madeley, C. R. (1991). Caliciviruses. *Rev. Med. Virol.*, **1**, 177–186.
24. Burroughs, J. N. and Brown, F. (1978). Presence of a covalently linked protein on calicivirus RNA. *J. Gen. Virol.*, **41**, 443–446.
25. Ray, R., Aggarwal, R., Salunke, P. N. *et al.* (1991). Hepatitis-E virus genome in stools of hepatitis patients during large epidemic in North India. *Lancet*, **338**, 783–784.
26. Goldsmith, R., Yarbough, P. O., Reyes, G. R. *et al.* (1992). Enzyme-linked immunosorbent assay for diagnosis of acute sporadic hepatitis E in Egyptian children. *Lancet*, **339**, 328–331.
27. Neurath, A. R., Kent, S. B., Strick, N. and Parker, K. (1986). Identification and chemical synthesis of a host cell receptor binding site on hepatitis B virus. *Cell*, **46**, 429–436.
28. Ou, J. H., Laub, O. and Rutter, W. J. (1986). Hepatitis B virus gene function: the precore region targets the core antigen to cellular membranes and causes the secretion of the e antigen. *Proc. Natl Acad. Sci. USA*, **83**, 1578–1582.
29. Jean Jean, O., Weimer, T., De Recondo, A. M. *et al.* (1989). Internal entry of ribosomes and ribosomal scanning involved in hepatitis B virus P gene expression. *J. Virol.*, **63**, 5451–5454.
30. Radziwill, G., Tucker, W. and Schaller, H. (1990). Mutational analysis of the hepatitis B virus P gene product: domain structure and RNase H activity. *J. Virol.*, **64**, 613–620.
31. Wu, J. Y., Zhou, Z.-Y., Judd, A. *et al.* (1990). The hepatitis B virus-encoded transcriptional *trans*-activator hbx appears to be a novel protein serine/threonine kinase. *Cell*, **63**, 687–695.
32. Ganem, D. and Varmus, H. E. (1987). The molecular biology of the hepatitis B viruses. *Annu. Rev. Biochem.*, **56**, 651–693.
33. Summers, J. and Mason, W. S. (1982). Replication of the genome of a hepatitis B-like virus by reverse transcription of an RNA intermediate. *Cell*, **29**, 403–415.
34. Lampertico, P., Malter, J. S. and Gerber, M. A. (1991). Development and application of an in vitro model for screening anti-hepatitis-B virus therapeutics. *Hepatology*, **13**, 422–426.
35. Howard, C. R., Stirk, H. J., Brown, S. E. and Steward, M. W. (1988). Towards the development of synthetic hepatitis B vaccines. In *Viral Hepatitis and Liver Disease*, A. J. Zuckerman (ed.), Liss, New York, pp. 1094–1101.
36. Okamoto, H., Imai, M., Tsuda, F. *et al.* (1987). Point mutation in the S gene of hepatitis B virus for a d/y or w/r subtypic change in two blood donors carrying a surface antigen of compound subtype adyr or adwr. *J. Virol.*, **61**, 3030–3034.
37. Wheeley, S. M., Tarlow, M. J. and Boxall, E. H. (1989). Chronic hepatitis B in male and female children of HBsAg carrier mothers. *J. Hepatol.*, **8**, 226–231.
38. Stevens, C. E., Toy, P. T., Tong, M. J. *et al.* (1985). Perinatal hepatitis B virus transmission in the United States: prevention by passive–active immunization. *JAMA*, **253**, 1740–1745.
39. Stevens, C. E., Taylor, P. E., Tong, M. J. *et al.* (1987). Yeast-recombinant hepatitis B vaccine: efficacy with hepatitis B immune globulin in prevention of perinatal hepatitis B virus transmission. *JAMA*, **257**, 2612–2616.
40. Carman, W. F., Zanetti, A. R., Karayiannis, P. *et al.* (1990). Vaccine-induced escape mutant of hepatitis B virus. *Lancet*, **336**, 325–329.

41. Harrison, T. J., Hopes, E. A., Oon, C. J. *et al.* (1991). Independent emergence of a vaccine-induced escape mutant of hepatitis B virus. *J. Hepatol.*, **13** (Suppl. 4), S105–S107.
42. McMahon, G., McCarthy, L. A., Dottavio, D. and Ostberg, L. (1991). Surface antigen and polymerase gene variation in hepatitis B virus isolates from a monoclonal antibody-treated liver transplant patient. In *Viral Hepatitis and Liver Disease,* F. B. Hollinger, S. M. Lemon and H. S. Margolis (eds), Williams & Wilkins, Baltimore, pp. 219–221.
43. Lieberman, H. M., LaBrecque, D. R., Kew, M. C. *et al.* (1983). Detection of hepatitis B virus DNA directly in human serum by a simplified molecular hybridization test: comparison to HBeAg/anti-HBe status in HBsAg carriers. *Hepatology*, **3**, 285–291.
44. Hadziyannis, S. J., Lieberman, H. M., Karvountzis, G. G. and Shafritz, D. A. (1983). Analysis of liver disease, nuclear HBcAg, viral replication, and hepatitis B virus DNA in liver and serum of HBeAg vs. anti-HBe positive carriers of hepatitis B virus. *Hepatology*, **3**, 656–662.
45. Vaudin, M., Wolstenholme, A. J., Tsiquaye, K. N. *et al.* (1988). The complete nucleotide sequence of the genome of a hepatitis B virus isolated from a naturally infected chimpanzee. *J. Gen. Virol.*, **69**, 1383–1389.
46. Carman, W. F., Jacyna, M. R., Hadziyannis, S. *et al.* (1989). Mutation preventing formation of hepatitis B e antigen in patients with chronic hepatitis B infection. *Lancet*, **ii**, 588–591.
47. Brunetto, M. R., Stemler, M., Bonino, F. *et al.* (1990). A new hepatitis-B virus strain in patients with severe anti-HBe positive chronic hepatitis-B. *J. Hepatol.*, **10**, 258–261.
48. Okamoto, H., Yotsumoto, S., Akahane, Y. *et al.* (1990). Hepatitis B viruses with precore region defects prevail in persistently infected hosts along with seroconversion to the antibody against e antigen. *J. Virol.*, **64**, 1298–1303.
49. Schlicht, H. J. and Schaller, H. (1989). The secretory core protein of human hepatitis B virus is expressed on the cell surface. *J. Virol.*, **63**, 5399–5404.
50. Brunetto, M. R., Giarin, M. M., Oliveri, F. *et. al.* (1991). Wild-type and e-antigen-minus hepatitis-B viruses and course of chronic hepatitis. *Proc. Natl Acad. Sci. USA*, **88**, 4186–4190.
51. Omata, M., Ehata, T., Yokosuka, O. *et al.* (1991). Mutations in the precore region of hepatitis-B virus DNA in patients with fulminant and severe hepatitis. *N. Engl. J. Med.*, **324**, 1699–1704.
52. Kosaka, Y., Takase, K., Kojima, M. *et al.* (1991). Fulminant hepatitis-B induction by hepatitis-B virus mutants defective in the precore region and incapable of encoding E-antigen. *Gastroenterology*, **100**, 1087–1094.
53. Kojima, M., Shimizu, M., Tsuchimochi, T. *et. al.* (1991). Post transfusion fulminant hepatitis-B associated with precore-defective HBV mutants. *Vox. Sang.*, **60**, 34–39.
54. Liang, T. J., Hasegawa, K., Rimon, N. *et al.* (1991). A hepatitis-B virus mutant associated with an epidemic of fulminant hepatitis. *N. Engl. J. Med.*, **324**, 1705–1709.
55. Carman, W. F., Fagan, E. A., Hadziyannis, S., *et al.* (1991). Association of a precore genomic variant of hepatitis-B virus with fulminant hepatitis. *Hepatology*, **14**, 219–222.
56. Beasley, R. P., Hwang, L. Y., Lin, C. C. and Chien, C. S. (1981). Hepatocellular carcinoma and hepatitis B virus: a prospective study of 22 707 men in Taiwan. *Lancet*, **ii**, 1129–1133.

57. Beasley, R. P. and Hwang, L.-Y. (1991). Overview on the epidemiology of hepatocellular carcinoma. In *Viral Hepatitis and Liver Disease,* F. B. Hollinger, S. M. Lemon and H. S. Margolis (eds), Williams & Wilkins, Baltimore, pp. 532–535.
58. Nagaya, T., Nakamura, T., Tokino, T. *et al.* (1987). The mode of hepatitis B virus DNA integration in chromosomes of human hepatocellular carcinoma. *Genes Dev.,* **1**, 773–782.
59. Wang, J., Chenivesse, X., Henglein, B. and Brechot, C. (1990). Hepatitis B virus integration in a cyclin A gene in a hepatocellular carcinoma. *Nature,* **343**, 555–557.
60. de The, H., Marchio, A., Tiollais, P. and Dejean, A. (1987). A novel steroid thyroid hormone receptor-related gene inappropriately expressed in human hepatocellular carcinoma. *Nature,* **330**, 667–670.
61. Hsu, T., Moroy, T., Etiemble, J. *et al.* (1988). Activation of c-myc by woodchuck hepatitis virus insertion in hepatocellular carcinoma. *Cell,* **55**, 627–635.
62. Kekule, A. S., Lauer, U., Meyer, M. *et al.* (1990). The preS2/S region of integrated hepatitis B virus DNA encodes a transcriptional transactivator. *Nature,* **343**, 457–461.
63. Rizzetto, M., Canese, M. G., Arico, S. *et al.* (1977). Immunofluorescence detection of new antigen–antibody system (delta/anti-delta) associated to hepatitis B virus in liver and in serum of HBsAg carriers. *Gut,* **18**, 997–1003.
64. Wang, C. J., Chen, P. J., Wu, J. C. *et al.* (1991). Small-form hepatitis-B surface antigen is sufficient to help in the assembly of hepatitis delta-virus-like particles. *J. Virol.,* **65**, 6630–6636.
65. Elena, S. F., Dopazo, J., Flores, R. *et al.* (1991). Phylogeny of viroids, viroid-like satellite RNAs, and the viroid-like domain of hepatitis delta virus RNA. *Proc. Natl Acad. Sci. USA,* **88**, 5631–5634.
66. Perrotta, A. T. and Been, M. D. (1992). Cleavage of oligoribonucleotides by a ribozyme derived from the hepatitis-delta virus RNA sequence. *Biochemistry,* **31**, 16–21.
67. Taylor, J. M. (1990). Hepatitis delta-virus: cis and trans functions required for replication. *Cell,* **61**, 371–373.
68. Luo, G. X., Chao, M., Hsieh, S. Y. *et al.* (1990). A specific base transition occurs on replicating hepatitis delta virus RNA. *J. Virol.,* **64**, 1021–1027.
69. Chang, F. L., Chen, P. J., Tu, S. J. *et al.* (1991). The large form of hepatitis-delta antigen is crucial for assembly of hepatitis-delta virus. *Proc. Natl Acad. Sci. USA,* **88**, 8490–8494.
70. Bradley, D. W., McCaustland, K. A., Cook, E. H. *et al.* (1985). Posttransfusion non-A, non-B hepatitis in chimpanzees: physicochemical evidence that the tubule-forming agent is a small, enveloped virus. *Gastroenterology,* **88**, 773–779.
71. He, L. F., Alling, D., Popkin, T. *et al.* (1987). Determining the size of non-A, non-B hepatitis virus by filtration. *J. Infect. Dis.,* **156**, 636–640.
72. Choo, Q. L., Kuo, G., Weiner, A. J. *et al.* (1989). Isolation of a cDNA clone derived from a blood-borne non-A, non-B viral hepatitis genome. *Science,* **244**, 359–362.
73. Kuo, G., Choo, Q. L., Alter, H. J. *et al.* (1989). An assay for circulating antibodies to a major etiologic virus of human non-A, non-B hepatitis. *Science,* **244**, 362–364.
74. Garson, J. A., Ring, C. J. A. and Tuke, P. W. (1991). Improvement of HCV genome detection with 'short' PCR products. *Lancet,* **338**, 1466–1467.
75. Miller, R. H. and Purcell, R. H. (1990). Hepatitis C virus shares amino acid sequence similarity with pestiviruses and flaviviruses as well as members of two plant virus supergroups. *Proc. Natl Acad. Sci. USA,* **87**, 2057–2061.

76. Hijikata, M., Kato, N., Ootsuyama, Y. *et al.* (1991). Gene mapping of the putative structural region of the hepatitis C virus genome by *in vitro* processing analysis. *Proc. Natl Acad. Sci. USA*, **88**, 5547–5551.
77. Bradley, D. W. (1985). The agents of non-A, non-B viral hepatitis. *J. Virol. Methods*, **10**, 307–319.
78. Fagan, E. A., Ellis, D. S., Tovey, G. M. *et al.* (1992). Toga virus-like particles in acute liver failure attributed to sporadic non-A, non-B hepatitis and recurrence after liver transplantation. *J. Med. Virol.*, in press.
79. Phillips, M. J., Blendis, L. M., Poucell, S. *et al.* (1991). Syncytial giant-cell hepatitis: sporadic hepatitis with distinctive pathological features, a severe clinical course, and paramyxoviral features. *N. Engl. J. Med.*, **324**, 455–460.

15 Clinical Treatment of Viral Hepatitis

STEPHEN A. LOCARNINI
Fairfield Hospital, Victoria, Australia

ANTHONY L. CUNNINGHAM
Westmead Hospital Institute of Clinical Pathology and Medical Research, Westmead, New South Wales, Australia

INTRODUCTION

Viral hepatitis is a common disease and a major global public health problem. Its primary aetiological agents are the enterically transmitted hepatitis A and hepatitis E viruses (HAV, HEV) and the parenterally transmitted hepatitis B virus (HBV), hepatitis D (delta) virus (HDV) and hepatitis C virus (HCV). For the past decade, the reported incidence of acute hepatitis in developed countries has continued to rise steadily (1) and the incidence of acute, symptomatic viral hepatitis has been estimated at approximately one per thousand population per year (2). The case mix in this setting comprises approximately 25% hepatitis A, 35% hepatitis B, 35% hepatitis C and, if present, 5% hepatitis D. Hepatitis E appears to be uncommon in developed countries such as the United States, Western Europe and Australia.

The major taxonomic features of the five agents of viral hepatitis and their nomenclature are shown in Table 15.1. All five forms of viral hepatitis can lead to acute disease, but only the parenterally transmitted hepatitis viruses are commonly associated with persistent infection and the development of chronic sequelae which include chronic active hepatitis, cirrhosis and primary hepatocellular carcinoma. Vaccines for the prevention of hepatitis A (3) and hepatitis B (4) are now available. However, for the millions of existing chronic carriers, there is no universally effective treatment to clear the virus and thereby limit the high risk of liver diseases associated with long-term carriage. The focus of this chapter is on antiviral chemotherapy and clinical treatment. An appreciation of its role in viral hepatitis should be based on an understanding of the natural history, clinical course and pathogenesis of the disease coupled with molecular insight into the unique nature of the virus–cell interactions in acute and chronic infections.

Antiviral Chemotherapy. Edited by D.J. Jeffries and E. De Clercq

Table 15.1. Classification and major features of the five agents of viral hepatitis

Virus	Family	Nucleic acid	Symmetry	Size	Type of hepatitis
HAV	Picornavirus	SS (+) RNA	Icosahedral	30 nm	Acute
HBV	Hepadnavirus	ds DNA	Isometric Enveloped	42 nm	Acute and chronic
HCV	Flavivirus	SS (+) RNA	Icosahedral Enveloped	40–50 nm	Acute and chronic
HDV	Virusoid	circular (−) RNA	Complex	37 nm	Acute and chronic
HEV	Calicivirus	SS (+) RNA	Isometric	35 nm	Acute

CLINICAL FEATURES AND GENERAL MANAGEMENT PRINCIPLES

The clinical features of the five forms of viral hepatitis cannot be readily distinguished from each other on the basis of symptoms and signs of disease or the profile of serum biochemistry tests alone. Sensitive and specific laboratory-based serological and virological assays are now available for each agent, thereby permitting a reliable diagnosis to be made in most cases. However, there have been recent reports of other viral-like agents involved in the aetiology of viral hepatitis (5), and as laboratory testing is further refined the number of agents of viral hepatitis will continue to grow.

ACUTE HEPATITIS

The major focus of antiviral chemotherapy for viral hepatitis has been the complications of acute disease. These complications include fulminant hepatitis, chronic hepatitis, and relapsing or reactivation hepatitis. For acute hepatitis, supportive and symptomatic measures combined with simple monitoring of patients are usually all that are required. In the case of acute hepatitis C, because of its propensity to develop chronicity, an argument can be made to treat the acute phase with appropriate antiviral chemotherapy (see below).

Typical symptoms of acute hepatitis include malaise, anorexia, nausea and vomiting, right upper quadrant pain and jaundice accompanied by dark urine and pale stools. An abrupt onset with fever, headache, weakness and myalgia is more typical of hepatitis A, while fever, rash (typically urticarial) and migratory non-deforming arthritis are sometimes seen with hepatitis B, and occasionally with other types, and are caused by immune complex deposition. Physical findings include jaundice, tender and firm hepatic enlargement, palpable splenomegaly and mild lymphadenopathy. A few vascular spider naevi may be transiently present.

Fulminant hepatitis can occur at any time during the course of the disease, and is accompanied by signs of hepatic encephalopathy: lethargy, sleepiness, personality change, cognitive impairment, hepatic foetor and hyperreflexia. Hepatic decompensation is revealed by prolonged prothrombin time, hypoglycaemia, hypoalbuminaemia, renal impairment and/or ascites. Fulminant hepatitis constitutes a medical emergency and has a high mortality despite intensive medical intervention including orthotopic liver transplantation (see below).

Acute viral hepatitis should be diagnosed with care (6a). The most important differential diagnoses are conditions requiring urgent specific treatment, such as ascending cholangitis, other types of severe sepsis, malaria and Wilson's disease. A 'golden rule' is that the febrile jaundiced patient has ascending cholangitis until proven otherwise. In patients aged over 50 years with no risk factors, an alternative diagnosis to viral hepatitis should be sought.

Confirming the diagnosis of acute viral hepatitis involves several steps:

1. The demonstration of acute hepatitis based largely on the pattern of serum biochemistry with dramatic (preferably at least 10-fold) elevations in serum aminotransaminase levels.
2. The exclusion of non-viral causes, usually on the basis of history, physical findings and associated laboratory data.
3. Identification of the responsible viral agent and, preferably, the source of infection.
4. If the clinical features or biochemical tests are in any way atypical, early ultrasound hepatic imaging should be arranged.
5. Accurate serological tests are now routinely available for diagnosis of hepatitis A, B, C, D and E as well as other uncommon viral causes of hepatitis such as the Epstein–Barr virus, cytomegalovirus, herpes simplex virus and human herpesvirus type 6 (6b).

Acute viral hepatitis is usually self-limiting and recovery is complete. As such, antiviral therapy of typical acute viral hepatitis is not usually indicated, although its role in acute hepatitis C is presently not clear (see below). Since there is no established antiviral therapy, management consists of supportive measures, symptom relief and avoidance of additional hepatic insult, combined with careful clinical and laboratory monitoring and follow-up. Supportive and symptomatic measures include adequate rest, good fluid intake and a generally nutritious diet. Frequent, small, low-fat, high-carbohydrate meals are preferred. Alcohol should be avoided during the acute symptomatic phase. Symptomatic relief may be required for nausea, pain, sleeplessness or pruritus. Although generally of little or no benefit unless cholestasis has been protracted, vitamin K supplementation is indicated if the prothrombin time is prolonged. Corticosteroids have not been shown to be of value in the treatment of acute viral hepatitis and their use in severe disease may even be hazardous.

Even though most patients with acute viral hepatitis can be managed at home, regular monitoring every two to three days is essential until clear-cut improvement occurs. There should be regular evaluation of symptoms, degree of jaundice and liver size. With evidence of hepatic decompensation blood should be drawn for transaminase, alkaline phosphatase, bilirubin levels and prothrombin times. Shrinking liver size in a patient with deepening jaundice is cause for serious concern. Once the patient is clearly improving, hepatic enzymes should be monitored every two weeks until normal levels are reached.

Hospitalization is indicated in those patients who are unable to attend regular follow-up, or who live alone, who have severe symptoms of volume depletion, or who have any evidence of hepatic decompensation.

FULMINANT HEPATITIS

Fulminant hepatitis represents the extreme end of the clinical spectrum of severity of acute viral hepatitis. The incidence of fulminant disease relates partly to the form of hepatitis, being highest in delta hepatitis and lowest in hepatitis A. Its incidence also relates to host factors such as age (more common in the elderly) and pregnancy if associated with hepatitis E virus infection. There is no specific treatment for fulminant hepatitis, although a relatively new approach to this dire syndrome is through emergency hepatic transplantation (253). Its high mortality rate (70–90%) makes antiviral chemotherapy an attractive therapeutic option. However, in the majority of cases, once hepatic failure occurs viral replication has usually ceased (254), and the marginal nature of the patient's hepatic reserve usually makes the addition of medications potentially dangerous.

CHRONIC HEPATITIS

Symptoms of hepatitis or carriage of specific viral markers for more than six months is usually designated as chronic infection (7). The two broad classes of chronic hepatitis, persistent and active, require liver biopsy for their differentiation. The enterically transmitted forms of viral hepatitis (A and E) are not associated with chronic hepatitis, or a carrier state, whereas the parenterally transmitted types (B, C and D) are major causes of chronic disease which is usually associated with persisting active viral replication.

In general, chronic persistent and chronic lobular hepatitis are benign entities which do not progress to fibrosis or cirrhosis and do not require therapy; symptoms are few. However, follow-up is needed to identify the uncommon patient who progresses to chronic active hepatitis. In chronic active hepatitis, the classical histological feature is piecemeal necrosis, involving the destruction of hepatocytes at the periphery of hepatic lobules and erosion of the limiting plate. This condition frequently progresses to cirrhosis and liver failure. The most common symptoms of chronic hepatitis are progressive fatigue and malaise, with or without fluctuating jaundice. In women, amenorrhoea is common.

Because clinical features do not distinguish between the various types of chronic hepatitis or their aetiologies, liver biopsy is an essential component of the diagnostic work-up of all patients. Liver function tests are invariably abnormal in chronic hepatitis, but this abnormality may consist solely of mild transaminase elevations and may not correlate with clinical or histological severity.

Laboratory tests indicate that chronic viral hepatitis is accompanied by persistence of viral replication. In hepatitis B, chronicity is invariably accompanied by persistence of HBV DNA in serum, or hepatitis B core antigen (HBcAg) with replicative intermediates of HBV DNA in the liver (8,9). In chronic delta hepatitis, HDV RNA can be demonstrated in serum and/or liver in almost all patients (10). Likewise, in chronic HCV infection HCV RNA can be found in the serum and liver of patients, with or without abnormal flares in serum biochemistry (11).

The major complication of chronic viral hepatitis is the development of liver cirrhosis with the associated problems of portal hypertension and loss of hepatocyte function. Once cirrhosis is present, patients are more likely to have symptoms of liver disease, the most common being chronic fatigue, poor appetite, wasting and weakness. The complications of portal hypertension include fluid retention, oedema and ascites, as well as variceal and gastrointestinal haemorrhage. In recent years, liver transplantation has greatly improved the prognosis of those patients with advanced cirrhosis.

A final complication of chronic viral hepatitis is primary hepatocellular carcinoma (HCC) (12). Both epidemiological and molecular biological evidence has firmly linked HCC with chronic HBV (12) and chronic HCV (13) infection. Worldwide, HBC is one of the major causes of cancer mortality in humans and chronic HBV and HCV infections are clearly involved as the major aetiological factors in the development of this tumour.

The essential management principles in chronic hepatitis are definition, aetiology and staging. Chronic persistent and lobular hepatitis require only observation and follow-up, whereas chronic active hepatitis depends on aetiological diagnosis (see below) as well as an assessment of the severity and stage of the disease. All patients should avoid consuming alcohol. Early diagnosis of treatable causes of chronic active hepatitis, including that due to HBV, HDV or HCV, is important. Thus, the major focus of therapy in chronic viral hepatitis has been prevention of progressive hepatic injury and cirrhosis. Since chronic viral hepatitis is accompanied by persistent active viral replication, antiviral therapy has been associated with remission at an early stage in some cases, thereby preventing and/or delaying the development of cirrhosis and possibly even HCC.

RELAPSING AND REACTIVATING HEPATITIS

A relapsing or polyphasic course of hepatitis (longer than eight weeks) has been observed in acute hepatitis A, hepatitis delta and hepatitis C (10,11,14). The relapses are almost certainly due to recurrence of viral replication during convalescence, thus making antiviral therapy a potentially useful approach for managing protracted or relapsing disease.

On the other hand, reactivation of viral replication is a well-recognized complication in patients with chronic viral infection receiving cytotoxic or immunosuppressive therapy. This has been well documented in HBV (15,16) and occasionally with fatal consequences on withdrawal of therapy (17). Since viral markers indicating active replication are usually found in these situations, selective inhibition of viral replication by antiviral chemotherapy could prove a useful therapeutic adjunct in oncology units with HBsAg-positive patients.

CLINICAL TREATMENT AND SPECIFIC ANTIVIRAL CHEMOTHERAPY OF VIRAL HEPATITIS

HEPATITIS A

Epidemiology

In most communities, 75–100% of persons aged over 50 years have detectable antibodies to HAV (anti-HAV). Hepatitis A is very contagious, the virus being transmitted by the faecal–oral route, often following close personal exposure or contamination of food or drinking water (14). Most infections in childhood are subclinical. The incubation period ranges from 15 to 45 days (average 25 days), with HAV detectable in the faeces from approximately two weeks before until about two weeks after the onset of dark urine (18,19).

Molecular virology

HAV is a non-enveloped virus which is ether resistant, stable at pH 3.0, and relatively resistant to inactivation by heat. It is inactivated by ultraviolet irradiation, formaldehyde and chlorine (20,21). The mature virion measures 27–32 nm in diameter, with a buoyant density of 1.32–1.34 g/cm^3 in caesium chloride and a sedimentation coefficient in sucrose of 160 S. It is classified as the type species of the genus Hepatovirus, within the family Picornaviridae (22).

The virion contains a linear genome of single-stranded positive sense RNA approximately 7500 nucleotides in length. A single open reading frame extends from nucleotide 735 at the 5′ terminal end to about 60 nucleotides in advance of the 3′ terminal poly(A) tract. This sequence encodes a protein with a molecular weight of about 250 000 Da (2200 amino acids). The genome organization of HAV is similar to that of other picornaviruses. A short genome-like protein (VPg) is covalently attached to the 5′ end of virion RNA, whilst the 3′ end terminates in a poly(A) tail (22). The 5′ region of the genome codes for the four major structural viral proteins (VP1–4) (14), with polymerase, helicase and proteinase motifs at the 3′ end (23). The precise cleavage junctions of most HAV proteins have yet to be determined.

Replication strategy

HAV survives the acid pH of the stomach, passes through the gastrointestinal mucosa by an unknown mechanism and spreads to the liver. The virus readily replicates in hepatocytes and in the mucosa of the small intestine during experimental infection of marmosets (24).

Once inside the hepatocyte, the HAV RNA genome is uncoated, and serves as both a template for translation of viral proteins as well as for transcription of negative RNA strand replicative intermediates. These intermediates subsequently serve as templates for the virion, genomic (+) RNA (25,26). The translation product from the polycistronic viral mRNA is a polyprotein which is cleaved into structural, proteolytic and synthetic enzymatic proteins including helicases and polymerases. The three major structural proteins (VP0, VP1 and VP3) assemble in the cytoplasm to form subviral particles, pentamers and procapsids (27) which then interact with newly synthesized viral genomic (+) RNA to form nucleocapsid particles (provirions). Finally, cleavage of the VP0 precursor into VP2 and VP4 produces the mature virion. Virus is then secreted in vesicles into bile as mature, infectious virions (22). In infected liver, most of the replication of HAV and associated changes in the hepatic parenchyma are predominantly periportal. Viral antigen is localized in the cytoplasm of hepatocytes and Kupffer cells and can be readily demonstrated by immunofluorescence (21).

Laboratory diagnosis

The typical serological and virological course of hepatitis A is very characteristic (28). Anti-HAV is usually present at the onset of disease, and by the time the patient seeks medical assistance significant titres of anti-HAV immunoglobulin M (IgM) can be detected (28). This HAV-specific IgM response is relatively short-lived and is usually no longer detectable 6–12 months after the onset of illness. In contrast, anti-HAV immunoglobulin G (IgG) rises slowly to peak at 6–12 months and is usually sustained for life (28).

Experimental models

HAV was first reported to be propagated in primary monolayer and explant cell cultures and in continuous cell strains of primate origin by Provost and Hilleman in 1979 (29). *In vitro*, the virus does not induce cytopathic changes under most conditions of culture, and tends to induce persistent, cell-associated infections. Cytopathic variant strains of HAV, which replicate faster and often to higher titre than the non-cytopathic wild-type strain, have been isolated (30). HAV can also infect marmosets (*Saguinus* sp.),. chimpanzees and other higher primates.

The successful propagation of HAV in cell culture has permitted an evaluation of its susceptibility to a wide range of antiviral agents *in vitro*. Vallbracht *et al.* (31) demonstrated that interferon α (IFN-α) inhibits replication of HAV, and this treatment can terminate persistent infections. Siegl and Eggers (32) showed that two anti-picornavirus inhibitors, guanidine-HCl and hydroxybenzyl benzimidazole (HBB), had little effect on HAV replication. More recently, Passagot and colleagues (33) screened a number of antiviral agents for anti-HAV activity and found seven agents which caused reductions in virus titre: ribavirin, amantadine, 2-deoxy-D-glucose, glucosamine, toxifolin, protamine and atropine. Widell *et al.* (34) evaluated 20 antiviral compounds and found significant inhibition of HAV replication with amantadine and ribavirin, but at doses where some cellular toxicity was noted. However, these *in vitro* studies have not identified an antiviral agent of sufficiently high therapeutic index to warrant trials in experimental animals or humans.

Clinical treatment of acute hepatitis A

In humans, hepatitis A infection causes an acute hepatitis only (14). The mechanisms underlying liver injury in hepatitis A are not fully understood. The initial non-cytopathic phase, during which HAV replicates and is released, is followed by decreased multiplication of the virus. The associated inflammatory cell infiltrate suggests that immune mechanisms are involved in the pathogenesis of acute hepatitis A, but little is known about the role of cell-mediated immune responses in the disease process (24).

Optimum management of patients with hepatitis A involves attention to personal hygiene, especially handwashing after toiletting and before eating, in order to reduce the risk of faecal–oral transmission. Patients with hepatitis A should avoid preparing food for others, and non-immune households and other close contacts should receive human immune globulin in a dose of 0.02 ml/kg intramuscularly as soon as possible after exposure. Immune globulin is 75–85% effective in preventing symptomatic hepatitis A infection if given before or within two weeks of exposure, and provides passive immunity for up to eight weeks following administration (6a).

Because of the normally benign outcome of hepatitis A, the need for specific antiviral therapy is restricted (22). However, there are clinical situations when treatment may be required, such as in prolonged or relapsing illness and in fulminant hepatitis A (35). In a very small number of hepatitis A cases, fulminant hepatic failure develops and can be fatal. Levin and Hahn (36) have treated one patient with fulminant hepatitis A, amongst a series of seven patients with sporadic fulminant hepatitis, with IFN-α. Five of the seven patients, including the single patient with fulminant hepatitis A, survived. This pilot study suggested that IFN-α therapy could improve the course of fulminant viral hepatitis, but further confirmatory studies will be required before useful guidelines can emerge. Although fulminant hepatitis A has a relatively good prognosis, orthotopic liver transplantation (OLT) may be required. Fagan *et al.* (37) have demonstrated that HAV can reinfect the donor liver after OLT. Recurrent hepatitis A in a transplanted liver does not jeopardize the patient's long-term survival after otherwise successful liver transplantation, and fulminant hepatitis A is not a contraindication to liver transplantation (38).

Another very unusual outcome of hepatitis A infection is a prolonged or relapsing course (39). These relapses can be severe and debilitating and have been associated with the reappearance of HAV excretion in the stools (40), implicating active viral replication in the disease process.

In conclusion, even though hepatitis A is regarded as a benign, self-limiting illness, there are occasional complications when infection results in a severe, prolonged, relapsing or even fatal outcome. Only limited studies on potential antiviral agents for use in hepatitis A are available and further investigations in this area are warranted. To date, IFN-α, ribavirin and amantadine have demonstrable *in vitro* activity against the virus, and as such may be indicated in severe or relapsing acute hepatitis A. Effective control and eventual elimination of hepatitis A will come with implementation of active immunization strategies using the new generation of HAV vaccines (22).

HEPATITIS E

Epidemiology

HEV is a major cause of epidemic and sporadic hepatitis in many developing countries of Africa, Asia, the Middle East and Central and South America. Epidemics are usually associated with faecal contamination of drinking water, and young adults are particularly affected. The incubation period is two to eight weeks, with a mean of 5.5 weeks (41–43). In developed countries, cases have usually been reported only in returned travellers. Hepatitis E is usually a self-limited hepatitis that is often cholestatic (41). Infection with HEV does not lead to chronic hepatitis or cirrhosis, and no carrier state has been identified. Its most striking clinical characteristic is the high mortality rate in pregnant women, with a case fatality rate of approximately 20%. This compares to a rate of less than 1% amongst men and non-pregnant women (42).

Molecular virology and replication strategy

HEV has only recently been recognized as the aetiological agent of enterically transmitted non-A, non-B hepatitis (43), and has not yet been successfully propagated *in vitro*. It appears to be extremely labile and does not tolerate exposure to high concentrations of salt, including caesium chloride. Pelleting of the virus from faecal specimens or gradient fractions frequently results in loss of recoverable virus. The majority of virus particles are 32–34 nm in diameter, with a size range of 27–38 nm. The particles are spherical and non-enveloped, with spikes and indentations visible on the surface. The sedimentation coefficient is 183 S, and the virus has a buoyant density in caesium chloride of 1.29 g/cm^3 (43).

The HEV genome is a single-stranded polyadenylated RNA of approximately 7500 nucleotides. Three open reading frames (ORFs 1, 2 and 3) have been identified with the structural protein (VP1) encoded at the 3′ end. Two strains of HEV, originating from Mexico and Burma, have been identified (43,44). The genomes of both have now been cloned and sequenced, with an unexpectedly high degree of nucleotide sequence divergence between the isolates, which is not reflected at the amino acid level (43). The Burma serotype is more common globally and, even though two different serotypes of HEV exist, cross-challenge studies conducted in cynomolgus macaques have shown that animals infected with the Burma strain are immune to reinfection by the Mexico isolate (43).

The largest open reading frame (ORF 1) extends approximately 5000 nucleotides from the 5′ end, and contains the RNA-dependent RNA polymerase and nucleoside triphosphate binding motifs. ORF 2 begins 37 bases downstream from the end of ORF 1 and extends for approximately 2000 nucleotides. It encodes the major structural protein of HEV, VP1. ORF 3 partially overlaps ORF 1 and ORF 2 and encompasses only 369 nucleotides. Its function is presently unknown.

In addition to the 7500 nucleotide full-length genomic transcript, two subgenomic, polyadenylated mRNAs of approximately 3700 and 2000 nucleotides have been detected in infected liver (43). The nature of the HEV genome and its organizational framework, the expression of viral mRNAs with two or more 3′ subgenomic species, and its biophysical properties most likely place HEV as the prototype human pathogen for a new class of RNA viruses, or perhaps as a separate genus within the family Caliciviridae.

Laboratory diagnosis

Immune electron microscopy (IEM) was first used to identify HEV and characterize the humoral immune response to it (45). HEV can usually be detected by IEM in the serum of patients with hepatitis during an outbreak. The humoral immune response, measured by IEM, immunofluorescence or enzyme immunoassay, is detectable within the first few days of onset of illness and rises steadily but slowly (47). The antibody response has been found to be variable in some studies and the exact duration of anti-HEV IgG is not known, but appears not to be as long lived as anti-HAV IgG. Anti-HEV IgM has been demonstrated during the acute phase but its reliability as a marker of acute infection has yet to be firmly established. The virus is found mainly in faeces in the late incubation period and disappears abruptly with the presentation of symptoms. HEV has also been detected in acute-phase faecal specimens and sera by using the polymerase chain reaction (PCR) assay (46). A wide range of commercially available assays using HEV recombinant antigens will be available in the very near future.

Experimental models

Transmission of HEV to non-human primates was first reported by Balayan and co-workers in 1983 (45) using cynomolgus macaques inoculated intravenously with faeces-derived virus. Other successful non-human primate studies have used African green monkeys, rhesus monkeys, marmosets (*Saguinis mystax*) and chimpanzees (43). To date, there has been no successful report of *in vitro* isolation of HEV from cell cultures.

Clinical treatment of acute hepatitis E

Hepatitis E is usually a self-limiting illness requiring no specific therapy. However, its severity in pregnant women argues strongly for an urgent search for appropriate antiviral drugs through characterization of HEV and its life-cycle. At present IFN-α would seem to be the most promising therapy for investigation in the treatment of this disease.

Since secondary spread of HEV from case to case is uncommon (43), prevention of hepatitis E infection requires attention to personal hygiene and access to biologically safe water and food during travel in developing countries (41). Not surprisingly, immunoglobulin prepared in developed countries does not confer protection against hepatitis E. Development of safe and effective vaccines with appropriate immunization protocols may eventually control hepatitis E.

HEPATITIS B

Introduction and epidemiology

HBV is largely transmitted by percutaneous and permucosal routes, with an incubation period ranging from 30 to 180 days. It is estimated that over 5% of the world's population, nearly 300 million people, are chronic carriers of HBV, and that about 25% of those infected early in life are likely to die of HBV-induced liver disease (4). Hepatitis B infection results in around two million deaths annually from cirrhosis and HCC. In most developed countries, the prevalence of HBV infection varies widely. Less than 0.1% of first-time volunteer blood donors are positive for hepatitis B surface antigen (HBsAg) but higher rates are found in male homosexuals (5%), intravenous drug users (9.0%), institutionalized mentally retarded children (15%) and migrants from southeast Asia (10–15%) and the Mediterranean region (3–5%) (4).

The critical determinant of the clinical outcome of HBV infection is the age at infection. If acquired early in life, the infection is usually subclinical, whereas in adults about one-third of infections result in clinical hepatitis. Conversely, the risk of HBV infection leading to the chronic carrier state is greater than 90% for infections acquired perinatally, but much lower for infections acquired after early childhood (5–10% overall and probably less than 5% for immunocompetent adults). The two principal forms of clinical expression of infection with HBV are acute hepatitis B and chronic hepatitis B. HBV is generally regarded as non-cytocidal to hepatocytes, and the lesion of hepatitis is the result of the interplay between the host's immune response and the virus–hepatocyte interaction (48).

Molecular virology

Human HBV is a spherical particle with a diameter of approximately 42 nm (Figure 15.1). It is a double-shelled DNA virus and is the prototype member of the family Hepadnaviridae (49). The virus has an outer envelope, approximately 8 nm in width, composed of protein, lipid and carbohydrate, and expresses a surface mosaic of antigens collectively called the hepatitis B surface antigen (HBsAg). The outer envelope surrounds a 27 nm, electron-dense, hexagonal inner core which is the nucleocapsid component of hepatitis B core antigen (HBcAg). Inside the core particle is an endogenous viral DNA polymerase, tightly associated with a single molecule of partially double-stranded circular DNA. Mature HBV particles have a buoyant density of 1.28 g/cm^3 in caesium chloride (49). Infection with HBV results in the

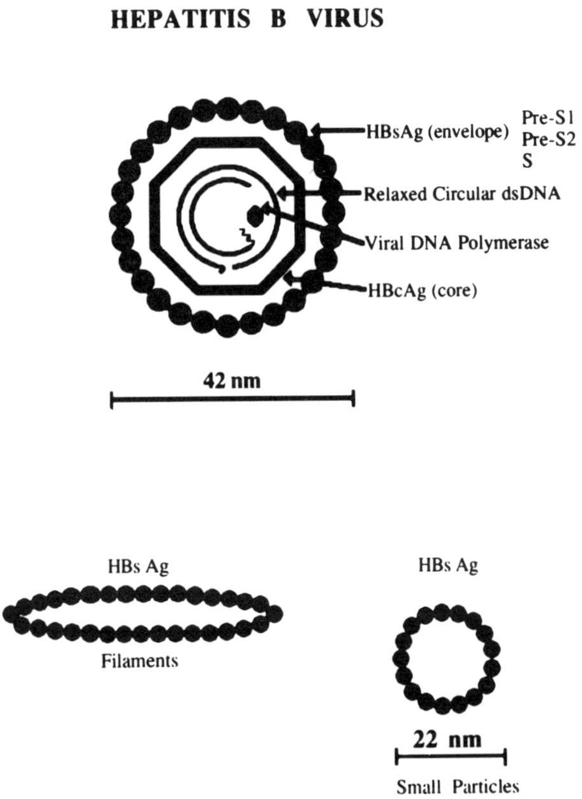

Figure 15.1. The structure and components of the hepatitis B virus and its major antigens

production of infectious virus particles (Dane particles) and two non-infectious forms: 22 nm spherical particles and 22 nm diameter filaments (Figure 15.1). The non-infectious particles are produced in vast excess and are composed entirely of HBsAg. Peak levels of HBsAg achieved during acute or chronic hepatitis can be as high as 200–500 μg/ml in serum, whereas the peak concentration of infectious HBV particles in serum rarely exceeds 10^8 per millilitre (50).

HBcAg is usually not detectable in serum unless special techniques are used to disrupt virions and remove HBsAg. However, it can be readily detected in liver, especially in chronic infections. A third antigen, the hepatitis B *e* antigen (HBeAg), is detectable in serum and usually correlates with the presence of HBcAg in the liver. Both HBV DNA and viral DNA polymerase can be detected in serum during the active replicative phases of HBV infection. These two markers are reliable means of assessing the activity of the infection as well as the level of viral replication and hence infectivity.

The HBV genome has an unusual and characteristic structure (Figure 15.2). It is a partially double-stranded, circularized DNA molecule which contains a variable, single-stranded region. Overall the genome is about 3200 nucleotide bases in length (51). The genome is made up of two strands of DNA: the long (L or minus) and short (S or plus) strand. The L strand is full length but is not a closed circle, and is interrupted by a nick at a unique site near the 5′ end of the S strand, which is fixed in location (nucleotide 1230). The molecule is held in a circular configuration because of overlapping base pairs on either side of the nick. The 5′ ends (or the

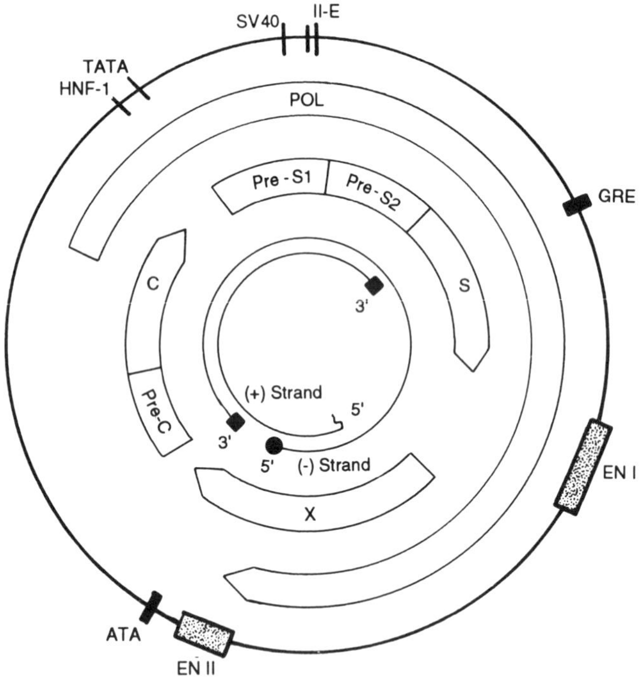

Figure 15.2. Physical and genetic map of HBV DNA. The broad arrows surrounding the genome represent the four open reading frames of the long minus strand. The positions of putative control elements are shown as solid vertical bars and stippled boxes. HNF-1 is the HNF-1 binding element located between nt 2719 and 2744. TATA is the TATA-like box at nt 2784 to 2790 which is a component of the SP-1 promoter. SV40 represents regions of sequence homology to the SV40 origin and late promoter. II-E shows a positive effect on SPII activity with an enhancer-like function. GRE is the glucocorticoid-responsive element. EN I, at nt 1074 to 1234, is the first enhancer which interacts with multiple proteins. EN II, at nt 1636 to 1741, is the second HBV enhancer. ATA, at nt 1755 to 1764, is an ATA box, a component of the core promoter. From Tiollais *et al.* (52) and Yuh and Ting (69)

cohesive region) of both strands are positioned near short (10–12 nucleotides) direct repeats, known as DR1 and DR2 (52). The 5′ end of the minus strand DNA is covalently attached to the terminal protein (TP) (53). The 3′ end of minus strand DNA has a 9–10-nucleotide terminal redundancy (r), which is believed to play a role during the template switch required for the synthesis of plus strand DNA (54). The 3′ end of the S strand is variable in location, so that the HBV DNA molecule has a single-stranded region that can vary from 10% to 60% of the genome. The 5′ end of the S strand is also modified with a 17–18 nucleotide-long capped RNA oligomer (55). The structure of this novel DNA reflects its complex replication strategy (see Figure 15.3) (54).

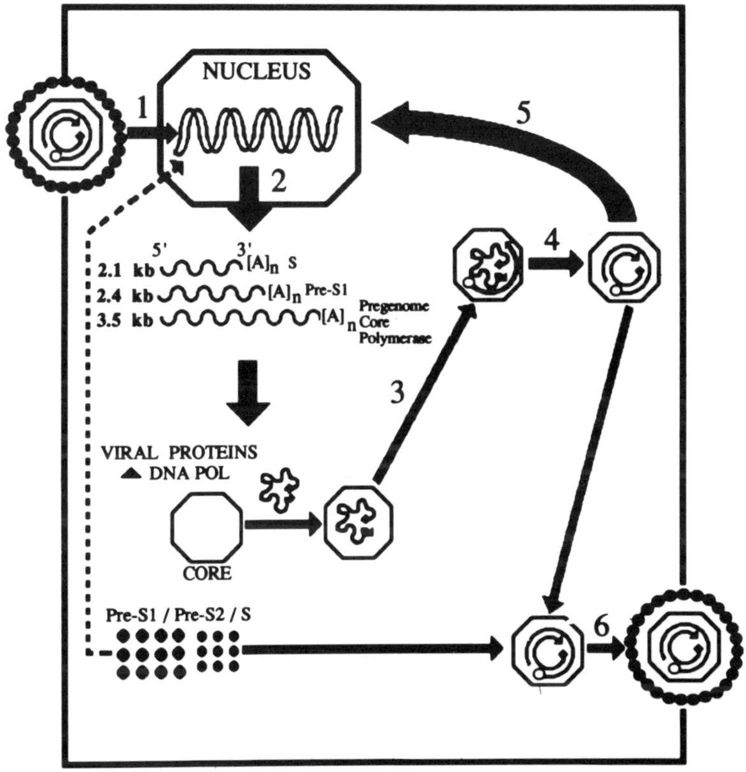

Figure 15.3. Replication cycle of HBV. Following attachment and uncoating, the life-cycle of the virus can be broken down into six major steps which are all potential targets for antiviral chemotherapy. Step 1: after nuclear transportation, the viral RC DNA is converted to an SC form. Step 2: the viral SC DNA acts as the transcriptional template producing viral RNA. Step 3: formation of the replicative complex and reverse transcription of the viral RNA into DNA. Step 4: second-strand synthesis via DNA polymerase. Step 5: amplification of viral SC DNA. Step 6: assembly of HBV. Modified from Summers and Mason (78) and Civitico *et al.* (91)

The minus strand carries the protein-coding capacity of the virus. This strand has four ORFs: pre-S/S, pre-C/C, P and X (Figure 15.2) (52). The four regions overlap with one another so that the minus strand is read one and a half times. This strategy enables HBV, the smallest of the known mammalian double-stranded DNA viruses, to use its coding capacity to the fullest (52,54).

The S gene has three different initiation codons that divide the gene into the pre-S1, pre-S2 and S regions (52) and three potential gene products, namely small, medium and large HBsAg. The HBsAg exists in glycosylated (gp) and non-glycosylated (p) forms. Small HBsAg (p24 and gp27) is the predominant form of HBsAg found in serum and is associated with the 22 nm small particle forms. Middle and large HBsAg are enriched on the surface of mature HBV particles. Both pre-S1 (gp42 and gp39) and pre-S2 (gp36 and gp33) are more immunogenic than small HBsAg (56). The pre-S1 specific domain possesses the HBV hepatocyte receptor binding site, located between amino acid residues 21 and 47 (57,58). The pre-S1 protein of all hepadnaviruses is myristoylated at the N-terminus (59), which is thought to play a key role in virus assembly, release and subsequent attachment to the hepatocyte receptor (60). All three forms of HBsAg are found together in the cytoplasm of infected hepatocytes (61).

The C gene has two initiation sites that divide it into pre-C and C regions, producing two molecular and antigenic forms HBeAg and HBcAg respectively. These are the nucleocapsid antigens of HBV. Initiation of translation at the first site (nucleotide 1814) produces a 212 amino acid polypeptide (p25), which has a signal peptide directing it to the endoplasmic reticulum where the signal piece is removed by a cellular signal peptidase. The polypeptide is further modified at the C-terminal end to be finally secreted as HBeAg (p15–p18) (62). HBeAg can be readily detected in sera of patients with high levels of viral replication. HBeAg is less readily detected in liver and can be demonstrated in a cytoplasmic and nuclear membrane pattern. The HBeAg is a soluble protein that is the product of the pre-C and C gene regions processed through the secretory pathway.

Initiation of translation of the C gene with the second start site (nucleotide 1901) produces a 183 amino acid polypeptide (p23), which after further modification self-assembles into core particles, which express the HBcAg polypeptide p19–21 (62). The HBcAg is usually nuclear in location, but in patients with active disease or extremely high levels of viral replication it is also detected in a diffuse cytoplasmic pattern. The HBcAg is an intracellular virion-associated nucleocapsid antigen that is the product of the C gene alone processed through the cytoplasmic pathway.

The P (or *pol*) gene is the longest ORF, occupying almost 80% of the genome. On the basis of sequence homology with the polymerase genes of several retroviruses, the middle and C-terminal portion of the gene encodes catalytic reverse transcriptase activity (63) and the C-terminal domain encodes RNase H activity (64). The terminal protein at the 5′ end of the minus strand DNA is encoded within the N-terminal end of the *pol* gene (65). The final HBV gene, X, specifies a polypeptide (HBxAg) of 145–154 amino acids in length with a molecular weight of 16–17 kDa (66). Transfection assays *in vitro* have demonstrated that the X protein has a *trans*-activating function which could have importance in regulation of viral replication (67).

The transcription of the four ORFs is controlled by at least four functionally defined promoters (reviewed in 68) in association with two enhancer regions (Figure 15.2) which display strong liver-specific and differentiated specific transcriptional activities (69). Enhancer I (EN I) is located in the upstream component (nt 1074 to 1234) of the X promoter and enhancer II (EN II) lies upstream (nt 1636 to 1741) of the C promoter (Figure 15.2). In addition, a glucocorticoid-responsive element (GRE) (70) stimulates S gene expression in conjunction with EN I (68).

Replication strategy: possible targets for antiviral chemotherapy

Hepadnaviruses replicate in a unique manner, but similar features are found in the retroviruses and other DNA virus life-cycles. Mason *et al.* (71) have suggested naming the hepadnaviral DNA genetic element 'retroid'.

Attachment, penetration and uncoating

The first stage of infection is attachment and penetration of infectious HBV into hepatocytes (Figure 15.3). Attachment is mediated by regions in the pre-S1 domain binding to a specific receptor(s) on hepatocytes. Neutralizing antibody and peptides homologous to either the attachment sites on the virus or on the receptor are potential candidates for blocking virus attachment (72). The exact method of penetration by the virus is unknown, but is thought to be via receptor-mediated endocytosis (72). The uncoating process of duck HBV (DHBV) has been blocked by lysosomotropic agents such as ammonium chloride and chloroquine, which increase the pH of the intracellular vesicles (73). Amantadine and rimantadine exert similar effects (74), and suramin is thought to block DHBV replication at this stage (75). Agents blocking this and earlier steps of infection would not eradicate infection alone, but rather prevent multiple rounds of reinfection with possible effects on horizontal transmission.

Nuclear translocation and nucleocapsid removal

The nucleocapsid is then translocated into the nucleus, with release of the virion DNA and subsequent generation of viral supercoiled DNA from the incoming virion DNA. It is possible that the nucleocapsids, or cores, enter the nucleus before the virion DNA is exposed, as HBcAg is frequently found in the nucleus during active HBV replication (76). A nuclear targeting signal has been identified on hepatitis B cores (77) and this could represent a prime target for antiviral intervention, as prevention of nucleocapsid transport to the nucleus would stop both initiation of infection and the intracellular amplification of viral supercoiled DNA from newly synthesized relaxed circular (RC) DNA. An equally important step is uncoating of hepatitis B cores (nucleocapsid disassembly) but no agent(s) have been found which act at these stages.

Viral DNA synthesis

The replication cycle of hepadnaviruses was first described by Summers and Mason (78) based on observations of the *in vivo* replication of DHBV. A similar replication pattern has since been confirmed for HBV (79) and involves asymmetric replication of the two DNA strands, rather than semiconservative replication (79).

There are four major steps in the replication of hepadnaviral genomes (Figure 15.3).

(i) Conversion of the asymmetric virion genomic DNA to symmetrical double-stranded, RC DNA in the nucleus (49). The RC DNA is then negatively twisted to form covalently closed circular or SC DNA (80,81). Viral SC DNA has been detected only in the nucleus of infected hepatocytes. It is not known whether the viral DNA polymerase or a cellular enzyme completes the synthesis of the viral DNA plus strand. Recent studies from Mason *et al.* (82) demonstrated that in the presence of phosphonoformate (foscarnet), viral SC DNA was synthesized following infection, but no new viral DNA was made until the drug was removed. Since the viral DNA polymerase is inhibited by phosphonoformate, repair of the incomplete virion DNA occurred by a cellular polymerase unaffected by the drug. The source of the enzymes responsible for the other activities involved in the conversion of viral RC DNA to viral SC DNA is unknown but is probably cellular. Inhibition of these steps could therefore result in unacceptable toxicity.

(ii) The SC DNA serves as a template for the synthesis of viral RNA (81,83) using host cell RNA polymerase II (84). Since viral transcription utilizes host cell RNA polymerase II, it might be considered an unsuitable target for chemotherapy. However, IFN-α has been shown to inhibit transcription of HBV RNA (85). This transcriptional inhibition was mediated through an indirect effort of IFN-α on the HBV enhancer via IFN-induced or modified cellular proteins which bind to the HBV enhancer and partially inhibit its activity.

While the translation process continues, the pregenomic RNA, newly synthesized viral DNA polymerase and the protein primer are all assembled with the major structural polypeptide of the viral core (86,87). This immature nucleocapsid complex is formed by spontaneous aggregation of translated core proteins in the cytoplasm with one of the greater than genome-length viral mRNAs also being encapsidated (88). IFN-α has recently been shown to inhibit HBV replication by blocking the pregenome RNA-primed assembly of core particles (89).

(iii) The minus strand is then synthesized by reverse transcription of the pregenome (78,79,83) using the endogenous viral reverse transcriptase. This occurs within the viral core particles in the cell cytoplasm (87). As reverse transcription proceeds, the RNA pregenome is degraded by the RNase H activity of the viral DNA polymerase (78). A capped, 18-base oligoribonucleotide remains after RNase H digestion (90). These steps are all potential targets for selective inhibition, but to date no compounds acting at these sites have been identified.

(iv) Synthesis of the second (plus) strand of DNA then occurs using the minus strand as the template (78,79) and the capped, 18-base oligoribonucleotide as the primer (90). The RNA oligomer which originates from the 5′ end of the pregenome contains DR1 and is transposed to base-pair with the DR2 site in the newly synthesized minus strand (76). Extension of the plus DNA strand by viral DNA polymerase follows (76). However, complete synthesis of this strand is not necessary for coating of the nucleocapsids and export of virus particles (52), explaining why infectious particles contain DNA with a single-stranded region.

Viral DNA synthesis has been the main focus in the HBV life-cycle targeted for selective antiviral inhibition. The major groups of compounds tested are the purine and pyrimidine nucleoside analogues and the pyrophosphate analogue phosphonoformate (see Table 15.2). All compounds evaluated which affect viral DNA synthesis also have associated cellular toxicity. Nucleoside analogues must be converted to nucleoside triphosphates by cellular enzymes (see below), in which form these inhibitors block HBV DNA synthesis by chain termination (91).

Post-translational modification: assembly and release

Assembly and release of mature HBV involves the coating of core particles by HBsAg and lipid-containing material derived from the cell membrane, and export from the cell (92). The exact mechanism of this is unclear (93) but the myristoylation site on pre-S1 appears vital (60,94).

No viral protein essential to the life-cycle of HBV is known to require proteolytic cleavage for activity or maturation. Thus, unlike the closely related retroviruses, proteinase inhibitors do not appear to offer potential

Table 15.2(a). *In vitro* tests of antiviral activity against hepadnaviruses

Analogue	Host system	Assay	Ref.
Phosphonoformate	Human	DNA pol	(157)
FIAC-TP BVUdR-TP ara-CTP ara-TPP	Human Woodchuck	DNA pol DNA pol	(158)
Suramin	Duck	DNA pol	(159) (160)
AZT-TP	Human	DNA pol	(161)
Phosphonoformate	Duck	DNA pol	(160)
Aphidicolin	Duck	DNA pol	(160)
TP of 5-propenyl derivatives (5-propenyl-2′-deoxyuridine)	Human Duck	DNA pol DNA pol RT	(162)
AZT-TP			(163)
Phosphonoformate ddCTP ddGTP ACVTP ddTTP FLT-TP AZTTP	Duck	DNA pol RT	(163)
TP of 3′-fluoropyrimidine derivatives	Human	DNA pol	(164)
ddCTP ddeCTP FdCTP ddMetCTP ddeMetCTP FMetdCTP FEtdcTP	Human	DNA pol	(165)
(*S*)ddC-TP enantiomers 3TC	Human	DNA pol	(166)

prospects for anti-hepadnaviral therapy. As discussed above, the envelope proteins are myristoylated (pre-S1) (59) and glycosylated (pre-S1, pre-S2 and S) (reviewed by Neurath and Kent (95)). Thus, inhibition of any of these modifications might reduce the levels of circulating virus, infectious virus or accumulated intracellular viral components. However, since post-

Table 15.2(b). *In vitro* tests of nucleoside analogues using intact cells

Analogue	Model System	Assay	Ref.
2′-CDG	Human: transfected cells (2.2.15)	DNA	(167)
IFN-α, IFN-β, ara-A, ara-C, ddA, ddC, AZT, ACV, oxetanocin-A	Human: transfected cells (HB611)	DNA	(126)
ACV, AZT	Human: transfected cells (2.2.15)	HBsAg HBeAg DNA pol	(168)
Fdd Thd, dde Thd, Fdd MeCyt, CI ddMeCyt, Add MeCyt	Human: transfected cells (2.2.15)	Core Ag DNA	(169)
ara-A, ara-AMP, AZT, ddC, ddA, ddG, ddDAPR, 2′-CDG, ACV, GCV, PMEA, HPMPC	Human: transfected cells (2.2.15)	DNA	(128)
ddG, ddI, AZT	Human: transfected cells (2.2.15)	DNA	(170)
ddC and related	Human: transfected cells (2.2.15)	DNA	(171)
ara-A, ara-AMP, AZT, ddC, d4T, 2′-CDG	Human: transfected cells	DNA	(172)
PMEDAP, PMEA, CS1-HPMPA, ddC, d4C	Human: transfected cells (HB611)	DNA	(173)
Dideoxy analogues from (169)	Human: transfected cells (2.2.15)	DNA Pre-S Ag	(174)
(*S*)ddC	Human: transfected cells (2.2.15)	DNA	(166)
ddA, ddG, ddT, ddDAPR, ddC, ddT	Duck: chronically infected primary hepatocytes	DNA	(175) (176)
ddC, ddA, AZT, BVdU, ACV, GCV, ribavirin	Duck: chronically infected primary hepatocytes	DNA Surface Ag	(91)
Penciclovir/famciclovir	Duck: chronically infected primary hepatocytes	DNA Surface Ag	(183a)
Cyclobut-A, cyclobut-G, AZT, ddC	Duck: acutely infected primary hepatocytes	DNA	(177)
(*S*)-HRMPA, PMEDAP, ddA, GCV, ddC	Duck: acutely infected primary hepatocytes	Core Ag DNA	(178)

Table 15.2(c). Tests in live animals

Analogue	Host system	Assay	Ref.
GCV ara-AMP	Ground squirrel: chronically infected	Serum DNA pol	(179)
ACV	Duck: chronically infected	Serum DNA	(159)
ara-A	Duck: chronically infected	Serum DNA Liver DNA	(180)
ddC	Duck: chronically infected	Serum DNA Liver DNA	(181)
AZT	Duck: chronically infected	Serum DNA Liver DNA	(182)
GCV	Duck: chronically infected	Serum DNA Liver DNA	(144)
Cyclobut-A Cyclobut-G AZT, ddC	Duck: chronically infected	Serum DNA	(177)
Various dideoxy derivatives	Duck: chronically infected	Serum DNA Serum pre-S Ag	(174)
Famciclovir	Duck: chronically infected	Serum DNA	(183b)
ddA, ddG, ddI, ddDAPR, ddC, ddI	Duck: acutely infected	Serum DNA Liver DNA	(175)
FIAC FMAU FEAU ara-AMP	Woodchuck: chronically infected	Serum DNA Serum DNA pol Liver DNA	(184)
Phosphonoformate	Woodchuck: chronically infected	Serum DNA	(185)
Phosphonoformate	Duck: chronically infected	Serum DNA	(186)

translational processing is mediated by host cell enzymes, selective inhibition poses some difficulties.

Generation and processing of viral SC DNA

In persistent infections, not all complete nucleocapsids are coated and exported, with some re-entering the replication cycle via an intracellular conversion pathway (Figure 15.3). This allows an amplification of SC DNA during the early stages of infection, before virus production (81). This 50-fold amplification enables the establishment of a pool of transcriptional templates in the cell without the need for semi-conservative replication or multiple rounds of reinfection (81). Selective inhibition of the generation and processing of viral SC DNA could result in eventual viral clearance (see below).

During a steady-state infection in persistently infected cells, it is likely that levels of HBV SC DNA in the nucleus are specifically regulated to maintain amounts that are sufficient for virus production but are not toxic to cells. Regulation could occur either through a cell-directed process or through a virus-directed negative feedback mechanism (81) (Figure 15.3). The viral envelope or surface proteins are not required for amplification of SC DNA during the early phase of infection, but are necessary for eventual suppression of amplification (96). Mutation of the pre-S envelope protein alone is sufficient to destroy both control of SC DNA amplification and the secretion of DNA-containing particles (96), with subsequent death of infected hepatocytes as a consequence of over-accumulation of viral SC DNA.

Cytopathology of HBV

The pathogenesis of liver damage in patients with acute and chronic HBV infection is generally believed to be immune-mediated (97). However, experimental evidence has been steadily accumulating that supports a direct cytotoxic role for HBV-mediated liver injury. Using a transgenic mouse model, Chisari *et al.* (98) have shown that high-level accumulation of intracellular pre-S1 protein is directly cytotoxic to hepatocytes. The 22 nm diameter S protein particles accumulate and block the endoplasmic reticulum. As the HBsAg filament (pre-S1) storage progresses, hepatocytes become ballooned, hydropic and eosinophilic, with the characteristic appearance of ground-glass cells, and undergo coagulative necrosis with time. Deletion of the myristoylation site on pre-S1 can overcome the block to secretion of HBV envelope proteins (94), thus bypassing the toxic effects of pre-S1 accumulation. In contrast, using HBV-transfected Hep G2 cells Roingeard *et al.* (99) have shown that high-level accumulation of intracellular HBcAg was also cytotoxic to the hepatoma cell line. More recently, Summers *et al.* (60,96) have demonstrated that mutants of DHBV with N-terminally truncated pre-S/S proteins displayed much higher levels of SC DNA. Hyper-amplification of viral SC DNA directly resulted in cell death. This effect was not mediated by the lack of the myristoylation signal on the pre-S/S protein.

In support of the experimental evidence, there are clinical situations when HBV appears to be cytopathic in its own right. High-level expression of HBV antigens has been described in fibrosing cholestatic hepatitis (FCH) (100), a syndrome developed as a result of severe HBV recurrence in patients undergoing OLT. The development of FCH is associated with rapidly progressive graft dysfunction resulting in mortality within six to eight weeks of clinical onset (101). Pre-C (102) and pre-S (102) mutants of HBV have now been isolated as the dominant virus population in patients with chronic liver disease in the Mediterranean region. Patients with pre-C mutants associated with chronic active hepatitis, often with cirrhosis, invariably displayed high levels of nuclear and cytoplasmic HBcAg on liver biopsy (104). Chronic carriers with deletions/defects in the pre-S2 protein often display higher viraemias ($> 10^6$ genome equivalents/ml) compared to wild-type HBV infected carriers (103), implying a higher level of viral SC DNA activity and possible hepatocyte toxicity.

Immunopathogenesis of acute and chronic hepatitis B

Recovery from HBV infection is dependent on the function and interrelationships of the patient's IFN and immune system. Chronic HBV infection arises when the virus exploits primary defects in these defences or neutralizes essential components of them (97).

In acute hepatitis B, the predominant infiltrating lymphocyte is the $CD8^+$ T cell (106). Since wild-type HBV is non-cytopathic (97,106) the injury of hepatocytes in acute hepatitis is thought to be mediated by $CD8^+$ cytotoxic T lymphocytes (Tc) recognizing peptides of the core protein presented in association with HLA class I proteins. This increase in HLA class I expression can be augmented by IFN-α (97). Recovery from acute hepatitis B therefore requires a normal IFN system, primed natural killer (NK) cells and primed T-helper (T_H) lymphocytes which then enhance the activity of cytotoxic T lymphocytes (Tc) and pre-B lymphocytes (97).

In chronic hepatitis B, the expression of HLA class I antigens is less than in acute disease. Correspondingly, the degree of lymphocyte infiltration and hepatocyte necrosis is less, suggesting that immune responses to the viral antigen(s) is not as great and that this blunted response may be responsible for the persistence of viral replication. Blunted responses in chronic hepatitis B may be mediated in part by the lack of increase in class I HLA expression as well as a deficiency in IFN-α production (106). Experimental systems using cloned HBV DNA transfected into different cell lines have suggested that the presence of HBV DNA and gene products inhibits both the production and intracellular effects of the IFNs (107,108). Chronic carriers of HBV often demonstrate immunological defects, especially in T_H, which result in inability to prime Tc such that infected clones are not eradicated. The T_H can also fail to prime pre-B cells, resulting in decreased production of neutralizing antibodies (97).

Thus, clinical treatment of hepatitis B requires strategies aimed at the key steps in the viral life-cycle (Figure 15.3) (103) in combination with immunological enhancement.

Laboratory diagnosis

The course and outcome of acute hepatitis B are variable (49,50). The serological and biochemical events that accompany a typical case of acute hepatitis B are shown in Figure 15.4. Acute hepatitis B infection can be divided into an early, replicative phase and a late, non-replicative phase. In the early phase, which includes the incubation period, HBsAg appears first, and is followed by HBeAg, HBV DNA and viral DNA polymerase. When serum aminotransferase activity begins to increase and symptoms first appear, the levels of HBV DNA and HBsAg are usually at their peak or starting to decline. At the time most patients seek medical attention, most are negative for serum HBV DNA and viral DNA polymerase. These markers of active viral replication disappear within one to eight weeks of the onset of symptoms, heralding the second, non-replicative phase, during which HBsAg is still present but without evidence of continuing viral replication. HBsAg usually remains detectable in serum throughout the clinical illness, disappearing in convalescence. Patients who clear HBsAg recover from their hepatitis and are left with no residual liver injury or viral persistence.

In some patients, HBsAg can still be detected some months after the onset

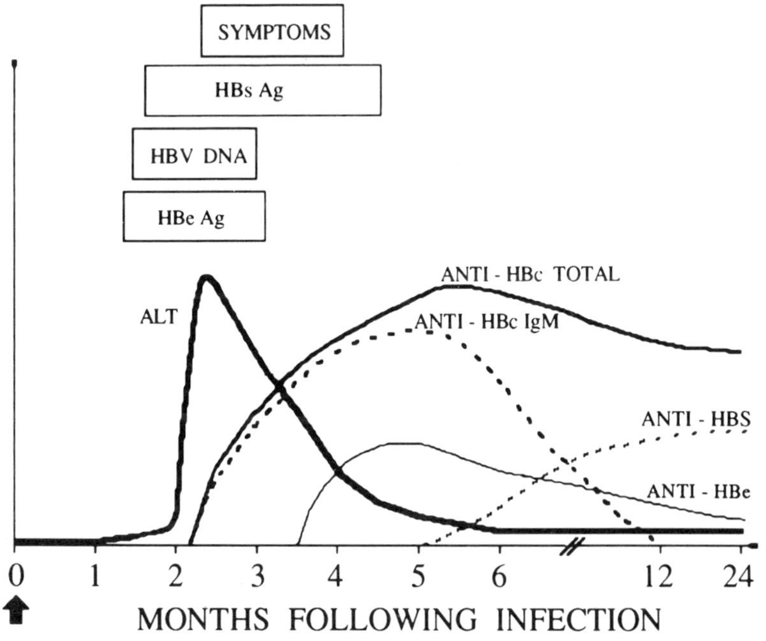

Figure 15.4. Diagrammatic representation detailing the clinical, serological and virological responses following a 'typical' acute hepatitis B virus infection. Modified from Locarnini and Gust (49)

of illness. This is usually because HBsAg is cleared slowly from blood, with a half-life of approximately eight days (109). Persistence of HBsAg in acute hepatitis B for more than 13 weeks is usually associated with the development of chronic infection (110).

The first antibody response in acute hepatitis B is to the HBcAg (anti-HBc), which occurs shortly before or at the time of the onset of illness (Figure 15.4) and invariably being present by the time jaundice is apparent (50). The initial response is primarily IgM, but with recovery IgG anti-HBc steadily increases whilst anti-HBc IgM declines and usually disappears within 3–12 months. Anti-HBc is a useful marker of past infection with HBV.

Antibody to the hepatitis B e antigen (HBeAg), anti-HBe, appears in most patients shortly after the loss of HBV DNA and HBeAg. Unlike anti-HBc, anti-HBe rarely reaches high titres in acute hepatitis and often disappears within a few months.

Antibody to HBsAg (anti-HBs) generally appears during recovery, after HBsAg has been cleared. There is often a window period between the disappearance of detectable HBsAg and the appearance of anti-HBs. Anti-HBs is a reliable marker of immunity and recovery from hepatitis B. However, patients in the convalescent phase of hepatitis B make only low levels of anti-HBs and up to 15% of patients never actually produce this antibody despite clearing HBV infection.

In chronic hepatitis B, a proportion of patients do not eliminate HBsAg and become chronic carriers of the virus (50). The carrier state is defined as the presence of HBsAg in serum for a period of six months or more (Figure 15.5). The initial pattern of HBV markers in patients who progress to chronic type B hepatitis is identical to that of patients with acute, self-limited disease. However, in chronic infection HBsAg titres do not decline as transaminase levels fall (Figure 15.5). The persistence of HBV DNA, viral DNA polymerase and high titres of HBeAg into the period of aminotransferase elevation heralds the establishment of chronic infection. Antibody response is usually restricted to anti-HBc, which arises at the onset of initial aminotransferase elevations or illness and then remains at high levels. Anti-HBs, if present, is detectable only in low titres.

The clinical course of chronic hepatitis B is variable, and the activity and severity of the disease can change markedly with time. In some patients, the disease is rapidly progressive, the virus remains detectable, and the patient develops cirrhosis within a few years of onset of infection. In other patients, periods of mild disease activity are followed by exacerbation of disease (abortive seroconversions) and the patient may develop cirrhosis after many years of infection (111). In other patients, the disease is mild or moderate, and ultimately the patient undergoes a spontaneous remission.

The 'typical' example of a carrier shown in Figure 15.5 demonstrates an important principle: the presence of disease activity correlates with the

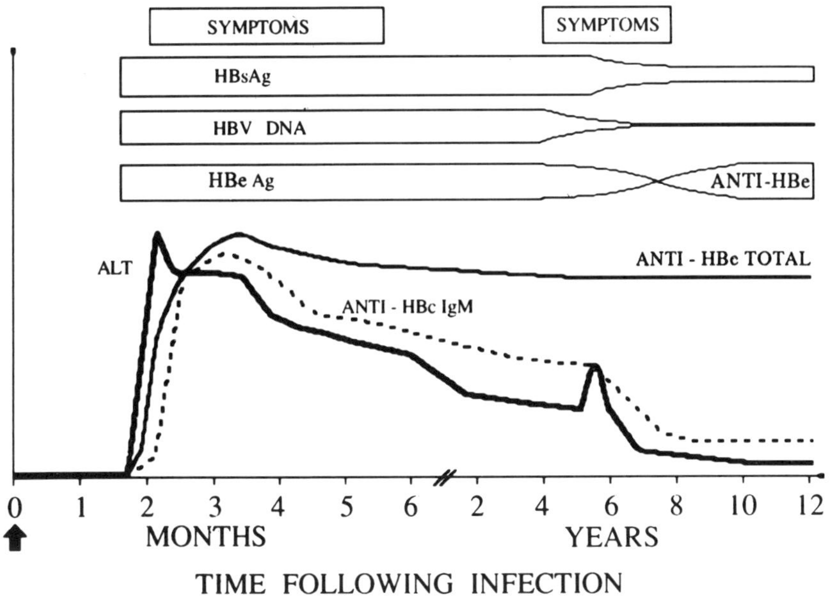

Figure 15.5. Diagrammatic representation detailing the clinical, serological and virological responses commonly seen in chronic type B hepatitis. Also shown is the eventual loss of HBeAg and resultant seroconversion to anti-HBe, six to eight years after exposure to HBV. Modified from Locarnini and Gust (49)

presence of markers of active viral replication. Like acute infection, chronic hepatitis B infection can be divided into two phases: a replicative and non-replicative phase. The replicative phase is characterized by the demonstration of HBV DNA, viral DNA polymerase, HBeAg and anti-HBc IgM (49). During this period, HBcAg can be found in the nucleus and cytoplasm of infected liver cells (112), and HBV DNA is extrachromosomal (113). During the non-replicative phase, chronic carriers of HBsAg lose HBeAg and develop anti-HBe at a rate of 5–25% per annum, depending on the population studied, with an overall rate of at least 50% of patients in longitudinal studies (114). The loss of HBeAg is usually accompanied by the disappearance of serum HBV DNA and viral DNA polymerase activity, a lowering of serum aminotransferase levels, and a marked improvement in liver histology (115). This switch from HBeAg to anti-HBe is often associated with a brief but significant flare-up of disease just prior to the seroconversion (the seroconversion illness) and heralds the non-replicative phase of the carrier state, where HBV DNA becomes integrated into the host cell genome (113). The seroconversion from HBeAg to anti-HBe has important clinical and virological implications. In the majority of cases, the loss of HBeAg from serum is associated with eradication of viral replication and patients become HBV DNA negative. These patients manifest a marked clinical improvement, with normalization of serum biochemical markers despite the continued presence of HBsAg. In a minority of cases, despite the apparent loss of HBeAg and production of anti-HBe, HBV DNA persists. These patients have been shown to be infected with precore mutants of HBV which have mutated and lost the ability to produce HBeAg (116). The appearance of these mutants of HBV is thought to be due to immune selection (116). Continued infection with these precore variants is often associated with more aggressive liver disease, higher viraemias and the rapid evolution of end-stage liver failure (116). In some cases, these variants have also been associated with the rapid development of fulminant hepatitis (116,117).

In the non-replicative phase of all carriers, serum HBsAg is still detected although active viral replication has stopped. The persistence of HBsAg is probably due to synthesis of HBsAg from molecules of HBV DNA that are integrated into host chromosomal DNA (113). Thus, in the majority of carriers, the termination of viral replication marks the onset of remission.

The final stage of the carrier state is marked by the disappearance of HBsAg from serum and occurs at a rate of approximately 1–2% per annum (118). It is generally associated with the development of anti-HBs and further normalization of liver function tests. For these reasons, the seroconversion from HBeAg to anti-HBe with the loss of HBV DNA and/or the disappearance of HBsAg from serum are used as successful therapeutic endpoint markers.

Experimental models: development of antiviral treatment strategies (see Table 15.2)

In vivo models

In the past few years, three models have been used to define the pathogenesis, natural history and carcinogenic properties of hepadnavirus infection and to test drugs for antiviral efficacy (119): the woodchuck hepatitis B virus (WHBV), the ground squirrel hepatitis B virus (GSHBV) and the duck hepatitis B virus (DHBV). Human HBV will infect chimpanzees, but this model is severely restricted due to ethical considerations.

Potential anti-hepadnaviral drugs have been tested *in vitro* for their ability to inhibit serum viral particle-associated DNA polymerase activity or *in vivo* for their capacity to reduce serum DNA polymerase or HBsAg. This approach clearly has limited application. In contrast, *in vivo* model systems in which HBV undergoes a complete life-cycle offer the advantage of being suitable for testing drug delivery methods, pharmacokinetics, drug toxicity and immune modulation, as well as for testing drugs targeted to all stages of the life-cycle. More limited *in vivo* models that might be useful in the future for drug testing are transgenic mice expressing complete virus (121) or specific viral antigens (98). These systems are not appropriate for testing drug action at targets preceding transcription, but allow selective inhibition of key steps in HBV which have been associated with direct pathogenic effects on hepatocytes.

In vitro models

Human HBV replicates poorly in cell culture. However, it has been shown to infect and replicate in primary cultures of both fetal and adult human hepatocytes (122,123). These studies have been difficult to reproduce but do allow investigators to evaluate fully the effects of antiviral compounds during the complete life-cycle of HBV from attachment through to release of virus.

Recently, other investigators have demonstrated HBV replication following transfection of human hepatoma cell lines with closed circular HBV DNA (124,125). Sells *et al.* (125) transfected the Hep G2 human hepatoma cell line with a plasmid containing two head-to-tail dimers of the HBV genome in a tail-to-tail orientation. The availability of these cells has allowed the study of viral replication from transcription through to virus release and thus they are useful for evaluating antiviral compounds which might affect viral reverse transcription and plus strand DNA synthesis (126–130). Improvements in primary liver cell culture preparation and survival have also enabled the establishment of antiviral screening systems for DHBV (91,131,132), WHBV and GSHBV (133).

Problems in clinical treatment of chronic hepatitis B

Nucleoside analogues for inhibition of HBV in hepatocytes

Following the discovery that the replicative cycle of HBV involved an obligate RNA intermediate and a cytoplasmic reverse transcriptase step (Figure 15.3) it seemed logical to test a range of nucleoside analogues, known to inhibit reverse transcriptase, for anti-hepadnavirus activity. In fact, reverse transcriptase inhibitors were generally found to be effective in cell-free systems and in transfected, continuous cell lines (Table 15.2) but the results were not usually reproducible in primary hepatocyte cultures or in live animals. Clinical trials of some of these nucleoside analogues have been disappointing (see Table 15.2). These apparently conflicting findings can be explained by certain features of hepatic nucleoside metabolism, which makes treatment of HBV extremely problematic.

Unlike the larger DNA viruses such as the herpesviruses, which encode their own pyrimidine nucleoside kinase, thymidylate synthetase and ribonucleotide reductase (134), HBV does not encode enzymes for deoxynucleoside salvage, synthesis or nucleotide reduction. Three important consequences of this lack of a virus-specific means of nucleotide production are a reliance on host cell enzymes for supply of nucleotides for DNA and RNA synthesis, a corresponding lack of selectivity for nucleoside analogues used as antiviral agents (due to the need for phosphorylation of these drugs via cellular kinases in contrast to acyclovir and ganciclovir), and virus-specific targets for antiviral nucleoside analogues are restricted to the viral nucleic acid polymerases.

Two further problems are posed by the liver being a major site for catabolism of nucleic acid precursors. Firstly, at least in the intact liver, exogenously supplied purine and pyrimidine nucleosides and nucleotides are rapidly catabolized, a process which apparently requires cooperation between the various cell types (135,136). Secondly, hepatocytes are able to recycle endogenous nucleotides, derived mainly from RNA turnover (137). Consequently hepatocytes contain high (millimolar) concentrations of these endogenous nucleotides (135) which compete with nucleotide analogues for binding to HBV DNA polymerase, effectively diluting the antiviral effect of the analogue.

Thus, if nucleoside chemotherapy for viral hepatitis is to be successful, nucleoside analogues must be found which will resist catabolism, gain entry to hepatic nucleic acid precursor pathways via the very limited cellular resources and be phosphorylated to produce nucleotides which are stable yet not recognized as substrates by cellular polymerases. Extrahepatic foci of infection present quite different problems which must also be faced.

Extrahepatic reservoirs

Hepadnaviruses have been found in a number of extrahepatic sites (120,138). Hosoda *et al.* (139) have demonstrated DHBV replication in kidney, pancreas and spleen with low levels in brain, lung, heart and intestine. Extrahepatic replication of WHBV has been found in bone marrow, thymus, spleen, pancreas, kidney, ovary and testis (140). Studies with human HBV have reported the presence of HBV DNA in cells from the lymphoid system but the DNA forms detected were not typical replicative intermediates (141). However, Korba *et al.* (142) found that a productive viral replication did occur following mitogenic stimulation of WHBV-infected woodchuck peripheral blood lymphocytes bearing non-replicative viral DNA. Thus, a number of extrahepatic tissues could act as a reservoir of HBV even if successful antiviral therapy eliminated HBV infection from the liver.

Viral SC DNA

As shown in Figure 15.3, the key intermediate in HBV replication is viral SC DNA. It is the transcriptional template but does not self-replicate like the papovaviruses (143). Most importantly, it is unaffected by treatment with compounds which normally inhibit viral DNA synthesis such as the purine and pyrimidine nucleoside analogues and phosphonoformate (144–146). These agents are effective in inhibiting the formation of mature viral DNA (147). However, when treatment with these nucleic acid synthesis inhibitors is stopped, HBV synthesis is resumed via a continued generation of viral mRNA from the unaffected nuclear viral SC DNA template. The problem of viral SC DNA resistance to conventional antiviral agents in patients and in the animal model systems is compounded by the observation that the number of viral SC DNA molecules per cell is amplified during persistent infection by the intracellular conversion pathway (see Figure 15.3) (81). The copy number is maintained at approximately 50 copies per cell in chronically infected liver (81) but it is not known how rapidly the viral SC DNA decays if viral replication, the intracellular conversion pathway and viral reinfection are fully arrested. However, studies have indicated that the half-life of DHBV SC DNA is approximately three to five days (145b). HBV SC DNA generation and processing have been inhibited *in vitro* using compounds known to interfere with DNA topology, including the intercalating topoisomerase II inhibitors and the DNA gyrase inhibitor nalidixic acid (91). These important studies have been confirmed in live duck experiments (145a), and because of its oral bioavailability nalidixic acid certainly warrants further investigation as a potentially useful anti-hepadnaviral agent.

HBV variants

As discussed previously, pre-C and pre-S mutants of HBV have been associated with more severe, and often fulminating, hepatitis B. The most likely mechanism is direct viral cytotoxicity due to over-accumulation of viral structural proteins (pre-S1 or HBcAg) in pre-C variants and the hyper-amplification of viral SC DNA in the case of pre-S2 mutants. Treatment of infections due to these viruses must be directed at blocking multiple steps in the viral replication cycle.

Integrated HBV sequences

Although integration of viral DNA is not part of the normal life-cycle of HBV, viral DNA integration does occur during chronic infection, most likely as a result of illegitimate recombination (148). There is no preferred site on the human chromosome for integration, although HBV DNA most likely integrates through its DR-1/DR-2 region (52,87). In long-term carriers, integrated HBV DNA is frequently the major viral DNA form present in the liver. The integrated viral DNA is commonly rearranged, with inversion and deletions. The genome is interrupted in such a way that generation of the complete pregenome needed to make infectious virus is not possible (148). The S ORF is usually intact and many individuals with integrated viral DNA make only small-particle HBsAg. The gene products of the integrated viral DNA are associated with pathogenesis. For example, in WHBV-infected woodchucks, the risk factors in the development of hepatocellular carcinoma appear to be persistent antigenaemia and the presence of viral DNA forms in the liver (149).

Fibrosis

Fibrosis is an important component of advanced chronic inflammatory liver disease and in cirrhosis fibrosis is accompanied by cell necrosis and nodular regeneration (150). These are key elements in the overall pathophysiology of chronic liver disease. Hepatic fibrosis is a complex process involving changes in the amount of extracellular matrix components, activation of cells capable of producing matrix materials, cytokine release and tissue remodelling (151). Compounds such as Catergen ((+)-cyanidanol-3), a non-toxic, naturally occurring flavenoid, have been shown to inhibit fibrogenesis (152). Catergen exerts its hepatoprotective effect by scavenging free radicals and inhibiting hepatocyte membrane lipid peroxidation (153). IFN-α therapy has recently been shown to reduce the fibrogenic and proliferative activity in patients with chronic hepatitis C by inhibiting the expression of transforming growth factor (TGF)-β1 mRNA in the liver (154). In addition to being an inhibitor of liver cell DNA synthesis, TGF-β1 is associated with hepatic fibrosis (155,156).

In summary, a strategy for the successful treatment of HBV infection could comprise:

1. Inhibition of viral DNA replication, including viral SC DNA generation and processing.
2. Stimulation of immunomodulatory activity in order to enhance NK and T_H, and orchestrate Tc and pre-B cell activity.
3. Removal of the excess HBsAg load, thereby reducing the immunosuppressive effect and minimizing the intracellular accumulation of the viral envelope proteins including pre-S1.
4. Possible inhibition or minimization of fibrogenesis through the use of hepatoprotective drugs.

This combined approach should eradicate infected hepatocytes and prevent further infection of susceptible cells (105,145).

Clinical treatment of chronic hepatitis B

Most efforts in antiviral therapy of hepatitis B, and of viral hepatitis in general, have been in the treatment of chronic infection.

Antiviral agents (Tables 15.2 and 15.3)

There have been a large number of trials of anti-HBV agents over the last 15–20 years (Table 15.3). Taken in the overall context of eliminating the hepatitis B carrier state, these trials have had only marginal success and have given cause for no more than guarded optimism.

Initial studies on antiviral therapy of chronic hepatitis B focused largely on adenine arabinoside (ara-A; vidarabine) and its water-soluble derivative, adenine arabinoside monophosphate (ara-AMP) (187). Both are potent DNA polymerase inhibitors, but were withdrawn from investigative use in the United States and Western Europe because of substantial neuromuscular toxicity and a relative lack of efficacy in most clinical studies (190). Several early European trials (192–194) demonstrated a statistically significant remission (loss of HBeAg within one year of starting therapy) following ara-AMP therapy when compared to untreated control patients. In contrast, studies from the United States (188–190) failed to show any benefit. The disparity in response rates may be related to differences in the populations studied. For example, patients infected in neonatal life who may be tolerant to HBV, and homosexual patients who have a secondary immune deficiency state, do not respond (213). Interestingly, most trials of antiviral agents conducted on Mediterranean populations have yielded higher response rates than trials on northern European and Asian populations (213,214). The reasons for these differences are unclear.

Fiume *et al.* (191) extended the earlier observations with ara-AMP by treating patients with a conjugate of ara-AMP and lactosaminated human

Table 15.3. Antiviral agents of potential use in chronic hepatitis B

Agent	Refs
ara-AMP	(187–194)
ACV	(195,196)
GCV	(197,198)
Famciclovir	(129,130,183a)
Azidothymidine	(199)
2′,3′-Dideoxy-3′-thiacytidine (3TC)	(166)
Foscarnet	(198–201)
Thymosin α	(203)
IFN-γ	(204–206)
IFN-β	(204,206)
IFN-α	(207–212)

serum albumin. These investigators demonstrated inhibition of viral DNA replication at significantly reduced doses (almost five-fold) of ara-AMP apparently because the conjugate selectively entered hepatocytes. However, further studies on drug targeting are clearly required to establish the longer term benefits of such an approach.

Acyclovir (ACV) (215) and ganciclovir (GCV) (216) are potent antiviral agents used to treat herpes simplex (215) and cytomegalovirus infections (216). In the triphosphate form, both inhibit the HBV DNA polymerase *in vitro* (Table 15.2). However, ACV has only very mild effects on HBV replication *in vivo*, and results of prolonged treatment have been disappointing (208). ACV has been evaluated in combination with IFN-α but with only limited success (195).

In contrast, GCV significantly inhibits HBV DNA in patients also infected with human immunodeficiency virus (HIV) (197). These observations have been extended using the duck HBV model (91,144), with 30- to 50-fold reductions in serum and liver viral DNA levels being achieved during therapy. More recently, Angus and colleagues (198) have successfully used the combination of GCV with phosphonoformate (foscarnet) to control the very high levels of viral replication following HBV recurrence in patients undergoing orthotopic liver transplantation for end-stage chronic hepatitis B. Between one and two orders of magnitude of inhibition of viral DNA replication was achieved (198), with a greater than 90% reduction in the level of intrahepatic HBsAg expression. These changes were directly associated with an improved clinical benefit. Further studies are clearly required to establish the usefulness of this therapeutic protocol.

Orally active forms of nucleoside analogues with demonstrated anti-HBV activity are presently under development. For example, penciclovir and its oral form famciclovir (129,130) have recently been shown to significantly inhibit hepadnaviral DNA replication both *in vitro* (183a) and *in vivo* (183b). The availability of such compounds will certainly provide a stimulus for improvement in existing therapeutic protocols in the management of chronic hepatitis B carriers.

Azidothymidine has no effect on HBV DNA replication *in vivo* (199), despite its potent *in vitro* activity against HBV DNA polymerase when in the triphosphate form (161–163).

Similarly, foscarnet monotherapy has demonstrated only a modest inhibition of HBV replication (202) which was transient at the dosages used.

The interferons

To date, the best-studied and most promising agent for the treatment of chronic hepatitis B is interferon (IFN) (207,217,218). The IFNs are a family of naturally synthesized proteins produced in response to viral infections and other stimuli (219). There are three major forms: IFN-α, derived from monocytes and transformed B lymphocytes; IFN-β, originating primarily from fibroblasts; and IFN-γ, produced by activated T_H lymphocytes. All three types have broad antiviral and immunomodulatory properties, with IFN-α and IFN-β having more antiviral than immunomodulatory activity when compared to IFN-γ.

IFN was first explored as a therapy for chronic hepatitis B in the mid-1970s (220). Initial studies were hindered by the limited supply and the relatively impure material derived from buffy-coat leucocytes together with a lack of information on the dose and duration of treatment needed for a response to therapy. However, in the early 1980s advances in recombinant DNA technology led to the commercial production of genetically engineered forms of IFN, resulting in numerous, exploratory clinical trials in chronic hepatitis B infection (221–225). These studies also laid the foundation for understanding the mechanism of action of IFN in chronic hepatitis B and defined three types of response or outcome of treatment:

(i) *A transient response,* where a lowering of HBV markers (serum HBV DNA and DNA polymerase) is not sustained once therapy is stopped (Figure 15.6). During therapy a decrease in serum viral DNA levels is observed but there is no accompanying improvement in liver disease or long-term remission of hepatitis.

(ii) *A partial response,* defined by the disappearance of serum HBV DNA and clearance of HBeAg which is also associated with an improvement in the accompanying liver disease (Figure 15.7). These patients often have an exacerbation of their hepatitis (a hepatitic flare) 8–12 weeks after commencement of therapy coincident with the loss of HBeAg and clearance of HBV DNA from serum. Unlike the transient response group the accompanying liver disease improves, despite serum HBsAg persistence. The patient's symptoms generally resolve, the remission in disease activity is usually sustained, and the patient has completed the transition from chronic active hepatitis B (replicative phase) to the healthy, asymptomatic hepatitis B carrier state (non-replicative phase) (208,209). Serum HBV DNA and liver HBcAg are no longer present and all the intrahepatic replicative intermediates of HBV DNA, the SC DNA, SS DNA and RC DNA can no longer be found. Presumably, the continued HBsAg-antigenaemia is derived from integrated molecules of HBV DNA (147).

(iii) *A complete response* to IFN therapy is heralded by a loss of HBV DNA, HBeAg and HBsAg from serum (Figure 15.8). As with the partial response patient, loss of markers of active hepatitis B replication coincides with the 'seroconversion illness' 8–12 weeks after therapy has started. The loss of HBsAg and HBeAg is followed by reversal of the liver disease and a normalization of the serum aminotransferases. A substantial number of complete responders develop anti-HBs. These patients have no HBcAg or HBV DNA replicative intermediates in their follow-up liver biopsies (147,226).

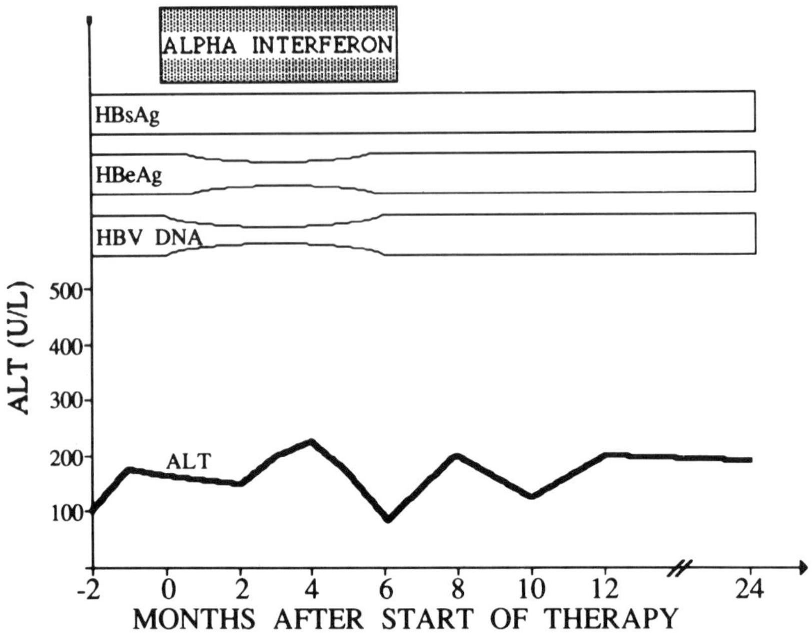

Figure 15.6. The clinical, serum biochemical, serological and virological course of a 'typical' patient with chronic hepatitis B who had only a transient response to therapy with IFN-α. During treatment, a slight decrease in serum viral DNA and HBeAg levels can be observed, but HBsAg persists with no change in the serum ALT pattern. Modified from Hoofnagle and Di Bisceglie (147). The dose of IFN is discussed in the text

These early investigations also provided valuable data on dose–response and safety and formed the basis for a number of multi-centred studies (207–210). The later studies confirmed that IFN-α can transform the replicating active phase of chronic hepatitis B infection to the non-replicative form. In summary, these studies have demonstrated:

(a) In highly selected groups of individuals infected with HBV (see below), 40–50% of those treated will permanently lose HBV DNA from serum and most of these will undergo seroconversion from HBeAg to anti-HBe (partial response, see Figure 15.7). This sustained suppression of HBV replication is associated with elimination of episomal HBV DNA from infected livers (226).

(b) More than half of the responders eventually lose HBsAg (217) and undergo virological cure of hepatitis B infection. Follow-up serum samples are HBV DNA negative (complete response, see Figure 15.8).

(c) Thrice weekly injections of IFN at doses of five million units or less

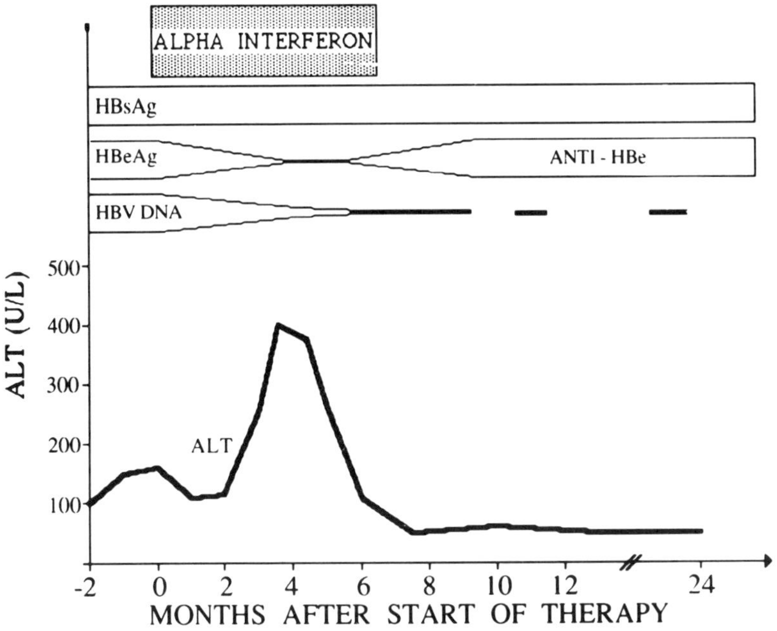

Figure 15.7. The clinical, serum biochemical, serological and virological responses of a 'typical' patient with chronic hepatitis B who had a partial response to therapy with IFN-α. During treatment, there is a steady decrease in serum HBV DNA and HBeAg, with HBV DNA only being detected by PCR, and HBeAg disappearing altogether, which is followed by the development of anti-HBe. This HBeAg seroconversion is associated with a flare in ALT (seroconversion illness), the patient remains positive for HBsAg and has a clinical remission in disease with serum ALT levels eventually falling to normal. Modified from Hoofnagle and Di Bisceglie (147). The dose of IFN is discussed in the text

inhibit viral replication as effectively and are better tolerated than higher, more frequent, dosing schedules. The side-effects of fatigue, muscle aching, changes in appetite and hair loss occur much less frequently at the lower dosage schedules.

(d) Successful therapy generally requires treatment for six months.

(e) As well as accelerating the transition from the replicative to the latent (non-replicative) phase, IFN also has a major impact on the associated liver disease. Over 80% of complete and partial responders normalize serum aminotransferase levels (207), and exhibit improved hepatic metabolic function (227) and histological features (207,210,218). These changes appear to be permanent (217).

(f) In patients demonstrating complete or partial responses following IFN therapy, the HBsAg clearance rate is approximately 15% per annum

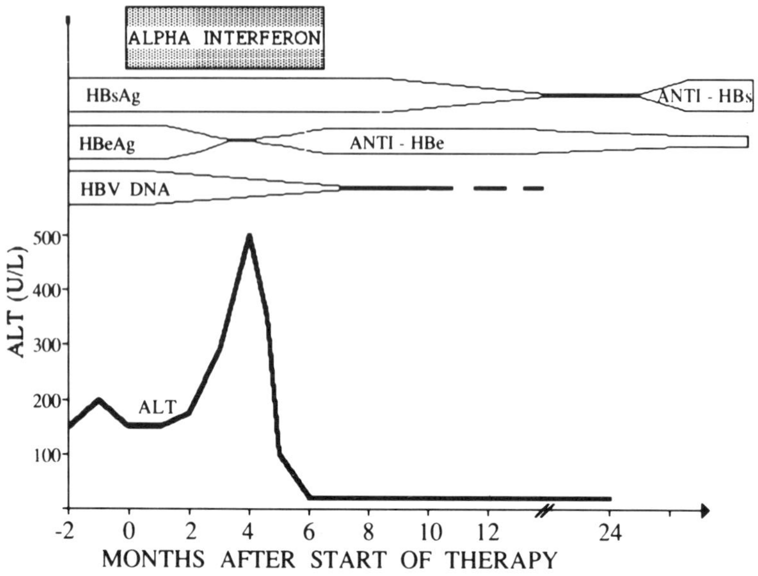

Figure 15.8. The clinical, serum biochemical, serological and virological responses of a 'typical' patient with chronic hepatitis B who had a complete response to therapy with IFN-α. During treatment, serum HBV DNA and HBeAg fall steadily as in a partial response and there is also a seroconversion illness during therapy. Following the development of anti-HBe, the titres of serum HBsAg begin to fall and eventually become negative and in some patients anti-HBs is produced. Serum HBV DNA is negative by PCR. Modified from Hoofnagle and Di Bisceglie (147) and Korenman *et al.* (217). The dose of IFN is discussed in the text

compared to the 2% annual clearance rate in untreated patients (217,228). The significantly accelerated clearance of HBV demonstrates that IFN therapy offers a true cure in many patients with chronic hepatitis B (218).

(g) All available forms of IFN-α, recombinant human IFN-αA (Roferon; Hoffman-La Roche, USA) (229,230), recombinant human IFN-α2b (Intron A; Schering Corporation, Kenilworth, USA) (207) and lymphoblastoid IFN (Wellferon; Burroughs Wellcome, Research Triangle Park, USA) (208) have a similar spectrum of activity and toxicity.

In summary, IFN therapy for chronic hepatitis B substantially alters what is otherwise a poor prognosis in many patients, especially those who have chronic active hepatitis B with cirrhosis (231). As well as antiviral and immunomodulating activity, IFN-α has recently been shown to inhibit fibrogenic activity in the liver (154) with beneficial effects on hepatic fibrosis.

Determinants of response: patient selection

The larger trials of interferon therapy in chronic hepatitis B have defined three major groups of patient responses:

Favourable outcome group Patients in this group demonstrate two major determinants: continuing HBV replication and underlying liver disease, usually chronic active hepatitis. Specifically, patients with low levels of serum HBV DNA (less than 100 pg/ml or 200 fmol/l) will have a better response rate to IFN compared to those with higher HBV DNA levels. Equally important, patients with an alanine aminotransferase (ALT) level greater than 150 U/l have a 50% chance of responding to IFN, but those with an ALT less than 100 U/l have less than a 20% chance of responding. Patients with a history of acute hepatitis or who have acquired hepatitis B infection within two years also have a good chance of responding, whereas those with lifelong infection usually do not respond. Unfortunately, this latter group includes most HBV carriers in the world, especially those born in the hyperendemic regions of Asia (207,226). Overall, only 40% (range 35–50%) of patients in this favourable group will respond (Figures 15.7 and 15.8) to IFN therapy.

Dubious outcome group Patients with more benign underlying liver disease (chronic persistent hepatitis) and with an ALT that is below 150 U/l but is more than 1.5 times the upper limit of normal usually have a much reduced response rate to IFN therapy. The response rate in this group is between 15% and 25% (232). Other patients in this category include those with high viraemias (HBV DNA greater than 100 pg/ml) including a subgroup who are infected with pre-C variants of HBV (233). During treatment of patients infected with pre-C mutants, the response rate is often higher than amongst HBeAg-positive patients (around 90%). However, as soon as treatment is completed almost every patient relapses or demonstrates reactivation (233). Brunetto *et al.* (234) have suggested that some of these patients benefit from therapy but require multiple courses.

Takeda *et al.* (235) were the first group to isolate precore mutants from patients undergoing IFN therapy. This phenomenon was confirmed by Gunther *et al.* (236) in six of nine patients, but emergence was not predictive of unsuccessful virus elimination. The emergence of the pre-C variants was paralleled by a drastic decrease of viraemia during treatment. The mutations appeared late after IFN therapy, coincident with anti-HBe seroconversion. Even more recently, Santantonio *et al.* (103) have described HBV variants with deletions in the pre-S2 region that appear not only during the natural course of infection, but also following IFN treatment. The exact pathological significance and clinical long-term outcome in these patients is presently unknown, but further detailed studies are clearly required.

Early studies suggested that male homosexuals and patients infected with HIV were less likely to respond to antiviral therapy than heterosexual patients (213). However, larger prospective studies have since failed to demonstrate a correlation between lack of response to treatment and sexual preference or even anti-HIV status (209). Thus, male homosexual patients who are HIV positive and who have high CD4 counts should not be excluded from IFN therapy if their chronic hepatitis B infection is severe. The response rate ranges between 15% and 30% in the short term, with longer-term follow-up demonstrating that some of these patients are prone to relapse and reactivation (147).

Studies in Asia, Europe and North America have revealed a strikingly lower response rate to IFN therapy amongst Oriental patients independent of HBV DNA levels (237,238). This probably reflects the fact that the majority of carriers in Asia acquired HBV perinatally, resulting in life-long carriage of the virus. It has been assumed that perinatal acquisition of HBV results in a degree of immunological tolerance to key epitopes of HBV required for clearance (111).

Low responses of antiviral therapy with IFN-α have also been reported in children. However, the majority of trials have been carried out in Asia (239). The difficulty in analysing results in children could be related to the observation that their chronic infection is usually mild, with low serum aminotransferase levels and high titres of HBV DNA. In this context Ruiz-Moreno *et al.* (240), in a prospective randomized control trial of IFN-α in Spanish children with chronic hepatitis B, demonstrated a partial response in almost 50% of them. The majority had acquired HBV postnatally, probably via intrafamilial spread, and all had abnormal ALT levels and active liver disease.

Unsuitable group Patients who are HBsAg positive but HBV DNA negative by dot blot hybridization, with ALT less than 1.5 times upper limit of normal, who are infected with HDV or who have severe cirrhosis with hepatic decompensation (serum albumin <30 g/l, prolonged prothrombin times and ascites), are unsuitable for IFN therapy because of the considerable risk of life-threatening IFN-induced decompensation. Patients with decompensated chronic hepatitis B have an extremely poor prognosis and currently can only be offered OLT, which itself has a poor relative outcome in this setting (241).

The major negative predictor of a response to IFN therapy is the presence of a complicating illness or immunosuppression. Very small numbers of patients with renal failure, immunological abnormalities, severe diabetes or concurrent immunosuppressive therapy (kidney, heart or liver transplants) have usually responded poorly to IFN-α therapy (147).

In summary, the three major positive determinants of response to IFN-α are high ALT, low HBV DNA (HBeAg positive), together with underlying chronic active hepatitis. Unfortunately, this represents only 20% of all patients with chronic infection (207,230). Even so, the positive long-term benefit of IFN-α therapy in these patients almost certainly represents a genuine cure (217,218) and should be pursued vigorously in the future.

Increasing the response rate: combination therapy

A more controversial aspect of the treatment of chronic hepatitis B has been the use of a short course or pulse of corticosteroids before starting antiviral therapy. Short courses of prednisone alone have been evaluated in controlled trials (242,243), and have led to transient decreases in aminotransferase levels but a marked increase in the titres of HBV DNA and HBsAg (244). HBV DNA contains a glucocorticoid responsive element (GRE) which interacts positively with the first enhancer to amplify HBV replication (Figures 15.2, 15.3). Thus, a pulse of prednisone could be dangerous. It is rarely followed by clearance of HBV DNA or HBsAg from serum and may actually be followed by a severe and prolonged exacerbation of disease activity (244). In patients with underlying cirrhosis, this hepatitic flare could have the undesirable and potentially fatal complications of variceal haemorrhage, hepatic encephalopathy or worsening of ascites (242,243).

Immunological priming provided by a short course of prednisone in combination with a subsequent course of IFN-α or ara-AMP has been evaluated in uncontrolled trials by several groups of investigators (189,223,245). Most studies claimed an enhancement of the response rate. Unfortunately none of these studies were adequately controlled. However, a recent randomized, controlled trial of steroid priming with IFN (207) established that in patients with low levels of ALT this approach could improve the otherwise poor response rate. In contrast, no extra benefit was observed in the group of patients with high levels of ALT. However, none of the data used to support this assertion reached statistical significance (232). Until a beneficial role for steroid priming is established, it is recommended to reserve this approach for patients who have already failed treatment with IFN-α alone or in patients who have mild disease (147).

Recombinant human IFN-β has been shown to inhibit HBV replication to a similar extent as IFN-α (204). IFN-β shares at least 70% homology with IFN-α, interacts with a common cell surface receptor and has a similar mechanism of action and toxicity profile (204). It is unlikely that a combination of IFN-α and IFN-β will offer any advantage over monotherapy. In contrast, IFN-γ has no homology with either IFN-α or IFN-β and acts on different cell surface receptors. In several studies in chronic hepatitis B, IFN-γ has less antiviral activity against HBV and more serious side-effects than IFN-α (204–206). The combination of IFN-γ and IFN-α did not offer any synergistic benefit over IFN-α alone (205).

A recent preliminary report has suggested that immunomodulatory thymosins, in particular thymosin α_1, may benefit patients with chronic active hepatitis B by permanently suppressing HBV replication (203). Thymosins are hormone-like polypeptides produced by thymus epithelial cells (246) and released into the peripheral circulation. Thymosin α_1 stimulates the *in vivo* production of IFN-α (247), and in the study of Mutchnick *et al.* (203) HBV DNA disappeared in responders after a transient increase in serum ALT. This observation suggests strongly that thymosin α_1, like IFN-α, precipitates the seroconversion illness that represents the immune-mediated clearance of HBV. Thymosin α_1 may prove to be as effective as IFN-α, with the advantage of being relatively free of significant side-effects (218).

Side-effects of interferons

The side-effects of IFN-α therapy in chronic hepatitis B fall into two patterns: effects occurring during the first days of therapy, and those that appear later (147).

At doses of IFN-α of 1 mU or greater, the first day of therapy is marked by the development of an influenza-like syndrome, 4–8 h after the first injection, which usually lasts 4–12 h. Associated fever, chills, muscle aches, headache and nausea can be ameliorated by paracetamol given a few hours before the expected onset of symptoms (248). These early side-effects decrease with subsequent injections, so that by the second week of therapy there are usually minimal amounts of muscle aches and low-grade fever (147).

The most troublesome side-effects of prolonged IFN-α therapy are fatigue, muscle aches and weight loss. These are usually dose-limiting. In up to 10% of patients, psychological side-effects can be severe enough to warrant altered dose or discontinuation of therapy (249). The major psychiatric side-effects are irritability and depression, which resolve within five days of cessation of therapy. Rarely, acute psychosis and severe depression can occur, but usually respond to discontinuation of treatment (250).

With IFN-α therapy in the dose range of 1–10 mU thrice a week some myelosuppressive effects can be expected. Neutropenia and thrombocytopenia are frequently observed in patients with cirrhosis and pre-existing bone marrow suppression. These toxic side-effects are reversed within a few weeks of discontinuing therapy (147). Probably as a consequence of the associated neutropenia, bacterial infections are the most important complication of IFN-α therapy. Urinary tract infections, sinusitis, bronchitis, septicaemia, lung and brain abscess and bacterial peritonitis have been reported during treatment (250).

Another important side-effect of IFN-α therapy is the development of autoantibodies with or without autoimmune disease (251). The most common is autoimmune thyroid disease, either hypo- or hyperthyroidism. Although more than 50% of patients develop autoantibodies, very few individuals develop clinical symptoms or signs of autoimmune disease. The appearance of autoimmunity with exacerbation of liver disease during IFN therapy may relate to an underlying autoimmune diathesis (252) and underscores the need for appropriate and thorough investigations of patients prior to commencement of treatment.

Summary

IFN-α has now been approved for use in hepatitis B in a large number of Western countries (232). A six-month course of IFN-α in doses of 5–10 mU three times a week results in a clinical, biochemical, serological and virological remission in 30–40% of patients with well-compensated liver disease who are serum HBeAg and HBV DNA positive (147,232). Careful case selection is imperative. Positive predictive factors for a response to treatment include high ALT and low levels of serum HBV DNA with underlying chronic active hepatitis. Pre-treatment of patients with low ALT using a corticosteroid is controversial, unproven and awaits the results of further controlled trials. Severe side-effects of IFN treatment amongst patients with chronic hepatitis B have been relatively infrequent, with few patients requiring dose reduction. Future studies will focus on newer immunomodulatory regimes such as thymosin α_1 (218) alone and in combination with newer antiviral agents targeted at key points in the replication life-cycle, including viral SC DNA (105,198).

Clinical treatment of fulminant hepatitis B

Fulminant viral hepatitis is a rare but serious complication of acute viral hepatitis B (200,201). The prognosis is grave, with only some 10–20% of patients surviving when grade IV coma is reached (253). The pathogenesis of fulminant hepatitis B is controversial. Brechot *et al.* (254) have shown that in the majority of cases multiplication of HBV has stopped by the time of onset of encephalopathy. However, in a subgroup of patients, HBV DNA can be detected in serum by dot blot hybridization (200). The only promising antiviral therapy to date has been infusions of phosphonoformate (201) (foscarnet), when three of four (75%) patients with fulminant hepatitis B who were HBV DNA positive on presentation survived (200). This outcome suggests that larger controlled studies of foscarnet should be undertaken.

Liver transplantation for hepatitis B

Hepatitis B virus-related liver disease may be an indication for OLT as a result of either cirrhosis due to chronic infection or, less commonly, fulminant hepatic failure due to acute infection (255). To date, the available evidence suggests that hepatitis B typically recurs following OLT for chronic hepatitis B and the long-term outcome is poor (256,257). In contrast, patients transplanted for fulminant acute hepatitis B appear generally to have a more benign course after recurrence of HBV infection (256,258).

The major determinant of the severity of recurrent hepatitis B post-transplantation appears to be the level of viral load prior to transplantation (258,259). Patients with chronic hepatitis B who are serum HBV DNA positive have more frequent and clinically more severe recurrences than patients without evidence of active viral replication (241). Therapeutic immunosuppression with high-dose steroids and cyclosporin A probably contributes to the enhanced severity of the HBV reinfection; HBV encodes a GRE which amplifies the enhancer activities of HBV DNA, and cyclosporin A has been shown to enhance WHBV replication (260).

A number of different approaches have been undertaken in an attempt to prevent or treat recurrent hepatitis B post transplantation. These have ranged from excluding HBV DNA positive patients from transplantation (259) to drug therapy aimed at suppressing hepatitis activity or viral replication in the graft. The use of IFN-α (261) and pooled human anti-HBs hyperimmune globulin (262) has met with very limited success. The immunological enhancement of HLA expression on the liver cells of the graft with the use of IFN poses a theoretical risk of graft rejection (255). Angus and colleagues (198) have recently described the use of combination chemotherapy with phosphonoformate and GCV to control very severe recurrence of HBV post transplantation. This treatment resulted in a greater than 30-fold reduction in serum HBV DNA and HBsAg levels, which was associated with the normalization of liver function and dramatic clinical improvement. If confirmed, such combination treatment offers a new therapeutic option in the management of severe HBV-induced disease.

HEPATITIS D

Introduction and epidemiology

Hepatitis D virus (HDV), also known as the hepatitis delta virus, is capable of replication only in persons who are also infected with HBV. Present evidence indicates that HDV needs the HBV envelope proteins to infect and exit hepatocytes, whilst the rest of its unusual life-cycle appears to be independent of HBV.

Transmission of HDV occurs by the same routes as for hepatitis B. Infection with HDV may occur either simultaneously with HBV (co-infection) or subsequent to HBV infection (superinfection), as either an acute or chronic illness (10). Both acute and chronic delta hepatitis tend to be severe, and HDV infection is generally considered to be the severest form of viral hepatitis and an important cause of fulminant hepatitis. In HDV-infected chimpanzees, the duration and magnitude of the hepatitis were directly related to the level and duration of hepatitis delta antigen (HDAg) expression (263). Thus, unlike HBV, HDV is directly cytopathic to hepatocytes, with recent evidence demonstrating that the p24 form of the delta antigen is the cytotoxic viral protein (264).

Hoofnagle (265) described the major epidemiological patterns of HDV infection: an endemic pattern which is found in certain populations where a high level of chronic hepatitis B carriage exists such as in the Mediterranean and Middle East, localized epidemics which have occurred amongst isolated communities where a high level of chronic hepatitis B carriers exist (i.e. superinfection) such as in Central America, and minor epidemics which occur in certain high-risk groups such as intravenous drug users and male homosexuals (mixed co-infection and superinfection). A fourth pattern has recently emerged in the setting of OLT, where HDV can establish a latent infection without the assistance of HBV (266). In this situation, HDV replication is independent of HBV in the first four to six months post OLT and the patient is asymptomatic. Then HBV replicative effects become apparent from six to eight months post OLT and the patient experiences severe hepatitis (241). Following transplantation, HDV seems to be neither directly pathogenic nor dependent on HBV for survival; cooperation with HBV is required only for the expression of disease.

Molecular virology

Rizzetto *et al.* (267) first discovered HDV whilst studying liver biopies from patients known to be infected with HBV but who presented with unexpectedly severe liver disease. Using antibodies derived from these patients these workers demonstrated the presence of a novel nuclear antigen not found in other individuals infected with HBV. This antigen, designated delta by Rizzetto *et al.* (267), was subsequently shown by transmission studies in chimpanzees to be part of an infectious agent that was superinfecting the hepatitis B carrier populations in Italy at the time (263). HDV is a 36 nm particle containing a 1.7 kb RNA molecule, the HDAg, surrounded by an envelope of HBsAg. Chimpanzee transmission studies determined that HDV was a defective virus which required a helper function provided by HBV for HDAg expression and HDV replication (263). Ponzetto *et al.* (268) subsequently transmitted HDV to woodchucks and demonstrated that the helper function and envelope can also be supplied by WHBV and WHBsAg respectively. In the serum of an infected host, the titre of HDV can be as high as 2×10^{11} infectious units per millilitre (269). The actual number of particles containing HDV RNA is similar, suggesting that the specific infectivity under optimal conditions is close to one (270).

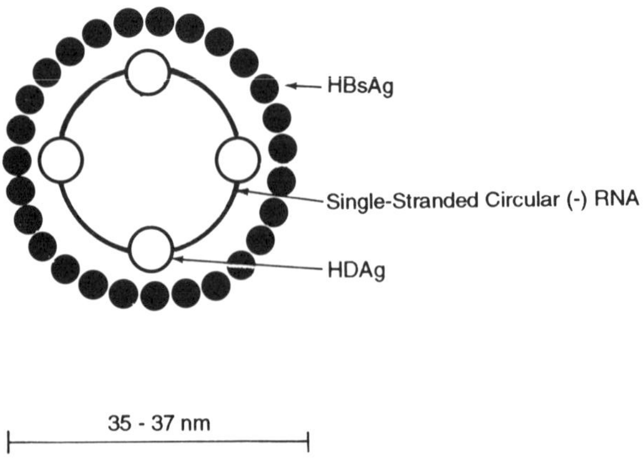

Figure 15.9. The structural components of the hepatitis delta virus. The outer envelope is comprised of HBsAg and the viral RNA is very closely associated with HDAg. Modified from Locarnini and Gust (49)

The virus

HDV particles can be distinguished from hepadnavirus particles by differences in density and sedimentation values (271,272). HDV particles lack a demonstrable core structure and are heterogeneous in diameter, with a mean of 36 nm (273) (see Figure 15.9).

The major interaction of HDV with HBV occurs during packaging, with HBV providing the final coat for HDV. Bonino *et al.* (272) have demonstrated differences in the relative amounts of the various related forms of HBV surface antigen in HDV as compared with HBV so the assembly process is selective. This analysis revealed values which are closer to the composition of the 22 nm form of HBsAg than to the complete HBV (Table 15.4).

Table 15.4. Distribution of HBV and HDV gene products in the various forms of HBV and HDV

HBV/HDV gene product	HBV and filaments	HBsAg (22 nm forms)	HDV
Pre-S1 [p39, gp42]	90%	Trace	Trace
Pre-S2 [gp33, gp30]	5%	Trace	Trace
S [p24, gp27]	5%	99%	Major
C [p22]	Yes	No	No
HDAg [p24, p27]	No	No	Major

Modified from Locarnini and Gust (49) and Bonino *et al.* (272).

HDV RNA

Inside HDV particles is a small single-stranded, circular RNA molecule of about 1700 bases (274) (see Figure 15.10). It does not contain poly(A) sequences and does not share homology with HBV DNA or host cell DNA (270). HDV RNA has a high degree of secondary structure and Wang *et al.* (274) have shown that it has the ability to fold onto itself by base-pairing to form an unbranched rod structure, similar to the plant viroids (275).

In infected cells, both HDV genomic RNA (minus sense) and antigenomic RNA (plus sense) can be detected. Analysis of the nucleotide sequences of both forms has revealed several potential ORFs (274,276,277). Only one ORF, ORF 5, expressed on the antigenomic RNA (Figure 15.10), functions during infection and encodes the HDAg.

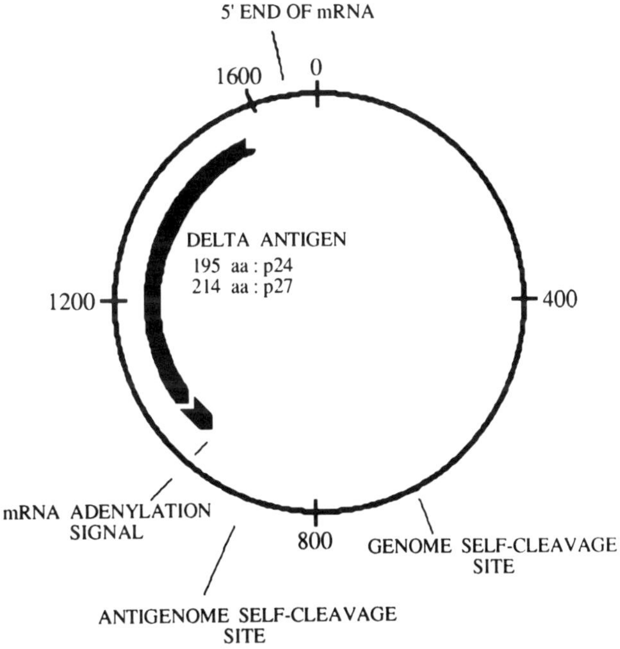

Figure 15.10. Physical and genetic map of HDV RNA. The 1679 nt sequence of Kuo *et al.* (299) is shown with the genome orientated clockwise. The coding regions for the small (1589–1010, 195 amino acids) and large (1598–953, 214 amino acids) forms of HDAg on the antigenome (counter-clockwise), along with the 5′ end (1631) and polyadenylation site (1934), are shown. The sites of self-cleavage on the genome-antigenome are indicated at 685/686 and 900/901 respectively. Modified from Taylor (270)

The delta antigen

Immunoblot analyses of liver and serum samples from HDV-infected animals have revealed two electrophoretic patterns of the HDAg p24 and p27 (272,278). This heterogeneity arises from a unidirectional mutation at a single nucleotide in the termination codon for delta antigen (codon: 196 UAG→UGG), which occurs during replication (279) and results in a truncated 195 amino acid long form (p24) and a full-length antigen (p27) which is identical in sequence except for an additional 19 amino acids at the C-terminus (see Figure 15.10). The HDV genome encoding p24 is referred to as the S (small) genome whilst the genome encoding p27 is referred to as the L (large) genome. Except for the single base change described above, there is no other difference between the two (280).

A number of important features have been derived from the predicted amino acid sequences of HDAg. Both the small and large forms contain the same RNA genome-binding domain (281) and act as RNA-binding proteins (282). Chao *et al.* (283) have noted a sequence with strong similarity to the nuclear localization signal of the glucocorticoid receptor protein. Lai *et al.* (284) have noted the presence of ordered leucines in HDAg consistent with a leucine zipper, to facilitate protein–protein interactions. The large form of HDAg has been shown by Chang *et al.* (281) to be modified *in vivo* by phosphorylation at serine residues. Recently, Glenn *et al.* (280) identified a prenylation fatty acid site at the C-terminus of large HDAg. This group also demonstrated that the large, but not the small HDAg produced secreted particles when co-expressed with HBV surface antigen, implicating this prenylation site as important in HDV morphogenesis.

Replication strategy

HDV replicates via RNA-directed RNA synthesis. An infected liver contains up to 300 000 copies of HDV RNA per cell, with approximately 80% genomic and 20% antigenomic RNA (270). In addition to these two major species of unit length, there are small amounts of multimeric forms. More than half of the unit length and multimeric forms are circular. Taken together, these observations strongly suggest that HDV, like RNA plant pathogens, replicates its RNA by a double rolling circle mechanism (285) (see Figure 15.11). In contrast to HBV, all of these RNA species are predominantly located in the nucleus of infected hepatocytes (286,287). However, a minor species of 800 bases and poly(A)+, the putative mRNA for HDAg, is largely localized to the cytoplasm (288,289).

For HDV RNA to produce unit-length circular RNA, a series of self-cleavage and self-ligation reactions that are specific (one site per molecule) and efficient are required (285) (see Figure 15.11). Sharmean *et al.* (290,291) demonstrated that HDV RNA has the ability to undergo *in vitro* self-cleavage

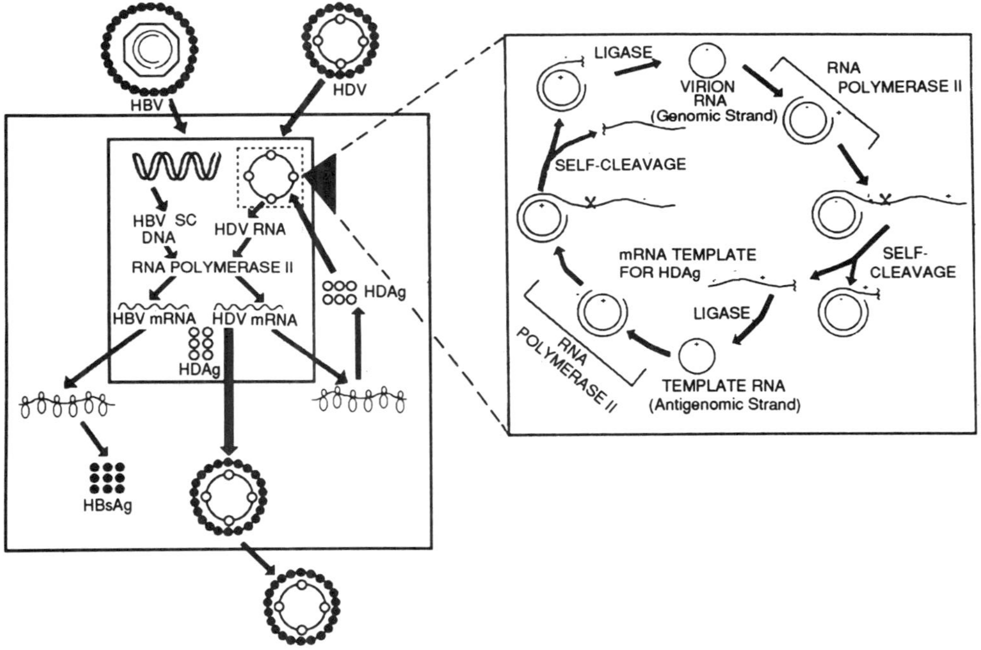

Figure 15.11. The replication cycle of HDV. A cell is co-infected with HDV and HBV or a HBV-infected cell is superinfected with HDV. The viruses are uncoated and both the genomes transported to the nucleus. The small HDAg is required for RNA replication and is shown attached to HDV RNA (see Figure 15.9). Viral mRNA is transcribed from both viral templates using host cell RNA polymerase II. Viral proteins are translated and HDAg is transported back to the nucleus. The HDV replicates its RNA by the rolling circle model; the endonuclease and ligase activities are non-enzymatic and are performed at the autocatalytic sites on the HDV genome. The new genomic HDV RNA, with HDAg attached, is transported to the cytoplasm and enveloped by HBsAg. Modified from Taylor (270) and Hoofnagle and Di Bisceglie (147)

and self-ligation reactions through *trans*-esterifications of the RNA. The two self-cleavage sites on HDV genomic and antigenomic RNA are very similar in sequence and have been mapped to positions 688/689 and 904/905 respectively (292) (see Figure 15.10). The self-cleavage of the antigenomic strand is downstream from the HDAg mRNA polyadenylation signal and mRNA adenylation site (270) (see Figure 15.10).

Viral RNA synthesis requires a host polymerase, RNA polymerase II—the same enzyme that utilizes the hepadnaviral transcriptional template. This was demonstrated by Macnaughton *et al.* (293), using an *in vitro* transfected cell model, who showed that HDV RNA replication was resistant to actinomycin D, but sensitive to 1.0 μg/ml of α-amanitin. Thus, RNA polymerase II must switch templates from double-stranded DNA to single-stranded RNA.

The HDAg, at 24–27 kDa, is too small to act alone as an RNA polymerase. The HDAg is a basic protein which is normally phosphorylated at serine residues (281) and binds HDV RNA. Even though HDAg is packaged, it does not form a capsid structure (Figure 15.10). The small HDAg is required for HDV RNA replication, whilst large HDAg is a potent *trans*-dominant inhibitor of this process (294). Evidence has now been obtained for specific HDV sequence changes occurring during genome replication that lead to the synthesis of the two species of HDAg. During HDV replication, S genomes (encoding p24) mutate to L genomes (encoding p27) through the codon change at position 196. At least two effects attributable to this mutation can be distinguished. The first is the conversion of an enhancer of genomic replication (small HDAg) into a potent *trans*-dominant inhibitor (large HDAg) (270,295). This dramatic difference in function is determined solely by the nature of the C-terminal amino acid, with proline being sufficient to confer enhancer activity (294). The second effect is the addition of a CXXX box to HDAg, which allows the protein to be prenylated (large HDAg) and presumably promote its incorporation into HBsAg-containing particles (280). The combined effects of the switch from production of small HDAg to large HDAg appear to have two roles: to suppress further genome replication and to promote the onset of packaging and HDV morphogenesis. Thus, during acute HDV infection, there is high-level expression of small HDAg (p24) with low levels of large HDAg (p27), whereas in chronic HDV infection this process is reversed.

Interaction with hepadnaviruses

Superinfection of hepatitis B carriers with HDV results not only in HDV expression and replication, but also a striking reduction in HBV replication (263). This interference of HDV with HBV replication is not fully understood but could be explained on the basis of more successful competition of HDV RNA for host cell RNA polymerase II and other key enzymes and substrates in the nuclei of infected cells. Whether HDV RNA has ribozyme activity or not is presently unclear (270,296). Also, the presence of HDV double-stranded RNA in infected cells could readily promote the RNase L and protein kinase pathways after IFN exposure. Importantly, viral double-stranded RNA in its own right is quite toxic to cells.

Potential targets for antiviral chemotherapy

HDAg is the major protein produced from HDV RNA. To date, there is no evidence for any other virus-specified proteins which could be potential targets for selective antiviral inhibition as the virus utilizes cellular RNA polymerase II to direct its RNA-dependent RNA synthesis (270). The cycle of HDV RNA replication includes several points at which double-stranded RNA is present (Figure 15.11), suggesting a possible role for IFN-α in therapy. The identification of a prenylation site on HDAg (280) has suggested several strategies to interfere with HDV, although the viral specificity of such compounds remains in doubt (280).

Laboratory diagnosis

Acute hepatitis delta co-infection and superinfection can be distinguished by clinical outcome and the use of specific serological markers (265,297). Acute delta co-infection is associated with acute hepatitis B virus infection and the serological course of a typical case is shown in Figure 15.12. Hepatitis B surface antigen followed by HDV RNA and HDV antigen are first detectable during the incubation period of the disease. Thereafter, serum aminotransferase levels begin to rise and clinical symptoms and jaundice appear. The pattern of elevations in serum aminotransferase levels is often biphasic. With the clearance of HBsAg, HDV replication and acute liver disease resolve. Antibody to HDV (anti-HDV) rises shortly after the onset of symptoms and is often of short duration and low titre. Several serum samples should be tested for anti-HDV IgM, and HDV antigen is usually only detectable in the early stages of infection. Patients with acute hepatitis delta co-infection will also have anti-HBc IgM in the acute-phase serum samples.

In contrast to delta co-infection, acute delta superinfection often leads to chronic hepatitis. Chronic HDV infection is often severe, and can lead to cirrhosis in up to 70% of patients (305). The progression to cirrhosis can be quite rapid and chronic hepatitis delta has a poor prognosis. It is also more easily recognized as most patients have rising titres of anti-HDV total and IgM (Figure 15.13). Since this form of infection occurs against a background of chronic HBV infection, the anti-HBc IgM is usually absent from acute-phase serum specimens. Chronic delta infection is easily diagnosed in those patients who have high titres of total anti-HDV in serum, but the detection

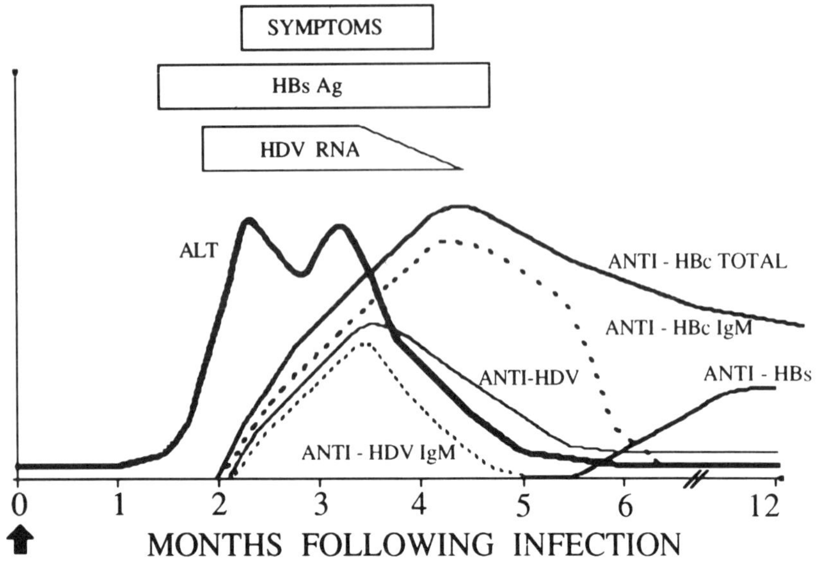

Figure 15.12. The clinical, serum biochemical, serological and virological responses of a 'typical' patient with acute delta co-infection. The ALT abnormalities can often be biphasic. The serological hallmark of delta co-infection is the presence of anti-HBc IgM, and transient anti-HDV IgM. Modified from Locarnini and Gust (49) and Hoofnagle (265)

of HDV RNA in serum is probably the most sensitive test of ongoing HDV infection. In assessing effects of antiviral therapy, tests for HDV RNA in serum are important and its rapid decrease from the serum is convincing evidence of effective therapy (298).

Experimental models

As discussed above, HDV infection occurs naturally in humans, and experimental transmission has been achieved in chimpanzees (263,305) and woodchucks (268). With these systems available, it has been possible to study the replication of HDV and the interactions between HDV and the helper hepadnavirus.

As with HBV, full-length cDNA clones of the HDV genome have been generated and multimers of this clone have been inserted into eukaryotic expression vectors. Kuo *et al.* (299) and Macnaughton *et al.* (282) have constructed trimers of HDV cDNA, which on transfection of liver and non-liver cell lines lead to synthesis of HDV genomes via RNA-dependent RNA synthesis. Such studies have provided evidence that there is no need for HBV functions in this process, thereby confining the role of HBV in the

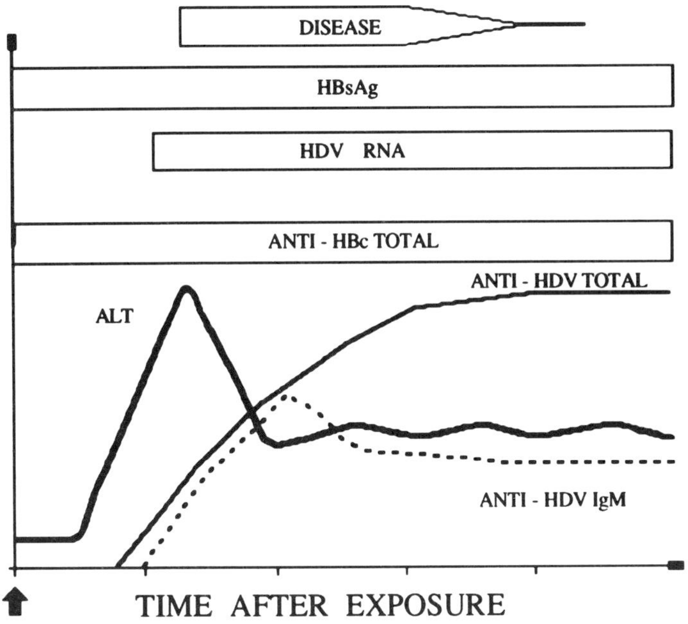

Figure 15.13. The clinical, serum biochemical, serological and virological responses of a 'typical' patient with acute delta superinfection. This patient has developed chronic delta infection. The serological hallmark of delta superinfection is the presence of anti-HBc IgG, and persistent anti-HDV IgM. Modified from Locarnini and Gust (49) and Hoofnagle (265)

life-cycle of HDV to packaging and virus entry (270). These studies also demonstrated that there is no requirement for liver-specific functions (283).

Primary cultures of woodchuck hepatocytes are susceptible to infection by HDV passaged through a woodchuck chronically infected with WHBV (300,301). Sureau *et al.* (302) have recently demonstrated that primary cultures of chimpanzee hepatocytes can also support HDV replication.

Using primary cultures of woodchuck hepatocytes, Petcu *et al.* (303) and Choi *et al.* (304) have shown that suramin acts on both HDV and HBV and blocks virus entry. Choi *et al.* (304) also studied the effects of α-amanitin, ACV and ribavirin and found that α-amanitin displayed weak inhibitory effects and ACV had no demonstrable effect. Interestingly, ribavirin inhibited HDV replication at a concentration of 10 μg/ml, but based on the current understanding of ribavirin's mechanism of action and HDV replication strategy, the antiviral effect of ribavirin was most likely indirect, possibly via cellular toxicity.

The recent availability of these model systems will provide ample opportunity in the future to evaluate a wider range of antiviral compounds and therapeutic treatment strategies for their effect(s) on HDV and HBV replication.

Clinical treatment of chronic hepatitis D

There is presently no established or effective therapy for either acute or chronic hepatitis D. Prednisone, azathioprine, levamisole and adenine arabinoside have been shown to be ineffective (305). The use of IFN-α has been most extensively studied (147).

A number of pilot studies with IFN-α have been undertaken (306,307) and each one has suggested that therapy decreases serum HDV RNA and HDAg levels and results in amelioration of disease in approximately 50% of patients. Serum levels of virus and serum aminotransferase activities also decrease rapidly. End of treatment liver biopsies revealed histological improvement and disappearance of hepatitis delta antigen from the liver. However, discontinuation of therapy, even after 12 months, was almost invariably followed by relapse of disease activity and reappearance of serum and liver markers of HDV replication (Figure 15.14).

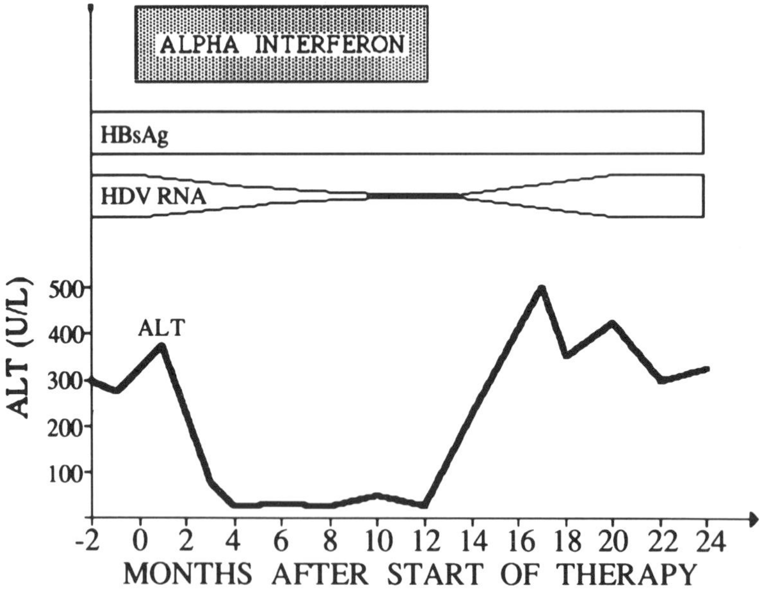

Figure 15.14. The clinical, serum biochemical, serological and virological responses of a 'typical' patient with chronic delta hepatitis who had been treated with a 12-month course of IFN-α. During therapy, there is an improvement in the serum aminotransferase abnormalities and a decrease in serum HDV RNA. However, on cessation of therapy a relapse in disease activity and viral replication is almost invariably observed. Modified from Hoofnagle and Di Bisceglie (147)

In conclusion, IFN-α therapy of chronic delta hepatitis appears to result in lowered serum aminotransferase levels in contrast to that occurring during treatment of chronic hepatitis B (Figures 15.7 and 15.8) and produces histological improvement in over 50% of patients. This is usually accompanied by temporary inhibition of HDV replication. However, this improvement is not sustained. This suggests that long-term or continuous therapy with IFN-α may be required in chronic delta hepatitis. The usefulness of this form of treatment may be limited by the side-effects of IFN, which may be particularly severe in those patients with advanced or decompensated liver disease.

Therapy should begin with a dose of 5 mU daily and continued for at least two months. If a beneficial effect on HDV RNA levels and serum aminotransferase activities is observed, therapy should be continued indefinitely (147). The dose of IFN-α should only be decreased if side-effects are intolerable. The decision to discontinue IFN-α should only be made if HBsAg becomes negative or if the liver biopsy shows no evidence of continued disease activity with or without markers of active HDV replication (147). The role of OLT for hepatitis D is emerging as an alternative approach to current antiviral treatment strategies (see below).

Clinical treatment of fulminant hepatitis D

Fulminant hepatitis is more likely if HBV occurs as a co-infection with HDV, or if HDV superinfects a chronic hepatitis B carrier, than when HBV is the sole aetiological agent of the severe hepatitis (308–310). Hedin *et al.* (200) successfully treated three of four cases of fulminant hepatitis B and D co-infection with continuous infusions of phosphonoformate. The 75% survival rate was a significant improvement over the untreated survival rate of less than 20% (311). These preliminary results are encouraging, but the mechanism of action of phosphonoformate in these cases is unclear.

Sanchez-Tapias *et al.* (312) treated nine patients with acute fulminant delta hepatitis with IFN-α. Only two survived, one of whom later developed chronic delta hepatitis and cirrhosis. Thus, it would appear that IFN had little effect in this disease. The present recommendation concludes that antiviral therapy of fulminant delta hepatitis should probably be used only in a situation where OLT is available if the disease progresses (147). Survival after liver transplantation for fulminant hepatitis delta is surprisingly good, ranging from 50% to 70% (241,313).

Liver transplantation for hepatitis D

The combined experience from North American and European centres (241,258,314,315) has suggested that hepatitis D probably recurs less often than HBV after liver transplantation. However, it is important to note that the interpretation of the findings in all these series has been confounded by the administration of hepatitis B immune globulin (HBIg) prophylaxis to all patients. Agnes *et al.* (316) described three patients not given HBIg in whom HDV and HBV infection recurred.

It is possible that failure to detect serum (or hepatic) markers of HBV infection whilst only HDV antigens are detected in the new graft (315) might reflect the effect of HBIg and does not signify complete clearance of HBV infection. This seemingly lower risk of recurrent HDV and HBV infection after OLT may reflect selective inhibition of HBV replication by HDV (265,266). Rizzetto *et al.* (266) have suggested that clinically significant HDV graft infection is found only with associated HBV reinfection and that, in the absence of HBV, HDV does not lead to graft dysfunction. Taylor (270) has further speculated that the reason for the better prognosis of OLT in patients with prior HDV infection is that the spread of HDV in the new graft provides enhanced resistance to infection with HBV. The possibility of using modified HDV (280) as a therapeutic agent will require extensive testing in suitable *in vitro* and *in vivo* models before clinical application is possible.

HEPATITIS C

Introduction and epidemiology

Hepatitis C virus (HCV) is the major cause of parenterally transmitted non-A, non-B hepatitis. There are at least 100 million HCV carriers in the world and the number of new cases each year has been estimated to be 175 000 in the United States and Western Europe collectively and 350 000 in Japan (13). Infection with HCV occurs predominantly by blood or blood products and also infrequently by sexual intercourse as well as vertically from infected mothers to their babies. However, in a significant proportion of cases, the mode of transmission is not defined. Clinically, classical hepatitis C resembles other forms of viral hepatitis (317,318) and at least 75% of cases are anicteric. A fluctuating course of aminotransferase activities (ranging from normal to 10-fold elevated) is typical. However, the most characteristic feature of the disease is its propensity to progress to chronic hepatitis. In prospective studies of cases following blood transfusion, 40–60% of cases infected with HCV develop biochemical or histological evidence of chronic liver disease (319,320) and half of these have chronic active hepatitis. Sporadic cases of hepatitis C are also likely to result in the development of chronic hepatitis (321). The incubation period ranges from 8 to 14 weeks (322).

Chronic hepatitis C is often mild or asymptomatic and its course can be prolonged and insidious. Most patients do not develop symptoms for more than 10 years after the onset of chronic infection. Unlike hepatitis B, the pathogenesis of the HCV-related liver disease appears to be due to the cytopathic effect of the virus rather than to the host immune response. Recent data have suggested that HCV-related cirrhosis is an important aetiological factor in HCC, especially in developed countries (323). It has been estimated that at least 20% of patients will develop cirrhosis, with a median time of 18 years, whilst the development of HCC will take a median of 24 years (13). Hepatitis C is clearly a significant cause of morbidity and mortality from liver disease and an effective treatment is needed.

Molecular virology

Only limited information is presently available on the structure, biochemical and biophysical properties of HCV. Filtration studies have shown that the diameter of infectious HCV is less than 80 nm (324), it exhibits a buoyant density of 1.09–1.11 g/cm^3 in sucrose density gradients (325) and has a sedimentation coefficient of approximately 150–200 S (326). HCV is an enveloped virus, and its infectivity is destroyed by extraction with chloroform (327,328) and by heating at 60 °C for 30 min (329).

A large number of HCV isolates have been cloned and sequenced (330). The virus contains a positive-stranded RNA genome comprising approximately 9400 nucleotides (nt) (331–333). This sequence contains a 340 nt long 5′ non-translated region (NTR), a single ORF which encodes a polyprotein of 3010/3011 amino acids (331,332) and a variable, short 3′ untranslated region (332,334). The 5′ terminal NTR represents the most highly conserved sequences (331–335), suggesting an important regulatory role during viral replication. The presence of a large polyprotein, the overall genetic organization, and sequence motifs indicating proteinase-helicase (NS-3) and viral polymerase (NS-5) activity, place HCV as a distant relative of the human flaviviruses and animal pestiviruses (336) probably occupying a third genus in the family Flaviviridae (337). The small 3′ NTR downstream from the large ORF contains between 27 and 55 nt depending on the HCV isolate (334). The presence of a poly(rA) tract at the 3′ terminus has not been confirmed (332–334).

A scheme for the genomic organization of HCV is shown in Figure 15.15. As for the flavivirus and pestivirus groups, HCV encodes a large polyprotein precursor from which individual viral proteins (both structural and non-structural) are processed co-translationally and/or post-translationally through the combined action of host-encoded and viral-encoded proteinases (330). The viral structural proteins are processed from the N-terminal end of the polyprotein, whilst the non-structural proteins are processed from the remaining polyprotein product. The structural proteins include a nucleocapsid (core or C) protein of 19 kDa which has RNA-binding properties (330) as well as two glycoproteins of approximately 33 kDa and 72 kDa. Comparison with the pesti- and flaviviruses indicates that gp33 corre-

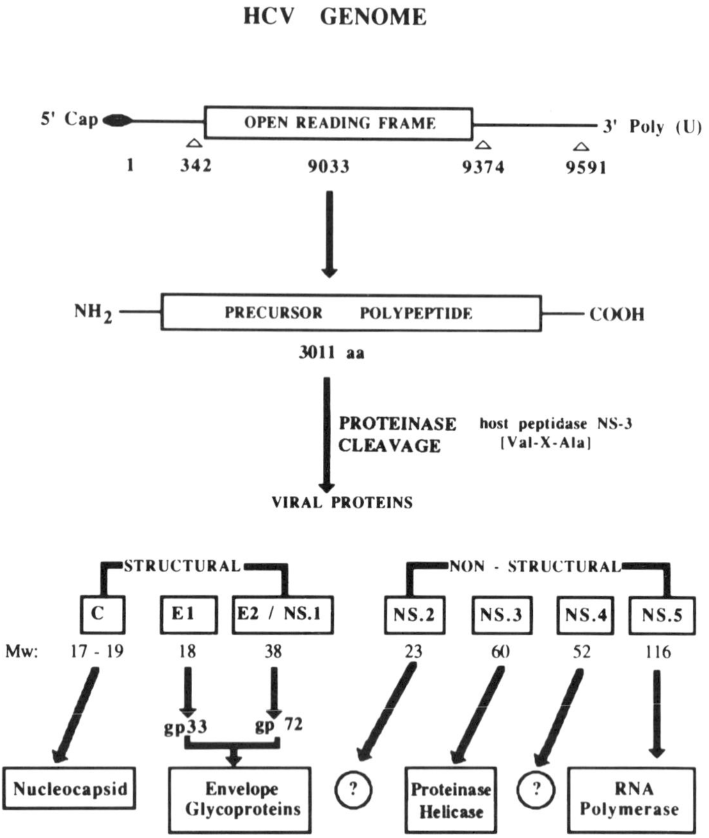

Figure 15.15. The physical and genetic map of HCV RNA. The observed and potential sizes of the viral proteins are shown in kilodaltons along with their proposed functions. The envelope proteins are heavily glycosylated (gp). Modified from Houghton *et al.* (330)

sponds to the matrix/envelope glycoprotein (E1) in the virion, whilst gp72 corresponds to the major viral envelope glycoprotein (E2/NS-1). There are 19 putative *N*-glycosylation sites, mostly clustered between amino acid 196 and 647 (338), corresponding to the envelope (E1/E2/NS-1) regions. The function of NS-2 is unknown but the protein is hydrophobic (331) and is found in association with cell membranes (330). The NS-3 protein contains a nucleoside triphosphate-binding helicase motif likely to be involved in unwinding the RNA genome for replication, and a serine proteinase involved in cleavage of the NS proteins from the polyprotein precursor (339). Like NS-2, the NS-4 protein is hydrophobic and probably membrane bound, but its function is not known. The NS-5 contains the RNA-dependent RNA polymerase motif that replicates RNA genomes.

Viral diversity

Comparison of the nucleotide sequences of several geographically distinct isolates indicates that HCV is heterogeneous, with sequence variability up to 40% (340,341). The E1 and E2/NS-1 envelope regions are particularly variable. Such heterogeneity is a feature of single-stranded RNA viruses (342). Based on these observations, HCV can be divided into at least three groups (330), with group I isolates (HCV-H) originating in the United States (343) and groups II and III circulating in Japan (332,341), with more genotypes being characterized presently.

Comparison of the different groups reveals a highly conserved 5′ NTR and a well-conserved core region. The E1 and E2/NS-1 domains demonstrate considerable heterogeneity, with conserved, moderately variable (V1, V2, V3), and hyper-variable (HVR-1 and HVR-2) sequence compartments alternating (330,338,344). Heterogeneity is also observed in the NS-3, NS-4 and NS-5 regions of the different HCV groups (330). This heterogeneity has implications not only for serological diagnosis but also for understanding the nature of the virus–host interaction, the evolution of chronic liver disease (345), host response to IFN-α therapy and development of effective vaccines. For example, Pozzato *et al.* (346) have found that with the Japanese type (groups II and III) HCV RNA is associated with more serious liver disease and with a poor response to IFN therapy.

Replication strategy: implications for pathogenesis and antiviral chemotherapy

Liver injury due to chronic infection with HCV is associated with characteristic alterations in the cytoplasm of infected hepatocytes in both humans and chimpanzees (325). These include dense reticular inclusion bodies, convoluted membranes derived from proliferated smooth endoplasmic reticulum, bundles of granular microtubules and characteristic tubular structures (from which HCV initially earned the name the tubule-forming agent) (329). Similar changes have been observed in cells infected with other RNA viruses (329) as well as a result of host cell-specific responses such as IFN (347).

The mechanism of HCV-associated liver injury is not fully understood, and factors other than cytocidal replication of HCV in hepatocytes may be involved. However, the pathogenesis of the HCV-related liver disease appears to be due mainly to the cytopathic effect of the virus rather than to the host immune response. The type, extent and distribution of HCV infection within the liver are presently unknown.

HCV has been cultured *in vitro* from primary hepatocytes derived from experimentally inoculated chimpanzees (348) and in the human T cell line MOLT-4 (349). While neither study was able to dissect the virus life-cycle in detail, Shimizu *et al.* (349) demonstrated intracellular minus strand HCV RNA replicative intermediates six days post infection, and the appearance of HCV core and NS-4 proteins seven days post infection. These data demonstrate that HCV is lymphotropic as well as hepatotropic, and confirm the suggestion of Hellings *et al.* (350), who demonstrated transmission of HCV to chimpanzees using leucocyte preparations.

In the hypothetical replication strategy of HCV shown in Figure 15.16, several potential antiviral targets emerge. Being an enveloped virus, lysosomotropic agents such as chloroquine, ammonium chloride, amantadine and suramin could significantly inhibit HCV if entry is via receptor-mediated endocytosis. Early translation produces a pool of viral non-structural proteins, including the NS-3 (proteinase-helicase) and NS-5 (RNA polymerase), required for viral protein processing (serine-proteinase) and RNA replication (helicase-replicase). These are unique viral proteins and suitable targets for selective antiviral inhibition.

Viral RNA replication most likely occurs in the smooth membranes (351) and is associated with a proliferation of these membranes as RNA replication proceeds (324). A key intermediate in RNA replication is the double-stranded RNA replicative form (RF). This form is recycled via helicase to produce a partially single-stranded, partially double-stranded replicative intermediate (RI) and eventually yields new progeny plus sense single-stranded RNA (351) (see Figure 15.16).

Ribavirin has been shown to be of some benefit in the management of chronic hepatitis C infection (352). Ribavirin inhibits IMP dehydrogenase (363), a key enzyme in the *de novo* biosynthesis of purine nucleotides resulting in a depletion of the purine nucleotide pools, dGTP and dATP. In this context, ribavirin would be expected to decrease HCV RNA replication but with associated toxicity.

A packaging signal on HCV RNA has not yet been identified and it is unknown if the HCV cores are phosphorylated. No myristoylation or prenylation sites have been described. However, the envelope proteins of HCV have 19 potential N-linked glycosylation sites, providing ample opportunity for inhibition of assembly and release of HCV through the use of glycosylation inhibitors and also IFN-α.

Interferon generally exerts its antiviral activity through the action of 2′,5′ oligo A synthetase and 2′,5′ oligo A, which activates specific enzymes RNase L and protein kinase. These enzymes depend on the presence of double-stranded RNA for their activity. The RNase L activity results in the enzymatic digestion of RNA not associated with ribosomes and the protein kinase phosphorylates elF-2b, thereby blocking initiation of any further translational events (219). In this context, the beneficial effect of IFN-α therapy for chronic hepatitis C can be understood to be predominantly antiviral rather than immunomodulating as is the case for chronic hepatitis B (147,354).

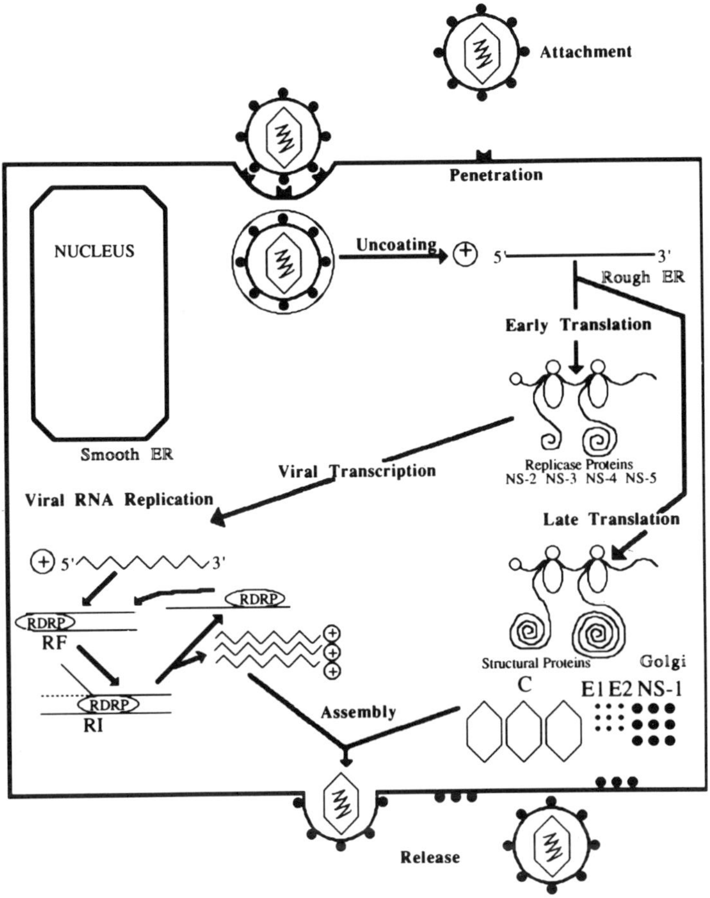

Figure 15.16. Hypothetical life-cycle of the HCV. Following attachment, penetration and uncoating the viral RNA is translated to produce a pool of replicase proteins required for genomic replication. Viral RNA replication almost certainly occurs in the smooth membrane compartment, associated with unusual tubular structures (324). The viral RNA is copied via the recycling of the double-stranded replicative form (RF) with the RNA-dependent RNA polymerase (RDRP) comprising helicase (NS-3) and polymerase (NS-5) activities. As the RF is unwound, a new strand is synthesized, producing the partially single-stranded, double-stranded replicative intermediate (RI). The new genomic RNA is released from RI and the RF then recycles back with the RDRP to commence the process again (351). In the later stages of replication more viral translation occurs, producing a pool of structural proteins which interact with the newly synthesized viral (+) RNA molecules and complete particles are formed. The life-cycle is based on the model of Chu and Westaway (351) for flaviviruses

Laboratory diagnosis

The typical serological course of acute hepatitis C virus infection is shown in Figure 15.17. HCV RNA, as detected by polymerase chain reaction (PCR), can almost always be detected at the time of presentation. It is the first marker to appear following infection and can be found as early as 10–14 days after exposure (355). Antibodies to HCV (anti-HCV) usually appear quite some time after peak aminotransferase elevations and not in all patients. First-generation assays detected antibodies to the NS-4 (C-100-3) region in up to one-third of cases of acute hepatitis C. These antibodies tend to appear late (mean 10 weeks after onset of dark urine) and not rise to high titre (356). Subsequent assays utilized other non-structural (NS-3 gene: 33c) and structural (core gene: c22) proteins, and antibody responses appeared earlier (median eight weeks) in more than half of patients with acute hepatitis C, and were higher in titre and lasted longer than responses to NS-4 (357). In acute hepatitis C, viraemia usually lasts less than four months. Detection of IgM antibody to HCV proteins (C-100-3) has now been described (358); it disappeared in those patients with a self-limited course but remained detectable in patients in whom chronic hepatitis C infection developed.

In chronic HCV infection, viraemia persists for more than six months. In most cases, HCV can be detected by PCR whether the serum aminotransferases are normal or not. The typical profile of chronic HCV infection is shown diagrammatically in Figure 15.18. Following the onset of acute hepatitis C, there is often a period of relatively rapid clinical recovery, followed by low to moderate levels of aminotransferase elevations with occasional exacerbations over the next decade. As in acute self-limited hepatitis C infection, anti-HCV can be detected within four to six weeks of onset of dark urine using second-generation assays. In chronic infection, antibody titres to the C-100-3 antigen are usually persistently elevated and only decrease or disappear when specific antiviral therapy is commenced (359). Virus can be demonstrated using PCR in serum and peripheral blood mononuclear cells over long periods of time (322). The most suitable marker for determining the response to antiviral therapy in chronic infection is the presence or absence of HCV from serum as determined by PCR. The disappearance of HCV is usually associated with a biochemical and histological improvement in the patient (360).

Experimental models: further implications for pathogenesis

HCV can be readily transmitted by parenteral injection to chimpanzees, and these animals have served as the primary model system for parenterally transmitted non-A, non-B hepatitis (PT-NANBH) (324). In transmission experiments, chimpanzees developed hepatitis after injection of factor VIII

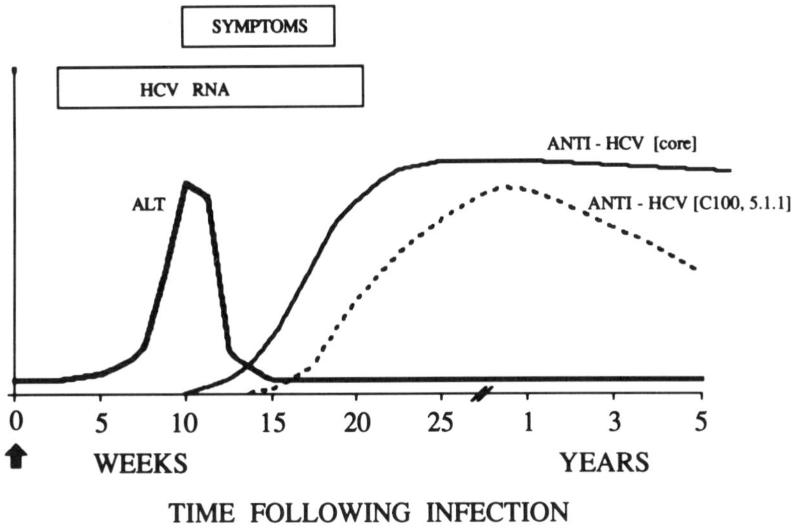

Figure 15.17. Diagrammatic representation describing the clinical, serological and virological responses commonly seen in a 'typical' case of acute hepatitis C. The HCV RNA can be detected by PCR as early as 14 days post infection. Antibodies to the C-100-3 region appear late after onset of illness, often 8–12 weeks, whilst antibodies to the core protein often appear much earlier. In the majority of cases, IgM to anti-C-100-3 appears during acute illness and disappears by 6–12 months after onset. The overall titre of anti-C-100-3 decreases with time in many patients. Modified from Beach *et al.* (357) and Farci *et al.* (322)

concentrate and factor IX complex implicated in PT-NANBH in human recipients, and NANBH has been serially transmitted by parenteral injection from chimpanzee to chimpanzee (324,361). The clinical disease in chimpanzees mimics that observed in humans, with the spectrum of responses being great.

Beach *et al.* (357) recently documented the antibody responses and virological parameters in eight chimpanzees experimentally inoculated with HCV. Five of eight animals produced IgG responses to core, and eight of eight to both 33c and C-100. When the three antigens were combined, at least one antibody response was measurable at or within three weeks of the major ALT peak. IgM responses were measurable in five of the eight chimpanzees, were of shorter duration, and usually appeared concomitantly with IgG responses. Viral RNA was detected four to seven days post infection, with the period preceding the ALT peak being characterized by fluctuating serum PCR positivity. Following the ALT peak, chronically infected animals with recurring ALT elevations were generally PCR positive, with intercedent PCR-negative periods. These studies indicate the need for a more stringent definition of HCV resolution.

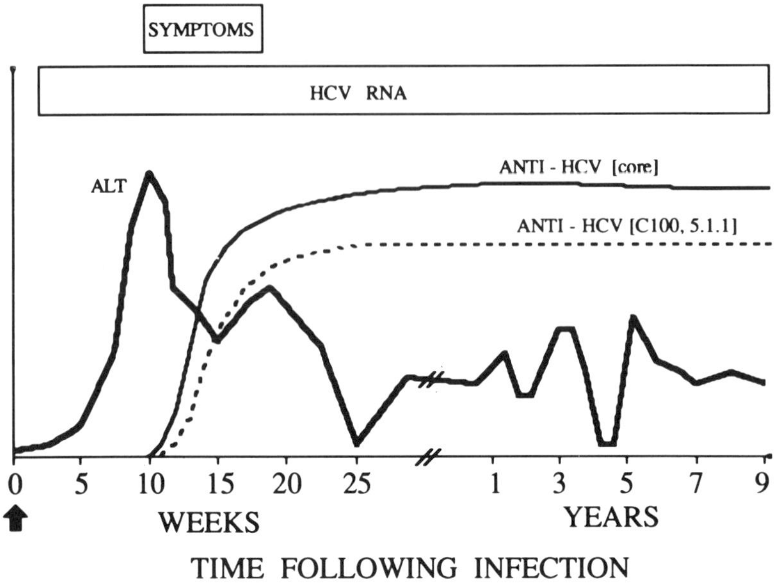

Figure 15.18. Diagrammatic representation detailing the clinical, serological and virological responses seen in a 'typical' patient who develops chronic hepatitis C following acute infection. In most cases, viral RNA in serum is detected invariably in serum by PCR. The failure to clear HCV RNA from the blood, 4–6 months after onset of acute illness, is almost invariably associated with chronic carriage. The persistence of IgM to anti-C-100-3 past 12 months is also associated with chronic carriage of HCV in many cases. The levels of antibody to both the core and C-100-3 are persistently elevated. Modified from Farci *et al.* (322) and Beach *et al.* (357)

This problem was further highlighted with the recent publication by Prince and colleagues (362) of 19 HCV cross-challenge episodes in chimpanzees. In this study, 59% of animals showed a seroconversion to HCV after challenge, 33% demonstrated the reappearance of HCV-associated hepatocellular ultrastructural changes, five animals not PCR positive at the time of challenge showed a return of PCR positivity, and 26% developed hepatitis after re-challenge. A total of 74% of the animals showed at least one of these signs of reinfection. In 10 animals the cross-challenge was done with heterologous strains and in nine with the originally infecting virus. There was no significant difference in the responses to homologous and heterologous challenges. These observations imply a particularly poor immune response and general host immunity to primary HCV infections. The implications for vaccine development are ominous.

Clinical treatment of hepatitis C

There have been several reports on the use of antiviral therapy for acute hepatitis C. Because of the very high risk for the development of chronic liver disease, the use of effective therapy, such as the IFNs, in acute hepatitis C might be expected to prove useful in preventing the development of chronic infection. Reports from Japan (363,364) have demonstrated that the use of short-term, low-dose IFN-β was effective in preventing the progression of acute NANBH to chronicity and eradicated HCV from peripheral blood (364). The results of these preliminary studies need to be interpreted cautiously before general recommendation of the use of IFN-β for acute hepatitis C can be considered.

The contribution of HCV to fulminant hepatitis has not been clarified. In developed countries, NANBH may account for about 40% of cases of fulminant hepatitis and has a particularly dismal prognosis, contributing disproportionately to deaths (365). As in other forms of hepatitis, OLT is currently offered as the best approach to improving the survival rate of fulminant hepatitis (241).

The use of ACV has shown no apparent short- or long-term beneficial effects on the serum aminotransferase levels or liver biopsy histology of patients with chronic NANBH (366). This study was performed before it was known that HCV was an RNA virus. More recently, Reichard *et al.* (352) evaluated oral ribavirin as therapy in 10 patients with chronic hepatitis C infection. In all patients a significant decrease in serum aminotransferase levels was observed during the 12-week treatment course. However, within six weeks of cessation of therapy the serum aminotransferase levels had returned to their pre-treatment level. The effects on serum anti-HCV or HCV RNA levels were not ascertained in this study. Thus, ribavirin therapy does show some promise in chronic hepatitis C and further studies alone or in combination with other agents such as IFN-α are required to assess its value in the management of chronic hepatitis C infection.

IFN-α therapy for chronic NANBH was first suggested by Hoofnagle *et al.* (367). Since then, a number of randomized controlled clinical trials of IFN-α for chronic hepatitis C have been published (368–371). All have indicated that prolonged therapy with IFN-α leads to decreases in serum aminotransferase levels and amelioration of the chronic inflammation and necrosis seen on liver biopsy specimens in up to 50% of patients with chronic hepatitis C (see Figure 15.19). Unfortunately, these studies have also demonstrated that at least 50% of the 'responders' relapse within eight weeks of stopping IFN therapy. On the other hand, the remainder appear to remain in biochemical and histological remission indefinitely. In addition, these patients usually become negative for HCV by PCR in the serum (360), implying a virological cure. Finally, some patients with severe liver disease who relapse after stopping IFN may be suitable for long-term

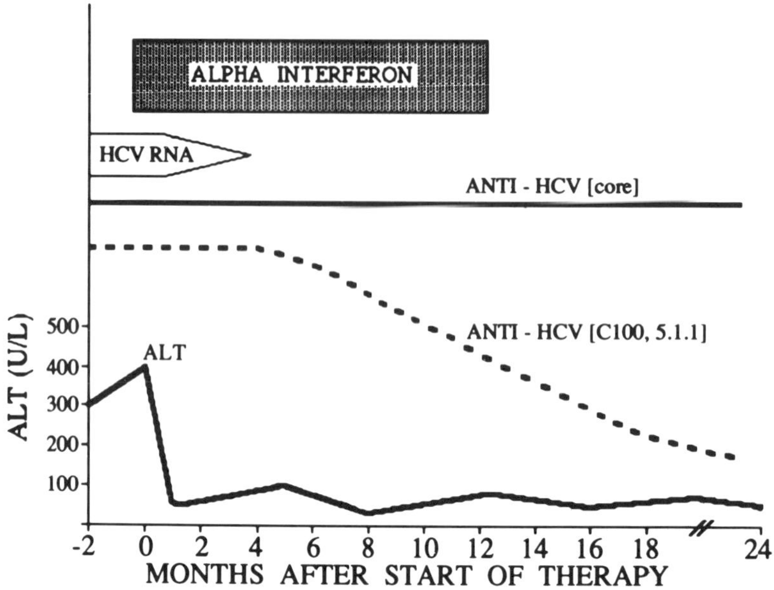

Figure 15.19. The clinical, serum biochemical, serological and virological responses of a 'typical' patient with chronic hepatitis C who had a complete response to therapy with IFN-α. During treatment, there is rapid improvement in serum aminotransferase which is permanent and a steady disappearance of HCV RNA from serum as shown by PCR. In responders, the serum HCV RNA is mostly negative 8–10 weeks after commencement of therapy. Responders also demonstrate a significant fall in the level of anti-C-100-3 during therapy. There is no change to the level of anti-core antibody. When treatment is completed, the HCV RNA does not return, serum ALT remains normal and the general clinical and histological improvement is maintained through the follow-up period. Modified from Hoofnagle and Di Bisceglie (147) and Lunel *et al.* (359). The dose of IFN is discussed in the text

treatment, since remission is usually induced with a second course and can be maintained by low-dose IFN treatment. The dose of IFN-α that produces these beneficial effects is much lower than that recommended for hepatitis B: 3 mU three times a week for six months is effective (232,373). A significant number of patients, between 40% and 60%, fail to show any response at all to treatment with IFN (Figure 15.20).

The role of corticosteroids in hepatitis C is not clear, but anecdotal evidence suggests they are not beneficial and may actually be detrimental (147).

Patient selection

Until recently, there has been no clinical feature, viral marker or other parameter identified that reliably predicted which patients would respond to

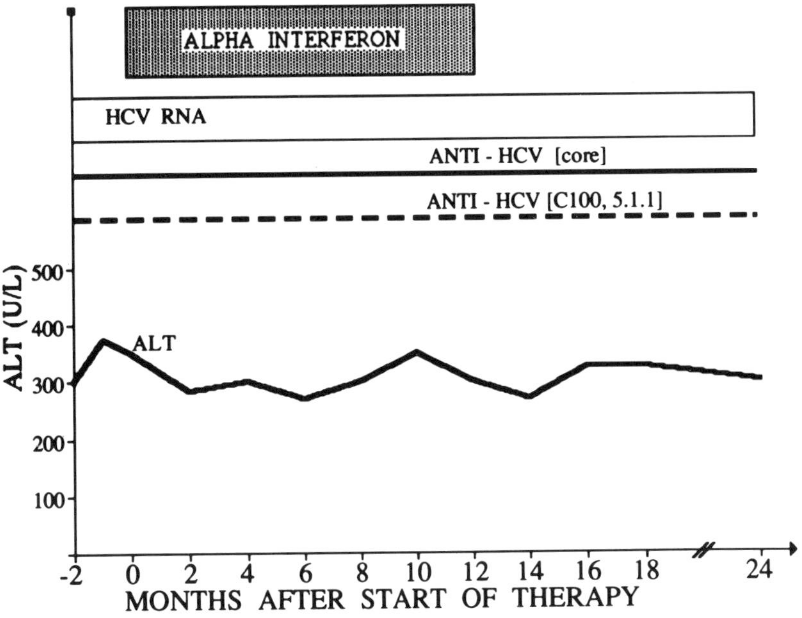

Figure 15.20. The clinical, serum biochemical, serological and virological profiles of a 'typical' patient with chronic hepatitis C who failed to demonstrate a response to therapy with IFN-α. During treatment, there was no effect on serum ALT or serum HCV RNA, and the anti-C-100-3 antibody level remained unchanged. The anti-core antibody pre-treatment serum level in this patient was of low titre. Modified from Lunel *et al.* (359)

treatment and have a subsequent long-term remission (369,372,374). However, the study by Lin *et al.* (374) demonstrated clearly that some groups of patients have a more favourable response to IFN treatment than others. Two major parameters have been identified as important: the method of acquisition and degree of liver disease. Patients who acquired HCV infection through needle-stick injuries (e.g. health care workers) or by injectable drug use have much higher response rates on initial IFN therapy (up to 80%, see reference 232) and 40% of these patients have a long-term response. These patients usually have mild chronic hepatitis C. In contrast, less than 40% of patients with severe liver disease, as characterized by extensive fibrosis or cirrhosis, responded during IFN therapy and all relapsed after stopping treatment. These findings have also been confirmed by Causse *et al.* (375). Lunel *et al.* (359) have demonstrated that very high antibody titres to C-22 on immunoblot (RIBA-11) before IFN-α treatment and significantly falling antibody titres to C-100-3 and C-33-C on immunoblot by the completion of treatment is associated with a positive response.

As discussed in the hepatitis B section, IFN-α therapy is associated with significant side-effects. At the doses used for hepatitis C (3 mU compared to 4.5 mU for hepatitis B), most patients tolerate the treatment well, but almost all have some degree of malaise, muscle aches, fevers, loss of appetite, sleep disturbances and poor concentration, especially during the first week of therapy. Probably the most serious side-effect of IFN-α is bone marrow suppression, particularly with thrombocytopenia and neutropenia (147).

A recently recognized side-effect of IFN-α therapy has been the induction of autoimmunity (252,376). In a high proportion of patients low levels of autoantibodies develop during therapy which are usually transient and not associated with illness (354). However, in 1–2% of patients a frank autoimmune condition arises which can manifest as thyroiditis (hypothyroidism or hyperthyroidism), Sjogren's syndrome, arthritis, idiopathic thrombocytopenic purpura or even haemolytic anaemia (377).

Infection with HIV should not be considered a contraindication to IFN therapy for chronic hepatitis C. Boyer *et al.* (378) have demonstrated that in patients with dual infection the response to, and tolerance of, recombinant IFN-α was not different from those usually observed in patients with chronic hepatitis C infection alone.

Patient evaluation

It is presently difficult to formulate recommendations for the use of IFN-α in hepatitis C mainly because of a lack of proven long-term effects in the majority of patients, the development of potentially serious side-effects and the high cost of treatment. The major focus of evaluation before IFN-α therapy begins should be to establish the diagnosis firmly. The patient should have biochemical and histological evidence of chronic hepatitis, virological (serum HCV positive by PCR) and possibly serological (anti-HCV) and epidemiological evidence of HCV infection, and no other potential causes of liver disease, including autoimmune chronic active hepatitis (autoantibody screen negative and normal immunoglobulin level, preferably).

Monitoring response

Patients should be seen at two- to four-week intervals while receiving IFN and have blood collected and tested for routine biochemical tests, serum aminotransferase activity and a full blood examination. Virological (HCV RNA by PCR) and serological (anti-C-100-3 and C-33-C) markers of viral replication should be followed during therapy. If no satisfactory response is evident after three months (greater than 50% drop in serum aminotransferase activities and/or HCV RNA by PCR negative) IFN should be stopped (354). If a response occurs, therapy should be continued for at least six months in the first instance, with adjustments of dose based on the degree of side-effects and changes in serum aminotransferase and HCV viraemia (232,354,371).

At the completion of treatment, a follow-up liver biopsy is probably not necessary because improvement is generally reflected by a decline in serum aminotransferase levels into the normal range. Once IFN is stopped, patients should be seen at regular intervals for at least 12 months to ascertain whether the response is sustained.

In those individuals that suffer a relapse of disease, the study of Hoofnagle *et al.* (367) demonstrated a benefit from a second course of recombinant IFN-α (rIFN-α) usually initiated at least six months after completion of the first. It might also be worth considering a course of lymphoblastoid IFN in those not responding to the first course of rIFN-α (379).

In summary, IFN-α is the first agent that has been clearly shown to have a beneficial effect in chronic hepatitis C and is a promising first step in the treatment of HCV. Future studies will need to consider combination chemotherapy with IFN-α and other antiviral agents as they are developed.

Liver transplantation for hepatitis C

As reviewed by Martin *et al.* (38), in patients transplanted for HCV-related cirrhosis, hepatitis C does recur in some patients and may lead to significant graft dysfunction, but this seems to be the exception rather than the rule. In this context HCV seropositivity in the recipient should not be regarded as a contraindication to OLT. However, anti-HCV-positive organ donors generally should be excluded from the donor pool based on the study of Pereira *et al.* (380), who found that acute hepatitis developed in almost half of the transplanted patients and the majority of these (12 of 14) developed chronic liver disease. The other two patients suffered subfulminant hepatic failure. This study also suggested that extrahepatic sites of HCV replication may exist, permitting transmission of HCV by solid organs other than the liver.

Presently, there have been no published trials of antiviral agents in order to control HCV replication in the post-transplantation period.

FUTURE PROSPECTS

The cornerstone of therapy for chronic viral hepatitis is IFN-α. It has significant benefit for a proportion of patients with chronic hepatitis B and C but unfortunately minimal benefit in chronic hepatitis D. Advances generally in antiviral drug development, based on rational screening and appropriate design to specific targets, are expected in the near future. Combination chemotherapy with the IFNs of agents with a high therapeutic index against HBV, HCV and HDV should promise improvements in overall management and patient well-being.

ACKNOWLEDGEMENTS

The authors gratefully acknowledge the contribution of Gilda Civitico for all the artwork and figure production. Also, our thanks are extended to Barbara Gray for her excellent editorial skills. Dr Scott Bowden, Stephen Williams, Chris Birch, Tim Shaw and Noreen Lehmann critically reviewed the manuscript and provided constructive changes.

REFERENCES

1. Margolis, H., Alter, M. and Krugman, S. (1991). Strategies for controlling hepatitis B in the United States. In *Viral Hepatitis and Liver Disease,* F. B. Hollinger, S. M. Lemon and H. S. Margolis (eds), Williams & Wilkins, Baltimore, pp. 720–722.
2. Morbidity and Mortality Weekly Report (May 1987). *Hepatitis Surveillance Report No. 51.* Centers for Disease Control, Atlanta.
3. Lim, W. L. and Yeoh, E. K. (1992). Hepatitis A vaccination. *Lancet,* **i**, 304.
4. Gust, I. D. (1992). Control of hepatitis B in Australia: the case for alternative strategies. *Med. J. Aust.,* **156**, 819–821.
5. Editorial (1990). The A to F of viral hepatitis. *Lancet,* **ii**, 1158–1160.

6a. Dienstag, J. L., Wands, J. R. and Koff, R. S. (1987). Acute viral hepatitis. In *Harrison's Principles of Internal Medicine,* 11th edn, E. Braunwald (ed.), McGraw-Hill, New York, pp. 1325–1338.

6b. Irving, W. L. and Cunningham, A.L. (1990). Serological diagnosis of infection with human herpesvirus type 6. *Br. Med. J.,* **300**, 156–159.

7. Wands, J. R., Koff, R. S. and Isselbacher, K.J. (1987). Chronic hepatitis. In *Harrison's Principles of Internal Medicine,* 11th edn, E. Braunwald (ed.), McGraw-Hill, New York, pp. 1338–1341.
8. Hadziyannis, S. J., Lieberman, H. M., Karvountzis, G. G. and Shafritz, D. A. (1983). Analysis of liver disease, nuclear HBcAg, viral replication, and hepatitis B virus DNA in liver and serum of HBeAg vs anti-HBe positive carriers of hepatitis B virus. *Hepatology,* **3**, 656–662.
9. Naumov, N. V., Portmann, B. C., Tedder, R. S. *et al.* (1990). Detection of hepatitis B virus antigens in liver tissue: a relation to viral replication and histology in chronic hepatitis B infection. *Gastroenterology,* **99**, 1248–1253.
10. Rizzetto, M. (1983). The delta agent. *Hepatology,* **3**, 729–737.
11. Farci, P., Alter, H. J., Wong, D. *et al.* (1991). A long-term study of hepatitis C virus replication in non-A, non-B hepatitis. *N. Engl. J. Med.,* **325**, 98–104.
12. Szmuness, W. (1989). Hepatocellular carcinoma and the hepatitis B virus: evidence for a causal association. *Prog. Med. Virol.,* **24**, 40–69.
13. Yano, M., Yatsuhashi, H., Inoue, O. and Koga, M. (1991). Epidemiology of hepatitis C virus in Japan: role in chronic liver disease and hepatocellular carcinoma. *J. Gastroenterol. Hepatol.,* **6** (Suppl. 1), 31–35.
14. Lemon, S. M. (1985). Type A viral hepatitis: new developments in an old disease. *N. Engl. J. Med.,* **313**, 1059–1067.
15. Hoofnagle, J. H., Dusheiko, G. M., Schafer, D. F. *et al.* (1982). Reactivation of chronic hepatitis B virus infection by cancer chemotherapy. *Ann. Intern. Med.,* **96**, 447–449.

16. Lok, A. S. F., Liang, R. H. S., Chiu, E. K. W. *et al.* (1991). Reactivation of hepatitis B virus replication in patients receiving cytotoxic therapy: report of a prospective study. *Gastroenterology*, **100**, 182–188.
17. Ouwubalili, J. K. (1988). Fulminant hepatic failure in nephrotic syndrome related to withdrawal of immunosuppressive therapy. *Postgrad. Med. J.*, **64**, 325–327.
18. Locarnini, S. A., Ferris, A. A., Stott, A. C. and Gust, I. D. (1974). The relationship between a 27 nm virus-like particle and hepatitis A as demonstrated by immune electron microscopy. *Intervirology*, **4**, 110–118.
19. Coulepis, A. G., Locarnini, S. A., Lehmann, N. I. and Gust, I. D. (1980). Detection of hepatitis A virus in the feces of patients with naturally-acquired infection. *J. Infect. Dis.*, **141**, 151–156.
20. Coulepis, A. G., Locarnini, S. A., Westaway, E. G. *et al.* (1982). Biophysical and biochemical characterization of hepatitis A virus. *Intervirology*, **18**, 107–127.
21. Gust, I. D., Coulepis, A. G., Feinstone, S. M. *et al.* (1983). Taxonomic classification of hepatitis A virus. *Intervirology*, **20**, 1–7.
22. Lemon, S. M. (1992). Hepatitis A virus: current concepts of the molecular virology, immunobiology and approaches to vaccine development. *Rev. Med. Virol.*, **2**, 73–87.
23. Cohen, J. I., Ticehurst, J. R., Purcell, R. H. *et al.* (1987). Complete nucleotide sequence of wild-type hepatitis A virus: comparison with different strains of hepatitis A virus and other picornaviruses. *J. Virol.*, **61**, 50–59.
24. Karayiannis, P., Jowett, T., Enticott, M. *et al.* (1986). Hepatitis A virus replication in tamarins and host immune response in relation to pathogenesis of liver damage. *J. Med. Virol.*, **18**, 261–276.
25. Locarnini, S. A., Coulepis, A. G., Westaway, E. G. and Gust, I. D. (1981). Restricted replication of human hepatitis A virus in cell culture: an intracellular biochemical study. *J. Virol.*, **37**, 216–225.
26. Anderson, D. A., Ross, B. C. and Locarnini, S. A. (1988). Restricted replication of hepatitis A virus in cell culture: encapsidation of viral RNA depletes the pool of RNA available for replication. *J. Virol.*, **62**, 4201–4206.
27. Anderson, D. A. and Ross, B. C. (1990). Morphogenesis of hepatitis A virus isolation and characterization of subviral particles. *J. Virol.*, **64**, 5284–5289.
28. Locarnini, S. A., Ferris, A. A., Lehmann, N. I. and Gust, I. D. (1977). The antibody response following hepatitis A infection. *Intervirology*, **8**, 309–318.
29. Provost, P. J. and Hilleman, M. R. (1979). Propagation of human hepatitis A virus in cell culture *in vitro*. *Proc. Soc. Exp. Biol. Med.*, **160**, 213–221.
30. Anderson, D. A. (1987). Cytopathology, plaque assay and heat inactivation of hepatitis A virus strain HM175. *J. Med. Virol.*, **22**, 35–44.
31. Vallbracht, A., Hofmann, L., Wurster, K. G. and Flehmig, B. (1984). Persistent infection of human fibroblasts by hepatitis A virus. *J. Gen. Virol.*, **65**, 609–615.
32. Siegl, G. and Eggers, J. H. (1982). Failure of guanidine and 2(alpha-hydroxybenzyl)-benzimidazole to inhibit replication of hepatitis A virus *in vitro*. *J. Gen. Virol.*, **61**, 111–114.
33. Passagot, J., Biziagos, E., Crance, J. M. and Deloince, R. (1988). Effect of antiviral substances on hepatitis A virus replication. In *Viral Hepatitis and Liver Disease*, A. Zuckerman (ed.), Liss, New York, pp. 953–955.
34. Widell, A., Hansson, B. G., Oberg, B. and Nordenfelt, E. (1986). Influence of twenty potentially antiviral substances on *in vitro* multiplication of hepatitis A virus. *Antiviral Res.*, **6**, 103–112.
35. Mijch, A. M. and Gust, I. D. (1986). Clinical, serological and epidemiologic aspects of hepatitis A virus infection. *Semin. Liver Dis.*, **6**, 42–45.

36. Levin, S. and Hahn, T. (1982). Interferon system in acute viral hepatitis. *Lancet*, **i**, 592–594.
37. Fagan, E., Yousef, G., Brahm, J. *et al.* (1990). Persistence of hepatitis A virus in fulminant hepatitis and after liver transplantation. *J. Med. Virol.*, **30**, 131–136.
38. Martin, P., Munoz, S. J. and Friedman, L. S. (1992). Liver transplantation for viral hepatitis: current status. *Am. J. Gastroenterol.*, **87**, 409–418.
39. Gordon, S. C., Reddy, K. R. and Sahiff, L. (1984). Prolonged intrahepatic cholestasis secondary to acute hepatitis A. *Ann. Intern. Med.*, **101**, 635–637.
40. Sjogren, M. H., Tanno, H., Fay, O. *et al.* (1987). Hepatitis A virus in stool during clinical relapse. *Ann. Intern. Med.*, **106**, 221–226.
41. Gust, I. D. and Purcell, R. H. (1987). Report of a workshop: waterborne non-A, non-B hepatitis. *J. Infect. Dis.*, **156**, 630–635.
42. Khuroo, M. S., Toli, M. R., Skidmore, S. *et al.* (1981). Incidence and severity of viral hepatitis in pregnancy. *Am. J. Med.*, **70**, 252–255.
43. Bradley, D. W. (1992). Hepatitis E: epidemiology, aetiology and molecular biology. *Rev. Med. Virol.*, **2**, 19–28.
44. Krawczynski, K. and Bradley, D. W. (1989). Enterically transmitted non-A, non-B hepatitis: identification of virus-associated antigen in experimentally infected cynomolgus macaques. *J. Infect. Dis.*, **159**, 1042–1049.
45. Balayan, M. S., Andjaparidze, A. G., Savinskaya, S. S. *et al.* (1983). Evidence for a virus in non-A, non-B hepatitis transmitted via the fecal–oral route. *Intervirology*, **20**, 23–31.
46. McCaustland, K. A., Shengli, B., Purdy, M. A. and Bradley, D. W. (1991). Application of two RNA extraction methods prior to amplification of hepatitis E virus nucleic acid by the polymerase chain reaction. *J. Virol. Methods*, **35**, 331–342.
47. Krawczynski, K., Bradley, D. W. and Kane, M. A. (1988). Virus associated antigen of epidemic non-A, non-B hepatitis and specific antibodies in outbreaks and in sporadic cases of NANB hepatitis. *Hepatology*, **8**, 1223.
48. Peters, M., Vierling, J., Gershwin, E. *et al.* (1991). Immunology and the liver. *Hepatology*, **13**, 977–994.
49. Locarnini, S. A. and Gust, I. D. (1988). Hepadnaviridae: hepatitis B virus and the delta virus. In *Laboratory Diagnosis of Infectious Diseases: Principles and Practice Volume II. Viral, Rickettsial and Chlamydial Diseases*, E. H. Lennette, P. Halonen and F. A. Murphy (eds), Springer-Verlag, New York, pp. 750–796.
50. Hoofnagle, J. H. and Schafer, D. F. (1986). Serologic markers of hepatitis B virus infection. *Semin. Liver Dis.*, **6**, 1–10.
51. Robinson, W. S. (1977). The genome of hepatitis B virus. *Annu. Rev. Microbiol.*, **31**, 357–377.
52. Tiollais, P., Pourcel, C. and Dejean, A. (1985). The hepatitis B virus. *Nature (London)*, **317**, 489–495.
53. Gerlich, W. H. and Robinson, W. S. (1980). Hepatitis B virus contains protein attached to the 5′-terminus of its complete DNA strand. *Cell*, **21**, 801–809.
54. Seeger, C., Summers, J. and Mason, W. S. (1991). Viral DNA synthesis. *Curr. Top. Microbiol. Immunol.*, **168**, 41–60.
55. Lien, J., Aldrich, C. E. and Mason, W. S. (1986). Evidence that a capped oligoribonucleotide is the primer for duck hepatitis B virus plus strand DNA synthesis. *J. Virol.*, **57**, 229–236.
56. Milich, D. R., Thornton, G. B., Neurath, A. R. *et al.* (1985). Enhanced immunogenicity of the pre-S region of hepatitis B surface antigen. *Science*, **228**, 1195–1199.
57. Pontisso, P., Petit, M. A., Bankowski, M. J. and Peeples, M. E. (1989). Human liver plasma membranes contain receptors for the hepatitis B virus pre-S1 region

and, via polymerized human serum albumin, for the pre-S2 region. *J. Virol.*, **63**, 1981–1988.
58. Pettit, M. A., Strick, N., Dubanchet, S. *et al.* (1991). Inhibitory activity of monoclonal antibody F35.25 on the interaction between hepatocytes (Hep G2 cells) and pre S1-specific ligands. *Mol. Immunol.*, **28**, 517–521.
59. Persing, D. H., Varmus, H. E. and Ganem, D. (1987). The pre-S1 protein of HBV is acylated at its amino terminus with myristic acid. *J. Virol.*, **61**, 1672–1677.
60. Summers, J., Smith, P. M., Huang, M. and Yu, M. (1991). Morphogenetic and regulatory effects of mutations in the envelope proteins of an avian hepadnavirus. *J. Virol.*, **65**, 1310–1317.
61. Thung, S. N., Gerker, M. A., Kasambalides, E. J. *et al.* (1986). Demonstration of pre-S polypeptides of hepatitis B virus in infected livers. *Hepatology*, **6**, 1315–1318.
62. Ou, J., Laub, O. and Rutter, W. (1986). Hepatitis B virus gene function: the precore region targets the core antigen to cellular membranes and causes the secretion of the e antigen. *Proc. Natl Acad. Sci. USA*, **83**, 1578–1582.
63. Toh, H., Hayashida, H. and Miyata, T. (1983). Sequence homology between retroviral reverse transcriptase and putative polymerase of hepatitis B virus and cauliflower mosaic virus. *Nature* (*London*), **305**, 827–828.
64. Radziwill, G., Tucker, W. and Schaller, H. (1990). Mutational analysis of the hepatitis B virus P gene product domain structure and RNase H activity. *J. Virol.*, **64**, 613–620.
65. Bartenschlager, R. and Schaller, H. (1988). The amino-terminal domain of the hepadnaviral P gene encodes the terminal protein (genome-linked protein) believed to prime reverse transcription. *EMBO J.*, **7**, 4185–4192.
66. Galibert, F., Chen, T. N. and Mandart, E. (1982). Nucleotide sequence of a cloned woodchuck hepatitis virus genome: comparison with the hepatitis B virus sequence. *J. Virol.*, **41**, 51–65.
67. Siddiqui, A., Jameel, S. and Mapoles, J. (1986). Transcriptional control elements of hepatitis B surface antigen gene. *Proc. Natl Acad. Sci. USA*, **83**, 566–570.
68. Schaller, H. and Fischer, M. (1991). Transcriptional control of hepadnavirus gene expression. *Curr. Top. Microbiol. Immunol.*, **168**, 21–39.
69. Yuh, C.-H. and Ting, L.-P. (1990). The genome of hepatitis B virus contains a second enhancer: cooperation of two elements within this enhancer is required for its function. *J. Virol.*, **64**, 4281–4287.
70. Tur-Kaspa, R., Shaul, Y., Moore, D. D. *et al.* (1988). The glucocorticoid receptor recognizes a specific nucleotide sequence in hepatitis B virus DNA causing increased activity of the HBV enhancer. *Virology*, **167**, 630–633.
71. Mason, W. S., Taylor, J. M. and Hull, R. (1987). Retroid virus genome replication. *Adv. Virus Res.*, **32**, 35–96.
72. Philipson, L. (1981). Virus receptors. In *Receptors and Recognition,* Series B, K. Longberg-Holm and L. Philipson (eds), Chapman & Hall, New York, pp. 11–36.
73. Offensperger, W.-B., Offensperger, S., Walter, E. *et al.* (1991). Inhibition of duck hepatitis B virus infection by lysosomotropic agents. *Virology*, **183**, 415–418.
74. Diana, G. D., Pevear, D. C., Otto, M. J. *et al.* (1989). Inhibitors of viral uncoating. *Pharmacol. Ther.*, **42**, 289–305.
75. Petcu, D. J., Aldrich, C. E., Coates, L. *et al.* (1988). Suramin inhibits *in vitro* infection by duck hepatitis B virus, Rous sarcoma virus, and hepatitis delta virus. *Virology*, **167**, 385–392.
76. Ganem, D. and Varmus, H. E. (1987). The molecular biology of the hepatitis B virus. *Annu. Rev. Biochem.*, **56**, 651–693.
77. Eckhardt, S. G., Milich, D. R. and McLachlan, A. (1991). Hepatitis B virus core

antigen has two unclear localization sequences in the arginine-rich carboxyl terminus. *J. Virol.*, **65**, 575–582.
78. Summers, J. and Mason, W. S. (1982). Replication of the genome of a hepatitis B-like virus by reverse transcription of an RNA intermediate. *Cell*, **29**, 403–415.
79. Fowler, M. J. F., Monjardino, J., Tsiquaye, K. N. *et al.* (1984). The mechanism of replication of hepatitis B virus: evidence of asymmetric replication of the two DNA strands. *J. Med. Virol.*, **13**, 83–91.
80. Miller, R. H. and Robinson, W. S. (1984). Hepatitis B virus DNA forms in nuclear and cytoplasmic fractions of infected human liver. *Virology*, **137**, 390–399.
81. Tuttleman, J. S., Pourcel, and Summers, J. (1986). Formation of a pool of covalently closed circular viral DNA in hepadnavirus-infected cells. *Cell*, **47**, 451–460.
82. Mason, W. S., Lien, J.-M., Petcu, D. J. *et al.* (1987). *In vivo* and *in vitro* studies on duck hepatitis B virus replication. In *Hepadnaviruses*, UCLA symposia on molecular and cellular biology, new series, Vol. 70, W. Robinson, K. Koike and H. Will (eds), Liss, New York, pp. 3–15.
83. Tagawa, M., Omata, M. and Okuda, K. (1986). Appearance of viral RNA transcripts in the early stage of duck hepatitis B virus infection. *Virology*, **152**, 477–482.
84. Seeger, C., Ganem, D. and Varmus, H. E. (1986). Biochemical and genetic evidence for the hepatitis B virus replication strategy. *Science*, **232**, 477–484.
85. Tur-Kaspa, R., Teicher, L., Laub, O. *et al.* (1990). Alpha interferon suppresses hepatitis B virus enhancer activity and reduces viral gene transcription. *J. Virol.*, **64**, 1821–1824.
86. Buescher, M., Reiser, W., Will, H. and Schaller, H. (1985). Characterization of transcripts and the potential RNA pregenome of duck hepatitis B virus: implication for replication by reverse transcription. *Cell*, **40**, 717–724.
87. Robinson, W. S., Miller, R. H. and Marion, P. L. (1987). Hepadnaviruses and retroviruses share genome homology and features of replication. *Hepatology*, **7**, 64s–73s.
88. Will, H., Reiser, W., Weimer, T. *et al.* (1987). Replication strategy of human hepatitis B virus. *J. Virol.*, **61**, 904–911.
89. Hayashi, Y. and Koike, K. (1989). Interferon inhibits hepatitis B virus replication in a stable expression system of transfected viral DNA. *J. Virol.*, **63**, 2936–2940.
90. Lien, J. M., Aldrich, C. E. and Mason, W. S. (1986). Evidence that a capped oligoribonucleotide is the primer for duck hepatitis B virus plus-strand DNA synthesis. *J. Virol.*, **57**, 229–236.
91. Civitico, G., Wang, Y., Luscombe, C. *et al.* (1990). Antiviral strategies in chronic hepatitis B infection: II. Inhibition of duck hepatitis B virus *in vitro* using conventional antiviral agents and supercoiled-DNA active compounds. *J. Med. Virol.*, **31**, 90–97.
92. Gudat, F. and Bianchi, L. (1977). Evidence for phasic sequences in HBcAg formation and cell membrane-directed flow of core particles in chronic hepatitis B. *Gastroenterology*, **73**, 1194–1197.
93. Pugh, J., Zweidler, A. and Summers, J. (1989). Characterization of the major duck hepatitis B virus core particle protein. *J. Virol.*, **63**, 1371–1376.
94. Prange, R., Clemen, A. and Streeck, R. F. (1991). Myristoylation is involved in intracellular retention of hepatitis B virus envelope proteins. *J. Virol.*, **65**, 3919–3923.
95. Neurath, A. R. and Kent, S. B. H. (1988). The pre-S region of hepadnavirus envelope proteins. *Adv. Virus Res.*, **34**, 65–142.
96. Summers, J., Smith, P. M. and Horwich, A. L. (1990). Hepadnavirus envelope

proteins regulate covalently closed circular DNA amplification. *J. Virol.*, **64**, 2819–2824.
97. Thomas, H. C. (1988). Hepatitis B viral infection. *Am. J. Med.*, **85** (Suppl. 2A), 135–140.
98. Chisari, F. V., Filippi, P., Buras, J. *et al.* (1987). Structural and pathological effects of synthesis of hepatitis B virus large envelope polypeptide in transgenic mice. *Proc. Natl Acad. Sci. USA*, **84**, 6909–6913.
99. Roingeard, P., Romet-Lemonne, J.-L., Leturcq, D. *et al.* (1990). Hepatitis B virus core antigen (HBcAg) accumulation in an HBV nonproducer clone of HepG2-transfected cells is associated with cytopathic effect. *Virology*, **179**, 113–120.
100. Lau, J. Y. N., Bain, V. G., Davies, S. E. *et al.* (1992). High level expression of hepatitis B viral antigens in fibrosing cholestatic hepatitis. *Gastroenterology*, **102**, 956–962.
101. O'Grady, J. G., Smith, H. M., Davies, S. E. *et al.* (1992). Hepatitis B virus reinfection after orthotopic liver transplantation: serological and clinical implications. *J. Hepatol.*, **14**, 104–111.
102. Santantonio, T., Jung, M. C., Miska, S. *et al.* (1991). Prevalence and type of pre-C HBV mutants in anti-HBe positive carriers with chronic liver disease in a highly endemic area. *Virology*, **183**, 840–844.
103. Santantonio, T., Jung, M. C., Schneider, R. *et al.* (1992). Hepatitis B virus genomes that cannot synthesize pre-S2 proteins occur frequently and as dominant virus populations in chronic carriers in Italy. *Virology*, **188**, 948–952.
104. Naumov, N. V., Schneider, R., Schneider, R. *et al.* (1992). Precore mutant hepatitis B virus infection and liver disease. *Gastroenterology*, **102**, 538–543.
105. Locarnini, S. (1991). Design of new antiviral agents for chronic hepatitis B virus infection. *J. Gastroenterol. Hepatol.*, **6** (Suppl. 1), 18–22.
106. Peters, M., Vierling, J., Gershwin, M. E. *et al.* (1991). Immunology and the liver. *Hepatology*, **13**, 977–994.
107. Twu, J. S., Lee, C. H., Lin, P. M. and Schloemer, R. H. (1988). Hepatitis B virus suppresses expression of human beta interferon. *Proc. Natl Acad. Sci. USA*, **85**, 252–256.
108. Onji, M., Lever, A. M. L., Saito, I. and Thomas, H. C. (1989). Defective response to interferons in cells transfected with the hepatitis B virus genome. *Hepatology*, **9**, 92–96.
109. Frosner, G. G. and Franco, E. (1984). New developments of open questions in the serology of hepatitis A and B. In *Viral Hepatitis and Liver Disease*, G. N. Vyas, J. L. Dienstag and J. H. Hoofnagle (eds), Grune & Stratton, New York, pp. 487–489.
110. Nielsen, J. O., Dietrichson, O. and Elling, P. (1981). Incidence and meaning of persistence of Australia antigen in patients with acute viral hepatitis: development of chronic hepatitis. *N. Engl. J. Med.*, **285**, 1157–1160.
111. Lok, A. S. F. and Lai, C.-L. (1990). Acute exacerbations in Chinese patients with chronic hepatitis B virus (HBV) infection: incidence, predisposing factors and etiology. *J. Hepatol.*, **10**, 29–34.
112. Naumov, N. V., Portmann, B. C., Tedder, R. S. *et al.* (1990). Hepatitis B virus antigens in liver tissue: a relation to viral replication and histology in chronic hepatitis B infection. *Gastroenterology*, **99**, 1248–1253.
113. Brechot, C. M., Hadchovel, J., Scotto, F. *et al.* (1981). Detection of hepatitis B virus DNA in liver and serum: a direct appraisal of the chronic carrier state. *Lancet*, **ii**, 765–768.
114. Sjogren, M. and Hoofnagle, J. H. (1985). Immunoglobulin M antibody to hepa-

titis B core antigen in patients with chronic type B hepatitis. *Gastroenterology*, **89**, 252–258.

115. Hoofnagle, J. H. and Alter, H. J. (1984). Chronic viral hepatitis. In *Viral Hepatitis and Liver Disease*, G. N. Vyas, J. L. Dienstag and J. H. Hoofnagle (eds), Grune & Stratton, New York, pp. 97–113.
116. Omata, M., Ehata, T., Yokosuka, O. *et al.* (1991). Mutations in the precore region of hepatitis B virus DNA in patients with fulminant and severe hepatitis. *N. Engl. J. Med.*, **324**, 1699–1704.
117. Liang, T. J., Hasegawa, K., Rimon, N. *et al.* (1991). A hepatitis B virus mutant associated with an epidemic of fulminant hepatitis. *N. Engl. J. Med.*, **324**, 1705–1709.
118. Alward, W. L. M., McMahon, B. J., Hall, D. B., *et al.* (1985). The long term serological course of asymptomatic hepatitis B virus carriers and the development of primary hepatocellular carcinoma. *J. Infect. Dis.*, **151**, 604–609.
119. Marion, P. L. (1991). Development of antiviral therapy for chronic infection with hepatitis B virus. *Curr. Top. Microbiol. Immunol.*, **168**, 167–183.
120. Marion, P. L. (1988). Use of animal models to study hepatitis B virus. *Prog. Med. Virol.*, **35**, 43–75.
121. Farza, H., Hadchouel, M., Scotto, J. *et al.* (1988). Replication and gene expression of hepatitis B virus in a transgenic mouse that contains the complete viral genome. *J. Virol.*, **62**, 4144–4152.
122. Rijntjes, P. J., Moshage, H. J. and Yap, S. H. (1988). *In vitro* infection of primary cultures of cryopreserved adult human hepatocytes with hepatitis B virus. *Virus Res.*, **10**, 95–109.
123. Gripon, P., Diot, C., Theze, N. *et al.* (1988). Hepatitis B virus infection of adult human hepatocyte cultures in the presence of dimethyl sulfoxide. *J. Virol.*, **62**, 4136–4143.
124. Sureau, C., Romet-Lemonne, J.-L., Mullins, J. I. and Essex, M. (1986). Production of hepatitis B virus by a differentiated human hepatoma cell line after transfection with cloned circular HBV DNA. *Cell*, **47**, 37–47.
125. Sells, M. A., Chen, M. L. and Acs, G. (1987). Production of hepatitis B virus particles in HepG2 cells transfected with cloned hepatitis B virus DNA. *Proc. Natl Acad. Sci. USA*, **84**, 1005–1009.
126. Ueda, K., Tsurimoto, T., Nagahata, T. *et al.* (1989). An *in vitro* system for screening anti-hepatitis B virus drugs. *Virology*, **169**, 213–216.
127. Price, P. M., Banerjee, R. and Acs, B. (1989). Inhibition of the replication of hepatitis B virus by the carbocyclic analogue of 2′-deoxyguanosine. *Proc. Natl Acad. Sci. USA*, **86**, 8541–8544.
128. Korba, B. E. and Gerin, J. L. (1992). Use of a standardized cell culture assay to assess activities of nucleoside analogues against hepatitis B virus replication. *Antiviral Res.*, **19**, 55–70.
129. Boyd, M. R., Bacon, T. H., Sutton, D. and Cole, M. (1987). Antiherpesvirus activity of 9-(4-hydroxy-3-hydroxy-methylbut-1-yl) guanine (BRL 39123) in cell culture. *Antimicrob. Agents Chemother.*, **31**, 1238–1242.
130. Vere Hodge, R. A., Sutton, D., Boyd, M. R. *et al.* (1989). Selection of an oral prodrug (BRL 42810: famciclovir) for the antiherpes agent BRL 39123 [9-(4-hydroxy-3-hydroxymethylbut-1-yl) guanine; penciclovir]. *Antimicrob. Agents Chemother.*, **33**, 1765–1773.
131. Tuttleman, J. S., Pugh, J. C. and Summers, J. W. (1986). In vitro experimental infection of primary duck hepatocyte cultures with duck hepatitis B virus. *J. Virol.*, **38**, 17–25.

132. Bishop, N., Civitico, G., Wang, Y. *et al.* (1990). Antiviral strategies in chronic hepatitis B virus infection. I. Establishment of an *in vitro* system using the duck hepatitis B virus model. *J. Med. Virol.*, **31**, 82–89.
133. Aldrich, C. E., Coates, L., Wu, T. T. *et al.* (1989). *In vitro* infection of woodchuck hepatocytes with woodchuck hepatitis virus and ground squirrel hepatitis virus. *Virology*, **172**, 247–252.
134. Frank, K. B. and Cheng, Y.-C. (1985). Mutually exclusive inhibition of herpesvirus DNA polymerase by aphidicolin, phosphonoformate and acyclic nucleoside triphosphates. *Antimicrob. Agents Chemother.*, **27**, 445–448.
135. Haussinger, D. (1989). Regulation of hepatic metabolism by extracellular nucleotides and eicosanoids: the role of cell heterogeneity. *J. Hepatol.*, **8**, 259–266.
136. Holstege, A., Gregenbacher, H. M., Jehle, L. and Hoppmann, J. (1991). Facilitated diffusion and sodium-dependent transport of purine and pyrimidine nucleosides in rat liver. *Hepatology*, **14**, 373–380.
137. Heydrick, S. J., Lardeux, B. R. and Mortimore, G. E. (1991). Uptake and degradation of cytoplasmic RNA by hepatic lysosomes: quantitative relationship to RNA turnover. *J. Biol. Chem.*, **266**, 8790–8796.
138. Omata, M. (1990). Significance of extra-hepatic replication of hepatitis B virus. *Hepatology*, **12**, 364–366.
139. Hosoda, K., Omata, M., Uchiumi, K. *et al.* (1990). Extrahepatic replication of duck hepatitis B virus: more than expected. *Hepatology*, **11**, 44–48.
140. Korba, B. E., Gowans, E. J., Wells, F. V. *et al.* (1988). Systemic distribution of woodchuck hepatitis virus in the tissues of experimentally infected woodchucks. *Virology*, **165**, 175–181.
141. Pontisso, P., Poon, H. C., Tiollais, P. and Brechot, C. (1984). Detection of hepatitis B virus DNA in mononuclear blood cells. *Br. Med. J.*, **288**, 1563–1566.
142. Korba, B. E., Cole, P. J., Shapiro, M. *et al.* (1989). *In vitro* production of infectious woodchuck hepatitis virus by lipopolysaccharide-stimulated peripheral blood lymphocytes. *J. Infect. Dis.*, **160**, 572–576.
143. Snapka, R. M. (1986). Topoisomerase inhibitors can selectively interfere with different stages of simian virus 40 DNA replication. *Mol. Cell. Biol.*, **6**, 4221–4227.
144. Wang, Y., Bowden, S., Shaw, T. *et al.* (1991). Inhibition of duck hepatitis B virus replication *in vivo* by the nucleoside analogue ganciclovir. *Antiviral Chem. Chemother.*, **2**, 107–114.
145a. Locarnini, S., Civitico, G., Wang, Y. *et al.* (1991). Mechanism of action of antiviral agents targeted against duck hepatitis B virus supercoiled DNA. In *The 1990 International Symposium on Viral Hepatitis and Liver Disease,* F. B. Hollinger, S. M. Lemon and H. Margolis (eds), Williams & Wilkins, Baltimore, pp. 669–671.
145b. Civitico, G. M. and Locarnini, S. A. (1994). The half-life of duck hepatitis supercoiled DNA in congenitally infected primary hepatocyte culture. *Virology*, **203**, 81–89.
146. Yokosuka, O., Omata, M., Imazeki, F. *et al.* (1985). Changes of hepatitis B virus DNA in liver and serum caused by recombinant leukocyte interferon treatment: analysis of intrahepatic replicative hepatitis B virus DNA. *Hepatology*, **5**, 728–734.
147. Hoofnagle, J. H. and Di Bisceglie, A.M. (1990). Antiviral therapy of viral hepatitis. In *Antiviral Agents and Viral Diseases of Man,* 3rd edn, G. J. Galasso, R. J. Whitley and T. C. Merigan (eds), Raven Press, New York, pp. 415–459.
148. Robinson, W. S., Klote, L. and Aoki, N. (1990). Hepadnaviruses in cirrhotic liver and hepatocellular carcinoma. *J. Med. Virol.*, **31**, 18–21.
149. Gerin, J. L., Cote, P. J., Korba, B. E. and Tennant, B. C. (1989). Hepadnavirus-induced liver cancer in woodchucks. *Cancer Detect. Prevent.*, **14**, 227–229.

150. Sherlock, S. (1989). Hepatic cirrhosis. In *Diseases of the Liver and Biliary System*, 8th edn, S. Sherlock (ed.), Blackwell Scientific, Oxford, pp. 410–424.
151. Bissell, M. (1990). Cell–matrix interactions and hepatic fibrosis. In *Progress in Liver Diseases*, Vol. 9, H. Popper and F. Schaffner (eds), Saunders, Philadelphia, pp. 143–155.
152. Suzuki, H., Yamamoto, S., Hirayama, C. *et al.* (1986). Cyanidanol therapy for HBe-antigen positive chronic hepatitis: a multicentre, double-blind study. *Liver*, **6**, 35–44.
153. Conn, H. O. (1983). Cyanidanol: will a hepatotrophic drug from Europe go West? *Hepatology*, **3**, 121–123.
154. Castilla, A., Prieto, J. and Fausto, N. (1991). Transforming growth factors β1 and α in chronic liver disease: effects of interferon alfa therapy. *N. Engl. J. Med.*, **324**, 933–940.
155. Fausto, N. and Mead, J. E. (1989). Regulation of liver growth: proto oncogenes and transforming growth factors. *Lab. Invest.*, **60**, 4–13.
156. Nakatsukasa, H., Evarts, R. P., Hsia, C.-C. and Thorgeirsson, S. S. (1990). Transforming growth factor β1 and type 1 procollagen transcripts during regeneration and early fibrosis of rat liver. *Lab. Invest.*, **63**, 171–180.
157. Nordenfelt, E., Oberg, B., Holgstrand, E. and Miller, E. (1980). Inhibition of hepatitis B Dane particle DNA polymerase activity by pyrophosphate analogs. *Acta Pathol. Microbiol. Immunol. Scand. B*, **88**, 169–175.
158. Hautz, O., Ooka, T., Vitvitski, L. *et al.* (1984). Comparison of properties of woodchuck hepatitis virus and human hepatitis B virus endogenous DNA polymerases. *Antimicrob. Agents Chemother.*, **25**, 242–246.
159. Tsiquaye, K. N., Collins, P. and Zuckerman, A. J. (1986). Antiviral activity of the polybasic anion, suramin and acyclovir in Hepadna virus infection. *J. Antimicrob. Chemother.*, **18**, 223–228.
160. Offensperger, W. B., Walter, E., Offensperger, S. *et al.* (1988). Duck hepatitis B virus: DNA polymerase and reverse transcriptase activities of replicative complexes isolated from liver and their inhibition *in vitro*. *Virology*, **164**, 48–54.
161. Nordenfelt, E., Lofgren, B., Chattopadhyaya, J. and Oberg, B. (1987). Inhibition of hepatitis B virus DNA polymerase by 3′-azido-3′deoxythymidine triphosphate but not its threo analog. *J. Med. Virol.*, **22**, 231–236.
162. Tao, P. Z., Lofgren, B., Lake-Bakaar, D. *et al.* (1988). Inhibition of human hepatitis B virus DNA polymerase and duck hepatitis B virus DNA polymerase by triphosphates of thymidine analogs and pharmacokinetic properties of the corresponding nucleosides. *J. Med. Virol.*, **26**, 353–362.
163. Lofgren, B., Nordenfelt, E. and Oberg, B. (1989). Inhibition of RNA- and DNA-dependent duck hepatitis B virus DNA polymerase activity by nucleoside and pyrophosphate analogs. *Antiviral Res.*, **12**, 301–310.
164. Meisel, H., Reimer, K., von Janta-Lipinski, M. *et al.* (1990). Inhibition of hepatitis B virus DNA polymerase by 3′-fluorothymidine triphosphate and other modified nucleoside triphosphate analogs. *J. Med. Virol.*, **30**, 137–144.
165. Matthes, E., Reimer, K., von Janta-Lipinski, M. *et al.* (1991). Comparative inhibition of hepatitis B virus DNA polymerase and cellular DNA polymerase by triphosphates of sugar-modified 5′-methyldeoxycytidines and of other nucleoside analogs. *Antimicrob. Agents Chemother.*, **35**, 1254–1257.
166. Chang, C.-N., Doong, S.-L., Zhou, J. H. *et al.* (1992). Deoxycytidine deaminase-resistant stereoisomer is the active form of (±)-2′,3′-dideoxy-3′-thiacytidine in the inhibition of hepatitis B virus replication. *J. Biol. Chem.*, **267**, 13938–13942.
167. Price, P. M., Banerjee, R. and Acs, G. (1989). Inhibition of the replication of hepa-

titis B virus by the carbocyclic analogue of 2′-deoxyguanosine. *Proc. Natl Acad. Sci. USA*, **86**, 8541–8544.

168. Galle, P. R. and Theilmann, L. (1990). Inhibition of hepatitis B virus polymerase activity by various agents: transient expression of hepatitis B virus DNA in hepatoma cells as novel system for evaluation of antiviral drugs. *Arzneimittelforschung*, **40**, 1380–1382.
169. Matthes, E., Langen, P., von Janta-Lipinski, M. *et al.* (1990). Potent inhibition of hepatitis B virus production *in vitro* by modified pyrimidine nucleosides. *Antimicrob. Agents Chemother.*, **34**, 1986–1990.
170. Aoki-Sei, S., O'Brien, M. C., Ford, H. *et al.* (1991). In vitro inhibition of hepatitis B virus replication by 2′,3′-dideoxyguanosine, 2′,3′-dideoxyinosine, and 3′-azido-2′,3′-dideoxythymidine in 2.2.15 (PR) cells. *J. Infect. Dis.*, **164**, 843–851.
171. Doong, S.-L., Tsai, C.-H., Schinazi, R. F. *et al.* (1991). Inhibition of the replication of hepatitis B virus in vitro by 2′,3′-dideoxy-3′-thiacytidine and related analogues. *Proc. Natl Acad. Sci. USA*, **88**, 8495–8499.
172. Lampertico, P., Malter, J. S. and Gerber, M. A. (1991). Development and application of an in vitro model for screening anti-hepatitis B virus therapeutics. *Hepatology*, **13**, 422–426.
173. Yokota, T., Mochizuki, S., Konno, K. *et al.* (1991). Inhibitory effects of selected antiviral compounds on human hepatitis B virus DNA synthesis. *Antimicrob. Agents Chemother.*, **35**, 394–397.
174. Matthes, E., von Janta-Lipinski, M., Will, H. *et al.* (1992). Inhibition of hepatitis B virus production by modified 2′,3′-dideoxythymidine and 2′,3′-dideoxy-5-methylcytidine derivatives: *in vitro* and *in vivo* studies. *Biochem. Pharmacol.*, **43**, 1571–1577.
175. Lee, B., Luo, W., Suzuki, S. *et al.* (1989). *In vitro* and *in vivo* comparison of the abilities of purine and pyrimidine 2′,3′-dideoxynucleosides to inhibit duck hepadnavirus. *Antimicrob. Agents Chemother.*, **33**, 336–339.
176. Suzuki, S., Lee, B., Luo, W. *et al.* (1988). Inhibition of duck hepatitis B virus replication by purine 2′,3′-dideoxynucleosides. *Biochem. Biophys. Res. Commun.*, **156**, 1144–1151.
177. Hung, L.-F., Brumbaugh, A. E., Bhatia, G. *et al.* (1991). Effects of purine nucleoside analogues with a cyclobutane ring and erythromycin A oxime derivatives on duck hepatitis B virus replication in vivo and in cell culture and HIV-1 in cell culture. *J. Med. Virol.*, **35**, 180–186.
178. Yokota, T., Kenno, K., Chonan, E. *et al.* (1990). Comparative activities of several nucleoside analogs against duck hepatitis B virus in vitro. *Antimicrob. Agents Chemother.*, **34**, 1326–1330.
179. Smee, D. F., Knight, S. S., Duke, A. E. *et al.* (1985). Activities of arabinosyladenine monophosphate and 9-(1,3-dihydroxy-2-propoxymethyl) guanine against ground squirrel hepatitis virus in vivo as determined by reduction in serum virion-associated DNA polymerase. *Antimicrob. Agents Chemother.*, **27**, 277–279.
180. Hirota, K., Sherker, A. H., Omata, M. *et al.* (1987). Effects of adenine arabinoside on serum and intrahepatic replicative forms of duck hepatitis B virus in chronic infection. *Hepatology*, **7**, 24–28.
181. Kassianides, C., Hoofnagle, J. H., Miller, R. H. *et al.* (1989). Inhibition of duck hepatitis B virus replication by 2′,3′-dideoxycytidine: a potent inhibitor of reverse transcriptase. *Gastroenterology*, **97**, 1275–1280.
182. Haritani, H., Uchida, T., Okuda, Y. and Shikata, T. (1989). Effect of 3′-azido-3′-deoxythymidine on replication of duck hepatitis B virus in vivo and in vitro. *J. Med. Virol.*, **29**, 244–248.

183a. Shaw, T. S., Amor, P., Civitico, G. *et al.* (1994). In vitro antiviral activity of penciclovir, a novel purine nucleoside analogue, against duck hepatitis B virus. *Antimicrob. Agents Chemother.*, **38**, 719–723.
183b. Tsiquaye, K. N., Slomka, M. J. and Maung, M. (1994). Oral famciclovir against duck hepatitis B virus. Replication in hepatic and non hepatic tissue of ducklings infected in ovo. *J. Med. Virol.*, **42**, 306–310.
184. Fourel, I., Hantz, O., Watanabe, K. A. *et al.* (1990). Inhibitory effects of 2′-fluorinated arabinosyl-pyrimidine nucleosides on woodchuck hepatitis virus replication in chronically infected woodchucks. *Antimicrob. Agents Chemother.*, **34**, 473–475.
185. Nordenfelt, E., Widell, A., Hansson, B. G. *et al.* (1982). No *in vivo* effect of trisodium phosphonoformate on woodchuck hepatitis virus producton. *Acta Pathol. Microbiol. Immunol. Scand.*, **90**, 449–451.
186. Sherker, A. H., Hirota, K., Omata, M. and Okuda, K. (1986). Foscarnet decreases serum and liver duck hepatitis B virus DNA in chronically infected ducks. *Gastroenterology*, **91**, 818–824.
187. Pollard, R. B., Smith, J. L., Neal, A. *et al.* (1978). Effect of vidarabine on chronic hepatitis B virus infection. *JAMA*, **239**, 1648–1650.
188. Hoofnagle, J. H., Hanson, R. G., Minuk, G. Y. *et al.* (1984). Randomized controlled trial of adenine arabinoside monophosphate for chronic type B hepatitis. *Gastroenterology*, **86**, 150–157.
189. Perrillo, R. P., Regenstein, F. G., Bodicky, C. J. *et al.* (1985). Comparative efficacy of adenine arabinoside 5′-monophosphate and prednisone withdrawal followed by adenine arabinoside 5′-monophosphate in the treatment of chronic active hepatitis type B. *Gastroenterology*, **88**, 780–786.
190. Garcia, G., Smith, C. I., Weissberg, J. I. *et al.* (1987). Adenine arabinoside monophosphate (vidarabine phosphate) in combination with human leukocyte interferon in the treatment of chronic hepatitis B: a randomized, double-blind, placebo-controlled trial. *Ann. Intern. Med.*, **107**, 278–285.
191. Fiume, L., Cerenzia, M. R., Bonino, F. *et al.* (1988). Inhibition of hepatitis B virus replication by vidarabine monophosphate conjugated with lactosaminated serum albumin. *Lancet*, **ii**, 13–15.
192. Weller, I. V. D., Lok, A. S. F., Mindel, A. *et al.* (1985). Randomized controlled trial of adenine arabinoside 5′-monophosphate (ara-AMP) in chronic hepatitis B virus infection. *Gut*, **26**, 745–751.
193. Ouzan, D., Chevallier, M., Laffranchi, B. *et al.* (1986). Therapeutic efficacy of ara-AMP in symptomatic HBeAg positive CAH: a randomized placebo controlled study in heterosexuals. *Hepatology*, **6**, 1151.
194. Marcellin, P., Ouzan, D., Degos, F. *et al.* (1989). Randomized controlled trial of adenine arabinoside 5′-monophosphate in chronic active hepatitis B: comparison of the efficacy in heterosexual and homosexual patients. *Hepatology*, **10**, 328–331.
195. Schalm, S. W., Heijtink, R. A., Van Buuren, H. R. and DeMan, R. A. (1985). Acyclovir enhances the antiviral effect of interferon in chronic hepatitis B. *Lancet*, **ii**, 358–360.
196. Alexander, G. J., Fagan, E. A., Hegarty, J. E. *et al.* (1987). Controlled clinical trial of acyclovir in chronic hepatitis B virus infection. *J. Med. Virol.*, **21**, 81–87.
197. Locarnini, S. A., Guo, K., Lucas, C. R. and Gust, I. D. (1989). Inhibition of HBV DNA replication by ganciclovir in patients with AIDS. *Lancet*, **ii**, 1225–1226.
198. Angus, P., Richards, M., Bowden, S. *et al.* (1993). Combination antiviral therapy controls severe post-liver transplant recurrence of hepatitis B virus infection. *J. Gastroenterol. Hepatol.*, in press.
199. Farraye, F. A., Maurish, D. M. and Zeldis, J. B. (1989). Preliminary evidence that

azidothymidine does not affect hepatitis B virus replication in acquired immunodeficiency syndrome (AIDS) patients. *J. Med. Virol.*, **29**, 266–267.

200. Hedin, G., Weiland, O., Ljunggren, K. *et al.* (1988). Treatment with foscarnet of fulminant hepatitis B and fulminant hepatitis B and D coinfection. In *Viral Hepatitis and Liver Disease,* A. J. Zuckerman (ed.), Liss, New York, pp. 947–952.
201. Price, J. S., France, A. J., Moaven, L. D. and Welsby, P. D. (1986). Foscarnet in fulminant hepatitis B. *Lancet*, **ii**, 1273.
202. Bain, V. G., Daniels, H. M., Chanas, A. *et al.* (1989). Foscarnet therapy in chronic hepatitis B virus E antigen carriers. *J. Med. Virol.*, **29**, 152–155.
203. Mutchnick, M. G., Appelman, H. D., Chung, H. T. *et al.* (1991). Thymosin treatment of chronic hepatitis B: a placebo controlled pilot trial. *Hepatology,* **14**, 409–415.
204. Bissett, J., Eisenberg, M., Gregory, P. *et al.* (1988). Recombinant fibroblast interferon and immune interferon for treating chronic hepatitis B virus infection: patients' tolerance and the effect on viral markers. *J. Infect. Dis.*, **157**, 1076–1080.
205. Di Bisceglie, A. M., Rustgi, U. K., Kassianides, C. *et al.* (1990). Therapy of chronic hepatitis B with recombinant alpha and gamma interferon. *Hepatology,* **11**, 266–270.
206. Caselmann, W. H., Eisenburg, J., Hofschneider, P. H. and Koshy, R. (1989). Beta and gamma interferon in chronic active hepatitis B: a pilot trial of short-term combination therapy. *Gastroenterology,* **96**, 449–455.
207. Perillo, R. P., Schiff, E. R., Davis, G. L. *et al.* (1990). A randomized, controlled trial of interferon alpha-2b alone and after prednisone withdrawal for the treatment of chronic hepatitis B. *N. Engl. J. Med.*, **323**, 295–301.
208. Alexander, G. J. M., Brahm, J., Fagan, E. A. *et al.* (1987). Loss of HBsAg with interferon therapy in chronic hepatitis B virus infection. *Lancet*, **i**, 66–68.
209. Hoofnagle, J. H., Peters, M. G., Mullen, K. D. *et al.* (1988). Randomized controlled trial of a four month course of recombinant human alpha interferon in patients with chronic hepatitis B. *Gastroenterology*, **95**, 1318–1325.
210. Brook, M. G., Karayiannis, P. and Thomas, H. C. (1989). Which patients with chronic hepatitis B virus infection will respond to alpha interferon therapy? A statistical analysis of predictive factors. *Hepatology*, **10**, 761–763.
211. McDonald, J. A., Caruso, L. and Thomas, H. C. (1989). A randomised controlled trial of recombinant interferon-α in treatment of HBV infection. *Gut*, **31**, 1116–1122.
212. Dusheiko, G., Di Bisceglie, A., Boyer, S. *et al.* (1985). Recombinant leukocyte interferon treatment of chronic hepatitis B. *Hepatology*, **5**, 556–560.
213. Novick, D. M., Lok, A. S. F. and Thomas, H. C. (1984). Diminished responsiveness of homosexual men to antiviral therapy for HBsAg-positive chronic liver disease. *J. Hepatol.*, **1**, 29–35.
214. Guardia, J., Esteban, R., Buti, M. *et al.* (1986). Prolonged inhibition of hepatitis B virus replication with vidarabine monophosphate in chronic active type B hepatitis. *Liver*, **6**, 118–122.
215. Furman, P. A., St Clair, M. H. and Spector, T. (1984). Acyclovir triphosphate in a suicide inactivation of the herpes simplex virus DNA polymerase. *J. Biol. Chem.*, **259**, 9575–9579.
216. Freitas, V. R., Smee, D. F., Chernow, M. *et al.* (1985). Activity of 9-(1,3-dihydroxy-2-propoxymethyl) guanine compared with that of acyclovir against human, monkey and rodent cytomegaloviruses. *Antimicrob. Agents Chemother.*, **28**, 240–245.
217. Korenman, J., Baker, B., Waggoner, J. *et al.* (1991). Long term remission of chronic hepatitis B after interferon therapy. *Ann. Intern. Med.*, **114**, 629–634.

218. Davis, G. L. (1991). Treatment of chronic hepatitis B. *Hepatology*, **14**, 567–569.
219. Samuel, C. E. (1988). Mechanisms of the antiviral action of interferons. *Prog. Nucleic Acid Res. Mol. Biol.*, **35**, 27–72.
220. Perrillo, R. P. (1989). Interferon therapy for chronic type B hepatitis: the promise comes of age. *Gastroenterology*, **96**, 532–536.
221. Davis, G. L. and Hoofnagle, J. H. (1986). Interferon in viral hepatitis: role in pathogenesis and treatment. *Hepatology*, **6**, 1038–1041.
222. Scully, L. J., Shein, R., Karayiannis, P. *et al.* (1987). Lymphoblastoid interferon therapy of chronic HBV infection: a comparison of 12 vs 24 weeks of thrice weekly treatment. *J. Hepatol.*, **5**, 41–58.
223. Perrillo, R. P., Regenstein, F. G., Peters, M. G. *et al.* (1988). Prednisone withdrawal followed by recombinant alpha interferon in the treatment of chronic type B hepatitis: a randomized, controlled trial. *Ann. Intern. Med.*, **109**, 95–100.
224. Lok, A. S. F., Weller, I. V., Karayiannis P. *et al.* (1984). Thrice weekly lymphoblastoid interferon is effective in inhibiting hepatitis B virus replication. *Liver*, **4**, 45–49.
225. Smith, C. I., Weissberg, J., Bernhardt, L. *et al.* (1983). Acute Dane particle suppression with recombinant leukocyte A interferon in chronic hepatitis B virus infection. *J. Infect. Dis.*, **48**, 907–913.
226. Lok, A. S. F., Ma, O. C. K. and Lau, J. Y. N. (1991). Interferon alfa therapy in patients with chronic hepatitis B virus infection: effects on HBV DNA in the liver. *Gastroenterology*, **100**, 756–761.
227. Williams, S. J. and Farrell, G. C. (1989). Serial antipyrene clearance studies detect altered hepatic metabolic function during spontaneous and interferon induced changes in chronic hepatitis B disease activity. *Hepatology*, **10**, 192–197.
228. Bortolotti, F., Cadrobbi, P., Crivellaro, C. *et al.* (1990). Long-term outcome of chronic type B hepatitis in patients who acquire hepatitis B virus infection in childhood. *Gastroenterology*, **99**, 805–810.
229. Dusheiko, G. M. (1991). Alpha-interferon treatment of chronic hepatitis B infection: predictors of responsiveness. *J. Gastroenterol. Hepatol.*, **6** (Suppl. 1), 7–12.
230. Williams, S. J., Craig, P. I., Cooksley, W. G. E. *et al.* (1990). Randomized controlled trial of recombinant human interferon αA for chronic active hepatitis B. *Aust. NZ J. Med.*, **20**, 9–19.
231. Weissberg, J. I., Andres, L. L., Smith, C. I. *et al.* (1984). Survival in chronic hepatitis B: an analysis of 379 patients. *Ann. Intern. Med.*, **101**, 613–616.
232. Farrell, G. C. (1992). Interferon treatment for chronic viral hepatitis in Australia: is it worth it? *Med. J. Aust.*, **156**, 873–876.
233. Pastore, G., Santantonio, T., Milella, M. *et al.* (1992). Anti-HBe-positive chronic hepatitis B with HBV DNA in the serum: response to a 6-month course of lymphoblastoid interferon. *J. Hepatol.*, **14**, 221–225.
234. Brunetto, M. R., Olivieri, F., Demartini, A. *et al.* (1991). Treatment with interferon of chronic hepatitis B associated with antibody to hepatitis Be antigen. *J. Hepatol.*, **13** (Suppl. 1), S8–S11.
235. Takeda, K., Akahane, Y., Suzuki, H. *et al.* (1990). Defects in the precore region of the HBV genome in patients with chronic hepatitis B after sustained seroconversion from HBeAg to anti-HBe induced spontaneously or with interferon therapy. *Hepatology*, **12**, 1284–1289.
236. Gunther, S., Meisel, H., Reip, A. *et al.* (1992). Frequent and rapid emergence of mutated pre-C sequences in HBV from e-antigen positive carriers who seroconvert to anti-HBe during interferon treatment. *Virology*, **187**, 271–279.
237. Lok, A. S. F., Lai, C. L., Wu, P. C. and Leung, E. K. Y. (1988). Long-term follow

up in a randomized controlled trial of recombinant alpha-interferon in Chinese patients with chronic hepatitis B infection. *Lancet*, **ii**, 298–302.
238. Lok, A. S. F. (1991). Alpha interferon therapy for chronic hepatitis B virus infection in children and Oriental patients. *J. Gastroenterol. Hepatol.*, **6** (Suppl. 1), 15–17.
239. Lai, C. L., Lok, A. S. F., Lin, H. J. *et al.* (1987). Placebo controlled trial of recombinant alpha interferon in Chinese HBsAg-carrier children. *Lancet*, **ii**, 877–880.
240. Ruiz-Moreno, M., Rua, M. J., Molina, J. *et al.* (1991). Prospective, randomized controlled trial of interferon alpha in children with chronic hepatitis B. *Hepatology*, **13**, 1035–1039.
241. Martin, P., Munoz, S. J. and Friedman, L. G. (1992). Liver transplantation for viral hepatitis: current status. *Am. J. Gastroenterol.*, **87**, 409–418.
242. Rakela, J., Redeker, A. G. and Weliky, B. (1983). Effect of short-term prednisone therapy on aminotransferase levels and hepatitis B virus markers in chronic type B hepatitis. *Gastroenterology*, **84**, 956–960.
243. Nair, P. V., Tong, M. J., Stevenson, D. *et al.* (1985). Effects of short-term, high-dose prednisone treatment of patients with HBsAg-positive chronic active hepatitis. *Liver*, **5**, 8–12.
244. Hoofnagle, J. H., Davis, G. L., Pappas, S. C. *et al.* (1986). A short course of prednisolone in chronic type B hepatitis: report of a randomized double-blind, placebo controlled trial. *Ann. Intern. Med.*, **104**, 12–17.
245. Yokosuka, O., Omata, M., Imazeki, F. *et al.* (1985). Combination of short-term prednisolone and adenine arabinoside in the treatment of chronic hepatitis B: a controlled study. *Gastroenterology*, **89**, 246–251.
246. Sztein, M. B. and Goldstein, A. L. (1986). Thymic hormones: a clinical update. *Springer Semin. Immunopathol.*, **9**, 1–18.
247. Huang, K.-Y., Kind, P. D., Jagoda, E. M. and Goldstein, A. L. (1981). Thymosin treatment modulates production of interferon. *J. Interferon Res.*, **1**, 411–420.
248. Gutterman, J. J., Fine, S., Quesada, J. *et al.* (1982). Recombinant leukocyte A interferon: pharmacokinetics, single dose tolerance and biologic effects in cancer patients. *Ann. Intern. Med.*, **96**, 549–556.
249. McDonald, E. M., Mann, A. H. and Thomas, H. C. (1987). Interferons as mediators of psychiatric morbidity: an investigation in a trial of recombinant alpha-interferon in hepatitis B carriers. *Lancet*, **ii**, 1175–1177.
250. Renault, P. F., Hoofnagle, J. H., Park, Y. *et al.* (1987). Psychiatric complications of long-term interferon alpha therapy. *Arch. Intern. Med.*, **147**, 1577–1580.
251. Burman, P., Totterman, T. H., Oberg, K. and Karlsson, F. A. (1986). Thyroid autoimmunity in patients on long-term therapy with leukocyte-derived interferon. *J. Clin. Endocrinol. Metab.*, **63**, 1086–1090.
252. Vento, S., Di Perri, G., Garofano, T. *et al.* (1989). Hazards of interferon therapy for HBV-seronegative chronic hepatitis. *Lancet*, **ii**, 926.
253. Peleman, R. R., Gavaler, J. S., Van Thiel, D. H. and Starzl, T. E. (1987). Orthotopic liver transplantation for acute and subacute hepatic failure. *Hepatology*, **7**, 484–489.
254. Brechot, C., Berneau, J., Thiers, V. *et al.* (1984). Multiplication of hepatitis B virus in fulminant hepatitis B. *Br. Med. J.*, **288**, 270–271.
255. Lake, J. R. and Wright, T. L. (1991). Liver transplantation for patients with hepatitis B: what have we learned from our results? *Hepatology*, **13**, 796–799.
256. Todo, S., Demetris, A. J., Van Thiel, D. *et al.* (1991). Orthotopic liver transplantation for patients with hepatitis B virus-related liver disease. *Hepatology*, **13**, 619–626.

257. O'Grady, J. G., Smith, H. M., Davies, S. E. *et al.* (1992). Hepatitis B virus reinfection after orthotopic liver transplantation: serological and clinical implications. *J. Hepatol.*, **14**, 104–111.
258. Samuel, D., Bismuth, A., Mathieu, D. *et al.* (1991). Passive immunoprophylaxis after liver transplantation in HBsAg-positive patients. *Lancet*, **337**, 813–815.
259. Levy, G. A., Sherber, A., Fung, L. S. *et al.* (1989). Relevance of hepatitis B viral DNA in assessment of potential liver allograft recipients. *Transplant. Proc.*, **21**, 3333–3334.
260. Cote, P. J., Korba, B. E., Steinberg, H. *et al.* (1991). Cyclosporin A modulates the course of woodchuck hepatitis virus infection and induces chronicity. *J. Immunol.*, **146**, 3138–3144.
261. Rakela, J., Wooten, R. S., Batts, K. P. *et al.* (1989). Failure of interferon to prevent recurrent hepatitis B infection in hepatic allograft. *Mayo Clin. Proc.*, **64**, 429–432.
262. Lauchart, Muller, R. and Pichlmayr, R. (1987). Immunoprophylaxis of hepatitis B virus reinfection in recipients of human liver allografts. *Transplant. Proc.*, **19**, 2387–2389.
263. Rizzetto, M., Hoyer, B., Canese, M. G. *et al.* (1980). Delta agent: association of delta antigen with hepatitis B surface antigen and RNA in serum of delta-infected chimpanzees. *Proc. Natl Acad. Sci. USA*, **77**, 6124–6128.
264. Cole, S. M., Gowans, E. J., Macnaughton, T. B. *et al.* (1990). Direct evidence for cytotoxicity associated with the expression of hepatitis virus delta antigen. *Hepatology*, **12**, 845–851.
265. Hoofnagle, J. H. (1989). Type D (Delta) hepatitis. *JAMA*, **261**, 1321–1325.
266. Rizzetto, M., Recchia, S. and Salizzoni, M. (1991). Liver transplantation in carriers of the HBsAg. *J. Hepatol.*, **13**, 5–7.
267. Rizzetto, M., Canese, M. G., Arico, J. (1977). Immunofluorescence detection of a new antigen-antibody system (δ-antiδ) associated to the hepatitis B virus in the liver and in the serum of HBsAg carriers. *Gut*, **18**, 997–1003.
268. Ponzetto, A., Cote, P. J., Popper, H. *et al.* (1984). Transmission of the hepatitis B virus-associated delta agent to the eastern woodchuck. *Proc. Natl Acad. Sci. USA*, **81**, 2208–2212.
269. Purcell, R. H., Satterfield, W. C., Bergmann, K. F. *et al.* (1987). Experimental hepatitis delta virus infection in the chimpanzee. In *Hepatitis Delta Virus and its Infection,* M. Rizzetto, J. L. Gerin and R. H. Purcell (eds), Liss, New York, pp. 27–36.
270. Taylor, J. M. (1991). Human hepatitis delta virus. *Curr. Top. Microbiol. Immunol.*, **168**, 141–166.
271. Bonino, F., Hoyer, W., Shih, J. W.-K. *et al.* (1984). Delta hepatitis agent: structural and antigenic properties of the delta-associated particles. *Infect. Immun.*, **43**, 1000–1005.
272. Bonino, F., Heermann, K.-H., Rizzetto, M. and Gerlich, W. H. (1985). Hepatitis delta virus: protein composition of delta antigen and its hepatitis B virus-derived envelope. *J. Virol.*, **58**, 945–950.
273. He, L.-F., Ford, E., Purcell, R. H. *et al.* (1989). The size of the hepatitis delta agent. *J. Med. Virol.*, **27**, 31–33.
274. Wang, K.-S., Choo, Q.-L., Weiner, A. J. *et al.* (1986). Structure, sequence and expression of the hepatitis delta viral genome. *Nature*, **323**, 508–513.
275. Sanger, H. L. (1987). Viroid replication. In *The Viroids,* T. O. Diener (ed.), Plenum, New York, pp. 117–166.
276. Wang., K.-S., Choo, Q.-L., Weiner, A. J. *et al.* (1987). Corrigendum: structure, sequence and expression of the hepatitis delta viral genome. *Nature*, **328**, 456.
277. Kuo, M. Y.-P., Goldberg, J., Coates, L. *et al.* (1988). Molecular cloning of hepatitis

delta virus RNA from an infected woodchuck liver: sequence, structure and applications. *J. Virol.*, **62**, 1855–1861.
278. Bergmann, K. F. and Gerin, J. L. (1986). Antigens of hepatitis delta virus in the liver and serum of humans and animals. *J. Infect. Dis.*, **154**, 702–705.
279. Luo, G., Chao, M., Hsieh, S.-Y. *et al.* (1990). A specific base transition occurs on replicating hepatitis delta virus RNA. *J. Virol.*, **64**, 1021–1027.
280. Glenn, J. G., Watson, J. A., Havel, C. M. and White, J. M. (1992). Identification of a prenylation site in delta virus large antigen. *Science*, **256**, 1331–1333.
281. Chang, M.-F., Baker, S. C., Soe, L. H. *et al.* (1988). Human hepatitis delta antigen is a nuclear phosphoprotein with RNA binding activity. *J. Virol.*, **62**, 2403–2410.
282. Macnaughton, T. B., Gowans, E. J., Reinboth, B. *et al.* (1990). Stable expression of the small polypeptide of hepatitis delta virus antigen in a eukaryotic cell line. *J. Gen. Virol.*, **71**, 1339–1345.
283. Chao, M., Hsieh, S.-Y., Luo, G. and Taylor, J. (1991). The antigen of human hepatitis delta virus: the significance of the two major electrophoretic forms. In *The Hepatitis Delta Virus*, J. L. Gerin, R. H. Purcell and M. Rizzetto (eds), Liss, New York, pp. 257–281.
284. Lai, M. M. C., Chao, Y. C., Chang, M.-F. *et al.* (1991). Functional studies of hepatitis delta antigen and delta virus RNA. In *The Hepatitis Delta Virus*, J. L. Gerin, R. H. Purcell and M. Rizzetto (eds), Liss, New York, pp. 283–292.
285. Taylor, J. M. (1990). Structure and replication of hepatitis delta virus. *Semin. Virol.*, **1**, 135–141.
286. Taylor, J. M., Mason, W., Summers, J. *et al.* (1987). Replication of human hepatitis delta virus in primary cultures of woodchuck hepatocytes. *J. Virol.*, **61**, 2891–2895.
287. Gowans, E. J., Baroudy, B. M., Negro, F. *et al.* (1988). Evidence for the replication of hepatitis delta virus RNA in nuclei after in vivo infection. *Virology*, **167**, 174–178.
288. Hsieh, S.-Y., Chao, M., Coates, L. and Taylor, J. (1990). Hepatitis delta virus genome replication: a polyadenylated mRNA for delta antigen. *J. Virol.*, **64**, 3192–3198.
289. Jilbert, A. R., Gowans, E. J., Macnaughton, T.B. and Burrell, C. J. (1991). Characterization of a subgenomic HDV-specific poly(A) + RNA species isolated from human hepatoma cells supporting HDV RNA replication. In *The Hepatitis Delta Virus*, J. L. Gerin, R. H. Purcell and M. Rizzetto (eds), Liss, New York, pp. 309–314.
290. Sharmeen, L., Kuo, M. Y.-P., Dinter-Gottlieb, G. and Taylor, J. (1988). The antigenomic RNA of human hepatitis delta virus can undergo self-cleavage. *J. Virol.*, **62**, 2674–2679.
291. Sharmeen, L. Kuo, M. Y.-P. and Taylor, J. (1989). Self-ligating sequences on the antigenome of human hepatitis delta virus. *J. Virol.*, **63**, 1428–1430.
292. Kuo, M. Y.-P., Sharmeen, L., Dinter-Gottlieb, G. and Taylor, J. (1988). Characterization of self-cleaving RNA sequences on the genome and antigenome of human hepatitis delta virus. *J. Virol.*, **62**, 4439–4444.
293. Macnaughton, T. M., Gowan, E. J., McNamara, S. P. and Burrell, C. J. (1991). Hepatitis delta antigen is necessary for access of hepatitis delta virus RNA to the cell transcriptional machinery, but is not part of the transcriptional complex. *Virology*, **184**, 387–390.
294. Glenn, J. G. and White, J. M. (1991). Trans-dominant inhibition of human hepatitis delta virus genome replication. *J. Virol.*, **65**, 2357–2361.
295. Taylor, J. M. (1990). Hepatitis delta virus: cis and trans functions required for replication. *Cell*, **61**, 371–373.

296. Hazelhoff, J. and Gerlach, W. L. (1988). Simple RNA enzymes with new and highly specific endoribonuclease activities. *Nature*, **334**, 585–591.
297. Di Bisceglie, A. M. and Negro, F. (1989). Diagnosis of hepatitis delta virus infection. *Hepatology*, **10**, 1014–1016.
298. Thomas, H. C., Lever, A. M. L., Scully, L. J. and Pignatelli, M. (1986). Approaches to treatment of hepatitis B virus and delta-related liver disease. *Semin. Liver Dis.*, **6**, 34–41.
299. Kuo, M. Y.-P., Chao, M. and Taylor, J. (1989). Initiation of replication of the human hepatitis delta virus genome from cloned DNA: role of the delta antigen. *J. Virol.*, **63**, 1945–1950.
300. Taylor, J., Mason, W., Summers, J. *et al.* (1987). Replication of human hepatitis delta virus in primary cultures of woodchuck hepatocytes. *J. Virol.*, **61**, 2891–2895.
301. Choi, S.-S., Rasshofer, R. and Roggendorf, M. (1988). Propagation of woodchuck hepatitis delta virus in primary woodchuck hepatocytes. *Virology*, **167**, 451–457.
302. Sureau, C., Jacob, J. R., Eichberg, J. W. and Lanford, R. E. (1991). Tissue culture system for infection with human hepatitis delta virus. *J. Virol.*, **65**, 3443–3450.
303. Petcu, D. J., Aldrich, C. E., Coates, L. *et al.* (1988). Suramin effectively inhibits in vitro infection by duck hepatitis B virus, Rous sarcoma virus and hepatitis delta virus. *Virology*, **167**, 385–392.
304. Choi, S.-S., Rasshofer, R. and Roggendorf, M. (1989). Inhibition of hepatitis delta virus RNA replication in primary woodchuck hepatocytes. *Antiviral Res.*, **12**, 213–222.
305. Rizzetto, M., Verme, G., Recchia, S. *et al.* (1983). Chronic HBsAg hepatitis with intrahepatic expression of delta antigen: an active and progressive disease unresponsive to immunosuppressive treatment. *Ann. Intern. Med.*, **98**, 437–441.
306. Rosina, F., Pintus, C., Meschievitz, C. and Rizzetto, M. (1991). A randomized controlled trial of a 12 month course of recombinant human alpha interferon in chronic delta (type D) hepatitis: a multicenter Italian study. *Hepatology*, **13**, 1052–1056.
307. Di Bisceglie, A. M., Martin, P., Lisker-Melman, M. *et al.* (1990). Therapy of chronic delta hepatitis with interferon alfa-2b. *J. Hepatol.*, **11**, 5151–5154.
308. Sagnelli, E. and Manzillo, G. (1983). Clinical aspects of delta agent infection in southern Italy. In *Viral Hepatitis and Delta Infection*, G. Verme, F. Bonino and M. Rizzetto (eds), Liss, New York, pp. 195–202.
309. Smedile, A., Farci, P., Verme, G. *et al.* (1982). Influence of delta infection on severity of hepatitis B. *Lancet*, **ii**, 945–947.
310. Lesbordes, J. L., Trep, C., Ravisse, P. *et al.* (1986). Infection with hepatitis delta virus. *N. Engl. J. Med.*, **314**, 517–518.
311. Sherlock, S. (1981). *Diseases of the Liver and Biliary System*, 6th edn, Blackwell Scientific Publications, Oxford.
312. Sanchez-Tapias, J. M., Mas, A., Costa, J. *et al.* (1987). Recombinant alpha 2a interferon therapy in fulminant viral hepatitis. *J. Hepatol.*, **5**, 205–210.
313. Marinucci, G., Valeri, L., Alfani, D. *et al.* (1986). Delta infection and liver disease recurrence in hepatic allografts. *Transplant. Proc.*, **18**, 1401–1404.
314. Rizzetto, M., Macagno, S., Chiaberge, E. *et al.* (1987). Liver transplantation in hepatitis delta virus disease. *Lancet*, **ii**, 469–471.
315. Grendele, M., Colledan, M., Gridelli, B. *et al.* (1990). Does the experience with liver transplantation suggest that hepatitis delta virus is not cytopathic? *Transplant. Proc.*, **22**, 1551–1553.
316. Agnes, S., Avolio, A. W., Magalini, S. C. *et al.* (1989). Results of liver transplan-

tation for delta hepatitis without HBIg immunoprophylaxis. *Transplant. Proc.*, **21**, 2426–2428.

317. Dienstag, J. L. (1983). Non-A, non-B hepatitis. I. Recognition, epidemiology and clinical features. *Gastroenterology*, **85**, 439–462.
318. Dienstag, J. L. (1983). Non-A, non-B hepatitis. II. Experimental transmission, putative virus agents and markers, and prevention. *Gastroenterology*, **85**, 743–768.
319. Koretz, R. L., Stone, O. and Gitnick, G. L. (1980). The long-term course of non-A, non-B post-transfusion hepatitis. *Gastroenterology*, **79**, 893–898.
320. Realdi, G., Alberti, A., Rugje, M. *et al.* (1982). Long-term follow-up of acute and chronic non-A, non-B post-transfusion hepatitis: evidence of progression to liver cirrhosis. *Gut*, **23**, 270–275.
321. Alter, M. J., Gerety, R. J., Smallwood, L. A. *et al.* (1982). Sporadic non-A, non-B hepatitis: frequency and epidemiology in an urban US population. *J. Infect. Dis.*, **145**, 886–893.
322. Farci, P., Alter, H. J., Wong, D. *et al.* (1991). A long term study of hepatitis C virus replication in non-A, non-B hepatitis. *N. Engl. J. Med.*, **325**, 98–104.
323. Kiyosawa, K., Tanaka, E., Sodeyama, T. *et al.* (1990). Transition of antibody to hepatitis C virus from chronic hepatitis to hepatocellular carcinoma. *Jpn. J. Cancer Res.*, **81**, 1089–1091.
324. Bradley, D. W., McCaustland, K. A., Cook, E. H. *et al.* (1985). Post-transfusion non-A, non-B hepatitis in chimpanzees: physicochemical evidence the tubule-forming agent is a small, enveloped virus. *Gastroenterology*, **88**, 773–779.
325. Bradley, D. W., McCaustland, K., Krawczynski, K. *et al.* (1991). Hepatitis C virus: buoyant density of the factor VIII-derived isolate in sucrose. *J. Med. Virol.*, **34**, 206–208.
326. Bradley, D. W. (1990). Hepatitis non-A, non-B viruses become identified as hepatitis C and E viruses. *Prog. Med. Virol.*, **37**, 101–135.
327. Bradley, D. W., Maynard, J. D., Popper, H. *et al.* (1983). Post-transfusion non-A, non-B hepatitis: physicochemical properties of two distinct agents. *J. Infect. Dis.*, **148**, 254–265.
328. Feinstone, S. M., Mihalik, K., Kamimura, T. *et al.* (1983). Inactivation of hepatitis B virus and non-A, non-B hepatitis by chloroform. *Infect. Immun.*, **41**, 816–821.
329. Bradley, D. W. (1985). The agents of non-A, non-B viral hepatitis. *J. Virol. Methods*, **10**, 307–319.
330. Houghton, M., Weiner, A., Han, J. *et al.* (1991). Molecular biology of the hepatitis C viruses: implications for diagnosis, development and control of viral disease. *Hepatology*, **14**, 381–388.
331. Choo, Q.-L., Richman, K. H., Han, J. H. *et al.* (1991). Genetic organization and diversity of the hepatitis C virus. *Proc. Natl Acad. Sci. USA*, **88**, 2451–2455.
332. Kato, N., Hijikata, M., Ootsuyama, Y. *et al.* (1990). Molecular cloning of the human hepatitis C virus genome from Japanese patients with non-A, non-B hepatitis. *Proc. Natl Acad. Sci. USA*, **87**, 9524–9528.
333. Takamizawa, A., Mori, C., Fuke, I. *et al.* (1991). Structure and organization of the hepatitis C virus genome isolated from human carriers. *J. Virol.*, **65**, 1105–1113.
334. Han, J. H., Shyamala, V., Richman, K. H. *et al.* (1991). Characterization of the terminal regions of hepatitis C virus: identification of conserved sequences in the 5′ untranslated region and poly(A) tails at the 3′ end. *Proc. Natl Acad. Sci. USA*, **88**, 1711–1715.
335. Okamoto, H., Okada, S., Sugiyama, Y. *et al.* (1990). The 5′-terminal sequence of hepatitis C virus genome. *Jpn. J. Exp. Med.*, **60**, 167–177.
336. Miller, R. H. and Purcell, R. H. (1990). Hepatitis C virus shares amino acid

sequence similarity with pestiviruses and flaviviruses as well as members of two plant virus supergroups. *Proc. Natl Acad. Sci. USA*, **87**, 2057–2061.

337. Plagemann, P. G. W. (1991). Hepatitis C virus: brief review. *Arch. Virol.*, **120**, 165–180.
338. Inchauspe, G., Zebedee, S., Lee, D.-H. *et al.* (1991). Genomic structure of the human prototype strain H of hepatitis C virus: comparison with American and Japanese isolates. *Proc. Natl Acad. Sci. USA*, **88**, 10292–10296.
339. Chambers, T. J., Weir, R. C., Grakovi, A. *et al.* (1990). Evidence that the N-terminal domain of nonstructural protein NS3 from yellow fever virus is a serine protease responsible for site-specific cleavages in the viral polyprotein. *Proc. Natl Acad. Sci. USA*, **87**, 8898–8902.
340. Enomoto, N., Takada, A., Nakao, T. and Date, T. (1990). There are two major types of hepatitis C virus in Japan. *Biochem. Biophys. Res. Commun.*, **170**, 1021–1025.
341. Okamoto, H., Kurai, K., Okada, S.-I. *et al.* (1992). Full-length sequence of a hepatitis C virus genome having poor homology to reported isolates: comparative study of four distinct genotypes. *Virology*, **188**, 331–341.
342. Holland, J., Spindler, K., Horodyski, F. *et al.* (1982). Rapid evolution of RNA genomes. *Science*, **215**, 1577–1585.
343. Choo, Q.-L., Kuo, G., Weiner, A. J. *et al.* (1989). Isolation of a cDNA clone derived from a blood-borne non-A, non-B viral hepatitis genome. *Science*, **244**, 359–362.
344. Weiner, A. J., Brauer, M. J., Rosenblatt, J. *et al.* (1991). Variable and hypervariable domains are found in the regions of HCV corresponding to the flavivirus envelope and NS1 proteins and the pestivirus envelope glycoproteins. *Virology*, **180**, 842–848.
345. Takada, N., Takase, S., Enomoto, N. *et al.* (1992). Clinical backgrounds of the patients having different types of hepatitis C virus genomes. *J. Hepatol.*, **14**, 35–40.
346. Pozzato, G., Moretti, M., Franzin, F. *et al.* (1991). Severity of liver disease with different hepatitis C viral clones. *Lancet*, **ii**, 509.
347. Schaff, Z., Hoofnagle, J. H. and Grimley, P. M. (1986). Hepatic inclusions during interferon therapy in chronic viral hepatitis. *Hepatology*, **6**, 966–970.
348. Jacob, J. R., Burk, K. H., Eichberg, J. W. *et al.* (1990). Expression of infectious viral particles by primary chimpanzee hepatocytes isolated during the acute phase of non-A, non-B hepatitis. *J. Infect. Dis.*, **161**, 1121–1127.
349. Shimizu, Y. K., Iwamoto, A., Hijikata, M. *et al.* (1992). Evidence for *in vitro* replication of hepatitis C virus genome in a human T-cell line. *Proc. Natl Acad. Sci. USA*, **89**, 5477–5481.
350. Hellings, J. A., Van der Veen du Prie, J., Snelting-Van Deusen, R. and Stute, R. (1985). Preliminary results of transmission experiments of non-A, non-B hepatitis by mononuclear leukocytes from a chronic patient. *J. Virol. Methods*, **10**, 321–326.
351. Chu, P. W. G. and Westaway, E. G. (1987). Characterization of Kunjin virus RNA-dependent RNA polymerase: reinitiation of synthesis *in vitro*. *Virology*, **157**, 330–337.
352. Reichard, O., Andersson, J., Schvarcz, R. and Weiland, O. (1991). Ribavirin treatment for chronic hepatitis C. *Lancet*, **i**, 1058–1061.
353. Streeter, D. G., Witkowski, J. T., Khare, G. P. *et al.* (1973). Mechanism of action of 1-β-D-ribofuranosyl-1,2,4-triazole-3-carboxamide (virazole), a new broad spectrum antiviral agent. *Proc. Natl Acad. Sci. USA*, **70**, 1174–1178.
354. Di Bisceglie, A. M. and Hoofnagle, J. H. (1991). Therapy of chronic hepatitis C with alpha-interferon: the answer? Or more questions? *Hepatology*, **13**, 601–603.

355. Weiner, A. J., Kuo, G. Bradley, D. W. *et al.* (1990). Detection of hepatitis C viral sequences in non-A, non-B hepatitis. *Lancet*, **335**, 1–3.
356. Kuo, G., Choo, Q.-L., Alter, H. J. *et al.* (1989). An assay for circulating antibodies to a major etiologic virus of human non-A, non-B hepatitis. *Science*, **244**, 362–364.
357. Beach, M. J., Meeks, E. L., Mimms, L. T. *et al.* (1992). Temporal relationships of hepatitis C virus RNA and antibody responses following experimental infection of chimpanzees. *J. Med. Virol.*, **36**, 226–237.
358. Quiroga, J. A., Campillo, M. L., Catillo, I. *et al.* (1991). IgM antibody to hepatitis C virus in acute and chronic hepatitis C. *Hepatology*, **14**, 38–43.
359. Lunel, F., Maisoneuve, P., Marcellin, P. *et al.* (1991). Relationship between anti-HCV antibodies measured by a quantitative RIBA assay and response to interferon in patients with chronic non-A, non-B hepatitis. *J. Hepatol.*, **13** (Suppl. 2), 547.
360. Chayama, K., Saitoh, S., Arase, Y. *et al.* (1991). Effect of interferon administration on serum hepatitis C virus RNA in patients with chronic hepatitis C. *Hepatology*, **13**, 1040–1043.
361. Bradley, D. W., Cook, E. H., Maynard, J. E. *et al.* (1979). Experimental infection of chimpanzees with anti hemophiliac (factor VIII) materials: recovery of virus-like particles associated with non-A, non-B hepatitis. *J. Med. Virol.*, **3**, 253–269.
362. Prince, A. M., Brotman, B., Huima, T. *et al.* (1992). Immunity in hepatitis C infection. *J. Infect. Dis.*, **165**, 438–443.
363. Ohnishi, K., Nomura, F. and Nakano, M. (1991). Interferon therapy for acute post-transfusion non-A, non-B hepatitis: response with respect to anti-hepatitis C virus antibody status. *Am. J. Gastroenterol.*, **86**, 1041–1049.
364. Omata, M., Yokosuka, O., Takano, S. *et al.* (1991). Resolution of acute hepatitis C after therapy with natural beta interferon. *Lancet*, **338**, 914–915.
365. Cuthbert, J. A. (1990). Hepatitis C. *Am. J. Med. Sci.*, **229**, 346–355.
366. Pappas, S. C., Hoofnagle, J. H. and Young, N. (1985). Treatment of chronic non-A, non-B hepatitis with acyclovir: pilot study. *J. Med. Virol*,. **15**, 1–9.
367. Hoofnagle, J. H., Mullen, K. M., Jones, D. B. *et al.* (1986). Treatment of chronic non-A, non-B hepatitis with recombinant human alpha interferon: a preliminary report. *N. Engl. J. Med.*, **315**, 1575–1578.
368. Di Bisceglie, A. M., Martin, P., Kassianides, C. *et al.* (1989). Recombinant interferon alpha therapy for chronic hepatitis C: a randomized double-blind, placebo-controlled trial. *N. Engl. J. Med.*, **321**, 1506–1510.
369. Davis, G. L., Balart, L. A., Schiff, E. R. *et al.* (1989). Treatment of chronic hepatitis C with recombinant interferon alpha. *N. Engl. J. Med.*, **321**, 1501–1506.
370. Jacyna, M. R., Brooks, M. G., Loke, R. H. T. *et al.* (1989). Randomised controlled trial of interferon-α (lymphoblastoid interferon) in chronic non-A, non-B hepatitis. *Br. Med. J.*, **298**, 80–82.
371. Marcellin, P., Boyer, N., Giostra, E. *et al.* (1991). Recombinant human α-interferon in patients with chronic non-A, non-B hepatitis: a multicenter randomized controlled trial from France. *Hepatology*, **13**, 393–397.
372. Davis, G. L. (1990). Recombinant α-interferon treatment of non-A, non-B (type C) hepatitis: review of studies and recommendations for treatment. *J. Hepatol.*, **11** (Suppl. 1), 572–577.
373. Farrell, G. C. (1991). Treatment of chronic hepatitis C with alpha interferon. *J. Gastroenterol. Hepatol.*, **6** (Suppl. 1), 36–40.
374. Lin, R., Schoeman, M. N., Craig, P. I. *et al.* (1991). Can the response to interferon treatment be predicted in patients with chronic active hepatitis C? *Aust. NZ J. Med.*, **21**, 387–392.

375. Causse, X., Godinot, H., Chevallier, M. *et al.* (1991). Comparison of 1 or 3 MU of interferon alfa-2b and placebo in patients with chronic non-A, non-B hepatitis. *Gastroenterology*, **101**, 497–502.
376. Mayet, W.-J., Hess, G., Gerken, G. *et al.* (1989). Treatment of chronic type B hepatitis with recombinant alpha-interferon induces autoantibodies not specific for autoimmune chronic hepatitis. *Hepatology*, **10**, 24–28.
377. Renault, P. F. and Hoofnagle, J. H. (1989). Side effects of alpha interferon. *Semin. Liver Dis.*, **9**, 273–277.
378. Boyer, N., Marcellin, P., Degott, C. *et al.* (1992). Recombinant interferon-alpha for chronic hepatitis C in patients positive for antibody to human immunodeficiency virus. *J. Infect. Dis.*, **165**, 723–726.
379. Cimino, L., Citarella, C., Nardone, G. and Budillon, G. (1991). Lymphoblastoid interferon in chronic hepatitis C patients, 'non-responders' to recombinant interferon-α (rIFN-α). *J. Hepatol.*, **13**, 419–420.
380. Pereira, B. J. G., Milford, E. L., Kirkman, R. L. and Levy, A. S. (1991). Transmission of hepatitis C virus by organ transplantation. *N. Engl. J. Med.*, **325**, 454–460.

Part F

PAPILLOMAVIRUS

Basic Research

16 Fundamental Research in Papillomavirus: Molecular Controls in Human Papillomavirus Infection

MIKAËL A. LE MOAL and FRANÇOISE THIERRY
Unité des Virus Oncogènes, Institut Pasteur, Paris, France

INTRODUCTION

GENERAL PRESENTATION AND CLASSIFICATION

The first papillomavirus, cottontail rabbit papillomavirus (CRPV), was described in 1933 by Richard Shope, as the aetiological agent for cutaneous papillomatosis in the rabbit (1). Papillomaviruses are widespread in nature and have been identified in many different species of higher vertebrates, most notably in humans or other primates, cattle, rabbits, horses, dogs, elk, deer and mice. This group of viruses, although known for over 80 years to be responsible for human warts, has remained refractory to standard methods of *in vitro* cultivation. Papillomaviruses are small, non-enveloped, double-stranded DNA viruses which replicate in the nucleus of infected cells. The icosahedral viral capsid is composed of 72 capsomers made of two structural proteins, one major capsid protein with a molecular weight of approximately 55 000 Da and one minor protein of 70 000 Da, which are encoded respectively by the L1 and L2 open reading frames (ORFs). The genomes of over 60 different papillomaviruses have been cloned in bacterial plasmids and the complete sequences of 15 of them are known.

The size of their genome (8000 bp versus 5000 bp) is one of the notable differences that distinguishes the papillomaviruses from the other members of the Papovaviridae family of small DNA viruses, which includes the simian virus SV40 and the murine polyomavirus. In addition, the characteristic genomic organization and biology of papillomaviruses are consistent with their belonging to a specific group containing only this class of viruses. A very distinct biological property of this class of viruses is their extreme tissue specificity. The papillomaviruses are highly species specific and there are very few known examples of cross-infection. They also often show specificity towards the location or type of tissue that they infect. Frequently,

Antiviral Chemotherapy. Edited by D.J. Jeffries and E. De Clercq

the lesions associated with papillomaviruses are benign. In humans, they are mainly represented by warts. In all cases, they show a preferred tropism for squamous epithelial cells. Expression of the complete virus cycle appears to be limited to the terminally differentiated cells of squamous epithelia. They are usually associated with epithelial (often cutaneous) proliferative lesions. Some animal papillomaviruses, such as bovine papillomavirus 1 (BPV1), also induce fibroblastic proliferation and are responsible for the formation of benign fibropapillomas.

Classification of papillomavirus isolates has been done by comparative hybridization of their genomes in liquid phase, under stringent conditions. Viruses that show less than 50% sequence homology have been classified into different subgroups. It should be noted that, with the generalization of sequencing methods, precise homologies can now be calculated for many viruses. So far 58 human papillomaviruses (HPVs) and 15 animal viruses have been isolated.

BIOLOGICAL PROPERTIES

This review will focus mainly on the subgroup of HPVs associated with lesions of the genital tract and more particularly with squamous cell carcinoma (Table 16.1). This type of cancer presents a serious medical problem, since worldwide it is the second commonest cause of cancer mortality for women after breast cancer. However, a large part of our knowledge of papillomavirus biology comes from studies involving the bovine papillomavirus, BPV1. This virus was one of the first genomes to be cloned in a bacterial plasmid and sequenced (2) and shown, in the early 1980s, to be able to transform rodent cells *in vitro*. An *in vitro* system for maintenance of the BPV1 genome in cell culture has thus been established (3) that allows a molecular analysis of viral gene expression. In this remarkable system, the viral genome was not only maintained by autonomous replication, but could also transform cells by expression of viral functions. Efforts to reproduce an analogous *in vitro* system with HPVs have not been successful for a long period of time. This situation is due to the very stringent keratinocyte specificity of HPV expression as mentioned above and the inherent difficulties in establishing differentiation of these cells *in vitro*.

Once the presence of HPV genomes in the majority of cervical carcinoma-derived cell lines or biopsies had been established, it seemed possible that such cell cultures could be used to study HPV viral expression. However, such experimental systems did not permit the analysis of viral replication since, in contrast to BPV1 in rodent cells, the HPV genomes are usually found integrated into the cellular chromosomes. Recently it has been shown that genital warts containing HPV genomes could grow *in vitro* in organotypic cultures also called raft cultures that allow terminal differen-

Table 16.1. Summary of lesions associated with human papillomaviruses. The location, type of lesions and the subtype of virus associated with each type of lesion are given according to information published elsewhere (121)

Location	Benign lesions	Neoplastic lesions	HPV type
Skin	Warts		**1, 2, 3, 4,** 7, **10,** 26–29, 41, 60, 65
	Epidermodysplasia verruciformis		**3, 5, 8,** 9, 12, 14, 15, 17, 19–25, 36, 38, 46, 47, 49, 50
		Invasive carcinoma or carcinoma *in situ*	**5**, 8, 14, 17, 20, 36, 47
Vulva, penis, anus	Condyloma acuminatum	Buschke–Loewenstein tumours	**6, 11**
	Papillomas		**6, 11**, 42
		Bowenoid papulosis	**16**, 18, 33, 34, 39
		Bowen's disease	**16**, 18, 33
		Invasive squamous cell carcinoma	**16**, 18
Uterine cervix, vagina	Condyloma acuminatum		**6, 11**
	Flat condyloma		6, 11, 16, 18, 42
		Intraepithelial neoplasia	**16, 18**, 30, **31, 33**, 34, 35, 39, 40, 43, 44, 45, 51, 52, 56–59, 61–64, 66, 67
		Invasive squamous cell carcinoma	**16, 18**, 31, 33, 35, 39, 45, 51, 52, 56, 58
		Adenocarcinoma	16,**18**, 35
Oral cavity	Focal epithelial hyperplasia (FEH)		**13, 32**
Larynx	Papillomatosis		**6, 11**

tiation of the keratinocytes at a liquid/air interface (4,5). The complete viral cycle has recently been obtained using this *in vitro* culture system, after treatment with 12-*O*-tetradecanoyl phorbol-13-acetate (TPA) with production of viral particles (6).

THE GENETIC MAP

The genome of papillomaviruses is composed of a circular double-stranded DNA as shown in Figure 16.1. Comparative analysis of complete or partial sequences of various genomes has indicated a very conserved organization (7). Large ORFs are organized with a remarkable similarity between human and animal papillomaviruses (Figure 16.2). The various ORFs are located on only one DNA strand, indicating that transcription is unidirectional. This observation was confirmed by the finding that viral RNAs found in BPV1-infected or CRPV-transformed cells are transcribed from the same DNA coding strand. It appears that this characteristic is shared by all the papillomaviruses.

The coding strand contains 8–10 translational ORFs. Among them, six to eight are designated as early (E) and two as late (L) (Figures 16.1 and 16.2).

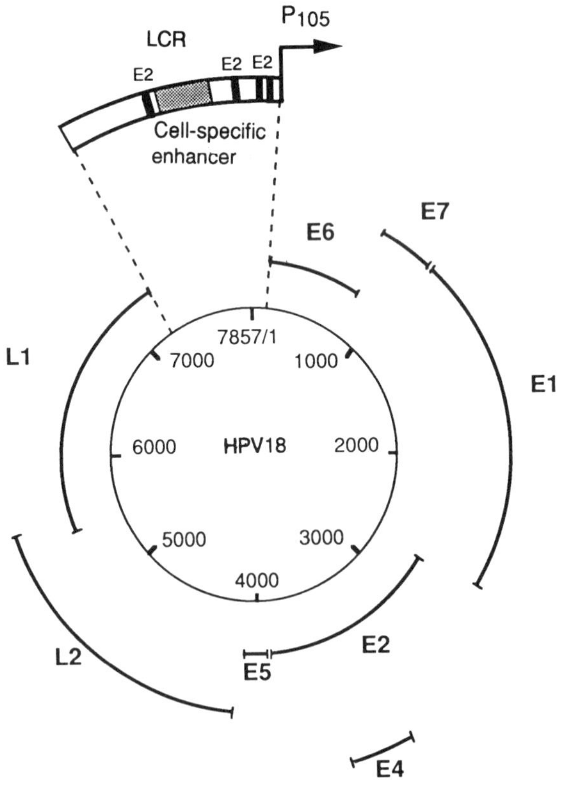

Figure 16.1. Genomic map of HPV18. The HPV18 genome is drawn according to nucleotide sequence numbering and location of the ORFs on the three different translational phases. E2 binding sites and the cell-specific enhancer within the long control region (LCR) are shown. The P_{105} promoter is denoted by an arrow

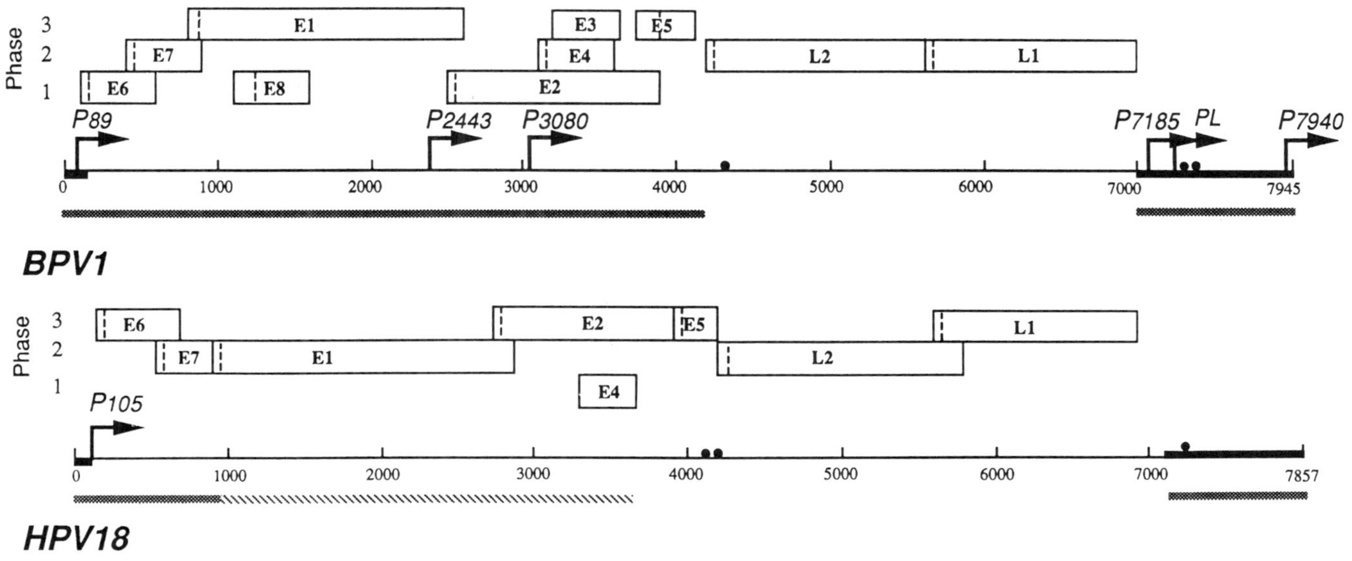

Figure 16.2. Comparative linear genetic maps of BPV1 and HPV18. The genomic organization of the bovine BPV1 and the human HPV18 viruses deduced from the primary DNA sequences. Genomes were linearized at a site corresponding to the Hpa I restriction site in BPV1. The various ORFs of the early and late regions are indicated on the three different translational frames. The LCR is indicated in bold and the various promoters are shown by arrows. The early and late polyadenylation sites are indicated by black spots. Grey lines under the genomic maps indicate the subfragments necessary for cellular transformation

This designation was based on the biological properties of the BPV1 genome. A portion of it (about 70%, shaded in Figure 16.2) was designated as 'early' since it was found to be sufficient to induce transformation and autonomous replication in rodent cells *in vitro* (8). Presence of the so-called 'late' region was necessary to permit the complete virus cycle with viral encapsidation. This distinction was later confirmed by the analysis of RNA from non-productive or productive infections. Messenger RNAs (mRNAs), coding for proteins involved in transformation and replication, terminate at the early polyadenylation site, while those coding for capsid structural proteins terminate at the late polyadenylation site (see Figure 16.2) (9). The same nomenclature has been used for human papillomaviruses based on sequence homologies of the designated ORFs. It appears, however, that certain ORFs, originally classed as early, such as E4 ORF of HPVs, may in fact be late genes.

A region of about 800 bp, known as the long control region (LCR) or upstream regulatory region (URR), is devoid of large ORFs and contains many *cis*-acting regulatory elements. The location and size of this region are well conserved amongst the papillomaviruses. It is located between the end of the L1 ORF and the beginning of the E6 ORF, as shown in Figure 16.1. The sequences are, however, quite divergent and, if common motifs are to be found, they consist of short sequences usually arranged in various combinations, specific to each genome. The transcriptional regulatory signals contained in this region have been well studied for the HPVs associated with genital tract infections. These analyses revealed the importance of transcriptional regulation of the expression of the transforming genes following HPV infection. In particular, they revealed that the HPVs contain a very strong epithelial cell-specific transcriptional enhancer, which is located in the regulatory region. Studies with the BPV1 system led to the identification of a short sequence which acts as an origin of replication. Some features of this sequence are relatively conserved as demonstrated by the comparison between BPV1 and HPV18 (Figure 16.9). The various functions of the regulatory region will be described in detail later.

ROLE OF THE OPEN READING FRAMES

Early open reading frames

The functions of several of the ORFs are now well known. This knowledge has been derived from the molecular analysis of different systems in which papillomavirus genomes have been expressed. Notably, BPV1 expression in transformed rodent cells and HPV expression in cervical carcinoma cell lines have been used and the known functions are listed in Table 16.2. Analysis of ORF function for the HPVs has been hampered by the inability of this class of virus to replicate *in vitro* in cell cultures. Cloning of the

Table 16.2. Roles of different ORFs. The ORFs for which some functional information is available are listed. The molecular weights are calculated from the sequence data. The virus type with which the function of the ORF has been primarily described is indicated. 'PVs' means that the function has been demonstrated for more than two viral subtypes

ORF	Approx. size	Function	Functions demonstrated for
E1	68–72 kDa	Replication	PVs
E2	48 kDa	Transcriptional regulator	PVs
		Replication	PVs
E2C	28/30 kDa	Transcriptional repressor	BPV1
E4	17 kDa	Viral maturation	HPV
E5	7 kDa	Transformation	BPV1,
	15 kDa	Transformation?	HPV16?
E6	18 kDa	Transformation	BPV1, HPV16/18
		Transcriptional activator	BPV1, HPV16
E7	16–20 kDa	Transformation	HPV16/18
		Transcriptional activator	HPV16/18
L1	56 kDa	Major capsid protein	PVs
L2	78 kDa	Minor capsid protein	PVs

ORFs in expression plasmids has therefore often been used to directly address this question. Transfection or co-transfection of such expression plasmids, into suitable cell lines, has revealed the functions of several of the ORFs, as listed in Table 16.2.

E2 is one of the best-studied ORFs. Since the original observation in 1985 (10) that the BPV1 E2 ORF encodes a transcriptional transactivator, many other E2s have been shown to share this property. The E2 protein binds as a dimer to a specific DNA sequence and is important for viral replication, as will be discussed below.

The E1 ORF is well conserved in its C-terminal moiety. It is essential for replication of papillomavirus DNA. Its function in replication has been mainly studied with BPV1. It binds to the viral origin of replication and to the E2 polypeptide.

Papillomaviruses contain three distinct transforming functions which are encoded by the E5, E6 and E7 ORFs. The transforming function of E5 has been studied mainly in BPV1 and homologous fibropapilloma viruses (11,12). It is a small polypeptide containing a hydrophobic domain at its amino-terminus, which is responsible for its association with the cytoplasmic membrane of infected cells. The amino acid sequences of E5 are very divergent among papillomaviruses. The BPV1 E5 protein is the smallest known oncoprotein (about 7 kDa). It is therefore unlikely that it possesses any intrinsic enzymatic activity. The BPV1 E5 protein may enhance the activity of the epidermal growth factor or colony-stimulating factor 1 receptors in NIH-3T3 cells via inhibition of receptor downregulation (13). Recently, E5 has been shown to interact with a 16 kDa cellular protein (14) which is a component of the vacuolar ATPases (15). This interaction may play a role in the function of the proton pumps interfering with the internalization and degradation of receptors. In HPVs, the E5 ORF is not well conserved and there are no sequence homologies with the BPV1 E5. The highly hydrophobic amino acid content (about 60%) is conserved. If cloned in a retroviral vector, the HPV16 E5 ORF appears to be able to transform murine keratinocytes *in vitro* (16). These results indicate that the E5 oncogenic function may well be conserved among papillomaviruses. It should be noted that in natural HPV cancers the transcriptional unit that gives rise to the E5 gene product is often disrupted during the process of viral integration into the host genome.

The products of the E6 and E7 ORFs are small polypeptides containing Cys-X-X-Cys motifs, which can bind zinc *in vitro* (17,18) suggesting zinc finger-like structures. They are found in the nucleus of infected cells. The BPV1 E6 ORF is another transforming function which cooperates with the homologous E5 gene to transform rodent cells *in vitro* (19). It has also been shown to be able to act as a transcriptional transactivator when linked to the DNA binding domain of E2 (20). Recently, the E6 and E7 polypeptides from the HPV types associated with high-risk genital infections, notably types 16 and 18, have been shown to cooperate in transforming human keratinocytes *in vitro* (21,22). Both of them are also transcriptional transactivators (23–25), although no homologous responsive elements have yet been found in the genomes of HPVs. The putative roles of the BPV1 E7 ORF and the HPV E5 ORF in the transformation process are less clear.

Late open reading frames

Expression of the early functions is detected in non-productive lesions, while expression of the late functions is necessarily linked to productive infections. Three polypeptides can be found to be expressed at high levels, in the terminally differentiated cells from productive lesions, encoded by the ORFs E4, L1 and L2. The latter polypeptides are the components of the viral capsid, while E4 is not. The presence of extremely high levels of E4 in warts, after HPV1 infection, was first demonstrated in 1986 (26) and 1987 (27). The exact role of this polypeptide is not yet understood but it seems to be intimately linked to the state of differentiation of the infected keratinocytes. In all the papillomaviruses, the E4 genes are contained within the E2 ORF but are translated from a different reading frame, as shown in Figures 16.1 and 16.2. Sequences of the various E4 ORFs are only partially conserved; some of them even lack an initiation codon. It seems therefore that the main E4 product would be translated from a spliced E1–E4 messenger RNA, using the E1 initiation codon. The E4 gene products of HPV1 as well as HPV16 are found associated with the cytokeratins of infected or transfected cells. Recent papers (28,29) suggest that E4 could perturb the very rigid cytoskeleton of terminally differentiated keratinocytes. This interaction even seems to lead to a complete collapse of the cellular intermediate filament network in epithelial cells (28). The role of these interactions in viral multiplication is not yet understood. Possibly, E4 helps to maintain the terminally differentiated cells in such a state that the maturation and final release of virus particles are facilitated.

HPVs AND CANCER

HPVs ASSOCIATED WITH ANOGENITAL INFECTIONS

We will focus mainly on a subclass of HPVs that has been found to be associated with lesions of the anogenital tract. This class of viruses has increasingly attracted attention over the past 10 years. They exclusively infect the mucous epithelium, mainly of the anogenital tract, but also of the pharynx or oral cavity. Most of the lesions associated with these viruses are benign, as indicated in Table 16.1. These 'genital' papillomaviruses are widespread in nature where they are venereally transmitted. With some of these viruses, notably type 16 or type 18, the risk of oncogenic transformation is important since 1–2% of the lesions can evolve into squamous cell carcinoma or invasive squamous cell carcinoma of the uterine cervix, as indicated in Table 16.1. Since the first demonstrations of the presence of the virus in a high percentage (more than 85%) (30) of cervical carcinomas, molecular analysis of viral expression has revealed that some of these viruses can indeed express oncoproteins. It is this carcinogenic conversion which has led to increasing interest in the papillomavirus field over the last few years.

STATE OF THE HPV GENOMES IN LESIONS

In benign genital productive lesions, HPV genomes are maintained in an episomal state and viral replication leads to the formation of mature virions. However, such lesions are much less productive than those formed in the skin (warts). Numerous virus types have been found associated with these benign or pre-malignant lesions, as listed in Table 16.1, and some of them are more frequent than others. The virus types 6, 11, 16 and 18 are the most frequently found and epidemiological studies indicate a uniform geographical distribution. HPV6 and HPV11 belong to a group of low oncogenic potential. They are associated with benign lesions of the anogenital tract, oral cavity or larynx and very few cases of association with squamous cell carcinoma have been reported. By contrast, HPV16 and HPV18 are the predominant types found in these cancers. While the benign or pre-malignant lesions, associated with any of these viruses, contain the viral DNA exclusively in the episomal form, in squamous cell carcinomas the viral genomes are found in both free and integrated states. Cell lines established from cancer biopsies only contain integrated viral DNA (31).

INTEGRATION

The integration of papillomaviruses in cervical carcinoma cell lines has been extensively studied. It appears from studies of cell lines containing the HPV16 or HPV18 genomes that there is a common pattern of viral integration. Notably, the integrated viral genome is often interrupted. The portion of the genome which is found integrated into the cellular DNA, and conserved among HPV-associated lesions, contains the regulatory and early sequences. The fragment of the genome which is integrated is indicated as a grey line under the linear map of HPV18 in Figure 16.2. Interruption occurs in the E1 C-terminal domain or E2 ORFs, before the early polyadenylation signal, as indicated in Figure 16.2. Therefore, the mRNAs transcribed from the integrated viral genomes will terminate in the flanking cellular sequences. On the other hand, the viral mRNAs are initiated from the promoter contained in the viral regulatory sequences (31–34). Interestingly, no specific sites for viral DNA integration in the cellular genome have been consistently found in HPV-associated lesions.

EXPRESSION OF THE INTEGRATED VIRAL GENOME

In all the HPV-associated cervical carcinoma cell lines studied so far, the integrated viral genomes are actively transcribed (31,35). Two major RNAs are produced that code for the E6 and E7 gene products, as shown in Figure 16.3. Putative shorter products from the E6 ORF, called E6* (two from the HPV16 and one from the HPV18 genome), could also be translated from the spliced viral mRNA shown in Figure 16.3, but their existence *in vivo* has never been proved and no function has ever been attributed to these putative products. It seems that the spliced RNA would be the preferential messenger for E7 translation, while the unspliced RNA would preferentially be used to translate the E6 gene product (25) (Figure 16.3). Both mRNAs are initiated at the same viral promoter contained in the viral regulatory region. The promoters are named after the nucleotide number at which the RNAs are initiated and are P_{105} in HPV18 (shown in Figures 16.1 and 16.2) and P_{97} in HPV16 (Figure 16.3). P_{105} and P_{97} are the main active promoters in the viral integrated HPV16 or HPV18 genomes in carcinoma

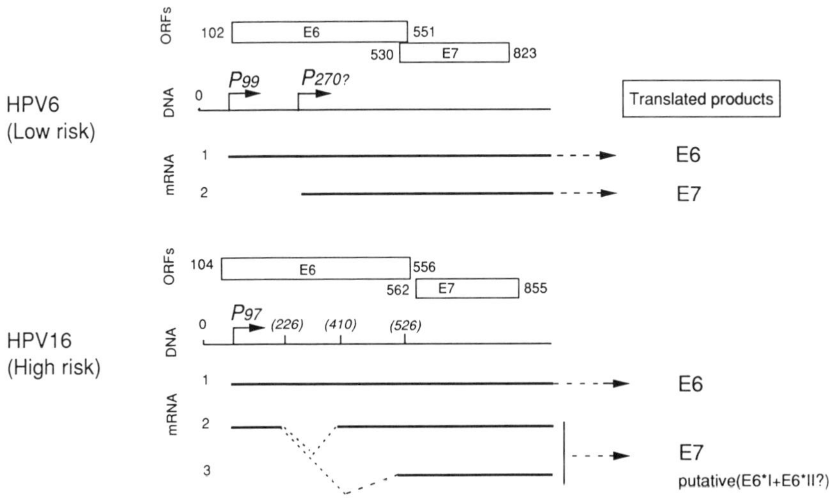

Figure 16.3. Transcription of the E6 and E7 ORFs in low- (HPV6) and high-risk (HPV16) viruses. Comparative transcriptional mapping of the E6 and E7 gene products of the low-risk genital papillomavirus type 6 and the high-risk type 16. Promoters are indicated by arrows, and mRNA by bold lines. Numbers in parentheses indicate the locations of splice donor and acceptor in the HPV16 E6 ORF. The two spliced RNAs could code for two putative fusion proteins within the E6 ORF (E6*I and E6*II) in addition to the full-length E7

cell lines. The transcriptional regulation of these promoters has been extensively studied and we will develop this point later on. Interestingly, the E6 and E7 ORFs of the non-oncogenic papillomavirus types HPV6 and HPV11 seem to be transcribed in a different manner: E6 is translated from an unspliced RNA containing the whole early region, while E7 is translated from an mRNA starting at a specific promoter in front of E7 (25,36) (Figure 16.3). These differences in expression could account in part for variations in the oncogenic potential of the two classes of viruses, as noted earlier. Both E6 and E7 are found in the nucleus of cervical carcinoma cell lines, while no other viral products seem to have been consistently found in these cells. These results point to the potentially crucial role of the E6 and E7 gene products in papillomavirus-induced transformation.

IN VITRO TRANSFORMATION

The E7 oncoprotein

HPV16 and HPV18 DNAs were initially shown to induce transformation of rodent cell lines, although at low efficiency, and could also transform baby rat kidney cells in conjunction with the activated *ras* oncogene. In these experimental systems, the transforming gene was shown to be encoded by the E7 ORF (reviewed in reference 37).

Recently, the genomes of HPV16 and HPV18 have been shown to transform human keratinocytes *in vitro* (38–42). Primary keratinocytes from human foreskin or normal cervix were transfected with the HPV16 or HPV18 viral DNAs. Cells in which the viral DNA had become integrated into the cellular genome were shown to be resistant to differentiation induced, notably, by high calcium concentrations in the culture medium. The transfected keratinocytes could then be established as cell lines. These cell lines have an extended life-span, are resistant to differentiation but are not tumorigenic in nude mice. They express the viral E6 and E7 gene products. Genetic analysis has indicated that these products are together necessary and sufficient to allow for keratinocyte immortalization *in vitro* (21,22). Interestingly, this situation is only found with the 'high-risk' HPVs, notably HPV16 or HPV18, but not with the 'low-risk' HPVs such as HPV6 or HPV11. These oncogenic characteristics seem to be linked to intrinsic properties of the E6 and E7 gene products themselves as well as to their transcriptional regulation.

The E7 oncoprotein is a short polypeptide of 98 amino acids which has not been shown to have any intrinsic enzymatic activities. The N-terminal 37 amino acids contain regions which are similar to the conserved domains 1 and 2 of adenovirus E1a protein. In E1a, these regions have been shown to be necessary for transformation and mediate interactions with the product of the retinoblastoma tumour suppressor gene (p105-RB). Related sequences in SV40 large-T antigen (T Ag) are also involved in binding to RB. It has been shown that, like E1a and T Ag, the HPV16 or HPV18 E7 proteins are able to bind p105-RB (43,44). A similar mechanism of action, involving interference of the viral oncoproteins with the function of RB in the control of normal cell proliferation, can thus be suggested for the three viral oncogenes, E1a, T Ag and E7. Binding of E7 to RB may explain its transcriptional transactivation property. The HPV16 E7 oncoprotein, like E1a or the SV40 T Ag, has been shown to be able to dissociate RB from a complex with the cellular E2F factor (45–47). This property of the E7 oncoprotein appears to be clearly linked to its ability to transactivate the adenovirus E2 promoter (24) and most certainly plays a crucial role in cellular transformation. Binding of RB to E2F or E7, as well as to E1a or T Ag, appears to be mutually exclusive and the interaction of RB with E2F has been shown to play an essential role in regulating cell proliferation. A possible role for the HPV E7 oncoprotein could be that the release of E2F from cellular complexes promotes activation of cellular genes (such as dihydrofolic reductase or DNA polymerase, for example, which contain E2F binding sites) whose activation might result in a favourable environment for viral DNA replication and completion of the viral cycle. In other situations, release of E2F could allow reactivation of cellular genes involved in continuous cellular proliferation (reviewed in reference 46).

The E6 oncoprotein

As noted before, the E6 oncoprotein is also necessary, in addition to the E7 protein, to transform keratinocytes *in vitro*. However, it has been more difficult to demonstrate its oncogenic potential. This small protein shares some structural features with E7 in that they both contain putative zinc finger structures as noted earlier (18). Mechanisms of *in vitro* transformation by adenoviruses involve not only E1a but also the E1B protein as a cooperative factor which interacts with the product of the cellular tumour suppressor gene p53. The E6 proteins of HPV16 and HPV18 have been shown to interact with p53 as well (48). Further characterization of this interaction has indicated that E6 could promote specific degradation of p53, by means of a process that involves the ubiquitin pathway, and is specific to the E6 products of the oncogenic HPV types, HPV16 and HPV18 (49).

In conclusion, while the roles of the E6 and E7 proteins in the *in vitro* transformation of human epithelial cells have now been clearly demonstrated, their exact roles *in vivo* remain puzzling. Cervical carcinoma cell lines established from carcinomas not associated with HPVs have been shown to harbour mutated RB and p53 cellular products in the absence of the viral oncoproteins E6 and E7 (50). It should be noted that the cellular transformation obtained *in vitro* with the combination of E6 and E7 does not totally reflect the oncogenic conversion seen *in vivo*, since the *in vitro* transformed cells are not tumorigenic in nude mice, while cervical carcinoma cell lines are highly tumorigenic in similar assays. The E6 and E7 ORFs are relatively well conserved among papillomaviruses whether or not they are associated with viruses with oncogenic potential *in vivo*. The oncogenic potential seems to correlate with some of the biochemical properties of the E7 proteins (51), although the E7 gene products of the HPV6 or HPV11 viruses, for example, have been shown to be able to bind p105-RB (44). This activity therefore does not seem to be necessarily linked to high oncogenic potential. It should be noted that the papillomaviruses induce cell proliferation in benign as well as pre-malignant lesions. This benign cell proliferation may be induced by mechanisms involving some of the oncogenic potentials of the E6 and E7 proteins.

TRANSCRIPTIONAL REGULATION

E2-MODULATED TRANSCRIPTIONAL REGULATION

The viral transcriptional modulator E2

As noted earlier, the product of the E2 ORF has been extensively studied. It is rather well conserved among papillomaviruses in its biochemical characteristics as well as structural features. It was first demonstrated to be a very efficient transcriptional activator of the BPV1 regulatory region (10). A similar transactivating potential has since been described for E2 gene products of various HPVs (52–55). The full-length product of the E2 ORF is a 50 kDa protein which presents a conserved predicted structure in three distinct domains, as shown in Figure 16.4. This structure is well conserved among papillomaviruses despite divergent primary sequences. For example, the amino acid homologies between the conserved N-terminal and the C-terminal domains of the BPV1 and HPV18 E2 proteins are only about 30%, while the hinge regions are totally divergent. The N-terminal part of

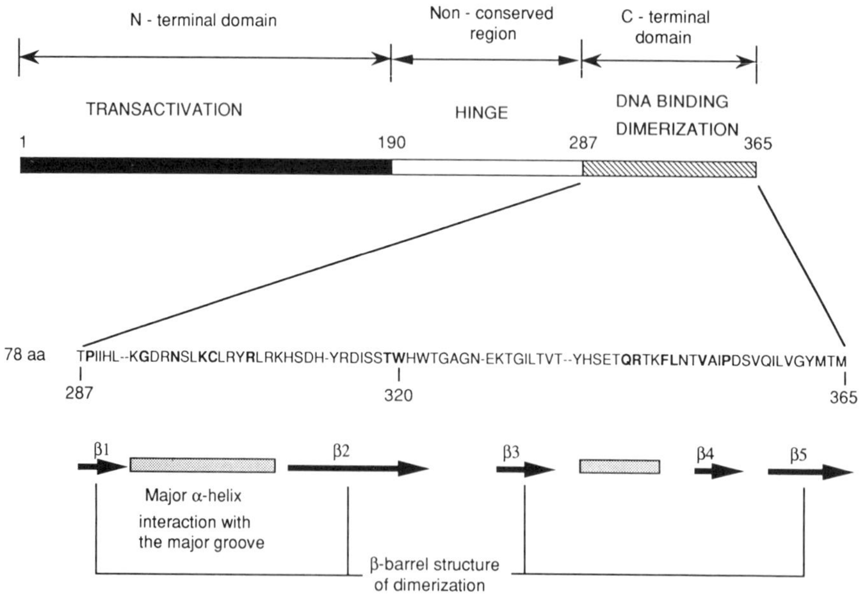

Figure 16.4. Structure and functional domains of the HPV18 E2. The three different domains defined by the amino acid sequence comparisons of the E2 proteins of 10 different papillomaviruses are indicated. The 78 amino acids which compose the C-terminal domain of the HPV18 E2 protein are given, the conserved amino acids among all E2 proteins are indicated in bold, β-sheets and α-helices of the C-terminal domain, schematized under the sequence, are from reference 122

the E2 polypeptide contains the transcriptional activation domain, while the C-terminal part contains the dimerization and DNA binding domain, as shown in Figure 16.4 (reviewed in references 56 and 57). This organization is therefore typical of the general structure of a eukaryotic transcriptional transactivator protein. It should be noted, however, that the transactivation as well as the dimerization/DNA binding domains do not obviously belong to any of the previously defined classes of transactivation or DNA binding/dimerization structures (58).

The crystal structure of the BPV1 E2 DNA binding domain (containing the C-terminal 84 amino acids of the protein), bound to its DNA target, has recently been published (59). It reveals novel types of interactions between the two E2 monomers which constitute, upon dimerization, an eight-stranded antiparallel β-barrel structure. This type of structure has never been observed before for a eukaryotic transcription factor. Furthermore, it is a rather unusual way for two monomers to interact and would explain the great stability of E2 dimers (which are only disrupted in 5 M urea). In addition, this study reveals a new structural scaffold for presenting recognition helices to successive major grooves of the specific DNA target. Interestingly, the results indicate that the amino acids conserved among E2s (revealed by sequence comparisons) are involved in the crucial interactions of the protein, as for instance tryptophan (W) at position 360 in BPV1 E2 (conserved at position 320 in HPV18 E2), which is essential for formation of the E2 dimers (Figure 16.4). It therefore appears from this study that E2 proteins from papillomaviruses constitute a novel class of eukaryotic DNA binding proteins.

E2-mediated activation

The papillomavirus E2 proteins have been shown to bind DNA specifically and recognize a short palindromic sequence ACCGNN·NNCGGT, which is present in multiple copies in all the regulatory regions of papillomaviruses (60). The E2 protein binds as a dimer to these sequences (61–63) and at least two of these sequences are necessary for efficient transactivation in transfected cells (64–66). This synergistic activation *in vivo* in transfected cells does not seem to correlate with a high cooperativity of DNA binding *in vitro* (61,67).

In conclusion, the E2 gene products of papillomaviruses are very potent transcriptional transactivators. They elicit a strong synergistic activation and cooperate with various cellular general transcription factors, such as SP1 or USF, to efficiently activate promoters in transfected cells (68,69).

E2-mediated repression

However, when studied in the context of transcription of the P_{105} promoter of HPV18 or the P_{97} promoter of HPV16, which are both promoters for the transforming functions, E2 repressed rather than activated transcription (32,52,70,71). This repression of transcription involved binding of the E2 protein to E2 binding sites close to the TATA box of P_{105} and P_{97} respectively (32,70) (Figure 16.5). The mechanism of E2 repression thus appears to involve steric hindrance at the site of formation of the transcriptional initiation complex. This hypothesis has been supported by recent *in vitro* experiments which indicated that E2 can activate heterologous promoters in *in vitro* transcription assays (although at a lower level than *in vivo*), while it represses the HPV18 P_{105} promoter. This repression can be relieved by mutation of the E2 binding site that is most proximal to the TATA box (72). These observations correlate well with results previously obtained in transient transfection experiments (32,70).

It therefore appears that for HPV18 and HPV16 one of the normal functions of the product of the E2 ORF is to repress transcription of the P_{105} and P_{97} promoters, which direct the synthesis of the E6 and E7 oncoproteins. As noted earlier, the integration of HPV16 or HPV18 genomes generally occurs in the E1 or E2 ORFs, with the consequence that the E2 transcriptional regulation circuit would be disrupted. This argues that one event, necessary for malignant progression, may be the deregulation of viral oncoprotein expression by disruption of the E2 ORF. Disruption of E1 and/or E2 may also play an important role in the negative control of viral replication, since both of these viral gene products are directly involved in this phenomenon.

CELLULAR TRANSCRIPTIONAL FACTORS

The non-coding regions of the HPV16 or HPV18 genomes have been shown to contain transcriptional enhancers which can only function in human epithelial cells (71,73–76). These sequences are contained within the non-coding segments of the viral genomes as indicated in Figure 16.5. They do not contain E2 binding sites and their regulation is independent of the expression of any viral gene products. Numerous cellular factors have been shown to interact with the regulatory regions of HPV16 or HPV18 by footprinting experiments as well as by gel shift experiments (77,78). Attempts to identify specific factors that interact with the enhancer subregion, which would be restricted to human epithelial cells, have long been unsuccessful. A recent report, however, suggested that a keratinocyte-specific factor interacts with a sequence that partially overlaps with an OCT1 binding element, located in the enhancer subregion of HPV18 (Figure 16.5) (79).

The regulatory regions of both HPV16 and HPV18 interact with a common subset of general transcription factors, such as CTF/NF1, SP1, AP1 and the glucocorticoid receptor, which are all positive regulation factors (77,78,80,81). Other factors like OCT1 or YY1 have also been described to interfere negatively with early gene expression (82,83). All these factors have been shown to participate to some extent in the transcriptional activi-

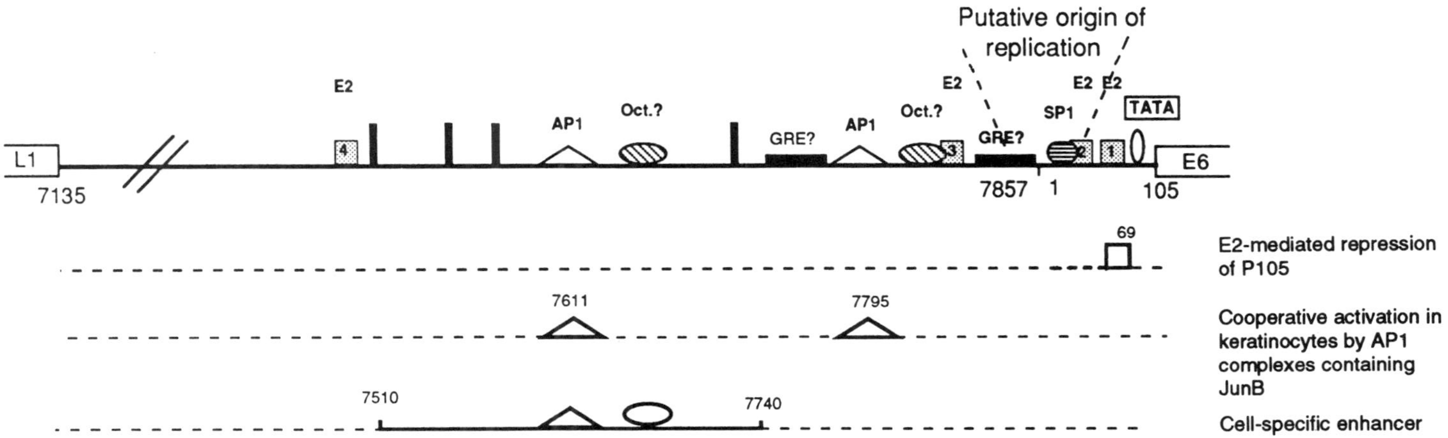

Figure 16.5. Schematic representation of the HPV18 LCR (long control region). The sites of interaction with cellular and viral transcription factors are indicated. The four E2 binding sites are represented by grey squares, NF1/CTF sites are represented by vertical black bars, SP1 site and the TATA box as well as the two AP1 binding sites are indicated. The two putative glucocorticoid responsive elements (GREs) are also indicated as horizontal black bars. The various known functions of the LCR are schematized below. The well-studied promoter P_{105} is indicated by an arrow. The E2 binding site, proximal to the P_{105} TATA box, to which binding of the E2 protein leads to transcriptional repression of P_{105}, is also indicated. The two AP1 binding sites have been shown to be essential for P_{105} activity in transfected keratinocytes. The cell-specific enhancer contained in a 230 bp fragment is necessary for transcriptional activation in human epithelial cells. The putative origin of replication, deduced by sequence comparison as described in Figure 16.9, is also shown

ties of these regions, although with some discrepancies among reports. These studies indicate that a very complex interplay of cellular and viral factors is involved in the tightly regulated transcription of HPVs. This transcriptional regulation appears dependent upon the differentiation state of the keratinocytes *in vivo* as well as exogenous signals, such as hormone induction. In this respect, it should be noted that the regulatory region of HPV18, as shown in Figure 16.6, contains potential binding sites for the glucocorticoid receptor or the nuclear hormone receptors with similar sequence specificities, such as the progesterone receptor. These sites are also present in the HPV16 regulatory region and there has indeed been some general indications of a functional regulation by hormones in HPVs. Interestingly, the same hormones are known to influence the differentiation state of the host keratinocytes. This situation is therefore creating a very intricate relationship between the viral and host cell regulation. The interconnections between these two control circuits in naturally occurring carcinomas as well as in experimental systems are not yet known.

Functional analysis of the potential AP1 binding sites present in the regulatory regions of HPV18 and HPV16 has indicated that these sites are indeed able to bind Jun/Fos heterodimers with high affinity (80,84). If these *cis*-elements are mutated in the HPV18 LCR, the keratinocyte-dependent activity of the P_{105} promoter is lost. *In vitro*, binding experiments with nuclear extracts from human keratinocytes have indicated that the major Jun component of the AP1 complex bound to HPV18 sequences is JunB.

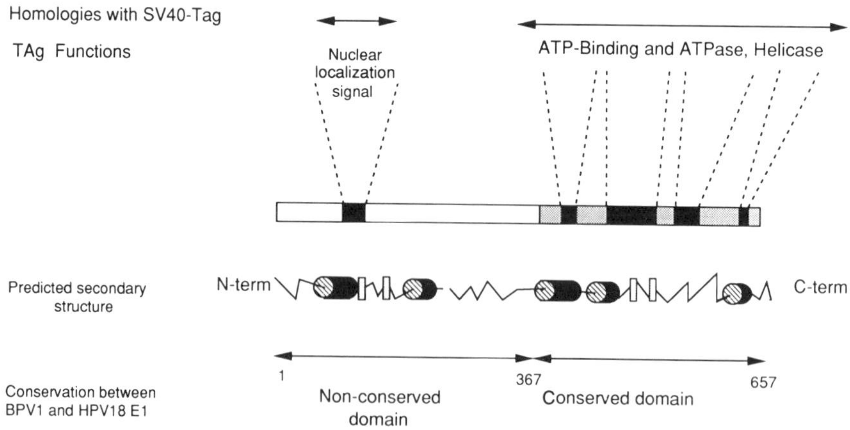

Figure 16.6. Predicted structure and functional domains of the HPV18 E1 protein. The predicted secondary structure of the HPV18 E1 protein is shown. The conserved and non-conserved domains, as defined by sequence comparisons among E1 polypeptides, are indicated: the C-terminal conserved domain is in grey and the N-terminal non-conserved domain in white. Regions within the conserved domain that show homologies with SV40 T Ag are represented by black boxes

This member of the Jun family is the major Jun protein expressed in keratinocytes and might be involved in the keratinocyte-specific transcription of HPV18 (84).

PAPILLOMAVIRUS REPLICATION

GENERAL FEATURES

Papillomavirus DNA replication has been studied for two main reasons. Firstly, an understanding of the complete viral cycle and the elements that control it would be useful for conceiving tools that would inhibit viral multiplication and spread and which could therefore be used in antiviral chemotherapy. The second reason stems from the observation that in infected cells papillomavirus genomes exist as mini-chromosomes with a chromatin structure identical to that of the cellular DNA. Viral replication takes place in the nucleus of infected cells and is dependent on the host cell nuclear machinery. Indeed, viral DNA replication has long been used as a model system for studying the basic enzymatic machinery required for replication of cellular replicons in higher eukaryotes (85–87). This has been especially true for small-DNA mammalian viruses (such as polyoma and SV40) which have provided our first insights into cellular DNA replication, and more precisely into how eukaryotic cellular DNA polymerases and their associated replication machinery are assembled at specific DNA sites to initiate replication.

In the early 1980s, the first studies of papillomavirus DNA replication led to the construction of tools for the molecular biologist, namely 'shuttle' vectors based on the genome of the bovine papillomavirus, BPV1 (reviewed in reference 88), that were able to replicate in bacteria as well as in mammalian cells. In fact the BPV1 chromosome can be maintained in rodent cells, such as mouse NIH-3T3 or C127 lines, as stable multi-copy nuclear plasmids, replicating in synchrony with the host cell DNA and being stably inherited. For human papillomaviruses host cells consist of epidermal keratinocytes for which no culture model has been available for a long time. However, some important advances have recently been made in the field of papillomavirus DNA replication which stemmed from the heterologous model system of BPV1 replication in rodent cell lines.

DISTINCTIVE CHARACTERISTICS OF PAPILLOMAVIRUS GENOME REPLICATION

The three steps in papillomavirus genome amplification

Three discrete modes of viral DNA replication can be distinguished in the infection cycle of a papillomavirus: (i) transient amplification (establishment) of the viral DNA, from one single infecting copy to a stable per-cell copy number; (ii) maintenance of this copy number during subsequent cell division, by means of a regulated replication coupled to cellular S phase; (iii) runaway vegetative multiplication leading to a massive amplification of viral genome, to capsid protein synthesis and viral maturation. This eventually leads to the release of infectious particles along with desquamation of the terminally differentiated keratinocyte.

Among non-lytic, small-DNA viruses, regulated copy number maintenance is unique to papillomaviruses and appears to involve genome replication mechanisms very similar to those occurring during cellular DNA replication. Such a regulated replication is also found for Epstein–Barr virus (89), which, however, possesses a much larger genome (175 kb). The papillomavirus maintenance phase is thus a model system of choice for replication studies. This situation contrasts with what is observed with lytic viruses such as mouse polyoma and simian SV40 which have also been extensively used as models for DNA replication studies (reviewed in reference 90), but differ markedly to what is encountered for the cellular genome since they lack a regulated proliferation step and replicate predominantly in an uncontrolled fashion.

Stringent relationship between papillomavirus genome replication and the differentiation state of the host epithelial cell

It is of importance to recall here the previously mentioned epitheliotropism of papillomaviruses, which largely results from their tissue-specific transcription. This tropism is maintained through their entire life-cycle, which is also intimately linked to, and modulated by, epidermal cell differentiation. These viruses primarily infect dividing, undifferentiated cells of the basal layer of the squamous epidermis, where they replicate to reach a stable copy number. In contrast, vegetative viral DNA replication and capsid maturation only occur within the upper cornified epidermal layers which consist of terminally differentiated, apoptotic keratinocytes (91–93). The tight association between papillomavirus gene expression pattern and keratinocyte differentiation probably means that the host cells produce signals (e.g. transcription factors?) able to modulate the expression of the viral genes responsible for viral DNA replication and viral particle maturation. The inability of standard culture methods to reproduce the various stages of epithelial differentiation *in vitro* explains the difficulties in establishing cellular models for the propagation of HPVs, and all the important recent definitive advances in our understanding of papillomavirus replication have been obtained with *in vivo* and *in vitro* studies using the BPV1 model. However, recent papers have reported the vegetative amplification of HPV31b (94) and HPV16 (95) in two different experimental systems. The first one makes use of the keratinocyte 'raft' culture system (4,5) and the second of grafting into nude mice of cells from the W12 line, previously isolated from a low-grade cervical intraepithelial neoplasia (96). Both systems support the formation of a differentiated, stratified epithelium. However, viral expression in these systems was investigated by *in situ* hybridization, which does not allow precise mechanistic studies. These systems remain very promising and the production of viral particles from raft cultures has recently been reported (97).

MOLECULAR PARTNERS INVOLVED IN PAPILLOMAVIRUS DNA REPLICATION

Experimental improvements

The recent experimental developments, which have enabled new insights into BPV1 replication, have included the setting up of highly efficient electroporation methods, where up to 20% of live cells could be transfected. This method could afterwards be used in short-term assays for the replication of BPV1 DNA co-transfected with expression vectors coding for BPV1 E1 and E2 (98). Another important development has been the utilization of eukaryotic (baculovirus (99,100) vaccinia virus (101)) as well as bacterial overproduction systems for E1 and E2 proteins (102,103), which were thereafter used either for *in vitro* binding studies or for *in vitro*-reconstituted replicative systems. In the latter, the efficiency of purified E1 and E2 proteins in supporting the replication of a BPV1 fragment-containing plasmid in a cell-free system was assessed (100). In both cellular and *in vitro* systems a similar experimental approach was used to distinguish between the input and the replicated DNAs: unreplicated viral DNA, which has been modified by bacterial methylases, is distinguished from the DNA synthesized in the eukaryotic cell by its sensitivity to Dpn I restriction enzyme digestion. Using progressive deletions of the viral sequence, replication origins (ORIs) of minimal length have also been determined in the viral genome.

The viral origin

The core origins of replication for the simian virus SV40 and the mouse polyomavirus genomes have been mapped to regions about 65 bp long. These regions include a 15–20 bp long A/T-rich stretch, which facilitates the initiation of DNA 'melting', a 23–34 bp long G/C-rich palindrome and a 14 bp long inverted repeat, potentially able to form a secondary structure required for the specific binding of various factors (reviewed in references 90 and 104). The minimal ORI of BPV1 has been defined by deletion analysis: its sequence is also 60 bp long, it spans the +1 nt position and encompasses the unique Hpa I site (see Figures 16.7 and 16.9). It consists of half the E2 binding site number 12, of an A/T-rich region and an 18 bp palindrome. The structure of this palindrome is conserved among papillomavirus subtypes (see Figure 16.8), and the insertion of a linker between the two inverted repeats disrupts ORI function (100,102). A similar organi-

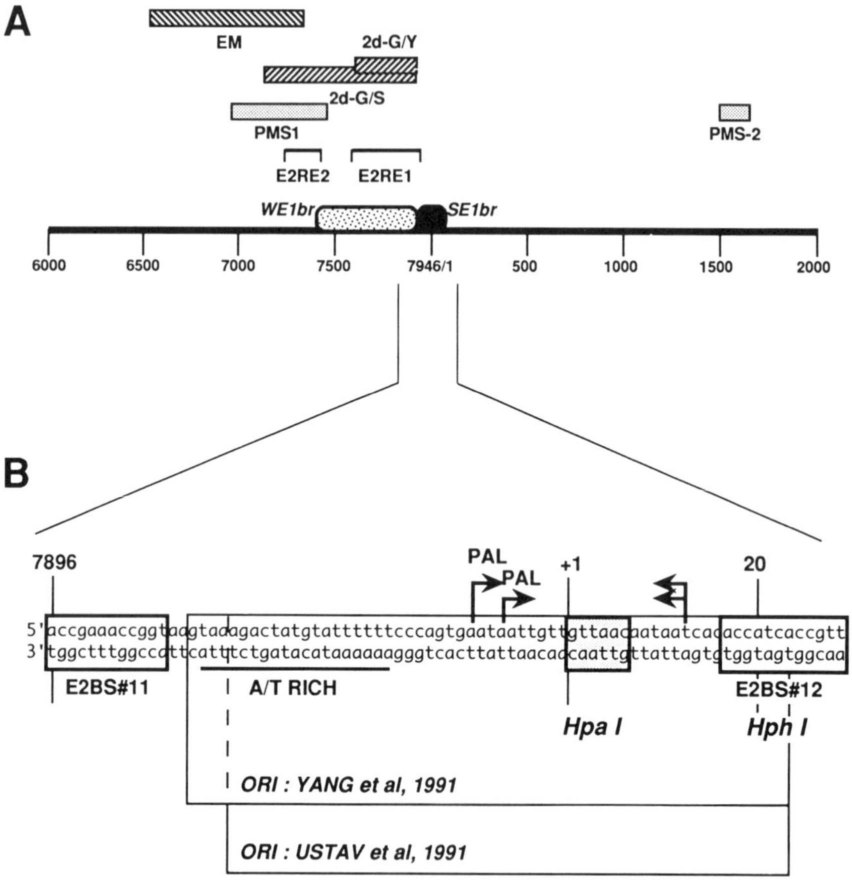

Figure 16.7. Schematic representation of the BPV1 sequence around the ORI. (A) Compilation of previous and current data on replication origins. The origin was mapped by electron microscopy (EM) at nt 6958 (± 400) (107), by two-dimensional electrophoresis between nt 7200 and 7800 (2d-G/S) (107) or between nt 7630 and 7830 (2d-G/Y). The plasmid maintenance sequences (105,106) are represented: PMS1 (nt 6945 to 7466) and PMS2 (nt 1514 to 1654). E2RE1 encompasses E2 binding sites 7–10 and E2RE2 sites 1–3. E1 binds weakly to the WE1br region and with strong affinity to SE1br. (B) Detail of the minimal ORI sequences originally defined by Yang *et al.* (100) and Ustav *et al.* (102) which are located between the two E2 binding sites (E2BS) number 11 (strong site) and 12 (weak site). The two A/T-rich palindromes centered on the Hpa I site and footprinted by E1 are depicted

```
BPV1    (+)ttttttcccagtgaataattgttGttaacaataatcacaccat
              :::   :    :  :::::: ::::: ::::  :    ::
HPV6b     (-)attttttaaaccaagattgttAttaactataagaaggaaat
              :::   :    :  :::::: ::::  ::::  :    ::
HPV11     (-)cttttttaaactaagattgttAttaagtataagaaggaaat
             ::::     ::::: ::::: ::: :  :: :: : :  :
HPV16     (-)ttttatacatgaattattgtaGtttagtattattatataag
                 :  :    ::: :: :  :::: : :  : :::
HPV18         (+)cacatactatacttttcAttaatacttttaacaattg
                          : ::  ::  ::: :::::::  :  ::
HPV31              (+)ctttttatacttAataataataatcttagtat
                      :     ::  : :: ::: :::::  ::   :
HPV33              (+)ttttatataataGtaaactataatgccaagtt
```

Figure 16.8. Alignment of putative ORI sequences from common HPVs. A 'dot-plot' sequence comparison program was used to determine the best homologies with BPV1 ORI, using a 25 nt window and a 15 nt stringency. Depending on the HPV type, the + or the – strand (as shown) gave the best result; the +1 nt positions are depicted and orientated accordingly (closed circle plus arrow). The unique Hpa I site of BPV1 is boxed

zation around the nt +1 position can be found in the human papillomavirus HPV18 (Figure 16.9).

These recent results contrast with (and show the limitations of) earlier studies now of little historical interest and mentioned thereafter: minimal plasmid maintenance sequences (PMS) had been defined (105,106), as well as sites of replication initiation, mapped by replication 'bubbles' identification under the electron microscope (107) or by migration pattern in two-dimensional agarose gel electrophoresis (108). The relative positions of these different regions is depicted in Figure 16.7. The requirement of these sequences for replication of the entire viral genome was never clearly demonstrated (reviewed in reference 109). Eventually, these early imprecise definitions did not collocate with the BPV1 minimal ORI recently defined.

Viral *trans*-elements

E1 is the main replication factor

The product of the E1 ORF is the longest and best-conserved viral protein among papillomaviruses (110). Two regions can be distinguished within its primary sequence (Figure 16.6): the C-terminal moiety (amino acids 300 onwards) is highly conserved within papillomavirus types, and we have found almost 40% amino acid sequence identity between papillomavirus types as distant as BPV1 and HPV18. The regions of strongest homology among E1 proteins are also those found conserved with respect to specific SV40 large-T regions (Figure 16.6) (111). E1 is a nuclear phosphoprotein

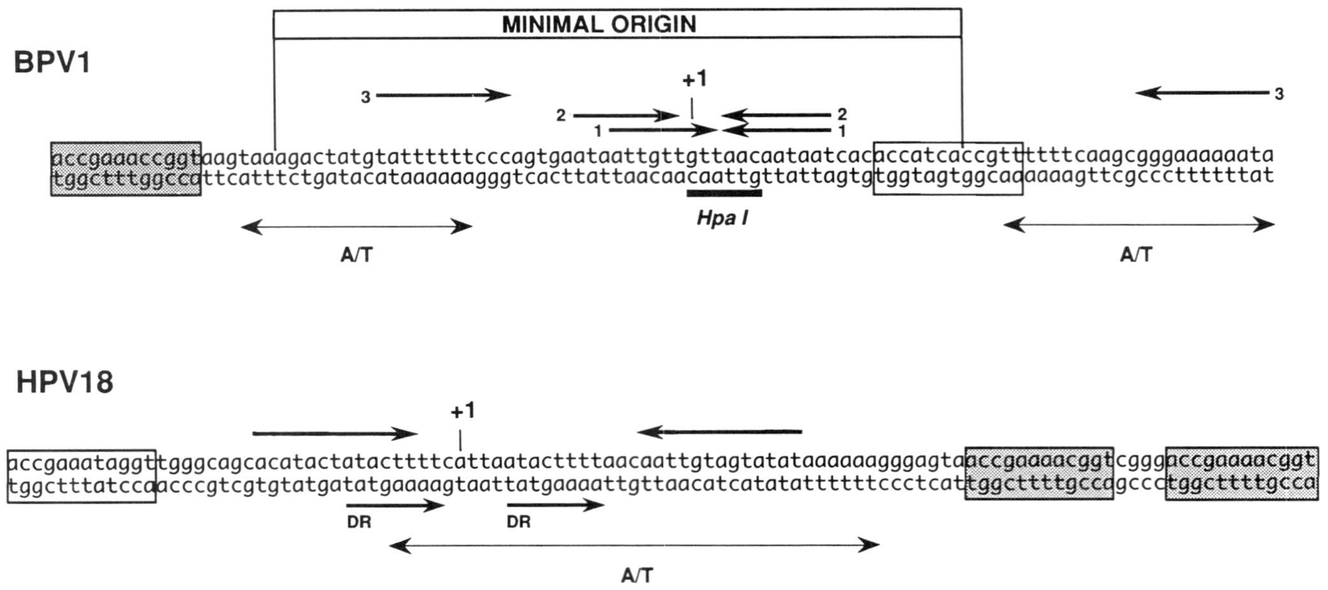

Figure 16.9. Major features of the BPV1 ORI region and of the putative HPV18 ORI region. The E2 binding sites are boxed (dark grey: strong site; light grey: weak site); their relevance for replication is discussed in the text. The inverted repeats, direct repeats (DR) and A/T-rich regions are indicated, as well as the +1 nt positions

(99,101,112); its nuclear localization signal is located in the N-terminal part around amino acids 102–108. An ATP binding region has been assigned within the broad C-terminal part of E1 (101); and a mutation at residue 434 abolishes this binding property (112).

As opposed to the E2 protein, little detail is known about the functional and biochemical properties of E1. In the mid 1980s, two distinct functions were genetically defined and mapped within the E1 ORF: the R (replication) and M (modulator) domains, corresponding to the 5′ and the 3′ moieties of E1, respectively (reviewed in references 88 and 109). However, this notion has recently been strongly challenged and E1 now appears to act as a single genetic unit. Accordingly, recent biochemical data demonstrate the production, in BPV1-transformed C127 cells, of a single 68–72 kDa protein corresponding to the full-length E1 ORF (101,112) that coincides with the replication-active form both *in vivo* (98) and *in vitro* (100).

BPV1 E1 is a DNA binding protein; this activity is carried by its N-terminal portion (101). Bacterially produced E1 binds to the viral region spanning nucleotides 7819–93 and footprints the two A/T-rich palindromes centered on the Hpa I site in the ORI sequence (102,103) (see Figure 16.7). The binding of E1 overproduced in eukaryotic cells infected by baculovirus (99,100) or vaccinia virus vectors (101) is enhanced by E2 and targeted close to the BPV1 ORI (100,113,114). The slight discrepancy between both forms of overproduced E1 may stem from differences in its phosphorylation state in bacteria versus the eukaryotic cell.

Involvement of the transcription factor E2

As reviewed earlier in this chapter, the product of the E2 ORF has been extensively studied and its function as a transcriptional activator is well described. It homodimerizes (Figure 16.4) and binds with very high affinity to DNA to the multiple $ACCG(N)_4CGGT$ palindromic sequences located in the non-coding regulatory regions of papillomaviruses.

In co-transfection experiments, E2 expression in *trans*, together with the full-length E1 protein, is necessary and sufficient to allow the replication of minimal BPV1-based replicons (98). This finding unravels new perspectives for the dual functions of E2 in replication as well as in transcription. The E2 gene product is directly involved in replication initiation; its activity is not conveyed through its transactivator role in E1 transcription as its function in replication is resistant to α-amanitin, a strong inhibitor of RNA polymerase II (100). The full-length E2 protein, and not the DNA binding, C-terminal moiety of E2 (Figure 16.4), is functional for replication (98,102,113).

Putative E1/E2 complex formation

The efficiency of E1 alone in initiating replication *in vitro* is weak and may depend on its effective concentration (100), while in co-transfection experiments E1 unequivocally requires complementation by E2 for efficient replication (98).

Direct interactions between E1 and E2 have been demonstrated in co-immunoprecipitation experiments (99,113,114). The requirement for E2 binding sites inside or close to the ORI has been recently evaluated: at least half of the E2 binding sequence located within the ORI region (Figures 16.7 and 16.9) is required for E1/E2 complex binding to DNA (Figure 16.7) (102,115). In this context, E2 may mostly stimulate and target E1 binding to the ORI through its own interaction with its DNA binding site (100).

Other roles have been suggested for E2 in replication (109): it might alter nucleosome structure over the viral ORI region, thus facilitating unwinding and melting of DNA (100). Since only under-phosphorylated E2 associates with E1 (113), it may also be a cell cycle-dependent regulatory element in the control of replication. Recently, E2 has been shown to interact with the cellular replication factor RPA (115).

Other viral and cellular (host) *trans* elements

Viral DNA replication also requires the various cellular functions involved in cellular DNA replication: recognition and targeting proteins, unwinding/helicase/topoisomerase activities, and leading- and lagging-strand processive synthesis by DNA polymerases α (primase), δ or ϵ (for recent reviews, see references 85–87 and 117). The involvement of viral products other than E1 and E2 has recently been re-evaluated and ruled out for BPV1 (98) as well as HPVs (118–121). The mean viral copy number is clearly a function of the cell type; its tight control, and the prevention of random, deregulated replication remains an enigma; is there some sort of *cis* mechanism mediated by the modification of the neo-synthesized DNA after each S to G2/M phase transition, or any *trans* control via a post-transcriptional modification of E1 or E2 (such as phosphorylation/dephosphorylation) that would be regulated during the cell cycle? This important point is a current research topic.

RECENT PROGRESS CONCERNING HPV REPLICATION

One of the most exciting aspects has been to assess that the HPVs follow a BPV1-analogous replication model (118–121). These studies show how well the E1, E2 and ORI elements are functionally conserved among papillomaviruses. Beyond the sequence comparison studies (Figures 16.8 and 16.9), there is a high degree of functional conservation between the ORI, the E1 and the E2 proteins of various papillomaviruses. Functional heterologous complementation studies, performed between the BPV1 *cis* and *trans* elements and their HPV counterparts, have clearly confirmed this functional conservation (117,120).

Such functional heterologous complementations do not indicate any specific requirement for tissue-restricted cellular factors. A key issue in HPV replication which therefore remains is the evaluation of the roles of cellular factors. The dependence of vegetative viral replication upon keratinocyte terminal differentiation is an example of obvious host cell factor involvement in viral replication.

GENERAL CONCLUSION

Despite the lack of a convenient homologous system for human papillomavirus expression, a number of the molecular aspects of their multiplication are well characterized today. The functions involved in the transcriptional regulation of their genes and in the cellular transformation that they induce *in vitro* are putative targets for the development of therapeutic tools to control viral infection and oncogenesis. The products of the E6 and E7 ORFs are among the rare viral oncogenes that have been shown to transform human cells in natural infections. They are also known to interact with two major tumour suppressors, p53 and p105-RB, respectively. In contrast, the product of the E2 ORF appears to negatively control the transcription of the transforming functions. All these viral proteins are therefore relatively well-defined targets for an antiviral chemotherapy designed to stop viral infection in pre-malignant as well as in malignant lesions.

Another promising field is the control of viral replication. It became clear recently that HPV replication uses the same molecular mechanisms as BPV1 replication. Consequently, another important target for antiviral chemotherapy would be the E1 protein. Any type of blockade introduced in one of the enzymatic activities or binding properties of this viral protein would interfere with viral replication and therefore with spread of virus.

Human keratinocytes are the specific susceptible host cell type for HPV infection *in vivo* as well as *in vitro*. Moreover, viral multiplication is linked to the terminal differentiation of these cells. It therefore seems that one potential way of interfering with viral spread would be to control epidermal differentiation. This point is particularly important with regard to the malignant conversion of genital lesions. Drugs that would be able to interfere temporarily with the terminal differentiation of genital epithelium could also prevent viral proliferation. Furthermore, in regard to this type of lesion, another important target is suggested by studies of the specific transcriptional regulation of the HPV types associated with pre-malignant lesions. Hormones such as steroids and retinoids take part in the control of viral genome expression as well as in keratinocyte differentiation. These hormonal controls could become useful tools to prevent cell transformation and viral multiplication.

ACKNOWLEDGEMENTS

We are grateful to Professor Moshe Yaniv and Dr Jonathan Ham for critical reading of the manuscript and David Sourdive for help in running the programs of protein structure analysis. This work was supported by grants from INSERM, Association pour la Recherche sur le Cancer, Ligue Nationale Française Contre le Cancer and the Fondation pour la Recherche Médicale.

REFERENCES

1. Shope, R. E. and Hurst, E. W. (1933). Infectious papillomatosis of rabbits with a note on the histopathology. *J. Exp. Med.*, **58**, 607–624.
2. Chen, E. Y., Howley, P. M., Levinson, A. D. and Seeburg, P. H. (1982). The primary structure and genomic organization of the bovine papillomavirus type 1 genome. *Nature*, **299**, 529–534.
3. Law, M. F., Lowy, D. R., Dvoretzky, I. and Howley, P. M. (1981). Mouse cells transformed by bovine papillomavirus contain only extrachromosomal viral DNA sequences. *Proc. Natl Acad. Sci. USA*, **78**, 2727–2731.
4. Asselineau, D., Bernard, B., Bailly, C. and Darmon, M. (1985). Epidermal morphogenesis and induction of the 67 kD keratin polypeptide by culture of human keratinocytes at the liquid–air interface. *Exp. Cell Res.*, **159**, 536–539.
5. Asselineau, D., Bernard, B. A. and Darmon, M. (1987). Three-dimensional culture of human keratinocytes on a dermal equivalent: a model system to study epidermal morphogenesis and differentiation *in vitro*. In *Models in Dermatology*, N. Lowe and H. Mailbach (eds), Karger, Basel, pp. 1–7.
6. Meyers, C., Frattini, M. G., Hudson, J. B. and Laimins, L. A. (1992). Biosynthesis of human papillomavirus from a continuous cell line upon epithelial differentiation. *Science*, **257**, 971–973.
7. Danos, O., Engel, L. W., Chen, E. Y. *et al.* (1983). Comparative analysis of the human type 1a and bovine type 1 papillomavirus genomes. *J. Virol.*, **46**, 557–566.
8. Lowy, D. R., Dvoretzky, I., Shober, R. *et al.* (1980). In vitro tumorigenic transformation by a defined sub-genomic fragment of bovine papilloma virus DNA. *Nature*, **287**, 72–74.
9. Baker, C. C. and Noe, J. S. (1989). Transcriptional termination between bovine papillomavirus type 1 (BPV1) early and late polyadenylation sites blocks late transcription in BPV1 transformed cells. *J. Virol.*, **63**, 3529–3534.
10. Spalholz, B. A., Yang, Y. C. and Howley, P. M. (1985). Transactivation of a bovine papillomavirus transcriptional regulatory element by the E2 gene product. *Cell*, **42**, 183–191.
11. Schiller, J. T., Vass, W. C., Vousden, K. H. and Lowy, D. R. (1986). E5 open reading frame of bovine papillomavirus type 1 encodes a transforming gene. *J. Virol.*, **57**, 1–6.

12. Schlegel, R., Wade, G. M., Rabson, M. S. and Yang, Y. C. (1986). The E5 transforming gene of bovine papillomavirus encodes a small, hydrophobic polypeptide. *Science*, **233**, 464–467.
13. Martin, P., Vass, W. C., Schiller, J. T. *et al.* (1989). The bovine papillomavirus E5 transforming protein can stimulate the transforming activity of EGF and CSF-1 receptors. *Cell*, **59**, 21–32.
14. Goldstein, D. and Schlegel, R. (1990). The E5 oncoprotein of bovine papillomavirus binds to a 16 kD cellular protein. *EMBO J.*, **9**, 137–145.
15. Goldstein, D. J., Finbow, M. E., Andresson, T. *et al.* (1991). Bovine papillomavirus E5 oncoprotein binds to the 16K component of vacuolar H(+)-ATPases. *Nature*, **353**, 347–349.
16. Leptak, C., Ramon y Cajal, S., Kulke, R. *et al.* (1991). Tumorigenic transformation of murine keratinocytes by the E5 genes of bovine papillomavirus type 1 and human papillomavirus type 16. *J. Virol.*, **65**, 7078–7083.
17. Barbosa, M. S., Lowy, D. R. and Schiller, J. T. (1989). Papillomavirus polypeptides E6 and E7 are zinc-binding proteins. *J. Virol.*, **63**, 1404–1407.
18. Cole, S. and Danos, O. (1987). Nucleotide sequence and comparative analysis of the human papillomavirus type 18 genome: phylogeny of papillomaviruses and repeated structure of the E6 and E7 gene products. *J. Mol. Biol.*, **193**, 599–609.
19. Schiller, J. T., Vass, W. C. and Lowy, D. R. (1984). Identification of a second transforming region in bovine papillomavirus DNA. *Proc. Natl Acad. Sci. USA*, **81**, 7880–7884.
20. Lamberti, C., Morissey, L. C., Grossman, S. and Androphy, E. J. (1990). Transcriptional activation by the papillomavirus E6 zinc finger oncoprotein. *EMBO J.*, **9**, 1907–1913.
21. Hawley-Nelson, P., Vousden, K. H., Hubbert, N. L. *et al.* (1989). HPV16 E6 and E7 cooperate to immortalize human foreskin keratinocytes. *EMBO J.*, **8**, 3905–3910.
22. Münger, K., Phelps, W. C., Bubb, V. *et al.* (1989). The E6 and E7 genes of the human papillomavirus type 16 together are necessary and sufficient for transformation of primary human keratinocytes. *J. Virol.*, **63**, 4417–4421.
23. Desaintes, C., Hallez, S., Van Alphen, P. and Burny, A. (1992). Transcriptional activation of several heterologous promoters by the E6 protein of human papillomavirus type 16. *J. Virol.*, **66**, 325–333.
24. Phelps, W. C., Yee, C. L., Münger, K. and Howley, P. M. (1988). The human papillomavirus type 16 E7 gene encodes transactivation and transformation functions similar to those of adenovirus E1A. *Cell*, **53**, 539–547.
25. Sedman, S. A., Barbosa, M. S., Vass, W. C. *et al.* (1991). The full-length E6 protein of human papillomavirus type 16 has transforming and trans-activating activities and cooperates with E7 to immortalize keratinocytes in culture. *J. Virol.*, **65**, 4860–4866.
26. Doorbar, J., Campbell, D., Grand, R. J. and Gallimore, P. H. (1986). Identification of the human papilloma virus-1a E4 gene products. *EMBO J.*, **5**, 355–362.
27. Breidburd, F., Croissant, O. and Orth, G. (1987). Expression of human papillomavirus type 1a E4 gene in warts. *Cancer Cells*, **5**, 115–122.
28. Doorbar, J., Ely, S., Sterling, J. *et al.* (1991). Specific interaction between HPV-16 E1–E4 and cytokeratins results in collapse of the epithelial cell intermediate filament network. *Nature*, **352**, 824–827.
29. Rogel-Gaillard, C., Breidburd, F. and Orth, G. (1992). Human papillomavirus type 1 E4 proteins differing by their N-terminal ends have distinct cellular localisations when transiently expressed in vitro. *J. Virol.*, **66**, 816–823.

30. Riou, G., Favre, M., Jeannel, D. J. *et al.* (1990). Association between poor prognosis in early-stage invasive cervical carcinomas and non-detection of HPV DNA. *Lancet*, **335**, 1171–1174.
31. Schwarz, E., Freese, U. K., Gissmann, L. *et al.* (1985). Structure and transcription of human papillomavirus sequences in cervical carcinoma cells. *Nature*, **314**, 111–114.
32. Romanczuk, H., Thierry, F. and Howley, P. M. (1990). Mutational analysis of cis elements involved in E2 modulation of human papillomavirus type 16 P97 and type 18 P105 promoters. *J. Virol.*, **64**, 2849–2859.
33. Schneider-Gädicke, A. and Schwarz, E. (1986). Different human cervical carcinoma cell lines show similar transcription patterns of human papillomavirus type 18 early genes. *EMBO J.*, **5**, 2285–2292.
34. Thierry, F., Heard, J. M., Dartmann, K. and Yaniv, M. (1987). Characterization of a transcriptional promoter of human papillomavirus 18 and modulation of its expression by simian virus 40 and adenovirus early antigens. *J. Virol.*, **61**, 134–142.
35. Smotkin, D. and Wettstein, F. O. (1986). Transcription of human papillomavirus type 16 early genes in a cervical cancer and a cancer-derived cell line and identification of the E7 protein. *Proc. Natl Acad. Sci. USA*, **83**, 4680–4684.
36. Smotkin, D., Prokoph, H. and Wettstein, F. O. (1989). Oncogenic and nononcogenic human genital papillomaviruses generate the E7 mRNA by different mechanisms. *J. Virol.*, **63**, 1441–1447.
37. Phelps, W. C., Münger, K., Yee, C. L. *et al.* (1989). Genital human papillomaviruses: transcriptional regulation and transformation. In *Common Mechanisms of Transformation by Small DNA Tumor Viruses*, L. P. Villarreal (ed.), American Society for Microbiology, Washington, DC.
38. Dürst, M., Dzarlieva-Petruskova, R. T., Boukamp, P. *et al.* (1987). Molecular and cytogenetic analysis of immortalized human primary keratinocytes obtained after transfection with human papillomavirus type 16. *Oncogene*, **1**, 251–256.
39. Kaur, P. and McDougall, J. K. (1988). Characterization of primary human keratinocytes transformed by human papillomavirus type 18. *J. Virol.*, **62**, 1917–1924.
40. McCance, D. J., Kopan, R., Fuchs, E. and Laimins, L. A. (1988). Human papillomavirus type 16 alters human epithelial cell differentiation in vitro. *Proc. Natl Acad. Sci. USA*, **85**, 7169–7173.
41. Pirisi, L., Yasumoto, S., Feller, M. *et al.* (1987). Transformation of human fibroblasts and keratinocytes with human papillomavirus type 16 DNA. *J. Virol.*, **61**, 1061–1066.
42. Schlegel, R., Phelps, W. C., Zhang, Y. L. and Barbosa, M. (1988). Quantitative keratinocyte assay detects two biological activities of human papillomavirus DNA and identifies viral types associated with cervical carcinoma. *EMBO J.*, **7**, 3181–3187.
43. Dyson, N., Howley, P. M., Münger, K. and Harlow, E. (1989). The human papillomavirus-16 E7 oncoprotein is able to bind to the retinoblastoma gene product. *Science*, **243**, 934–937.
44. Münger, K., Werness, B. A., Dyson, N. *et al.* (1989). Complex formation of human papillomavirus E7 proteins with the retinoblastoma tumor suppressor gene product. *EMBO J.*, **8**, 4099–4105.
45. Chellapan, S. P., Hiebert, S., Mudryj, M. *et al.* (1991). The E2F transcription factor is a cellular target for the RB protein. *Cell*, **65**, 1053–1061.
46. Nevins, J. R. (1991). Transcriptional activation by viral regulatory proteins. *Trends Biochem. Sci.*, **16**, 435–439.

47. Phelps, W. C., Bagchi, S., Barnes, J. A. *et al.* (1991). Analysis of transactivation by human papillomavirus type 16 E7 and Adenovirus 12S E1A suggests a common mechanism. *J. Virol.*, **65**, 6922.
48. Werness, B. A., Levine, A. J. and Howley, P. M. (1990). Association of human papillomavirus type 16 and 18 E6 proteins with p53. *Science*, **248**, 76–79.
49. Scheffner, M., Huibregtse, J. M., Vierstra, R. D. and Howley, P. M. (1993). The HPV16 E6 and E6-AP complex functions as ubiquitin-protein ligase in the ubiquitination of p53. *Cell*, **75**, 495–505.
50. Scheffner, M., Münger, K., Byrne, J. C. and Howley, P. M. (1991). The state of the p53 and retinoblastoma genes in human cervical carcinoma cell lines. *Proc. Natl Acad. Sci. USA*, **88**, 5523–5527.
51. Münger, K., Yee, C. L., Phelps, W. C. *et al.* (1991). Biochemical and biological differences between E7 oncoproteins of the high and low risk human papillomavirus types are determined by amino-terminal sequences. *J. Virol.*, **65**, 3943–3949.
52. Bernard, B. A., Bailly, C., Lenoir, M. C. *et al.* (1989). The human papillomavirus type 18 (HPV18) E2 gene product is a repressor of the HPV18 regulatory region in human keratinocytes. *J. Virol.*, **63**, 4317–4324.
53. Hirochika, H., Broker, T. R. and Chow, L. T. (1987). Enhancers and trans-acting E2 transcriptional factors of papillomaviruses. *J. Virol.*, **61**, 2599–2606.
54. Hirochika, H., Hirochika, R., Broker, T. R. and Chow, L. T. (1988). Functional mapping of the human papillomavirus type 11 transcriptional enhancer and its interaction with the trans-acting E2 proteins. *Genes Dev.*, **2**, 54–67.
55. Phelps, W. C. and Howley, P. M. (1987). Transcriptional trans-activation by the human papillomavirus type 16 E2 gene product. *J. Virol.*, **61**, 1630–1638.
56. Dostatni, N., Giri, I., Sousa, R. *et al.* (1989). Mechanisms of activation or repression of viral transcription by the E2 product of papillomaviruses. In *Common Mechanisms in Transformation by Small DNA Tumor Viruses*, L. P. Villarreal (ed.), American Society of Microbiology, Washington, DC, pp. 169–183.
57. Ham, J., Dostatni, N., Gauthier, J. M. and Yaniv, M. (1991). The papillomavirus E2 protein: a factor with many talents. *Trends Biochem. Sci.*, **16**, 440–444.
58. Mitchell, P. J. and Tjian, R. (1989). Transcriptional regulation in mammalian cells by sequence-specific DNA binding proteins. *Science*, **245**, 371–378.
59. Hegde, R. S., Grossman, S. R., Laimins, L. A. and Sigler, P. B. (1992). Crystal structure at 1.7 A of the bovine papillomavirus-1 E2 DNA-binding domain bound to its DNA target. *Nature*, **359**, 505–511.
60. Androphy, E. J., Lowy, D. R. and Schiller, J. T. (1987). Bovine papillomavirus E2 trans-activating gene product binds to specific sites in papillomavirus DNA. *Nature*, **325**, 70–73.
61. Dostatni, N., Thierry, F. and Yaniv, M. (1988). A dimer of BPV-1 E2 containing a protease resistant core interacts with its DNA target. *EMBO J.*, **7**, 3807–3816.
62. McBride, A. A., Byrne, J. C. and Howley, P. M. (1989). E2 polypeptides encoded by bovine papillomavirus type 1 form dimers through the common carboxyl-terminal domain: transactivation is mediated by the conserved amino-terminal domain. *Proc. Natl Acad. Sci. USA*, **86**, 510–514.
63. McBride, A. A., Schlegel, R. and Howley, P. M. (1988). The carboxy-terminal domain shared by the bovine papillomavirus E2 transactivator and repressor proteins contains a specific DNA binding activity. *EMBO J.*, **7**, 533–539.
64. Hawley-Nelson, P., Androphy, E. J., Lowy, D. R. and Schiller, J. T. (1988). The specific DNA recognition sequence of the bovine papillomavirus E2 protein is an E2-dependent enhancer. *EMBO J.*, **7**, 525–531.

65. Spalholz, B. A., Lambert, P. F., Yee, C. L. and Howley, P. M. (1987). Bovine papillomavirus transcriptional regulation: localization of the E2-responsive elements of the long control region. *J. Virol.*, **61**, 2128–2137.
66. Thierry, F., Dostatni, N., Arnos, F. and Yaniv, M. (1990). Cooperative activation of transcription by bovine papillomavirus type 1 E2 can occur over a long distance. *Mol. Cell Biol.*, **10**, 4431–4437.
67. Gauthier, J. M., Dostatni, N., Lusky, M. and Yaniv, M. (1991). Two DNA-bound E2 dimers are required for strong transcriptional activation and for cooperation with cellular factors in most cells. *New Biologist*, **3**, 498–509.
68. Ham, J., Dostatni, N., Arnos, F. and Yaniv, M. (1991). Several different upstream promoter elements can potentiate transactivation by the BPV1 E2 protein. *EMBO J.*, **10**, 2931–2940.
69. Spalholz, B. A., Vande Pol, S. B. and Howley, P. M. (1991). Characterization of the cis elements involved in basal and E2-transactivated expression of the bovine papillomavirus P2443 promoter. *J. Virol.*, **64**, 743–753.
70. Thierry, F. and Howley, P. M. (1991). Functional analysis of E2-mediated repression of the HPV18 P105 promoter. *New Biologist*, **3**, 90–100.
71. Thierry, F. and Yaniv, M. (1987). The BPV1-E2 trans-acting protein can be either an activator or a repressor of the HPV18 regulatory region. *EMBO J.*, **6**, 3391–3397.
72. Dostatni, N., Lambert, P. F., Sousa, R. *et al.* (1991). The functional BPV1 E2 trans-activating protein can act as a repressor by preventing formation of the initiation complex. *Genes Dev.*, **5**, 1657–1671.
73. Cripe, T. P., Haugen, T. H., Turk, J. P. *et al.* (1987). Transcriptional regulation of the human papillomavirus-16 E6–E7 promoter by a keratinocyte-dependent enhancer, and by viral E2 trans-activator and repressor gene products: implications for cervical carcinogenesis. *EMBO J.*, **6**, 3745–3753.
74. Gius, D., Grossman, S., Bedell, M. A. and Laimins, L. A. (1988). Inducible and constitutive enhancer domains in the noncoding region of human papillomavirus type 18. *J. Virol.*, **62**, 665–672.
75. Gloss, B., Bernard, H. U., Seedorf, K. and Klock, G. (1987). The upstream regulatory region of the human papillomavirus-16 contains an E2 protein independent enhancer which is specific for cervical carcinoma cells and regulated by glucocorticoid hormones. *EMBO J.*, **6**, 3735–3743.
76. Thierry, F., Garcia-Carranca, A. and Yaniv, M. (1987). Elements that control the transcription of genital human papillomavirus type 18. *Cancer Cells*, **5**, 23–32.
77. Garcia-Carranca, A., Thierry, F. and Yaniv, M. (1988). Interplay of viral and cellular proteins along the long control region of human papillomavirus type 18. *J. Virol.*, **62**, 4321–4330.
78. Gloss, B., Chong, T. and Bernard, H. U. (1989). Numerous nuclear proteins bind the long control region of human papillomavirus type 16: a subset of 6 of 23 DNase I protected segments coincides with the location of the cell specific enhancer. *J. Virol.*, **63**, 1142–1152.
79. Mack, D. H. and Laimins, L. A. (1991). A keratinocyte-specific transcription factor, KRF-1, interacts with AP1 to activate expression of human papillomavirus type 18 in squamous epithelial cells. *Proc. Natl Acad. Sci. USA*, **88**, 9102–9106.
80. Cripe, T. P., Alderborn, A., Anderson, R. D. *et al.* (1990). Transcriptional activation of the human papillomavirus-16 P97 promoter by a 88-nucleotide enhancer containing distinct cell-dependent and AP1-responsive modules. *New Biologist*, **2**, 450–463.
81. Gloss, B. and Bernard, H. U. (1990). The E6/E7 promoter of human papilloma-

virus type 16 is activated in the absence of E2 proteins by a sequence-aberrant SP1 distal element. *J. Virol.*, **64**, 5577–5584.
82. Bauknecht, T., Angel, P., Royer, H. D. and zur Hausen, H. (1992). Identification of a negative regulatory domain in the human papillomavirus type 18 promoter: interaction with the transcriptional repressor YY1. *EMBO J.*, **11**, 4607–4617.
83. Hoppe-Seyler, F., Butz, K. and zur Hausen, H. (1991). Repression of the human papillomavirus type 18 enhancer by the cellular transcription factor Oct-1. *J. Virol.*, **65**, 5613–5618.
84. Thierry, F., Spyrou, G., Yaniv, M. and Howley, P. M. (1992). Two AP1 sites binding JunB are essential for HPV18 transcription in keratinocytes. *J. Virol.*, **66**, 3740–3748.
85. Gasser, S. M. (1991). Replication origins, factors and attachment sites. *Curr. Opin. Cell Biol.*, **3**, 407–413.
86. Hübscher, U. and Thömmes, P. (1992). DNA polymerase ϵ: in search of a function. *Trends Biochem. Sci.*, **17**, 55–58.
87. So, A. G. and Downey, K. M. (1992). Eukaryotic DNA replication. *CRC Crit. Rev. Biochem. Mol. Biol.*, **27**, 129–155.
88. Howley, P. M. (1991). Papillomavirinae and their replication. In *Fundamental Virology*, B. N. Fields, D. M. Knirpe *et al.*, Raven Press, New York, pp. 743–768.
89. Adams, A. (1987). Replication of latent Epstein–Barr virus genomes in Raji cells. *J. Virol.*, **61**, 1743–1746.
90. Fanning, E. and Knippers, R. (1992). Structure and function of simian virus 40 large tumor antigen. *Annu. Rev. Biochem.*, **61**, 55–85.
91. Fuchs, E. (1990). Epidermal differentiation. *Curr. Opin. Cell Biol.*, **2**, 1028–1035.
92. Fuchs, E. (1990). Epidermal differentiation: the bare essentials. *J. Cell Biol.*, **111**, 2807–2814.
93. Turyk, M. E., Golub, T. R., Wood, N. B. *et al.* (1989). Growth and characterization of epithelial cells from normal human uterine ectocervix and endocervix. *In Vitro Cell Dev. Biol.*, **25**, 544–556.
94. Bedell, M. A., Hudson, J. B., Golub, T. R. *et al.* (1991). Amplification of human papillomavirus genomes in vitro is dependent on epithelial differentiation. *J. Virol.*, **65**, 2254–2260.
95. Sterling, J., Stanley, M., Gatward, G. and Minson,T. (1990). Production of human papillomavirus type 16 virions in a keratinocyte cell line. *J. Virol.*, **64**, 6305–6307.
96. Stanley, M. A., Browne, H. M., Appleby, M. W. and Minson, A. C. (1989). Properties of a non-tumorigenic human cervical epithelial cell line. *Int. J. Cancer*, **43**, 672–676.
97. Meyers, C., Frattini, M. G., Hudson, J. B. and Laimins, L. A. (1992). Biosynthesis of human papillomavirus from a continuous cell line upon epithelial differentiation. *Science*, **257**, 971–973.
98. Ustav, M. and Stenlund, A. (1991). Transient replication of BPV-1 requires two viral polypeptides encoded by the E1 and E2 open reading frames. *EMBO J.*, **10**, 449–457.
99. Blitz, I. L. and Laimins, L. A. (1991). The 68-kilodalton E1 protein of bovine papillomavirus is a DNA binding phosphoprotein which associates with the E2 transcriptional activator in vitro. *J. Virol.*, **65**, 649–656.
100. Yang, L., Li, R., Mohr, I. J. *et al.* (1991). Activation of BPV-1 replication in vitro by the transcription factor E2. *Nature*, **353**, 628–632.
101. Santucci, S., Androphy, E. J., Bonne, A. C. and Clertant, P. (1990). Proteins

encoded by the bovine papillomavirus E1 open reading frame: expression in heterologous systems and in virally transformed cells. *J. Virol.*, **64**, 6027–6039.
102. Ustav, M., Ustav, E., Szymanski, P. and Stenlund, A. (1991). Identification of the origin of replication of bovine papillomavirus and characterization of the viral origin recognition factor E1. *EMBO J.*, **10**, 4321–4329.
103. Wilson, V. G. and Ludes, M. J. (1991). A bovine papillomavirus E1-related protein binds specifically to bovine papillomavirus DNA. *J. Virol.*, **65**, 5314–5322.
104. Eckhart, W. (1991). Polyomavirinae and their replication. In *Fundamental Virology*, B. N. Fields, D. M. Knirpe *et al.*, Raven Press, New York, pp. 727–741.
105. Lusky, M. and Botchan, M. R. (1984). Characterization of the bovine papilloma virus plasmid maintenance sequences. *Cell*, **36**, 391–401.
106. Lusky, M. and Botchan, M. R. (1986). Transient replication of bovine papilloma virus type 1 plasmids: cis and trans requirements. *Proc. Natl Acad. Sci. USA*, **83**, 3609–3613.
107. Waldeck, W., Rosl, F. and Zentgraf, H. (1984). Origin of replication in episomal bovine papilloma virus type 1 DNA isolated from transformed cells. *EMBO J.*, **3**, 2173–2178.
108. Schvartzman, J. B., Adolph, S., Martin, P. L. and Schildkraut, C. L. (1990). Evidence that replication initiates at only some of the potential origins in each oligomeric form of bovine papillomavirus type 1 DNA. *Mol. Cell Biol.*, **10**, 3078–3086.
109. Lambert, P. F. (1991). Papillomavirus DNA replication. *J. Virol.*, **65**, 3417–3420.
110. Giri, I. and Danos, O. (1986). Papillomavirus genomes: from sequence data to biological properties. *Trends Genet.*, **2**, 227–232.
111. Clertant, P. and Seif, I. (1984). A common function for polyoma virus large-T and papillomavirus E1 proteins? *Nature*, **311**, 276–279.
112. Sun, S., Thorner, L., Lentz, M. *et al.* (1990). Identification of a 68-kilodalton nuclear ATP-binding phosphoprotein encoded by bovine papillomavirus type 1. *J. Virol.*, **64**, 5093–5105.
113. Mohr, I. J., Clark, R., Sun, S. *et al.* (1990). Targeting the E1 replication protein to the papillomavirus origin of replication by complex formation with the E2 transactivator. *Science*, **250**, 1694–1696.
114. Le Moal, M. A., Yaniv, M. and Thierry, F. (1994). The bovine papillomavirus type 1 (BPV1) replication protein modulates transcriptional activation by interacting with BPV1 E2. *J. Virol.*, **68**, 1085–1093.
115. Li, R. and Botchan, M. R. (1993). The acidic transcriptional activation domains of VP16 and P53 bind to the cellular replication protein A and stimulate in vitro BPV1 DNA replication. *Cell*, **73**, 1207–1221.
116. Ustav, E., Ustav, M., Szymansky, P. and Stenlund, A. (1993). The bovine papillomavirus origin of replication requires a binding site for the E2 transcriptional activator. *Proc. Natl Acad. Sci. USA*, **90**, 898–902.
117. Linn, S. (1991). How many Pols does it take to replicate nuclear DNA? *Cell*, **66**, 185–187.
118. Chiang, C. M., Dong, G., Broker, T. R. and Chow, L. T. (1992). Control of human papillomavirus type 11 origin of replication by the E2 family of transcription regulatory proteins. *J. Virol.*, **66**, 5224–5231.
119. Chiang, C. M., Ustav, M., Stenlund, A. *et al.* (1992). Viral E1 and E2 proteins support replication of homologous and heterologous papillomavirus origins. *Proc. Natl Acad. Sci. USA*, **89**, 5799–5803.
120. Del Vecchio, A. M., Romanczuk, H., Howley, P. M. and Baker, C. C. (1992). Transient replication of human papillomavirus DNAs. *J. Virol.*, **66**, 5949–5958.
121. Remm, M., Brain, R. and Jenkins, J. R. (1992). The E2 binding sites determine

the efficiency of replication for the origin of human papillomavirus type 18. *Nucleic Acids Res.*, **20**, 6015–6021.
122. Hegde, R. S., Grossman, S. R., Laimins, L. A. and Sigler, P. B. (1992). Crystal structure at 1.7 A of the bovine papillomavirus-1 E2 DNA-binding domain bound to its DNA target. *Nature*, **359**, 505–512.

Index

Note: Page references in *italics* refer to Figures; those in **bold** refer to Tables

Index compiled by Annette Muster